LABOR AND DELIVERY: IMPACT ON OFFSPRING

EMANUEL A. FRIEDMAN, M.D., Sc.D.

Professor of Obstetrics and Gynecology
Harvard Medical School and
Obstetrician-Gynecologist-in-Chief
Beth Israel Hospital, Boston

RAYMOND K. NEFF, Sc.D.

Associate Professor of Biostatistics
School of Public Health and
Assistant Vice Chancellor
Information Systems and Technology
University of California, Berkeley

PSG PUBLISHING COMPANY, INC.
LITTLETON, MASSACHUSETTS

Library of Congress Cataloging-in-Publication Data

Friedman, Emanuel A., 1926-
  Labor and delivery.

  Includes index.
    1. Labor (Obstetrics)—Longitudinal studies.
2. Childbirth—Longitudinal studies. 3. Children—
Health and hygiene—United States—Longitudinal studies.
4. Medical care—United States. I. Neff, Raymond K.
II. Title. [DNLM 1. Delivery. 2. Labor. 3. Outcome
and Process Assessment (Health Care) WQ 300 F862L]
RG652.F74 1986   362.1′984′0973021   86-8876
ISBN 0-88416-553-1

Published by:
PSG PUBLISHING COMPANY, INC.
545 Great Road
Littleton, Massachusetts 01460

1987. PSG PUBLISHING COMPANY, INC.

This is a publication of the Collaborative Perinatal Project, National Institute of
Neurological and Communicative Diseases and Stroke, National Institutes of
Health, Contract N01-NS-8-2381. Based on data collected by the Perinatal
Research Branch of the National Institute of Neurological and Communicative
Diseases and Stroke.

Printed in the United States of America.

International Standard Book Number: 0-88416-553-1

Library of Congress Catalog Card Number: 86-8879

Last digit is the print number: 9 8 7 6 5 4 3 2 1

Dedicated to the memory of Rudolph F. Vollman
· Physician, scientist, scholar, and educator,
whose foresight, dedication, commitment, and
friendship made this work possible
1912-1985

Contents

Foreword

"Labor and Delivery: Impact on Offspring" is a major report based on data from the Collaborative Perinatal Project (NCPP) of the National Institute of Neurological and Communicative Disorders and Stroke (NINCDS). One of the primary objectives of the NCPP was to develop the association between labor and delivery factors and outcome of the child. In 1973, a Comprehensive Plan for Analysis and Interpretation of Collaborative Perinatal Project Data was devised. An extensive bibliography exists reporting on analyses proposed in the plan and now completed. The focus of the analyses in this book emanate from labor and delivery variables.

The NCPP data collection began in 1958 when the first mothers were registered in the study and ended with the last follow-up examinations on the children in 1974. The data collection period lasted some 16 years. The Comprehensive Plan for Analysis and Interpretation of Collaborative Perinatal Project Data was designed to be responsive to the original objectives of the study as well as those developed during the years of data collection. This volume publishes the results of analyses supported by the Public Health Service research contract N01-NS-8-2381 which was awarded in 1978 to Boston's Beth Israel Hospital with Dr. Emanuel A. Friedman as principal investigator. The general concepts for the analyses that Dr. Friedman and Dr. Neff have completed had their beginning in the Obstetrical Task

Force of the Collaborative Perinatal Project. Dr. Friedman is particularly familiar with the NCPP data as he participated in the planning phase for the NCPP and served as the obstetrical coordinator of the project in the field unit at Columbia University.

The time interval from the planning of the collaborative study in the mid-1950s to the publication of this monograph is over 30 years. The entire project—beginning with planning in the mid-1950s, the data collection between 1958 and 1974, and in recent years the analytic and interpretative phases—could only have been completed with the cooperation, collaboration, and continued commitment of many people including the parents and their children, the professionals of many disciplines, and the support staff. All these people helped forge the plans into reality and each report from the NCPP gratefully acknowledges their contributions.

This volume presents a risk assessment for a large number of labor and delivery factors and provides a factual basis for discussion of the risk-benefit relationship of many labor and delivery practices. Dr. Friedman and Dr. Neff have made an important contribution to the literature assessing labor and delivery factors. This report meets one of the objectives of the Collaborative Perinatal Project and provides data to stimulate further research on identification and delineation of risk to the baby during labor and delivery.

Joseph S. Drage, MD
Bethesda, Maryland

Preface

The material in this book represents the culmination of a professional lifetime of interest in labor and delivery phenomena. A series of very fortunate circumstances led me to this point. They began with a formal association *ab initio* in 1957 with the National Collaborative Perinatal Project (which we will henceforth refer to as the Project or NCPP) as obstetric coordinator of the field unit at Columbia University and continuing for 30 years in various consultative roles with several NCPP task forces created specifically to address data gathering and analysis. Simultaneously, related research activities over the years have concentrated on exploration of the labor process in some depth, yielding several hundred relevant publications.

What my foregoing clinical research admittedly lacked was the wherewithal to provide meaningful long-term follow-up data on surviving infants. In this regard, the Project data were unique. Not only was there information available pertaining to those children, but the numbers of cases were very substantial and the depth and uniformity of the material were impressive.

In a previous monograph dealing with analysis of NCPP data on pregnancy hypertension,* I waxed eloquent (and prolix) on the virtues and special attributes of the Pro-

---

*Friedman EA, Neff RK: *Pregnancy Hypertension: A Systematic Evaluation of Clinical Diagnostic Criteria.* Littleton, Mass, PSG Publishing Co, 1977.

ject. It would not be appropriate to repeat that exercise here, but I do feel some mention, however brief, is fitting to the conception, development, and the implementation of this enormous program. They recognized that the resource to be produced would have far-reaching potential. We owe them much.

Acknowledgments of appreciation and thanks are due to all the stalwarts who contributed so much of their time and effort to this investigation, including Marlene R. Sachtleben-Murray and Audrey Landay in the Department of Obstetrics and Gynecology at the Beth Israel Hospital; Frederick Pratter, John Schoenherr, Elizabeth Allred, Katherine Taylor-Halvorsen, Donald C. Olivier, David Eaglesfield, Jane Soukup, and Peggy Morrison at the Health Sciences Computing Facility of the Harvard School of Public Health; and Bill Williams and Irene B. Ross at the Perinatal Research Branch (PRB) of NINCDS. Particular gratitude is due to Joseph S. Drage, MD, Chief, PRB, for his unflagging support and much appreciated encouragement.

Special comment is warranted to ensure that the data are fully appreciated in context. It is too easy to denigrate the importance of a study based on a clinical experience that is not current. Indeed, it could not be current if evaluation of long-term infant results is the objective. The paradox of requiring today's practices to be applicable to children who are being studied for late neurologic and developmental deficiencies should be obvious.

Obstetric practices have changed over the years, of course, in terms of diminished frequencies of difficult and potentially traumatic operative vaginal procedures, increased cesarean sections, less analgesia and anesthesia, less uterotonic stimulation, and the introduction of electronic fetal heart rate monitoring, among many others. Merely because the mixture of activities has been modified (that is, the relative proportions in the composite of overall practice), it does not mean that we cannot examine the effects of each specific practice in a meaningful way.

If anything, a case could be made for studying such effects before the recent changes were made to ascertain if the changes in clinical practice were actually justifiable. To examine the results afterward risks confounding the analysis by the effects of other changes introduced concurrently or subsequently.

Of greater concern to me are those who detract simply because the database is a product of the NCPP. Over the years, some individuals have regularly deprecated these data without justification. Of course, there were problems at the outset in regard to accuracy and uniformity of definitions, but diligent training of observers, measures imposed to ensure quality control, and exhaustive editing operations corrected such recognized deficiencies. Skeptics (and I include myself among them, at least in the early years) were unwilling to accept as reliable the massive accumulated material that ultimately constituted the data bank of the Project now estimated to exceed 2 billion items of information.

Having worked closely with these data and personally examined and cross-verified several exhaustive samplings of raw clinical observations and recordations against magnetic tape information, I feel I can speak with authority on the subject. I am able to provide assurances as to reliability. Accuracy and completeness are far superior to that which can be expected from much smaller studies, even many carried out within a single institution. That in itself is a special tribute to the army of coordinated observers and editors who functioned so effectively to this end. They can be justifiably proud of their achievement, particularly since it provided the means whereby studies such as this one could be carried out in the interest of assessing and improving obstetric practices.

Emanuel A. Friedman, MD, ScD
Boston, Massachusetts

CHAPTER 1

Introduction

Summary

The shortcomings of past experimental studies and the pitfalls inherent in most comparative clinical investigations are highlighted. Examples are offered of the kinds of specious arguments that so often find their way into clinical practice. A broader, more encompassing investigation appears to be justified that will take confounding factors into account and weigh the effects of those variables simultaneously acting to influence outcome. The NCPP data resource makes such an in-depth study feasible.

Attributed to an apocryphal philosopher is the adage, "Man's most dangerous journey is his passage through the birth canal." He or she was incorrect, of course, because the zygote's trip through the fallopian tube takes a far greater toll. This inaccuracy aside (and discounting the rhetorical chauvinism reflected in "man" and "his"), no one will deny that the processes of labor and delivery can be inherently hazardous.

Despite current justifiable and laudatory emphasis on the normal and physiologic (as opposed to the pathologic) aspects of birthing and the consumeristic movement fostering a return to "nature," it is clear to anyone willing to examine the past dispassionately that the birthing experience has never been harm-free to mothers and babies. In fact, notwithstanding the strident antagonism of some women who lament against the unfeeling technology that has been applied for surveillance of today's fetuses during labor, the survival rates have never been better and there are additional acknowledged benefits in the quality of life achieved by surviving infants.

Historically, the further back in time one goes—and, therefore, the closer to nature one gets—the worse the outcome results one finds. The same applies to data from primitive societies, strongly suggesting that more natural is not necessarily better. This is not to imply that technology is all good (or even any good) and, therefore, is to be mandated to the exclusion of humanism. Nothing could be further from a desired objective. We should be trying to determine which specific aspects of technological advances are valuable in terms of objective contributions to fetal and maternal well-being, under what circumstances they are best applicable, and how they can be best integrated into programs of care so that they will not be intrusive, demeaning, or dehumanizing.

Too much of past obstetric practice was based on dogma; too much of current practice is based either on scientific tools introduced without clearly documented scientific foundation or, by contrast, on raw emotion and intuition. Neither extreme can be fully justified; in the absence of factual data to show benefit or adverse effect, prevailing arguments about why one or the other is preferable cannot be taken as definitive or even defensible.

Clinical studies to date, as applied to such obstetric practices are in the main experiential reports ranging from testimonials attesting to the author's prowess, skill, or luck to descriptions of relevant maternal and short-term infant results. The latter are usually limited to perinatal mortality and Apgar scores for the babies and febrile morbidity for the mothers. All are constrained by at least three sets of serious shortcomings. First is the matter of experimental design which usually does not allow the writer (and certainly not the reader) to draw valid conclusions pertaining to how the results differ from those of other reported series. Second, the control or referent data, if any, cannot be relied upon to be comparable. Third, internal confounding by selection factors or concurrent changes in practices is ignored (perhaps unrecognized or if recognized, unacknowledged).

We do not intend to be hypercritical by pointing out these deficiencies. We accept the obvious fact that budget, personnel, and time are all in short supply in even the most dedicated academic departments. Moreover, ethical considerations prevail to prevent application of scientific, laboratory-type experimental designs to clinical investigations of this type. In addition, there is generally limited patient material to permit one to apply more sophisticated analytical techniques to the problems at hand.

Apparently false conclusions abound in the obstetric literature. (We feel it essential to add here that the problem is not exclusively ours but cuts across all medical specialties equally). Some become ingrained by custom and usage; others are replaced in time by gratifyingly substantive concepts or, regrettably, by "truths" that may be just as flimsy. Pitfalls of logic ensnare us if we are not careful to appreciate possible specious relationships that uncritical analytic approaches may create. Let us examine several types of these to illustrate our recurrent dilemma.

Take the example of the effect of membrane rupture on labor: many thoughtful obstetricians hold that amniotomy stimulates labor and they cannot be disabused of this strongly held clinical impression. Today the issue is not terribly important—indeed it is essential moot—because amniotomy is done so frequently for purposes of applying a scalp electrode for internal fetal heart rate monitoring. For the sake of argument, however, it has to be stated that scientific (that is, objective) documentation of a beneficial effect does not yet exist. Most attempts to provide such documentation have shown neither benefit nor harm—that is to say, the subsequent labor progression was neither enhanced nor inhibited. Further, it should be noted that physicians of an earlier era were very much concerned about "dry labor," a condition of poor labor progress allegedly resulting from amniotomy, the very same procedure so many use today to augment labor.

The clinical impression of accelerated labor following membrane rupture appears to derive from the physiologic acceleration of labor that occurs normally in all labors. It is easy to appreciate the logic of an assumption that the acceleration results from the procedure; it is much more difficult to translate the objective data that show that same acceleration with and without amniotomy into clinically acceptable terms, particularly when the "mindset" is unwilling to consider this alternative explanation.

Perhaps another less emotion-laden example is in order to illustrate a similar difficulty, this time as related to confounding factors. Our British colleagues have long recognized an apparent association between induction or stimulation of labor by oxytocin and the development of subsequent neonatal jaundice. This simple observation does hold up in many studies, but not all. Not done, however, was any attempt to determine if some other factor might be causative instead.

Suppose oxytocin use is merely a marker (a flag, so to speak) for aggressive obstetric interventive management. If correct, perhaps these cases are more likely to be managed by operative delivery procedures which are potentially traumatic. Trauma causes bleeding into tissues and tissue spaces; absorption of such blood enhances neonatal jaundice. This turns out to be the case. When instances of oxytocin usage are stratified (that is, divided or grouped) accordingly, the adverse effect of such procedures becomes immediately evident in the frequency of jaundice.

A third type of error concerns illogical conclusions based on comparisons between dissimilar populations of cases. For example, there has been much concern and chagrin over the apparently poor showing of the United States in overall perinatal mortality statistics vis-à-vis similar data from countries such as Sweden. This is interpreted to reflect relatively poor obstetrical care here.

However, when births are statified by infant weights, our data come out the same; actually, in some weight categories, our results are quite a bit better. How then can the overall results turn out worse? The answer lies in the make-up of our baby population: we deliver proportionally many more small or premature infants. Because such infants have higher mortality rates than term-sized babies, it follows that our overall mortality rate will be higher than a country where fewer small babies are born.

The labor and delivery processes consist of many different component events and influences. In sheer numbers, these factors comprise a complex constellation that challenges even the most sophisticated analytical minds. Many foregoing published studies pertaining to the fetal and infant effects of labor and delivery factors must be considered to have only limited validity. Studies in which no attempt was made to control for relevant factors or in which control was only superficial are suspect.

Nonetheless, the findings of such studies may serve to alert clinicians and to suggest to clinical investigators that further clarification is needed. We do not seriously fault prior studies for their shortcomings. Indeed, we have contributed large numbers to the literature ourselves. In the past, constraints of patient population size and, more critically, limitations of analytical capabilities (especially in the precomputer era) proved insurmountable obstacles.

While statistical methods and expertise may have been available, they have generally not been brought to bear for a variety of quasi-legitimate reasons. The numbers of qualifying patients under close observation were often too small to satisfy the technical needs of applicable testing methods. In addition, the enormous effort required and the expense that that effort would entail precluded such analyses.

The unique opportunity to explore important relevant questions concerning the wide range of factors in and around the birth phenomenon and to assess the impact of those factors on the fetus and surviving infant was provided through the vehicle of the NCPP data bank. The impressively large numbers of patients studied, the wealth of recorded observations, and the intensity of follow-up material made this resource especially well-suited for our needs. We recognize it is likely that such a treasury of information may never again be available as a consequence of increasingly stringent budgetary limitations imposed on matters relating to broad health care research.

Despite its size, the data resource is found inadequate at times to provide sufficient numbers of cases to permit study of the rarer conditions or the more esoteric combinations of factors. Indeed, the larger the number of factors studied, the greater the probability that one will encounter problems relating to small sample sizes.

We believe the material developed from these data and the conclusions derived from the resulting analytical findings should be of more than academic interest because they are clinically valuable and applicable to practice. Nonetheless, we are aware that not only are we unable to answer all the questions we have posed (and many we could not explore because of limited support), but many of the answers we give may require modification in the immediate or distant future as new skills and technological modalities are introduced. Even as this is being written, the discipline of obstetrics is rapidly changing. It is gratifying to believe that some of our findings will benefit current and future generations of gravidas and their offspring; but it is more realistic to consider the likelihood that they may serve as foundational material upon which future investigations may be built.

CHAPTER 2

Program Objectives

Summary

The specific aims of the study are outlined as related to determining the effects on the fetus and surviving infant of the course of labor, the drugs used, intrinsic prelabor factors, and delivery events and procedures. Identifying risk factors would then facilitate recognition of the gravida-at-risk whose fetus may be in jeopardy. The sequence of investigational approaches to accomplishing these ends is briefly addressed.

Given the complexity of the labor and delivery phenomena and the many factors that need to be studied individually and collectively, we recognized how essential it was for a systematic approach to be used. We sought to ascertain which factors might adversely or beneficially affect the fetus and the surviving infant. Once such factors could be identified, their interrelationships with one another had to be defined. Moreover, we felt it necessary to determine whether combinations of factors were additive or synergistic in their effects or were instead subtractive (that is, counterbalancing).

Thus, the effect on offspring of a range of factors had to be assessed first. Then the dependence of one or more factors on each other needed elucidation. Finally, how the coexistence of factors altered their impact required investigation. These three basic considerations were principal guiding objectives. To illustrate, we wanted to learn the precise impact of specific types of forceps operations on offspring, appreciating the common association of some midforceps procedures with an antecedent disordered labor, which in itself might have an unfavorable fetal effect and thereby enhance the adverse influence of the instrumental delivery.

There was little doubt at the outset that the problem confronting us was not simple to solve. Indeed, there was no small concern that it might be insoluble within the constraints of available data and support resources. Conceptually, we proposed to determine the effects on the fetus and the surviving infant of clinically definable labor factors, a range of labor disorders, and the spectrum of delivery procedures. Our aim was thus to identify and quantitate the specific risk factors in labor and delivery that contribute to perinatal mortality and to the development of long-term neurologic and developmental disorders in children.

Projects

Our approach dealt with numerous categories of identifiable variables. Our proposed analyses were designed to encompass a series of delimited projects. They included the following:

1. We desired to ascertain the effects on outcome of specific clinical features, including incremental durations and rates of progression of the several component parts of labor as defined by the cervical dilatation and fetal descent patterns of labor.

2. We wanted to learn the effects on the fetus and the child of disordered or dysfunctional labor as defined by distribution data for the durations and slopes of the labor progression patterns.

3. We desired to study the effects of adjunctive pharmacologic agents used in labor for sedation, tranquilization, analgesia, anesthesia, uterotonic stimulation for induction or augmentation of labor, and others as encountered.

4. We felt it essential to investigate the effects of intrinsic conditions, such as race, advancing maternal age, gravidity, parity, gestational duration, birth weight, discordance between birth weight and gestational age, membrane status, the duration of ruptured membranes, cephalopelvic relationships, fetal presentation, position, station,

attitude, synclitism, and a host of other related variables.

5. We wanted to ascertain the effects of specific labor and delivery procedures on the offspring, such as amniotomy, manual and forceps rotations, the several types of forceps application and delivery, breech maneuvers, version, cesarean section, and other procedural processes.

6. We desired to incorporate the dynamic factor of time in labor, with specific reference to predefined phases of labor progression, into all the foregoing factors so as to try to identify adverse effects as related to the occurrence or application of the risk factors within a given time frame in the course of the labor.

7. We felt it important to try to identify those constellations of labor and delivery factors that place the fetus and infant in jeopardy, thereby to establish criteria for defining high-risk labor and delivery based on objective data.

8. We desired to detect features in the gravida associated with or contributing to the development of high-risk labor and delivery constellations, as aforementioned, thereby to provide data to alert physicians to the identification of specific gravidas-at-risk who are likely to have such problems and to jeopardize their offspring as a consequence.

9. Finally, we wanted to provide the wherewithal to establish meaningful standards of care as recommendations for the practice of obstetrics in regard to the management of labor and delivery, aiming toward reducing or eliminating avoidable fetal and infant death and damage.

Rationale

Our rationale for embarking on these extensive and often frustrating investigations reflected our desire to improve obstetrical care by examining collective experience and objectively determining, if possible, what is good and what is bad (in simple, if not simplistic terms). Over the course of three decades, the senior author has been intimately involved in clinical and laboratory studies dealing with labor and delivery phenomena.

During this time, it has become increasingly clear that clinical investigations in this area have been seriously hampered by severely constraining databases. Usually, the numbers of homogeneously grouped cases have been necessarily small. Even where approaching substantive numbers, long-term follow-up information is essentially nonexistent or fragmentary at best in such studies.

The limitations inherent in published reports, heretofore based on such limited material, are transparent because they focused on the specific issues as applied to very delimited sets of labor and delivery variables. They did not take into account the many possibly confounding factors that were likely to be at play. Indeed, they were unable to take such factors into account because of the aforementioned constraints.

Data Bank

The data collected for the NCPP are unique in regard to their potential for providing answers to critical questions posed with reference to risk factors that may be acting. This applies especially as they relate to disease states or high-risk situations that may give rise to fetal and infant morbidity. The available data, collected prospectively on the myriad factors relating to labor and delivery, were expected to prove far more significant in helping to define the relative significance of risk factors than any clinical investigations heretofore conducted.

The scope of the NCPP data bank and the extent of available information with regard to labor and delivery events, coupled with the depth of detail in regard to long-erm infant follow-up, make this material especially relevant to solving problems pertaining to the intrinsic effects of obstetrical phenomena. Moreover, it should be feasible to solve problems relating to the confounding effects of the large number of variables that may be acting by virtue of the large

numbers of cases that have been studied. As a consequence, it is believed that sophisticated statistical analytic techniques can be effectively applied.

Overview

Using this singular resource, we proposed to study the impact on outcome of a host of clinical factors relating to labor and delivery. These factors were to be studied singly and in combination. Where relevant, they were to be investigated as they related to their appearance or occurrence over the course of the labor progression. This was expected to provide a means for studying the significance of various dynamic patterns of change as well. We anticipated undertaking a series of analytic studies to ascertain which groups of factors were interrelated in terms of risk, thereby reducing the number of risk factors that were to be subsequently considered. We planned to pursue discriminant function and logistic regression analyses to determine those specific risk factors having the greatest impact on adverse fetal and infant results. Such information, when obtained, was to provide means for identifying those combinations of risk factors of greatest concern to us by virtue of their collective effects on the offspring. These were expected to constitute the criteria for defining the highest risk labor and delivery situations.

Once we had defined high-risk labor and delivery based on outcome events, we intended to pursue investigations to provide concise characterization of the gravida who is likely to develop these conditions. This was to be accomplished by detailing relevant contributory factors in her actuarial, socioeconomic, family health history, and medical and obstetrical background. If these objectives were to be achieved, we felt they would collectively contribute much to clinical practice. They would help to define clinical patterns of labor and delivery conditions that could be expected to yield high fetal and infant hazard. Moreover, they would help us to describe the gravida who can be expected to place her fetus at risk as pregnancy advanced. This information would serve to alert clinicians to their presence.

CHAPTER 3

Data Collection Resource

Summary

The history and objectives of the NCPP are reviewed. The collaborating field units are identified and the methods used for ensuring complete and accurate data collection are detailed. Sample frame selection techniques and the wide spectrum of information collected from the study population are outlined. The content of the data collection forms and information processing measures are also provided.

The foundation for the study reported in this monograph was the database produced by the NCPP.* The Project was begun in 1958 after 4 years of intensive planning. Patients were studied in depth at 14 university hospital settings under the aegis of the Perinatal Research Branch of NINCDS. The initial intent of the NCPP was to provide prospective clinical data for purposes of focusing upon associations between perinatal events and adverse effects in the fetus

---

Some of the details outlined in Chapters 3-5 are modified from those we published earlier in Friedman EA, Neff RK: *Pregnancy Hypertension: A Systematic Evaluation of Clinical Diagnostic Criteria.* Littleton, Mass, PSG Publishing Co, 1977.

* The NCPP was originally entitled "The collaborative investigation on clinical-pathologic correlation in cerebral palsy, mental retardation, and other neurological disorders having their origin in the perinatal period." It was renamed to reflect its broader goals as "The collaborative study on cerebral palsy, mental retardation, and other neurological and sensory disorders in infancy and childhood." The National Institute of Neurological and Communicative Diseases and Stroke (NINCDS) was originally called the National Institute of Neurological Diseases and Blindness, and subsequently the National Institute of Neurological Diseases and Stroke, before assuming its current name.

and child. The effects of particular concern were organic neurologic defects in surviving offspring. The early years were involved in matters related to determining procedures for patient selection, developing meaningful forms, and establishing uniform procedures for recording the data.

Aims

The intention of the project planners was to provide a broad prospective, multidisciplinary epidemiologic study for purposes of examining the causes of bad outcomes. They designed the study as a prospective examination of antepartum, intrapartum, and postdelivery observations coupled with extended and extensive follow-up of the offspring. The data derived can be considered unique from three distinctive points of view: they were collected prospectively, they deal with a very large population group, and they provide unmatched, long-term, carefully conducted and recorded assessments of the children.

As noted above, the NCPP began to accumulate the massive array of important objective data that form the basis for this study in 1958. Input continued until the end of 1965 for registration of obstetrical patients. Eight more years elapsed for purposes of ensuring long-term follow-up of surviving children. Details of the NCPP—including its design, population, procedures, protocol, and data processing procedures—have been presented elsewhere.*

Collaborating Institutions

Implementation of the Project was an herculean undertaking because of the intricate collaboration required. Patient selec-

---

*Niswander KR, Gordon M (eds): *The Collaborative Perinatal Study of the National Institute of Neurological Diseases and Stroke: The Women and Their Pregnancies.* Philadelphia, WB Saunders Co, 1972; Hardy JB, Drage JS, Jackson EC: *The First Year of Life.* Baltimore, John Hopkins University Press, 1979.

tion procedures had to be determined, forms had to be developed, and procedures for recording the data uniformly had to be evolved by means of manuals, workshops, meetings, and pretesting.

A total of 14 university hospital institutions participated, including:

> Boston Lying-in Hospital and Children's Hospital Medical Center, Boston
> Buffalo Children's Hospital
> Charity Hospital of Louisiana, New Orleans
> Columbia-Presbyterian Medical Center, New York
> The Johns Hopkins Hospital, Baltimore
> Medical College of Virginia, Richmond
> New York Medical College and Metropolitan Hospital Center
> Pennsylvania Hospital and Children's Hospital, Philadelphia
> Providence Lying-in Hospital
> University of Minnesota Health Sciences Center, Minneapolis
> University of Oregon Medical School, Portland
> University of Tennessee and Gailor Hospital, Memphis

Coordination was provided by the Perinatal Research Branch (PRB) of the NINCDS. It not only directed the collaborative effort but served as a repository and processing facility for the NCPP data collected at each of the collaborating field units and remitted to it.

Data Collection Approach

The data were first collected and recorded as uniformly as possible and as soon as feasible after a relevant event had occurred. The completed protocols upon which the results of all examinations and interviews were recorded were submitted to the PRB for editing, coding, and processing.

Many of the forms used for data collection were structured to facilitate precoding. Personnel were hired, trained, and supervised so that at each institution a coterie of specially trained and highly skilled interviewers and examiners were engaged in the collection and recording of the information that was later to be encoded.

In order to maintain accuracy, uniformity, and reliability of data, detailed instructional manuals were created and series of workshops were periodically provided for training new personnel and reenforcing essential requisites of conduct for others.

Within each institution, teams were established to pursue relevant matters relating to obstetrics, pediatrics, pediatric neurology, child psychology, pathology, and speech, language, and hearing. In addition, within each participating institution, a central administrative staff coordinated the activities of these diverse groups and served as liaison with the PRB.

Patient Selection

The gravid population selected for inclusion in the NCPP was meant to represent a broad spectrum of pregnancy conditions, as free as possible from biases interjected on the basis of special interests. Samples were chosen in a manner that would not interfere with the routine operations of a maternity service. For each institution, restrictions were placed to provide a case load that could be handled comfortably by the personnel involved. Numbers ranged from about 300 to 2000 patients annually per institution. Selection ratios within the hospital units ranged from 10% to 100% of registered prenatal patients.

Selection criteria were rigorously monitored to ensure an appropriate sample frame essentially free from the introduction of concentrations of special pregnancies based on referral patterns or institutional interests. Selection methods varied widely from the systematic selection of every nth pregnancy to selection based on the terminal digits of the history number, the day of birth, or other device.

Spectrum of Data Collection

Once a patient was registered into the Project, a sequence of interviews and examinations was undertaken. At each prenatal clinic visit, she was interviewed concerning her medical history (or interval history). Also, considerable socioeconomic and genetic information was obtained about the gravida, her family, the baby's father, and the father's family. The obstetrician recorded the results of physical examinations, histories, and laboratory determinations.

Customarily, antepartum clinic visits were scheduled on a monthly basis during the first 7 months of pregnancy, every 2 weeks during the eighth month, and weekly thereafter. When the patient was admitted into the hospital for labor and delivery, her physical status was reevaluated and all the events of labor and delivery were recorded in detail by a trained observer. A summary of the labor and delivery was completed by the obstetrician responsible for the patient's care.

The placenta was examined carefully by NCPP pathologists who also conducted postmortem examinations of stillbirths and neonatal deaths, whenever applicable. Puerperal events were detailed as well. Additionally, any antepartum hospital admission was appropriately recorded.

The neonate was observed initially in the delivery room and examined periodically by the NCPP pediatrician at 24-hour intervals in the newborn nursery. A detailed neurologic examination was done at two days of age. Much information from the nursery period was included, such as nurses' observations and the results of all laboratory determinations. A diagnostic summary of the nursery period was written by a NCPP pediatrician.

Subsequently, the child was followed for up to 8 years. At each specific follow-up examination, the mother was interviewed to obtain the child's interval history and a physical examination was done to record

11

the child's physical measurements. Pediatric examination was made at 4 months.

Psychological examinations to determine mental and motor development were done at 8 months, 4 years, and 7 years of age. Extensive neurologic examinations were given at 1 and 7 years, respectively, and speech, language, and hearing examinations at 3 and 8 years.

Interval histories were updated at 18 months and at 2, 5, and 6 years. The family and social history was obtained again at the 7-year examinations. All supplementary information from special examinations of children with problems was obtained from hospital or physician records. Diagnostic summaries were prepared at 1 year and at 7 years of age.

Information Processing

The data were entered on specially designed forms for later encoding and compilation into a data bank. As stated earlier, procedure manuals were developed to ensure uniformity of data collection and nomenclature throughout the various collaborating institutions. It was recognized that detailed and comprehensive information was necessary for meaningful etiologic studies. Moreover, it was deemed essential to eliminate ambiguities in terminology and to assure comparability of information collected over the long duration of the Project by many different examiners at the several institutions. Without such assurances, reproducibility and pooling would be unacceptable.

Finally, it was necessary to simplify and standardize the processing of information at all stages of data collection and handling. Most of the items of information on the structured Project forms were arranged with check boxes for both positive and negative answers, ensuring that there would be no confusion between a negative response and an omission. This approach was meant to facilitate direct key punching and to diminish the opportunity for coding errors.

Narrative information could also be entered as needed, particularly for describing events taking place in and around the delivery process. Data collection and processing was complicated somewhat by the need to restructure forms from time to time when it became obvious that such changes were essential for greater accuracy or internal consistency or to provide more detail than was previously available.

The specific forms utilized in this study are tabulated below, together with annotations to indicate the kind of information contained on each so as to help familiarize those who are not knowledgeable about the Project with their content.* Specific items were collected from each of these forms, as needed, for evolving a composite integrated data file of workable size for the current investigations.

---

* Copies of all forms and their instructional manuals are available on request from the Developmental Neurology Branch, Neurological Disorders Program, NINCDS, NIH, Bethesda, MD 20014.

Project Forms and Their Content*

AR-1 Obstetrical Administrative Record
  Identification of patient, institution, dates of registration, of last menstrual period, and of birth, marital status, and race
OB-2 Reproductive History
  Review of past pregnancy outcomes
OB-3 History Since Last Menstrual Period
  Symptom review, illnesses, operations, radiation, work, smoking
OB-4 Gynecologic History
  Menarche, menstrual pattern, infertility history, contraception
OB-5 Recent Medical History
  Details of recent illnesses, disabilities, medications

OB-6   Past Medical History
       Prepregnancy hospitalizations, radiologic examinations or treatment, transfusions

OB-7   Infectious Disease and System Review
       Childhood illnesses, infectious and parasitic disease

OB-8   Repeat Prenatal History
       Interval symptom review since last visit, completed at each visit and at delivery

OB-9   Prenatal Record
       Menstrual history, obstetrical experience, details of complete physical examination

OB-10   Laboratory Data
       Blood type, Rh, Rh titer, hemoglobin, hematocrit, Coombs' test, serology, urinalysis, Papanicolaou smear, blood sugar, glucose tolerance test, etc

OB-15   Drugs in Pregnancy
       All medications taken, gestational age, and duration of administration

OB-33   Delivery Room Events
       Type of delivery, details of forceps application, traction, delivery of head and body, cord clamping, and placenta delivery

OB-34   Obstetrician's Summary of Labor and Delivery
       Details of labor including durations of stages, fetal presentation, position, rotation, instrumentation, degree of difficulty, placental abruption, placenta previa, induction, stimulation, bleeding, dysfunction, dystocia, and cord problems

OB-35   Anesthetic Agents
       Type, time, route given, level attained, and response for each agent

ADM-49   Labor Data
       Abstracted information on vital signs and progression of dilatation and descent in labor

ADM-50   Labor Data
       Observations of fetal heart and meconium in labor as well as bleeding and rupture of membranes

ADM-51   Labor and Delivery Drugs
       Same as OB-15 for drugs given in labor

OB-42   Past Medical History
       Replaced OB-9 effective April 1962

OB-43   Initial Prenatal Examination
       Replaced OB-9 effective April 1962

OB-44   Prenatal Observations
       Replaced OB-10 effective April 1962

OB-45   Laboratory Record
       Replaced OB-10 effective April 1962

OB-51 and OB-52   Admission Examination
       Internal examination findings for hospital admission before delivery

OB-55   Delivery Report
       Replaced OB-34 effective April 1962

OB-57   Anesthetic Agents
       Replaced OB-35 effective April 1962

OB-58   Summary of Puerperium
       Weight, blood pressure, and temperature data

OB-60   Obstetric Diagnostic Summary
> Encoded details of diagnoses for all systems, pregnancy outcomes, and complications

PATH-1   Gross Placental Examination
> Morphology of placenta, cord, vessels; pathologic conditions, infarcts, thromboses, hemorrhages

PATH-2   Microscopic Placental Examination
> Vessels, amnion, chorion, thrombosis, necrosis, infiltrations, infarctions

PATH-3   Autopsy Protocol
> Details of postmortem findings

PED-1   Delivery Room Examination of the Neonate
> Sex, weight, times to first breath and first cry, resuscitation measures, physical findings, reflexes, Apgar score details at 1, 2, 5, 10, 15, and 20 minutes

PED-2   Neonatal Examination
> Body, head, and chest measurements, cyanosis, jaundice, respirations, heart rate, brief neurologic and physical examination

PED-3   Nursery History
> Incubator, humidity, oxygen needs, weight changes, feeding, activity, cry and respirations, pallor, seizures, etc

ADM-44 and PED-4   Report of Fetal or Infant Death

PED-5   Results of Tests Done on Neonate
> Blood type, Rh, Coombs' test, bilirubin determinations, and hemoglobin

PED-6   Neonatal Neurologic Examination
> Detailed neurologic findings

PED-7   Summary of Hospital Course of Neonate
> Hospital duration, neuromuscular problems, dysmaturity, etc

PED-8   Newborn Diagnostic Summary
> Encoded details of diagnoses for all systems
> PED-10   Four-Month Pediatric Examination
> Physical findings and detailed neurologic examination

PED-11   One-Year Neurologic Examination
> Complete physical and detailed neurologic examination

PED-12   Summary of First Year of Life
> Same as PED-8 for subsequent period till age 1 year

PED-14   Physical Growth Measurements
> Weight, length, head and chest circumference for each examination

PED-75   Seven-Year Visual Examination

PED-76   Seven-Year Neurologic Examination

ADM-88 and IDC-77   Years 1-to-7 Summary

PS-1-5   Eight-Month Psychological Examination
> Details of findings at age 8 months, stressing both mental and motor performance (Bayley scales of infant development)

PS-10-17   Three-Year Speech, Language, and Hearing Examination
> Details of language reception, expression, hearing, speech mechanisms, and memory

PS-20-25   Four-Year Psychological Examination
> Details of IQ battery using Stanford-Binet intelligence scale, Graham-Ernhart block sort, motor test, and behavior profile

PS-26 Four-Year Psychological Examination
 Contains mother's IQ as well
PS-30-38 Seven-Year Psychological Examination
 Full battery of IQ testing using Bender-Gestalt test, Wechsler intelligence
 scale, achievement, Goodenough, abstract, tactile, and behavior studies
PS-40-45 Final Speech Language and Hearing Examination
 Eight-year study of hearing and auditory memory, language comprehen-
 sion and expression, and speech mechanism and production
FHH-1 Family Health History
 Data on religion, birthplace, education, employment, housing, and income of
 gravida and father of baby
FHH-9 Family Health History Review
SE-1 Socioeconomic Interview
 Confirmatory information on birthplace, education, employment, religion,
 housing, income, etc
GEN-5-8 Family History Interview

CHAPTER 4

Database

Summary

The core study population of 58,806 gravidas is characterized superficially by race, age, parity and gestational age at the time they first presented for obstetrical care. Loss to follow-up is addressed. Criteria for a study cohort of gravidas are applied to yield a more homogeneous index population. This group of 45,142 patients is examined to show its similarity to the population from which it was derived. Working data files are developed for detailed study. The files are refined to ensure sufficient information and eliminate obvious errors. Labor progression data are similarly cleansed by a rectification process to ensure accuracy and reliability. Screening criteria are applied for analysis of labor progression. Overall outcome data are reviewed for reference.

A total of 58,806 women registered in the NCPP during their antepartum course. They constituted a cross-sectional sampling (44.5%) of more than 132,000 who met the basic criteria for acceptance at the collaborating institutions and who constituted the collective obstetrical experience at these hospital units.

Although most of these women constituted the "core" population, having been sampled appropriately by random means, some were specifically selected for study (and designated noncore) because of special interests at several of the institutions. One institution served as a referral center for pregnant diabetics, for example. These noncore cases (4.5% of the study population and 2.0% of the base population from which they were derived) were not meant to be included in studies such as this.

Patient Characteristics

The make-up of the core group has been

detailed extensively in a previous publication.* Superficially characterized, their racial distribution was:

46.0% white
46.2% black
6.8% Puerto Rican
1.0% other

The socioeconomic and ethnic composition of the core NCPP population reflected that of the populations from which they were derived. For example, marital status was as follows:

73.1% married
18.1% single or never married
8.8% widowed, divorced, or separated

The median age was 23.6 years. The age breakdown was:

25.7% under age 20 years
35.8% aged 20-24 years
20.0% aged 25-29 years
11.0% aged 30-34 years
5.9% aged 35-39 years
1.6% aged 40 years and older

A total of 40,273 (68.5%) patients were entered into the Project for the first time; the remaining 31.5% were reregistered for one or more subsequent pregnancies as well.

Parity distribution in the NCPP population was about as expected:

36.0% para 0
20.5% para 1
14.0% para 2
16.5% para 3-4
10.5% para 5 or greater

Not all pregnancies, needless to say, resulted in viable fetuses. A total of 649

* Niswander KR, Gordon M (eds): *The Collaborative Perinatal Study of the National Institute of Neurological Diseases and Stroke: The Women and Their Pregnancies.* Philadelphia, WB Saunders Co, 1972.

gravidas (1.1%) aborted fetuses weighing less than 500 g or had an ectopic implantation or hydatidiform molar degeneration of the conceptus. Singletons were produced in most of the NCPP pregnancies, but there were multiple pregnancies in 445 (0.8%).

Patients registered for care and observation over a wide range of gestational ages:

8.3% up to 12 weeks
13.2% from 13 to 16 weeks
18.0% from 17 to 20 weeks
15.6% from 21 to 24 weeks
12.1% from 25 to 28 weeks
19.8% over 28 weeks

Thus, more than 80% of patients had registered by the 28th week. Unfortunately, some (0.5%, designated "walk-in" patients) received no antepartum care and were seen for the first time at term or in labor. For those registering early, observations were recorded at each subsequent visit.

Follow-Up Losses

A small number (3.9%) were lost to follow-up during the index pregnancy by virtue of the fact that they did not return for their expected periodic antepartum visit and/or were not delivered at a collaborating institution. Attempts were made to continue Project observations and recordings whenever it was known that a patient was relocating to an area in which another NCPP institution could carry on, thereby ensuring that that individual would be retained within the population under study. These efforts notwithstanding, some patients were either not traceable or were found too late to recoup the missing information concerning delivery and fetal outcome.

Inevitably, others were lost to follow-up after delivery, so that important data concerning growth and development of their offspring were not available for inclusion in the data files. Patient losses were minimized by the major efforts that were made to prevent attrition of the Project population, and the high rate of successful follow-up is illustrated by the fact that more than 85% of Project children were examined at the prescribed 1-year interval for neurologic evaluation and more than half were still enrolled after 8 years.

Index Population

Seeking a reasonably homogeneous population of gravidas for our investigation, we limited ourselves to a cohort of core NCPP registrants who were entering the Project for the first time. This eliminated the possible bias of noncore patients (2637 in all), whose special problems were likely to confound any future analysis; it also reduced the anticipated difficulties attendant upon reentering the same woman into the series on one or more occasions with succeeding pregnancies (9161 gravidas). Those 281 designated walk-in, and the 135 with indeterminate gestational age because the date of their last period was unknown or unrecorded or grossly unreliable were excluded, as were gravidas who had ectopic pregnancy or who were aborting a mole or a fetus weighing less than 500 g (649 in number).

Moreover, we desired to examine only those providing sufficient information to permit a dynamic study of the clinical diagnostic features of concern to us, namely the labor and delivery events. Accordingly, those without such data on file (3139) were summarily eliminated. The series was further constricted by deleting 445 women carrying multiple pregnancies, 2313 lost to follow-up, and 2637 aforementioned who were not part of the Project core group. Exclusions are summarized in Table 4-1.

Characteristics of Index Group

The residual 45,142 gravidas formed the population base from which we obtained the essential data for this study. That they were truly representative was indicated by the high degree of concurrence in distribution of actuarial data. For example, racial distribution was similar to that of the parent population from which they were derived:

48.0% white
41.5% black
10.5% other

Age distribution was also comparable:

27.8% under age 20 years
66.3% aged 20-34
 5.8% aged 35 and older

Table 4-1
Study Population

	No.
Total enrolled NCPP gravidas	58,806
Exclusions*	
Repeat pregnancy	9,161
Multiple pregnancy	445
Walk-in (no antepartum care)	281
Ectopic, abortion, or hydatidiform mole	649
Unknown data of last menstrual period	135
Non-core case	2,637
Lost to study	2,313
Residual study gravidas	45,142
Labor observations	275,632

* Exclusions are not additive because one or more reasons for deletion may apply to a given patient.

18

Parity distribution was likewise similar:

43.3% para 0
48.1% para 1-4
 8.6% para 5 or more

Gestational duration at delivery was also normally distributed:

 0.5% under 28 weeks
 1.4% between 28 and 31 weeks
 5.3% between 32 and 35 weeks
16.8% between 36 and 38 weeks
55.0% between 38 and 41 weeks
20.8% over 41 weeks

Data Files

Working data files were constructed for these index cases from the massive data bank originally compiled from the raw NCPP input information described earlier (see chapter 3) to include relevant information deemed likely to be useful in our analyses. In addition to identification and actuarial items (such as age, race, and parity), we included all recorded labor-delivery observations. Our master file was made up of 5,701,183 cards of data (on 80-column key-punch cards). Labor data relating only to the 45,142 index cases totaled 275,632 cards.

It was felt essential to ensure that every case provided an essential minimum amount of information for our study purposes. Thus, cases in which there were no pediatric data on the surviving infant could not be considered useful; the 725 cases without such records were, therefore, set aside. Similarly, 139 had no record of when labor began, 3139 had no recorded observations during labor, and 417 were duplicate files. That left a residual of 40,722 gravidas and 146,059 data cards.

For labor progression information alone, this represented more than 200,000 recorded observations, distributed as follows:

5,396 gravidas had 1 recorded

examination in labor
 4,583 had two examinations
 5,405 had three examinations
 5,328 had four examinations
 4,867 had five examinations
 3,862 had six examinations
11,281 had seven or more examinations
40,722 total gravidas

Further refinement was needed for providing enough data for analyzing the course of labor. Dating and timing errors of obvious nature (eg, onset of labor or observations in labor incorrectly timed to have occurred after the delivery) were encountered in 2453 records. By deleting the entire file for these gravidas at this time, we were left with 38,269 gravidas and their 189,830 recorded examinations.

Rectification Process

Reliability of data (aside from the issue of error analysis; see chapter 6) was of concern, of course. All nonregressive points were considered acceptable. The principle, which has been previously detailed,* defines those observations that are considered most likely to be correct when sequential discrepancies are encountered as those which do not regress (although those remaining unchanged are acceptable, of course). For example, any estimate of cervical dilatation followed by a smaller estimate is probably inaccurate and, therefore, can be ignored. To illustrate, let us examine the sequence of dilatation that runs:
3.0, *5.0*, 3.5, 4.0, *6.0*, 4.5, *10.0*, 9.5, 10.0
Regressive points, shown in italics, can be eliminated to provide a much more utilitarian (and probably more correct) plot of nonregressive observations:
3.0, 3.5, 4.0, 4.5, 9.5, 10.0
This rectification process deleted a total of 16,124 unacceptable (or at least unusable) recordings of observations from 38,269

---

* Friedman EA: *Labor: Clinical Evaluation and Management*, ed 2. New York, Appleton-Century-Crofts, 1978, pp 47-48.

gravidas. This was done without affecting the number of gravidas, of course, leaving 173,706 examinations for analysis.

Criteria for Labor Analysis

A requirement for pursuit of the analysis of labor progression was the ability to reconstruct the pattern of cervical dilatation. Minimum criteria had to be met, including (1) known time of onset of labor, (2) known time of delivery, (3) at least one documented nonregressive recorded observation of dilatation (and its associated time) between 3.0 and 6.0 cm dilatation, and (4) at least one comparable reading between 6.5 and 9.0 cm. The last two items were needed for reconstructing the active phase by providing enough information to calculate the maximum slope of dilatation accurately. Extrapolations forward and backward in time also allowed one to determine the beginning of the deceleration phase and the end of the latent phase, respectively (see chapter 8).

These criteria could not be met, so that a maximum slope of dilation could not be calculated, in 20,334 cases. This left an index population of 17,935 gravidas with ample information for reconstructing the entire dilatation process by means of a sophisticated computer program. Although all case material was retained for later examination, it was this subset that we utilized preliminarily for the main thrust of our investigation because it offered us the most complete data of its kind.

A similar approach rectified fetal descent data to yield 38,066 gravidas with 171,944 acceptable recordings of fetal station. For purposes of reconstructing the descent pattern, we needed at minimum some means for assessing when the deceleration phase of dilatation began (at which time

descent should be at its maximum, of course). Because such information was not always available or capable of being reconstructed from the dilatation pattern, the index population was reduced to 15,853 gravidas with 96,994 recorded labor examinations (Table 4-2). Among these cases, 1496 did not permit calculation of the maximum slope of descent (usually because two acceptable observations during the interval from beginning of the deceleration phase to delivery were not recorded), leaving a residual index population of 14,357 in all.

Compiling Labor-Delivery and Outcome Data

At the outset, data relating to the labor and delivery and to specific outcomes, particularly concerning the fetus, were compiled. These latter included such obviously important outcomes as death or survival (expressed as fetal death, neonatal death, and combined perinatal mortality); neonatal depression as reflected in low Apgar scores (less than six) at one and five minutes after birth; psychologic and neurologic abnormality at 8 months of age (as determined by abnormally low Bayley mental, motor, and global scores); abnormal findings at the 1-year neurologic examination; abnormal speech, language and hearing results at 3 years of age; and abnormally low four-year and seven-year IQ results (less than 70).

The frequencies of these critical outcome variables in our study population are shown in Table 4-3. Subsequently, many other items of interest were added to our files for study, particularly those variables that might serve to augment or confound the outcome relationships or to predict the development of the disease processes under surveillance.

Table 4-2
Case Selection

		Gravidas
CERVICAL DILATATION		
NCPP master file	5,701,183 cards	58,806
Study cohort	275,632 cards	45,142
No pediatric information		725
Labor onset unrecorded		139
No recorded dilatation observations		3,139
Duplicate record		417
Residual cohort	146,059 cards	40,722
Date or time discrepancy		2,453
Residual	189,830 examinations	38,269
Regressive dilatation recordings	16,124 examinations	
Residual	173,706 examinations	38,269
Maximum slope of dilatation		
not calculable or unacceptable		20,334
Residual index population (dilatation study)		17,935
FETAL DESCENT		
Residual cohort	146,059 cards	40,722
No station observations		1,259
Date or time discrepancy		1,397
Residual	190,825 examinations	38,066
Regressive station recordings	18,881 examinations	
Residual	171,944 examinations	38,066
Onset of deceleration unknown		22,213
Residual	96,994 examinations	15,853
Maximum slope of descent		
not calculable or unacceptable		1,496
Residual index population (descent study)		14,357

Table 4-3
Referent Outcome Data

Variable	Frequency, %
Fetal death	0.83
Neonatal death	0.84
Perinatal mortality	1.67
Depressed 1-minute Apgar score (< 6)	13.2
Depressed 5-minute Apgar score (< 6)	2.6
Abnormal 8-month global evaluation	1.50
Abnormal 8-month Bayley motor score (< 20)	0.60
Abnormal 8-month Bayley mental score (< 56)	0.62
Abnormal 1-year neurological examination	1.60
Abnormal language reception	7.4
Abnormal language expression	5.8
Abnormal hearing	2.2
Abnormal speech mechanism	3.7
Abnormal speech production	2.0
Low 4-year IQ (< 70)	4.3
Low 7-year IQ (< 70)	4.0

CHAPTER 5

Definitions of Variables

Control or Stratification Variables

Collaborating institution: The university hospital at which the gravida received her antepartum care and was delivered; one of the cooperating units whose obstetric population was systematically enrolled for study.

Race: Designation of race of gravida, based on mother's response to inquiry during her first antepartum interview.

Age: Chronological age of gravida at time of registration into the Project, in years completed.

Parity: Number of prior pregnancies terminated at or after 20 weeks of gestational duration, without consideration of the number of infants (eg, twins) or their survival.

Outcome Variables

Livebirth: Delivery of a living, viable infant weighing at least 500 g, and demonstrating spontaneous respirations and/or heart beat.

Stillbirth, fetal death: Intrauterine death of fetus weighing 500 g or more before or during labor, subsequently delivered with no objective evidence of life at birth.

Neonatal death: Demise of a liveborn infant up to and including the 28th day of life.

Infant death: Death of a liveborn infant after 28 days but prior to its first birthday.

Perinatal mortality: Rate of death (per

This chapter provides brief explanatory descriptions of many of the major variables explored in these investigations. It is by no means a complete listing of all the variables studied, however.

1000) based on the sum of fetal and neonatal deaths divided by the total number of infants born, multiplied by 1000.

Birth weight: First weight recorded for the newborn infant, usually obtained within 30 minutes of birth, expressed in grams.

Apgar score: Summation of scores for the vital signs of the newborn infant (heart rate, respiratory effort, muscle tone, reflex irritability, and skin color) at one and at five minutes after birth, respectively, ranging from 10 (best condition) to 0 (poorest condition); neonatal depression considered to be present with scores of 5 or less. Data for Apgar scores were also trichotomized into (1) severe depression, 0-4; (2) moderate depression, 5-7; (3) not depressed, 8-10.

Mental score: Score on Bayley mental scale of infant development derived from standardized psychological examination administered at 8 months of age; scores below 56 considered abnormal.

Motor score: Bayley motor scale results obtained at 8 months of age; abnormal if below 20.

Global score: Summary of the psychological results of extensive examination performed at age 8 months.

Neurological abnormality: Overt disorder diagnosed at 1 year of age on detailed neurologic examination.

Speech, language, and hearing examination: Comprehensive testing of language reception, language expression, hearing, speech mechanism, and speech production at 3 and 8 years of age.

Intelligence quotient: Stanford-Binet intelligence scale summary score obtained at age 4 and 7 years; considered abnormally low if below 70. IQ scores were also standardized by race and sex for this study, using cut points (at two standard deviations below the mean) based on stratified race-sex specific distributions of scores, as follows for 4- and 7-year scores:

White males	70	76
Black males	62	64
White females	73	75
Black females	65	67

Children scoring below these cut points were deemed abnormal. The cut points for suspect cases were:

White males	86	90
Black males	76	77
White females	90	89
Black females	78	79

Risk Variables

Gestational age: Duration of pregnancy at the time of delivery as calculated from the first day of the last menstrual period prior to conception, expressed in weeks completed.

Labor course: A series of derived variables based on reconstruction of the pattern of cervical dilatation and fetal descent, with specific quantitation of durations of latent phase, active phase, deceleration phase, and total first and second stages plus maximum slopes of dilatation and descent.

Type of delivery: Designation of delivery process as to vaginal versus abdominal delivery and further differentiation according to presentation (vertex versus breech), instrumentation (spontaneous versus forceps or vacuum extraction), type of operative approach (low forceps, midforceps, forceps rotation, axis traction, version, etc), and degree of difficulty. Ancillary procedures, such as fundal (Kristeller) pressure, are included here.

Fetal position: Spatial relationship of fetal presenting part with reference to the maternal pelvis (left occiput anterior, direct sacrum posterior, etc.), stratified by degree of flexion or extension and asynclitism.

Labor induction: Process for attempting to initiate labor, usually by amniotomy and/or uterotonic stimulation, whether successful or not. A similar designation exists for labor augmentation. The indication for the induction or augmentation, if any, is always specified. Details of drug, dosage, and mode of administration, and reactions are noted.

Membrane status: Condition of the chorioamniotic membranes, that is, intact or ruptured, at various time frames such as before labor, at onset of labor, in active phase, or during second stage.

Obstetrical attendant: Person directly responsible for the actual delivery procedure, specifically staff physician, resident, intern, nurse, midwife, or medical student.

Shoulder dystocia: Impeded delivery of the fetal shoulders following successful vaginal delivery of the head.

Cord complication: Prolapse of the umbilical cord, both overt and occult, as well as short cord, nuchal cord, or true knot in cord.

Abruptio placentae: Premature separation of the normally implanted placenta, generally diagnosed on the basis of characteristic clinical manifestations.

Placenta previa: Forelying placenta at or over the internal os of cervix, usually presenting with painless vaginal bleeding.

Drugs in labor: Agents used for sedation, tranquilization, analgesia, anesthesia, uterotonic stimulation, etc, to which parturients are exposed in the course of labor; they are specified as to type, dosage regimen, time given, route, and reaction.

Predictor or Modifier Variables

Marital status: Married, single, common-law, etc, as recorded in response to query in early antepartum interview.

Patient status: Clinic or private; patients at all but one institution were exclusively sampled from the clinic service population.

Prior pregnancies: Number of precedent conceptions regardless of outcome.

Prior viable pregnancies: Number of foregoing pregnancies carried to viability, 20 weeks of gestational age, regardless of outcome to fetus or number of fetuses resulting.

Outcome of last prior pregnancy: Reported result to fetus, whether abortion, surviving livebirth, stillbirth, neonatal death, or late infant death.

Birth weight of last prior pregnancy: As recorded, in grams.

Smoking history: Recorded duration in years, largest amount smoked per day, current amount in number of cigarettes per day.

Length of time to conceive, contraception, sterility investigation: As recorded.

Medical, surgical, and psychiatric conditions: Extensive survey based on information encoded in the NCPP data files.

Symptom survey: Review of subjective manifestations considered possibly relevant.

Blood type: Landsteiner typing group (O, A, B, and AB), determined early in pregnancy.

Rh factor: Presence or absence of D-antigen coating the maternal erythrocytes.

Lowest hemoglobin, hematocrit: Minimal value obtained on periodic blood analyses done during the course of pregnancy.

Prepregnancy weight: Maternal weight prior to conception, in pounds, as reported to interviewer early in pregnancy.

Maternal height: Height, in inches, as obtained at first antepartum physical examination.

Religion: Gravida's religion, as recorded, in major denominations.

Place of birth: Geographic area and generic designation as to urban, rural, etc.

Education: Completed formal schooling of gravida.

Family income: Annual income as reported to interviewer early in pregnancy.

Housing density: Number of rooms in living quarters divided by number of occupants.

Socioeconomic index: Combined mean of scores based on education and occupation of head of household, together with that for total annual income, range 0-93:

Education:

1 year of college or more	90
High school graduate	70
10th-11th grade	40
7th-9th grade	10
Less	0

Annual family income:

$7000 or more	100
$6000-6999	90
$5000-5999	80
$4000-4999	70

$3000-3999	50	Craftsman	50
$2000-2999	30	Operative	40
$1000-1999	10	Domestic	30
Less	0	Other service	20

Occupation:

		Laborer (including farm)	10

Professional (and college student)	90
Proprietor or manager	80
Clerical	70
Sales	60

None (including noncollege student) 0

Infant sex: Phenotype as determined at time of birth.

CHAPTER 6

Error Surveillance and Analysis

Summary

Extensive examination of the original patient hard-copy records was carried out to verify magnetic tape entries pertaining especially to labor progression information contained therein. The overall error rate was quite small. Whereas frequencies varied among institutions, none was found to have an unacceptably high rate. The analysis clearly showed the data files to be suitably complete and accurate for our investigational purposes.

Because so much depended on the data reliability, we felt compelled to determine completeness and accuracy before embarking on these studies. Further, we felt an obligation to ensure that any information we might eventually derive about relationships between labor-delivery factors and outcome could be relied upon as valid. Toward this end, we concentrated on variables critical to our needs, seeking among them entries that carried a high probability of being erroneous. We cross-checked the NCPP stored magnetic tape entries against those in the original hard-copy patient records written at the bedside when the observations were first made and recorded.

This entailed extensive hand operations. As stated, we concentrated on variables pertaining to the labor process, including such important items of information as date, time, cervical dilatation and fetal station. Patient records were preselected by a specially designed computer program devised as a means for data screening and case selection. All observations entered in a case selected in this manner were surveyed validated.

Record Selection

We especially sought out cases in which recordings were likely to be spurious. To accomplish this, the program first sorted and ordered the sequence of all recorded observations of dilatation and station for all patients by clock time and date, the date having been converted to Julian calendar for uniformity and continuity (ie, May 13 is Julian day 133, except in leap year). Next, the rates of progression were calculated for each pair of adjacent sequential recordings. A negative rate was deemed suspect because it was likely to represent an error (of observation, entry, coding, or key punching) since regression of dilatation or descent is not expected in nature, even under the most abnormal or pathologic circumstances. Similarly, positive rates in excess of acceptable limits (which we arbitrarily set at 10 cm/h at the outset) were felt to warrant confirmation because, while they did occur in nature, they were sufficiently unusual to justify verification. Thus, although they were not necessarily errors, by definition, such rapid rates of change occurred so seldom in clinical practice that we felt they represented a phenomenon with a high probability of being wrong.

From among the quarter million recorded labor observations (see chapter 4), we were able to identify 24,927 as potentially spurious by this computer-selection technique. They were found to have been incorporated into the records of 17,021 women. Less than 40% (9921) were of the more serious negative-rate variety; they involved 6982 gravidas. Within the Project records of the 17,021 patients, there were a total of 137,235 examinations recorded (including the possible spurious ones, of course); there were 54,620 recorded examinations in the files of the subpopulation of 6982 women who were of greatest interest to us because of the more dubious observations entered for them.

Institutional Distribution

Distribution by institution is shown in Table 6-1. The overall frequency ranges from 21.9% to 89.2% of core cases, but the more critical negative-rate "error" falls between 4.8% and 22.7%. Except for cases from Institution 31, in which both types of

Table 6-1
Distribution of Gravidas with Potentially Spurious Entries by Institution

Institutional Code	Total NCPP Core Cases No.	Total Error Series No.	%	Negative-Rate Entries No.	%	Rapid-Rate Entries No.	%
05	12,915	3,630	28.1	1,488	11.5	2,142	16.6
10	2,928	931	31.8	140	4.8[b]	791	27.0[a]
15	2,590	568	21.9[b]	205	7.9[b]	363	14.0
31	1,578	967	61.3[a]	358	22.7[a]	609	38.6[a]
37	3,766	1,198	31.8	575	15.3	623	16.5
45	3,243	1,074	33.1	462	14.2	612	18.9
50	3,127	1,123	35.9	416	13.3	707	22.6
55	1,912	1,706	89.2[a]	136	7.1[b]	1,570	82.1[a]
60	3,181	1,136	35.7	613	19.3[a]	523	16.4
66	9,970	2,566	25.7	1,771	17.8[a]	795	8.0[b]
71	2,777	737	26.5	486	17.5[a]	251	9.0[b]
82	3,553	1,385	39.0[a]	332	9.3[b]	1,053	29.6[a]
Total	51,540	17,021	33.0	6,982	13.5	10,039	19.5

a   Statistically significant increase, p less than 0.01.
b   Statistically significant decrease, p less than 0.01.

entries were seen rather often (22.7% negative-rate and 38.6% rapid-rate entries), no apparent correlative trend was uncovered. By contrast, the records from five institutions (10, 55, 66, 71 and 82) showed paradoxically counterbalancing high frequencies of one type of entry and low frequencies of the other. It seems likely, on this basis, that these data did not necessarily reflect the quality of the record entries.

Other factors were perhaps at play here. One could conjecture that the population make-up at several institutions favored precipitate labors (eg, large numbers of high-parity gravidas) or that their obstetrical practices fostered rapid cervical dilatation and fetal descent (eg, frequent use of uterotonic augmentation of otherwise normal labors). Negative-rate entries could reflect activities at a teaching program in which medical or nursing students or inexperienced interns or residents may have misinterpreted observations. While the latter constitute errors insofar as the patient is concerned, they could not be considered recording errors from our viewpoint. It was clear from these data, nevertheless, that closer analysis of the data was in order.

Types of Errors

When the 17,021 cases with suspicious entry sequences were examined in more detail, it was found that observations of cervical dilatation were involved much more often than those of fetal station (61.4% versus 37.3%, and 1.4% in which both were involved concurrently). Since there were about the same number of dilatation and station recordings in the NCPP files (see chapter 4), the frequency of dilatation entry errors thus identified far exceeded the expected proportion.

Moreover, breakdown by both the type of entry and the variety of potential error (Table 6-2) illustrated that both kinds of errors occurred more commonly with dilatation recordings. Negative-rate entries involved more than 1.6 times the number of dilatation observations than station observations (23.8% versus 14.7%); rapid-rate entries involved more than 1.7 times the dilatation records (37.6% versus 22.6%).

Institutional data (Table 6-2) was quite consistent in this regard as well. In only one hospital (15) was the aforementioned relationship not encountered. The descent data

Table 6-2
Types of Potentially Spurious Entries by Institution*

Institution Code	Rapid Dilatation	Rapid Descent	Negative Dilatation	Negative Descent	Both Negative
05	38	21	31	9	1
10	46	39	8	7	0
15	20	44	14	20	2
31	39	24	20	17	0
37	46	6	33	15	0
45	45	12	24	17	2
50	48	15	28	6	3
55	55	37	5	3	0
60	28	18	33	20	1
66	19	12	42	26	1
71	27	7	34	25	7
82	40	36	13	11	0
Total	38	23	24	15	1

* Data presented in percentages across rows for each institution.

there inexplicably proved to contain more potential errors than the dilatation recordings, although as noted earlier, the absolute prevalence of such observations at that institution was small.

As we have just seen, cases identified as having a possible labor entry error totalled 33.0% of the NCPP core population. Nearly two thirds related to excessively rapid rates of change. These were examined first because the broad range of institutional frequencies (see above) made us skeptical about their validity. Preliminary survey did indeed verify that the rapid-rate criterion for case selection was a poor one because nearly all the file data relating to those sequences were correct. Our subsequent analytic efforts in regard to entry errors, therefore, concentrated almost exclusively on a sampling of the 6982 gravidas who had been identified as having negative-rate entries in their records.

Data Verification

Our first full-scale error analysis dealt with examination of the records of a sampling of 200 gravidas delivered at one institution (05). This hospital unit was specifically chosen because it was the facility at which a plurality of NCPP infants were delivered, namely 25.1%; its Project population, therefore, could be considered representative of the whole. The 200 cases constituted 5.5% of the 3630 preselected cases with identifiable errors or 13.4% of the 1488 with negative-rate errors. Among the latter, they were a 1:7 sampling—that is, every seventh listed record arranged by registration identification number was selected for detailed study.

Examination of these 200 records yielded 8644 data items for corroboration. Each of these was verified by hand with the original hard-copy patient record, including 2154 calendar date entries, 2154 clock time entries, 2163 cervical dilatation entries, and 2173 fetal station entries. A total of 88 true errors were uncovered for an overall error rate referable to these data items of 1.02%.

This was considered to be an acceptable and creditable finding.

These 88 errors included seven date entries or 0.32% of the 2154 date recordings we examined in this phase of the analysis; 26 time entries or 1.21% of the time recordings we studied; 27 cervical dilatation entries or 1.25%; and 28 station entries or 1.29%. All appeared to have resulted from key-punch mistakes. All proved to be correctable in the sense that the correct datum could be readily fed back into the Project magnetic tapes for purposes of substitution for the erroneous item of information.

Among 187 computer-identified sequencing "errors" involving dilatation recordings, only three were verified as having actually been incorrect, or 1.60%; for 63 station recordings thus identified, three were indeed incorrect, or 4.76%; 2 of 253 time values associated with erroneous sequences were confirmed to be wrong, or 0.79%.

We also examined those recordings in the case records that had not been flagged as possibly spurious. We did this in order to learn whether comparable frequencies of error occurred in observations that appeared essentially correct. Among 1764 dilatation recordings that were not suspected of being problematical in any way, we found six or 0.34% to have been incorrectly entered onto the magnetic tape, plus 13 or 0.74% that had been omitted, and 3 or 0.17% that could not be found in the original hard-copy record. This yielded a total error rate for "correct" dilatation data of 1.25%. Similarly, for 1925 "correct" station data, six or 0.31% were in error, 15 or 0.78% omitted, and two or 0.10% not verifiable, for a total error rate of 1.19%. For 1901 "correct" time entries, seven or 0.37% were wrong and 17 or 0.89% had been omitted, totalling 1.26% errors. There were no identifiable errors of this nature within the date entries.

Finally, we surveyed "blank" entries, specifically seeking to determine if any data that had been omitted from the magnetic tape sequences did actually exist in the original patient records. Among 212 such omissions in dilatation sequences, two were located in the records, or a 0.94% error rate; similarly, two were found among 185 blank station entries, or 1.08%.

Frequency of Errors

In all, therefore, there were 88 errors: 38 true errors (of commission) in the entered data (0.44%); 45 items that had been inadvertently omitted (0.52%); and five items that could not be verified from the source documents (0.06%). This tallied to a total error rate of 1.02% among the 8644 items of data that were surveyed.

Interestingly and of critical concern, in only two instances among the 200 patient records that we studied could any of these 88 errors be considered to have been at all serious in terms of their possible impact on a clinical assessment of the labor course. One of them would have resulted in the

failure to diagnose an arrest of dilatation had the error not been uncovered. The other would have incorrectly caused a failure of descent to be diagnosed. In no other case could the error have influenced either diagnosis or management in any discernible way. The error analysis for the data surveyed in the records derived from Institution 05 is summarized in Table 6-3.

Expanded Survey

We expanded this form of analysis to assess uniformity across other institutional data. An additional 267 case records were surveyed in an attempt to examine a reasonable number of recordings from the other collaborating hospitals. The cases were selected on a proportional basis according to population size, taking into account the relative frequency of identified potential errors, concentrating particularly on the negative-rate type as before. The propor-

Table 6-3
Error Analysis Based on Review of Institution 05 Data

Information Surveyed	Total No.	Confirmed No.	Confirmed %	Error[a] No.	Error[a] %	Omission[b] No.	Omission[b] %	Unverified[c] No.	Unverified[c] %
Cervical dilatation									
Routine entries	1,764	1,742	98.75	6	0.34	13	0.74	3	0.17
Identified "errors"	187	184	98.40	3	1.60	0	0.00	0	0.00
Blank entries	212	210	99.06	2	0.94	0	0.00	0	0.00
Total	2,163	2,136	98.75	11	0.51	13	0.60	3	0.14
Fetal Station									
Routine entries	1,925	1,902	98.81	6	0.31	15	0.78	2	0.10
Identified "errors"	63	60	95.24	3	4.76	0	0.00	0	0.00
Blank entries	185	183	98.92	2	1.08	0	0.00	0	0.00
Total	2,173	2,145	98.71	11	0.51	15	0.69	2	0.09
Time designation									
Routine entries	1,901	1,877	98.74	7	0.37	17	0.89	0	0.00
Identified "errors"	253	251	99.21	2	0.79	0	0.00	0	0.00
Total	2,154	2,128	98.79	9	0.42	17	0.79	0	0.00
Date designation									
Total	2,154	2,147	99.68	7	0.32	0	0.00	0	0.00
Grand total	8,644	8,556	98.98	38	0.44	45	0.52	5	0.06

[a] Entry in magnetic tape incorrect when compared with hard-copy recording.
[b] Recording in original hard-copy file omitted from magnetic tape.
[c] Entry in magnetic tape not found in hard-copy record.

tional sampling approach we used yielded a 1:36.5 sampling of computer-identified cases overall, ranging from a low yield for an institution (such as 55) with a rather high frequency of the inconsequential rapid-rate "errors" (92.0%) to high ratios for those (such as 66 and 71) with high frequencies of the more serious negative-rate errors (69.0% and 65.9%).

Based solely on the incidence of negative-rate errors identified in each institution's records, the sampling technique provided an overall ratio of 1:15.0 and relative homogeneity with regard to selection by institution, ranging from 1:13.6 to 1:23.9 (of case records examined to records preselected because they contained an identifiable "error" of this type), for all institutions, except 05 which had been previously studied in greater depth (1:7.4 ratio). The sampling distribution is displayed in Table 6-4.

Among the 467 case records we surveyed by the method detailed above, we validated 17,916 data entries in all (Table 6-5). These were derived from 4462 recorded labor examinations pertaining to 4488 observations and entries of cervical dilatation, 4504 of station, 4462 of clock time, and 4462 of calendar date. In total, only 188 actual errors could be found for an overall error rate of 1.05%. This was almost identical with the 1.02% rate disclosed by our earlier more limited review of Institution 05 records, and equally gratifying.

Observations of cervical dilatation, numbering 4488 in all, were found to be erroneous 50 times, or 1.11%. Fourteen of these were expectedly concentrated in the data group (totalling 352) that had been specifically identified as a negative-rate error by our case selection program, or 3.98%; 34 occurred in routine survey of 3788 entries not suspected to be in error (0.90%), and the remaining two in 348 blank entries (0.57%). Comparable findings were encountered among the 4504 fetal station recordings of which 56 or 1.24% were wrong.

Again as anticipated, the greatest frequency of true errors occurred in those previously identified as possible errors (14 of 207, or 6.76%); fewer errors occurred in routinely surveyed station data (40 of 3955, or 1.01%) and least in blank entries (two of 342, or 0.58%). Time and date entries were relatively more accurate, overall error rates of 0.87% (39 of 4462 time designations) and 0.96% (43 of 4462 date recordings) being found. As to time designations, the error rate was the same whether associated with an identified error (five of 562, or 0.89%) or not (34 of 3900, or 0.87%). Table 6-5 summarizes this aspect of our analysis.

Table 6-4
Case Sampling for Error Analysis by Institution

Institution Code	Core Cases (A)	Total Errors (B)	Negative-rate Errors (C)	Cases Sampled (D)	Ratio to Core (D:A)	Ratio to Error (D:B)	Ratio to Neg. Rate (D:C)
05	12,915	3,630	1,488	200	1:61	1:18.2	1:7.4
10	2,928	931	140	9	1:325	1:103.4	1:15.6
15	2,590	568	205	14	1:185	1:40.6	1:14.6
31	1,578	967	358	19	1:83	1:50.9	1:18.8
37	3,766	1,198	575	28	1:135	1:42.8	1:20.5
45	3,243	1,074	462	23	1:141	1:46.7	1:20.1
50	3,127	1,123	416	20	1:156	1:56.2	1:20.8
55	1,912	1,706	136	10	1:191	1:170.6	1:13.6
60	3,181	1,136	613	29	1:110	1:39.2	1:21.1
66	9,970	2,566	1,771	74	1:135	1:34.7	1:23.9
71	2,779	737	486	23	1:121	1:32.0	1:21.1
82	3,553	1,385	332	18	1:197	1:76.9	1:18.4
Total	51,540	17,021	6,982	467	1:110	1:36.5	1:15.0

Institutional Differences

Stratification by institution (Table 6-6) showed a spectrum of overall error rates ranging from 0.19% for Institution 60 to 3.38% for Institution 55. No special attributes of the institutions at either extreme of the distribution could be identified to ex-

Table 6-5
Error Analysis for All Project Data Reviewed

Information Surveyed	Entries Verified	Errors Encountered	Overall Rate %	Corrected Rate* %
Cervical dilatation				
Routine entries	3,788	34	0.90	0.03
Identified "errors"	352	14	3.98	0.85
Blank entries	348	2	0.57	0.00
Total	4,488	50	1.11	0.09
Fetal station				
Routine entries	3,955	40	1.01	0.03
Identified "errors"	207	14	6.76	0.48
Blank entries	342	2	0.58	0.00
Total	4,504	56	1.24	0.04
Time designation				
Routine entries	3,900	34	0.87	0.04
Identified "errors"	562	5	0.89	0.36
Total	4,462	39	0.87	0.04
Date designation				
Total	4,462	43	0.96	0.02
Grand total	17,916	188	1.05	0.05

* Corrected by deleting errors without significant clinical impact on labor-delivery evaluation and management.

Table 6-6
Error Analysis by Institution

Institution Code	Cases Reviewed	Examinations Surveyed	Observations Verified	True Errors Encountered	Overall Rate %	Corrected Rate* %
05	200	2,154	8,644	88	1.02	0.02
10	9	80	320	1	0.31	0.00
15	14	97	390	7	1.80	0.00
31	19	208	834	2	0.24	0.00
37	28	200	803	10	1.25	0.12
45	23	235	944	26	2.75	0.21
50	20	227	928	22	2.37	0.11
55	10	111	444	15	3.38	0.45
60	29	259	1,036	2	0.19	0.00
66	74	533	2,135	9	0.42	0.05
71	23	166	668	4	0.60	0.00
82	18	192	770	2	0.26	0.00
Total	467	4,462	17,916	188	1.05	0.05

* Corrected by deleting errors of no apparent clinical significance.

plain the differences thus uncovered. It was deemed unlikely that we were observing any intrinsic differences in attention to details of record keeping or diligence in editing at the source institution because most of the true errors we detected were of the key-punch entry type (see above). Since all operations related to coding, key punching, and data entry onto magnetic tape stores were handled in a uniform manner at the central NCPP headquarters in Bethesda, it follows that institutional record-keeping activities could not be faulted (except perhaps insofar as neatness and legibility were concerned since such factors might influence a key-punch operator's ability to transfer hard-copy information accurately).

The institutional differences were reflected in the error rates for each of the variables of information surveyed (Table 6-7). The frequency of true errors seen in recording of cervical dilatation, which averaged 1.11% overall, ranged from 0.00% at three hospitals (Units 10, 31, and 60) to 4.22% at one (Institution 50). Fetal station entries were wrong 1.24% of the time with the same range of 0.00% (at Institutions 55 and 60) to 4.22% (again at Institution 50). Timing errors averaged 0.87%, with a very wide spread from 0.00% in eight of the 12 collaborating units to 9.01% in one (at Hospital 55). Dates were wrong in 0.96% over-

all, with a range of 0.00% in six units to 8.94% in one (Unit 45).

As can be seen, some institutions yielded consistently good data across the gamut of variables (eg, Units 10, 31, 60, 66, 71, and 82), but none was comparably consistent at the bad end of the scale. Most of the recording errors in the data from Institution 55, for example, were concentrated in the time entries, with dating errors trailing behind; both dilatation and station recordings were creditably accurate. By contrast, almost all the errors at Institution 45 were dating mistakes, whereas at Institution 50 nearly all were dilatation and station misreadings.

The inconsistencies inherent in these observations make it impossible for us to offer logical generalizations as to possible cause. We do not intend this comment to stress the differences but rather to emphasize that there did not seem to be any identifiable area of data resource that could be considered substandard or unworthy. As we noted, the overall true error rate was very small and we found no institution with unacceptable data in terms of pervasively high error rates across the range of variables.

Impact of Errors

Furthermore, the errors we uncovered appeared to have negligible significance in

Table 6-7
Error Analysis by Institution and Variable

Institutional Code	Total No.	%	Cervix No.	%	Station No.	%	Time No.	%	Date No.	%
05	8,644	1.02	2,163	1.25	2,173	1.29	2,154	1.21	2,154	0.32
10	320	0.31	80	0.00	80	1.25	80	0.00	80	0.00
15	390	1.80	98	2.04	98	1.02	97	0.00	97	4.12
31	834	0.24	208	0.00	210	0.95	208	0.00	208	0.00
37	803	1.25	201	1.49	202	1.49	200	0.00	200	0.00
45	944	2.75	236	0.85	238	1.26	235	0.00	235	8.94
50	928	2.37	237	4.22	237	4.22	227	0.44	227	0.44
55	444	3.38	111	1.80	111	0.00	111	9.01	111	2.70
60	1,036	0.19	259	0.00	259	0.00	259	0.77	259	0.00
66	2,135	0.42	534	0.19	536	0.93	533	0.00	533	0.56
71	668	0.60	168	1.19	168	1.19	166	0.00	166	0.00
82	770	0.26	193	0.52	193	0.52	192	0.00	192	0.00
Total	17,916	1.05	4,448	1.11	4,504	1.24	4,462	0.87	4,462	0.96

terms of their possible impact on clinical evaluation and management of the labor in which they occurred (see above). All but nine of the 188 errors identified among the 17,916 items of information we verified had no recognizable adverse effect, leaving a corrected rate of 0.05% overall (Table 6-5). Four of them were dilatation errors (0.09% of 4488 recordings); two were station errors (0.04% of 4504 entries); two were timing errors (0.04% of 4462); and one was a dating error (0.02% of 4462 recordings). Six of these nine clinically important recording errors had been identified by our computer selection program on the basis of a negative-rate trend (three dilatation, one station, and two timing errors). If the aforementioned total error rates were considered good at the 1% level, these must be deemed especially fine at rates consistently less than 0.1%.

Corrected error rates by institution were equally favorable (Table 6-6). No such meaningful errors were found at six of the hospitals surveyed; one each occurred at three hospitals, and two each at three others. The highest frequency (at Institution 55) was only 0.45%, still quite acceptable, reflecting two such errors in 444 observations.

These findings indicate that the magnetic tape files can be relied upon as a valid resource because they contain highly accurate data pertaining to the labor events. Despite the fact that we set out specifically and deliberately to examine data entries that had a high likelihood of being wrong, we were favorably impressed with the very small error rates we encountered. Moreover, the huge task of collecting data from different institutions as observed and recorded by different personnel should work against uniformity, accuracy, and reliability; nonetheless, we have confirmed the exemplary high standards of completeness and accuracy achieved by these data.

CHAPTER 7

Research Design

Summary

The study as conceptualized is designed to utilize outcome measures to identify adverse and beneficial labor and delivery risk factors. The latter in turn would flag intrinsic characteristics of the gravida to serve as predictors. Stepwise sequences are presented for dealing with labor progression variables as a group, then adjunctive drugs, intrinsic factors, and finally delivery-related variables. The statistical methods to be used are specified.

As outlined earlier (chapter 2), our aim was to determine the influence of labor-delivery factors on fetal and infant outcome, with particular concentration on long-term effects. Toward this end, we wanted to try to identify specific risk factors contributing to perinatal death and to the development of neurologic and developmental disorders. Once such factors were identified, we felt it important to quantitate their impact. Then it would be necessary to describe the constellation of factors that place the fetus and infant in special jeopardy. This would allow us to define high-risk labor and delivery. It would also permit us to describe the gravida-at-risk who is likely to develop those specified labor-delivery constellations later in the course of her pregnancy. Finally, such information might prove clinically useful in providing means for making meaningful recommendations for standards of care designed to optimize outcome.

Proposed Analyses

The components of the series of analyses

that formed the sequence of activities we envisioned to accomplish these objectives were as follows:

1. Error analysis (chapter 6)
2. Labor progression data patterns (chapters 8-14)
3. Adjunctive pharmacologic agents (chapters 15-18)
4. Intrinsic maternal, fetal, and pelvic factors (chapters 19-21)
5. Delivery variables (chapters 22-24)
6. Aggregation of risk factors (chapter 25)
7. Predictor variables (chapter 28)
8. Gravida-at-risk (chapter 29)
9. Obstetrical standards (chapter 30)
10. Practice recommendations

This stepwise approach is detailed here to help guide the reader in tracing the path we took. While we never lost sight of our ultimate goal, tangential explorations proved necessary at times, making the road we travelled appear somewhat circuitous. Moreover, these steps did not always actually take place seriatim, even though they are presented here chapter by chapter as if they had. Temporarily insoluble data manipulation or analytical problems in a given area did not prevent us from moving on to areas more amenable to solution, while continuing to work concurrently on the knottier issues still pending. Mention will be made of these problems in passing for completeness.

Design Overview

An overview of the design might make it easier to comprehend the flow and logic in these programmatic steps (Figure 7-1). We expected that bad outcomes (A) would help identify adverse labor-delivery risk factors (B). In other words, those labor-delivery variables carrying the most deleterious effects will be flagged as hazardous. Once we have been able to identify such risk factors associated with the labor and delivery process, those predictor variables (C) that are determined to lead most often to the aberrant labor-delivery constellation (B) can be defined. The relevant predictor variables (C) describe the gravida-at-risk who is most likely to develop the deleterious labor-delivery pattern. Thus, the outcome (A) defines the labor-delivery risk (B) and the latter then defines the predictive factors (C).

To this end, we addressed the issue of assessing the effects of potential risk factors on outcome first (B-to-A relationship in Figure 7-1). Because more than 2000 variables (ultimately 2441 in all) were to be considered within the risk-variable category, we divided the material into four logical groups, namely (1) labor factors, (2) adjunctive drugs and anesthetics, (3) intrinsic maternal and fetal factors, and (4) delivery-related factors. Each of these groups of variables was examined in turn both for the individual isolated effect of every variable on outcome as well as for the

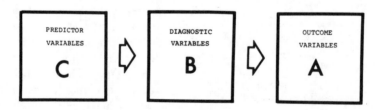

Figure 7-1. Design overview concept. The outcome variables (A) in fetus and infant help identify those diagnostic entities (B) in labor and at delivery that place the offspring at risk. These conditions in turn help to define predictor variables (C) in the pregnancy that may prove useful for identifying the gravida-at-risk.

collective effects of all items in the group acting simultaneously. This is represented pictorially in Figure 7-2. Those variables in each of the four major groups proving to have a significant impact on the fetus were then to be aggregated for purposes of determining their interrelational effects on outcome, that is, the effect of each variable when all others were being simultaneously taken into effect.

Later, it will be necessary to reconsider the risk effects of the residual factors first having deleted those designated "intrinsic" in order to determine whether any of the latter were functioning as predictor variables (C-to-B pathway in Figure 7-1). Analyses were then to be carried out to weigh the relationship between these (and other) possible predictors and the constellation of labor and delivery factors found to affect the fetus and infant, bringing us full circle back to fulfill the objectives of the original proposed design (Figure 7-3).

Editing and Creating Data File

Preliminarily, data editing had to be completed and an appropriate data file established. The details of these operations are neither critical to the material that follows nor germane to the central theme. This should not be interpreted to signify that such foundational activities are unimportant; on the contrary, without them, little could have been accomplished (that is to say, little that could be considered meaningful). The extensive error analysis, reported in detail in chapter 6, verified that our data file was both complete (for our needs) and accurate.

Analysis of Labor Data

Labor progression data were to be investigated next to determine which aspects of the patterns of labor progression might be associated with bad outcomes. In this

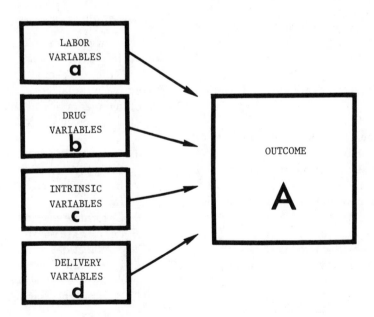

Figure *7-2.* Detailed examination of risk factor to outcome pathway (B-to-A relationship) depicted in Figure 7-1. Potential risk factors are divided into four logical groups. The outcome effects of all variables in each group are examined separately and collectively: a-A, chapter 14; b-A, chapter 18; c-A, chapter 21; d-A, chapter 24.

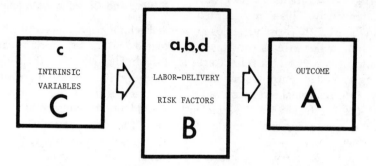

Figure 7-3. Rearrangement of grouped variables to permit assessment of the possible predictor effects of intrinsic variables (c, Figure 7-2) in the constellation of residual labor-delivery factors (a, b, and d, Figure 7-2) found to have significant outcome effects. This provides a means for evaluating the C-to-B pathway in Figure 7-1; the analysis is detailed in chapter 26.

regard, we had strong leads based on foregoing studies.* Nevertheless, we did not wish to be influenced by preceding observations. Instead, we felt it important to allow the data on outcome to define those variables relating to labor progression that placed the fetus and infant at risk (see above). Accordingly, we devised a series of logical steps to accomplish this objective:

1. Formulate dilatation and station file.
2. Rectify data.
3. Screen for minimum standards of acceptability.
4. Construct dilatation and descent pattern sequences.
5. Compute relevant durations and slopes.
6. Determine distributions.
7. Define disordered patterns.
8. Relate increments of durations and slopes to outcomes.

9. Relate disordered patterns to outcomes.
10. Identify labor course risk variables.
11. Quantitate degree of risk.

Analysis of Adjunctive Agents

Adjunctive pharmacologic agents administered to women in labor were to be studied in the next phase of this project, encompassing analgesics, anesthetics, and uterotonic agents, among many others. We expected to proceed as follows:

1. Compile data file encompassing all drug exposure.
2. Incorporate route, dosage, and time factors.
3. Determine distributions by agents, categories of agents, and combinations.
4. Enumerate drug usage and dosage patterns by phase of labor.
5. Select agent-usage combinations.
6. Relate agents to outcomes.
7. Relate agents to outcomes by phase of labor.
8. Relate agents to outcomes by time administered before delivery.
9. Identify drug risk variables.
10. Quantitate degree of risk.

---

* Friedman EA: Patterns of labor as indicators of risk. *Clin Obstet Gynecol* 1973; 16:172, Friedman EA, Sachtleben MR, Bresky PA: Dysfunctional labor: XII. Long-term effects on infant. *Am J Obstet Gynecol* 1977; 127:779; Friedman EA, Sachtleben-Murray M, Dahrouge D, Neff RK: Long-term effects of labor and delivery on offspring: A matched-pair design analysis. *Am J Obstet Gynecol* 1984; 150:941.

Analysis of Intrinsic Factors

Subsequently, the impact of intrinsic obstetrical factors was to be determined by a similar series of steps. Before proceeding, however, it was essential to spell out potentially relevant maternal and fetal factors that could be considered to constitute the spectrum of variables that are known to have or are suspected of having adverse effects on the fetus or surviving infant. The following is an admittedly incomplete list giving the several general categories of intrinsic variables and examples of each:

Demographic variables: Race, marital status, hospital status, age, gravidity, parity, height, prepregnancy weight, socioeconomic index

Gestational variables: Pregnancy duration, membrane status, duration of ruptured membranes, prelabor cervical preparation and fetal station, labor induction

Pelvic variables: Cephalopelvic relationship, pelvic architecture, pelvic capacity, disproportion at inlet, midplane or outlet

Fetal variables: Presentation, position, station, flexion, synclitism, birthweight, weight-gestational age relationship, meconium, hydramnios, sex

Historical variables: Obstetrical experience, prior abortion, prior premature delivery, prior stillbirth, smoking, education, employment, housing, income, birthplace, maternal IQ

Intercurrent disorders: Heart disease, thromboembolic disease, pulmonary disease, blood disease, diabetes mellitus, thyroid disease, venereal disease, etc

These were to be incorporated into the data file for evaluation as to their possible individual and collective effects on the infant according to the following sequence:

1. Designate maternal and fetal variables of potential relevance.
2. Establish variable file.
3. Determine distribution.
4. Determine distribution by phase of labor.
5. Ascertain duration of existence.

6. Relate intrinsic variables to outcomes.
7. Identify intrinsic obstetrical risk variables.
8. Quantitate degree of risk.

Analysis of Delivery Factors

Analysis of delivery variables followed along the same lines. First, we had to specify those variables relating to the delivery process that deserved inclusion on the basis of possible adverse impact on the fetus or infant, choosing from the long list of such variables included in the master files. The following served as a preliminary working list:

Delivery type: Spontaneous delivery, low forceps, midforceps (by fetal station and position), vacuum extraction, assisted breech, breech extraction, cesarean section

Ancillary procedure: Amniotomy, manual rotation, forceps rotation, forceps flexion, external cephalic version, internal podalic version, manual or forceps conversion, forceps to aftercoming head, axis traction

Indication for procedure

Difficulty of procedure

Complication: Abruptio placentae, placenta previa, cord prolapse, vasa previa, marginal sinus rupture, uterine rupture, shoulder dystocia

These delivery-related variables were to be studied in much the same manner as the others, specifically entailing the following:

1. Define relevant delivery variables.
2. Construct delivery variable data file.
3. Determine distributions.
4. Relate delivery variables to outcomes.
5. Identify delivery risk variables.
6. Quantitate degree of risk.

To this point, we will have been able to flag a series of variables on labor course, pharmacologic agents, and intrinsic obstetrical and delivery conditions that are associated with a high risk of bad outcome. The types of outcomes we will study have already been provided (chapter 4), ranging from immediate intrauterine and neonatal death to long-term follow-up into early school years and encompassing 35 different dichotomized outcome variables as well as two collective indices of outcome.

Statistical Methodology

Relating the various study factors to outcome required techniques applicable to both continuous variables (eg, duration of latent phase of labor) and categorical variables (eg, membranes ruptured versus intact). To begin with, we undertook to use the most widely accepted technique for relating continuous and categorical variables to outcomes (the latter considered as dichotomous variables—that is, bad outcome present or absent), namely logistic regression analysis.*

Logistic regression analysis was to be pursued in order to provide critical insights concerning the relative impact of each of the continuous variables, specifically the derived labor variables, on fetal and infant outcomes. We were encouraged to develop this process when we determined we could transform the statistical distributions of labor progression measurements into distributions that very closely follow the gaussian (normal) distribution by means of rather simple transformation processes. For example, the latent phase duration distributions could be linearized on a gaussian scale by transforming the latent phase data by its square root. The fourth root transform satisfied the needs for linearizing the distribution of the slope of dilatation. All the classical statistical analytic machinery associated with the gaussian distribution is applicable on the transform scale.

However, when we undertook to relate outcome events to these transformed varia-

bles (chapter 11), we learned that the risk factors did not follow a symmetrical sigmoid curve as specified by the logistic model. Instead, it tended to yield an asymmetric Gompertz function. We concluded reluctantly, therefore, that the logistic function was a poor mathematical model for purposes of deriving a risk function. Despite the great effort we had expended in this pursuit, the results were unsatisfactory, so that a different approach had to be sought.

Nonparametric Analysis

Greater success was achieved by a nonparametric analysis to evaluate the null hypothesis that a labor progression parameter, for example, was unrelated to the risk of an abnormal outcome. Under this hypothesis, we generated the expected number of abnormalities for each quantum of every labor variable. We assessed the deviation of each observed value from its expected value, using the Freeman-Tukey deviate.* The Freeman-Tukey deviate z is defined as:

$$z = \sqrt{\Phi + 1} + \sqrt{\Phi} - \sqrt{4E - 1}$$

where E, the expected frequency, is computed from the total number with the adverse outcome divided by the grand total (total for normal outcome plus total for bad outcome), all multiplied by the number with the specific increment of variable under surveillance; and Φ is the actual number of adverse outcomes for that particular variable increment. The Freeman-Tukey deviates (FTD) are asymptotically distributed as the standard gaussian distribution. Thus, an FTD value of 1.96 or -1.96 can be interpreted to mean that the expected incidence of an adverse outcome differed from the observed incidence with a total probability (two-sided) of 5%; an FTD of 2.58 or -2.58 signifies a 1% probability (two-sided) of chance occurrence under the null

*Cox DR: Some procedures connected with logistic qualitative response curve, in David F N (ed.): *Research Papers in Statistics.* London, John Wiley & Sons, 1966, pp 55-71.

* Bishop YMM, Fienberg SE, Holland PE: *Discrete Multivariate Analysis: Theory and Practice.* Cambridge, Mass, The MIT Press, 1975, p 130.

hypothesis.

This approach proved very satisfactory for highlighting those levels of both continuous variables (made discontinuous by grouping) and categorical variables that are likely to be associated with bad outcomes. The technique thus provided a means for designating the risk factors of special interest to us. Incremental data (continuous variables made discontinuous by grouping) were especially well handled because we were able to examine sequences of FTD values to determine levels of relevance. Runs of substantially *negative* FTD values, for example, indicated zones (incremental segments) of a given parameter in which there was a clear *deficit* of observed bad outcomes; zones with substantially *positive* FTD values indicated regions of *excess* abnormal outcomes. In this way, we could define levels of potential adverse risk as well as levels at which the fetus or infant were apparently protected.

Risk Assessment

Relative risk and odds ratio statistics were to be assessed as well. The basic analytical method to be used was the two-way contingency table that relates each potential risk factor to each outcome being studied. Point and interval estimates of the relative risk and odds ratio statistics will be computed for each two-by-two table.* In tables larger than two-by-two, a reference cell will be identified for each table and these statistics computed in relation to the referent cell. Significance testing will be accomplished by the Mantel-Haenszel chi-square test of the null hypothesis that the potential risk factor is not associated with the outcomes.† For a stratified series of two-by-two tables, where the odds ratio is uniform over all the tables, the Mantel-Haenszel chi-square test is optimal; however, it is also used in the case of nonuniform odds ratios. Zelen's test for nonuniformity of the odds ratio will be used to detect nonuniformity.‡ For tables with more than two categories of the potential risk factor, Mantel's extension will be used.ξ We planned also to estimate the relative risk from multidimensional contingency tables using hierarchical log-linear models and the principle of maximum-likelihood.‖ The probability distribution for the "cross-sectional" data collected in this study, as summarized in the two-by-two tables, is the multinomial distribution. For continuous outcome variables, we expected to use multiple regression analysis, both linear and nonlinear as appropriate to the hypothesis under consideration.

We will define high risk variables as those variables with significantly high relative risk or odds ratio values. We will also seek to identify relevant low-risk variables on the basis of relative risk or odds ratio values that are significantly lower than unity. We will use the Seigel-Greenhouseζ method and the multiple logistic regression model of Prenticeδ for estimating relative risk and odds ratio with multiple stratification variables. In this way, multiple factors can be studied simultaneously. The rationale for studying variables in combination includes the possibility that factors may be acting synergistically or antagonistically, or the presence of one factor may modify the effect of another on the outcome. We anticipate beginning our investigations by con-

* Gart JJ: Point and interval estimation of the common odds ratio in the combination of 2x2 tables with fixed marginals. *Biometrika* 1970; 57:471; Thomas DT: Exact and asymptotic methods for the combination of 2x2 tables. *Comput Biomed Res* 1975; 8:423; Gart J J: The comparison of proportions: A review of significance tests, confidence intervals and adjustments for stratification. *Rev Int Stat Inst* 1971; 39:148.

† Mantel N, Haenszel W: Statistical aspects of the analysis of data from retrospective studies of disease. *J Nat Cancer Inst* 1959; 22:719.

‡ Zelen M: The analysis of several 2x2 contingency tables. *Biometrika* 1971; 58:129.

ξ Mantel N: Chi-square tests with one degree of freedom: Extensions of the Mantel-Haenszel procedure. *J Am Statist Assoc* 1963; 58:690.

‖ Basic methods are contained in Bishop YMM, Fienberg SE, Holland PW: *Discrete Multivariate Analysis: Theory and Practice*. Cambridge, Mass, The MIT Press, 1975.

ζ Seigel DG, Greenhouse SW: Multiple relative risk functions in case control studies. *Am J Epidemiol* 1973; 97:324.

δ Prentice R: Use of the logistic model in retrospective studies. *Biometrics* 1976; 32:599.

sidering potential risk factors singly, thus identifying those potential risk factors likely to be related to the outcomes under study. Combinations of variables thus identified will then be studied as related to synergism/antagonism or effect modification.

Cluster Analysis

Given these effective methods for designating risk variables, perhaps in large numbers, we felt we would be able to focus on groups with distinctive profiles that could be related to high fetal and infant risk. Aggregative hierarchical clustering techniques* were to be brought to bear to improve the set of variables, by which we meant to try to identify analytic variables that are very similar in informational content. Those that are similar contain much the same information insofar as they relate to bad outcome, each reflecting a comparable kind of adverse impact. By studying one of them (that is, one item in a cluster) as an indicator of risk, we would be studying all of those having comparable degrees of similarity.

For these purposes, a large matrix of similarity scores was to be established for variables or for gravidas. This would permit us to take items for which we had some measure of similarity and aggregate them into subgroups of similar items. The similarity between a pair of variables was defined as the absolute value of their Pearson (product-moment) correlation. The absolute value was used so that two variables with correlation near -1 would be considered to be as closely associated as a pair with correlation near +1 rather than maximally dissimilar.

The aggregative hierarchical clustering method was used in order to produce not just one cluster but a whole hierarchy of different clusterings of the group of variables under study. This began with the trivial clusterings of the group of n variables into n one-variable clusters. Then it proceeded step-by-step, merging the pair of most similar clusters into a single new cluster at each step. Finally, all variables have been merged into a single cluster.

The result of this process can be represented as a diagrammatic tree in which each twig represents one of the individual variables and each branching point represents the joining of a pair of clusters into a new cluster of variables. From among the number of different criteria proposed for choosing the pair of clusters to merge at each step, we chose to use the mean intercluster similarity criterion. At each succeeding step, clusters are joined where the mean intercluster similarity is largest, signifying that the mean correlation between the variables in one cluster and the variables in the other cluster is highest.

Our principal objective in pursuing hierarchical clustering in this investigation was not strictly to construct groups of variables, but rather to condense the information that we expected would be forthcoming from all the aforementioned analyses. From the sheer numbers of studies we had anticipated, it was fully expected that large numbers of ostensible risk variables would be generated (if only by chance relationships). Thus, we could foresee the need to reduce the numbers of variables to be studied by some logical means while at the same time ensuring that we would not discard variables of real interest. If we could identify labor and delivery factors that were closely interrelated, only one such factor from a well-defined cluster needed to be considered in successive multivariate analyses. Logically, inclusion of an entire set of highly intercorrelated variables in a multivariate procedure for estimating the effect of a specific labor-delivery factor on offspring will reduce the efficiency of the resultant estimates.*

Control of Confounding

The basic method of controlling for con-

---

* Hartigan JW: *Clustering Algorithms*. New York, John Wiley & Sons, 1975; Anderberg MR: *Cluster Analysis for Applications*. New York, Academic Press, 1973.

founding will be to cross-classify the relevant study series by each confounding factor, creating a stratified series of two-way contingency tables of outcome by potential risk factor relating to labor-delivery event. There are a number of methods in principle for controlling for confounding. These specifically include (1) restriction of the study series to homogeneously defined groups; (2) matching a series of cases with specific labor outcome to a series without that outcome on the values of the confounding factors to be controlled† (both individual and frequency-matching may be used); (3) stratification by one or more cross-classified variables*; or (4) multivariate modeling. Modeling usually takes the form of multiple logistic regression functions.

Additional aid for determining potential confounding factors is provided by the aforementioned cluster analyses. Confounding factors are perforce related to both the adverse outcome (to the offspring) and some specific labor-delivery factors being investigated. Thus, if such factors are found together with a specific labor-delivery variable within a given cluster (related by virtue of similarity of effect with regard to bad outcome), it follows that those factors can be identified as potential confounding factors.

Multivariate Analysis

Modeling by multivariate analysis will be used to identify the most meaningful potential risk factors culled from the foregoing analytical methods. It will enable us to take into account all of those variables deemed relevant by virtue of an association with bad outcome, while simultaneously controlling the influences of independent variables relating to such factors as actuarial, demographic, or institutional influences. The linear discriminant function† and logistic regression analysis are both widely used as multivariate analysis methods. Among those techniques employed in situations in which random variation in several variables has to be studied simultaneously, they have proved especially helpful for ascertaining the extent to which populations overlap with or diverge from each other. We felt we could use the linear discriminant function and the logistic regression function to determine which variables are most effective in distinguishing between parturients who place their offspring at serious risk and those who do not.

These multivariate techniques involve applying separate discriminant function analyses and logistic regression analyses to previously identified risk variables singly and in combination, while controlling for various possible confounding factors. From the total series of variables studied in this way, we felt we would be able to derive extreme t statistics with associated low p values to designate those variates that are likely to add significant information to the information provided by all other variates already in the model. As each variate is added, better distinction is expected to be provided between at-risk and not-at-risk labor-delivery constellations. The composition of such constellations should eventually be clarified by this definitive approach.

Risk-modifying factors were also to be studied, stratifying the multivariate analysis on each level of the modifying factor (that is, we shall perform separate analyses for each value of the factor). By modifying factor we mean one that appears to change the effect (that is, the risk) of a given labor-delivery variable over its range of values.

†Miettinen OS: Matching and design efficiency in retrospective studies. *Am J Epidemiol* 1970; 91:111; Miettinen OS: Individual matching with multiple controls in the case of all-or-none responses. *Biometrics* 1969; 25:339; Miettinen OS: Estimation of relative risk from individually matched series. *Biometrics* 1970; 26:75.

*Cochran WG: The effectiveness of adjustment by subclassification in removing bias in observational studies. *Biometrics* 1968; 24:295.

†Dempster AP: *Elements of Continuous Multivariate Analysis.* Reading, Mass, Addison-Wesley, 1969.

The modifying factor need not itself cause the variation in effect, but merely be associated with effect variation. In general, modifying factors can be identified on the basis of subject matter knowledge. Separate analyses are to be performed for each possible category. In addition, identification will be empirical, separate analyses being run preliminarily to assess whether the measure of effect varies over the categories of the potential modifying factor. Under certain circumstances of no fourth (or higher) order interactions among variables, one can test for effect modification as follows: If the ratio of the difference of the two effect estimates over corresponding standard error of the difference exceeds the value of two ($p < .05$), then we have empirical evidence that there is modification of labor-delivery risk by this stratifying variable. If high-order interactions exist in the data, then log-linear analysis* is the analytical method of choice.

All candidates for inclusion as risk factors for the multivariate analyses must themselves be risk factors of bad outcome when considered in isolation—that is, in bivariate analysis, the factor is associated with such adverse outcome effect. It would be an obvious waste of resources to consider variables in multivariate analysis which are not themselves individual risk factors. The peril this poses from an investigational point of view is, of course, the possibility that important risk factors will be ignored because their deleterious (or protective) effects were masked by some overriding factor with equal or larger magnitude of effect that happened to arise concurrently but may not actually have been associated in the data at hand.

This situation can be detected in the bivariate analysis of each individual risk factor. When a factor is dropped from a multivariate analysis conducted in a step-down manner (deleting the least significant variable until all individual variables attain a minimal significance level, say $p \leq .05$), it is possible that the deleted factor is individually significant, but it shares too much variability (covariation) with a more significant factor. To carry along the less significant factor is not wrong, but it is inefficient. Carrying along a great many such factors can vitiate the multivariate analysis altogether.

Multivariate analysis of a set of potential risk factors proceeds by creation and examination of the marginal distribution of each variable. These distributions are computed when all the case selection and omission criteria are invoked. All coded values must be verified for allowable ranges and legitimacy; extraneous values are noted for eventual special treatment. Further, each variable must have any missing or exceptional values noted, again for later treatment. Illegitimate variables are dropped from the analysis; unacceptable values of variables are noted for special treatment along with their relative frequencies.

It should be stressed that multivariate analysis requires that all cases have values entered for all variables; if they do not, the case is omitted. However, for a data set such as that provided by the NCPP files, complete case data are generally not always available. In fact, NCPP cases often do not have all variables present with legitimate values. Thus, use of multivariate analysis may prove inefficient if large numbers of cases have to be deleted as a consequence of missing data. It is critical, therefore, that we provide a method for treating variables which have missing value codes in order to ensure successful pursuit of multivariate analyses. We adopted the rule that the value of each variable should always be considered to be present; thus, the missing value is not taken to be an indication of no information, but rather as a positive statement for another category or categories of the discrete variable (called "missing" and/or "exceptional").

Another interpretation of the rule is needed for use with continuous, nondis-

* Bishop YMM, Fienberg SE, Holland PE: *Discrete Multivariate Analysis: Theory and Practice.* Cambridge, Mass, The MIT Press, 1975, p 130.

crete variables. For the type of risk factors considered in this study, all variables will be handled as if they were discrete, with suitable recoding and use of cut points (incremental divisions) for continuous variables. Thus, the values missing and exceptional are then merely other values, and no case will have to be omitted because some variables have missing values.

Many forms of multivariate analysis are based on the use of a linear model which implies that the outcome—or a monotone function of it (outcome metameter)—is related to a linear combination of the risk factors. We recognize that little in biology or medicine varies linearly over any appreciable range—that is, much of the variation in biological phenomena is nonlinear. Thus, we shall have to adopt a multivariate model which can take account of nonlinear relationships. The most flexible and simplest or fundamental is that based on the use of indicator or binary (zero/one) variables. A variable, such as inlet pelvic capacity, for example, has the following possible values: code 0, adequate; code 1, contracted; code 2, borderline; code 9, unknown. These four values are transformed into four indicator variables:

$X_1 = 1$ if code 0; else $X_1 = 0$
$X_2 = 1$ if code 1; else $X_2 = 0$
$X_3 = 1$ if code 2; else $X_3 = 0$
$X_4 = 1$ if code 9; else $X_4 = 0$

It is apparent that knowing the values of any three X values gives the fourth. Thus, only three are "independent," the fourth being logically dependent on the other three, allowing us to omit one of them. In principle, any one may be dropped, but we adopt the rule to drop only the most "normal" or typical value, designated the referent value. The X that is set to 1 for the referent value is dropped from the list. In general terms, if a variable has K categories, then only K-1 independent indicator variables are used in multivariate analysis.

Other details are equally important in forming a set of indicator variables. For example, no indicator should be formed if there are no actual data with that category value. No indicator should be formed if it is coincident with another indicator for another variable in the data set—that is, if the actual data make two indicators synonymous, then either one or the other must be dropped. Multivariate analysis does not tolerate any redundancy in the set of variables to be used. Redundancy is not uncommon because missing values occur in clumps so that when one value is missing, other variables also have missing values. One missing value indicator variable should be used for the subset of variables in place of one missing value indicator for each raw variable. Another situation occurs when a series of variables has no values because they are describing an underlying event which is not applicable to that case. Again, one overall indicator of "nonapplicability" should be used for that particular subset of raw variables.

Modeling complex and interrelated biological variables is acknowledged to be difficult. This is so because (1) not all cases should be used, (2) not all variables have values, (3) the basic phenomenon is generally nonlinear even when the model is mathematically linear, and (4) the actual data may have built-in patterns of missing or not-applicable codes. In each case, experience with these modeling techniques shows the way. Often, only actual trial and error with the real data will reveal the successful modeling after several (or many) false starts.

The aim of multivariate analysis, as stated above, is quantification of the effect of one or more variables on the outcome variables. For this investigation of labor-delivery factors, all outcome variables were designed to be dichotomous (normal versus abnormal). This would allow us to utilize multivariate modeling techniques for such outcomes, concentrating on the two currently most prevalent techniques, namely linear discriminant function analysis and logistic regression analysis. For valid statistical inferences to be drawn, linear discriminant function requires data for each outcome to be distributed as the multivariate normal or gaussian distribution. In fact, the requirement of "gaussianity" is more demanding: the distribution for both normal and abnormal outcomes must each be gaussian. However, all of the variables in this study are themselves indicator variables which do not jointly follow the multivariate gaussian distribution. In some cases, the linear combination of a series of indicators (equivalent to a score of the sum of weighted indicator variables) can approximate a univariate gaussian distribution. It becomes important to ensure that the linear discriminant function is appropriate to use. Methods are available for detecting problematic situations in which it will not work well enough.* Inspection of the zero-order correlation coefficients is useful, for example; if they are all positive, the linear discriminant function should not be expected to serve well.

Logistic Regression Analysis

An alternative to linear discriminant function is logistic regression analysis, which does not have the problem associated with validity of inferences that pertains to use of multivariate indicators. Therefore, it should always be applicable, at least in theory. It proved particularly valuable for our needs, as will be seen. As a practical matter, however, the volume of computation of the logistic regression goes up geometrically with increasing numbers of variables. Large numbers of indicator variables thus produce a very substantial computational burden, even for very fast computers. The computation of the linear discriminant function, by contrast, only goes up as the square of the number of variables; it is, therefore, incomparably less work to compute. Some packaged programs compute the linear discriminant function first and then use it to do the logistic regression analysis.

We had expected to use linear discriminant function analysis to select the proper model, that is, to search for a meaningful subset of risk variables. Then we would utilize logistic regression analysis on only those final selected variables for purposes of obtaining estimates of effects from the model, together with applicable standard errors. In actuality, however, we found it necessary to use the aforementioned nonparametric bivariate method for screening, proceeding directly to logistic regression for multivariate analysis.

The estimate of effect for each indicator variable controlling for all other risk factors was taken to be the relative risk (RR, risk ratio, or rate ratio). We expected to use the odds ratio as the estimator of relative risk when the incidence of a bad outcome is less than 10% (as it is for most of the outcomes we will be studying). The odds ratio is estimated by the principle of maximum likelihood from the antilog (to base e) of the logistic regression coefficient for the indicator variable whose effect is to be assessed.

Evaluation of the effect of multiple factors will be done by the standardized morbidity ratio, which is calculated as the observed number of abnormalities (bad outcomes) divided by the expected number of abnormalities. This latter number is, in turn, computed from the logistic regression analysis. Thus, the relative risk is the effect parameter for single factors and the standardized morbidity ratio is the comparable effect parameter for multiple factors. Important risk factors will be defined when the relative risk or standardized morbidity ratio parameter estimates are non-null according to statistical tests of significance (specifically, likelihood ratio tests). The estimated ratios will enable us to quantitate the level of risk for the various labor-delivery factors under surveillance.

Procedures and techniques are thus available to be pursued for carrying out the full sequence of multivariate analyses from raw data to case selection to formation of a valid multivariate model. The model can be expected to yield effect estimates for each

---

*Gilbert ES: On discrimination using qualitative variables. *J Am Statist Assoc* 1968; 63:1399; Moore DH: Evaluation of five discrimination procedures for binary variables. *J Am Statist Assoc* 1973; 68:342.

factor individually, controlling for all other factors, while for subsets of factors, controlling for complementary sets.

CHAPTER 8

Labor Data Development

Summary

An index population of 17,925 gravidas was shown to have ample labor progression data to permit reconstruction of utilitarian cervical dilatation patterns; 14,357 has sufficient observations recorded for reproducing the descent patterns. Programmatic means were developed to recreate the labor progression sequence in each case for purposes of dissection and detailed measurement of its component parts. In addition to various duration and slope quantitations, arrest of progress was diagnosable and the duration of an arrest measurable. Supplementary data were also obtained from cases with incompletely evolved labors.

Our first explicit task in regard to exploring the Project data resource for the impact of labor on the fetus was to describe the labor data pool and its limitations. Error analysis (chapter 6) had already demonstrated the reliability of this resource. At this point, our objective was to determine its scope.

Selecting Index Data Pool

From the total NCPP population of 58,806 gravidas, we culled 45,142 cases (chapter 4) that met all criteria of preselection as core study cases (first study pregnancies and appropriate cohort). These cases contained 275,632 labor observation recordings. Deleting those without pediatric information and those with absent or clearly erroneous date and time entries left 38,269 cases with 189,830 recorded examinations. Rectification of labor progression data (explained in chapter 4) reduced the number of valid observations to 173,706. Reconstruction of adequate patterns of cervical dilatation was feasible for 17,925 women; among them, it was possible to develop usable patterns of fetal descent in 14,357.

Because the proportion of "lost" cases in this initial investigational thrust was relatively large (75.6% of the total or more appropriately, 68.2% of the core population), we felt it important to ensure that the deleted cases did not represent a special group of cases that differed in any important way from the index group. If they did, it would follow that one could not draw valid conclusions about the population from which the index group was drawn (nor, of course, about gravid populations at large) merely by studying the index sample. If substantive differences existed, such selection biases would have to be considered in all future analyses.

Accordingly, we examined both the used and the unused cases for a large variety of relevant factors, such as distribution among the collaborating hospitals, outcomes (and outcomes by institution), parity, race, age, and a host of others. Close review of this material satisfied us that there were no outstanding differences between the material we selected for further study and that which we had tentatively tabled. Further, we recognized the latter was not truly lost because it was still available for later study. Indeed, we intended to return all the cases to the main body of the investigation in such aspects of study as the logistic regression analysis planned to encompass the full data set, for example, when it became necessary to determine predictive factors of the gravida-at-risk.

Graphing Dilatation Patterns by Computer

Once the major effort of case selection and data editing was completed, we embarked directly on investigations dealing with labor assessment. Our initial undertaking was to recreate the clinical capacity to trace dilatation and descent patterns by means of computer algorithms. First, as stated earlier (chapter 4), patterns were smoothed by a rectification process which recognizes unphysiologic—and therefore, unacceptable—regressive points and rejects them. Second, minimal standards of acceptability were applied to ensure that it would be possible to reconstruct the labor pattern. These minimal requirements included documented and recorded clock times of labor onset (t_0) and labor conclusion (t_4), a point (with known dilatation, time, and date) between 2.5 cm and 6.0 cm (b_1), and another between 6.0 cm and 9.0 cm (b_2). In regard to the last two items, it was felt necessary for purposes of meaningful calculation of maximum slope that the points be at least 1 cm apart from each other.

Given these four points of data at minimum (Figure 8-1), we found we could derive all the essential quantifiable features of the dilatation pattern. We felt the reconstructed pattern based on these items of information alone would permit us to calculate those phase durations and slopes of special interest. In sequence, we examined the two selected dilatation observations (b_1 and b_2), each of which offered both magnitude of dilatation and designation of the time the observation was made (D_1T_1 and D_2T_2). From these, the maximum slope of active phase dilatation was calculable from:

$$b = \frac{D_2 - D_1}{T_2 - T_1}$$

The line representing the maximum slope of the active phase is defined by the equation:

$$y = a + bx$$

where a is the y intercept and b is the maximum slope as just derived.

Retrograde projection can be done to approximate the end of the latent phase if additional observations are unavailable to permit one to reconstruct that point in time

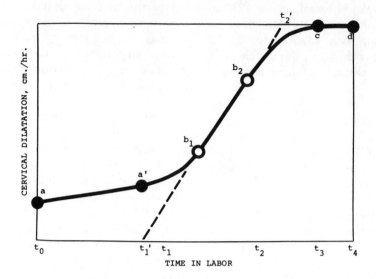

Figure 8-1. Schematic representation of algorithm for computer reconstruction of the cervical dilatation pattern in labor. Minimum criteria for acceptability for this process are known time of labor onset (t_0) and time of delivery (t_4) plus two points in the active phase (b_1 and b_2) to define the maximum slope of dilatation. Antegrade and retrograde extrapolation of the maximum slope line derived from points b_1 and b_2 make it possible to quantitate all critical components of the dilatation curve (see text for details). A comparable algorithm was developed for the analysis of the fetal descent pattern.

more accurately. The latent phase of dilatation ends and the active phase begins (t_1) where the retrograde extrapolation of the maximum slope line crosses the last dilatation value recorded for the latent phase at a'. This is done, of course, by solving the last equation for that value of x which represents cervical dilatation at the end of the latent phase to obtain t_1. Alternatively, the forward projection of the latent phase slope can be used in the event there are more than one dissimilar rectified dilatation recordings in the latent phase. If no latent phase is recorded, extrapolation back to 2.5 cm yields the average earliest probable end of latent phase (t_1').

Forward projection of the maximum slope along the time scale will cross full cervical dilatation (10 cm by convention, accepting the inherent error of this common clinical assumption) at the earliest probable time for the end of the active phase and the beginning of second stage (t_2'). If onset of second stage is known (t_3), it can be used to advantage to reconstruct the time of onset of the deceleration phase (t_2), unless this point in time is also known. If there are no recordations at 8.5-9.0 cm to help establish t_2 empirically, the projection of maximum slope forward to 8.5 cm will serve as an adequate approximation. The time interval from this point to full cervical dilatation can be considered the maximum duration of the deceleration phase. Second stage duration is calculated from the first known 10-cm recording (t_3) to the time of delivery (t_4) or from projected t_2' to delivery if the time full dilatation was first achieved is unknown.

In this way, we can derive a series of phase durations and slopes of special interest (hereinafter referred to as "derived labor variables"):

Total duration of labor, $t_4 - t_0$
Duration of first stage, $t_3 - t_0$
Duration of latent phase, $t_1 - t_0$ or $t_1' - t_0$
Duration of active phase, $t_3 - t_1$, $t_2' - t_1$, $t_3 - t_1'$ or $t_2' - t_1'$
Duration of deceleration phase, $t_3 - t_2$ or $t_2' - t_2$
Duration of second stage, $t_4 - t_3$
Maximum slope of active phase dilatation, b

Defining Arrest Pattern by Computer

Arrest of progression presented a special problem. The clinical diagnosis heretofore has required documentation of the cessation of progressive dilatation in the active phase (or cessation of progressive descent, usually in the second stage) by two consecutive vaginal examinations spaced a minimum time interval apart (two hours for dilatation, one hour for descent). We did not wish to impose these older definitions in order to try to let the data and their relations to outcome dictate the correct cut points. Thus, rather than merely making the assumption that two hours of arrested progress was significant in terms of adverse fetal impact, we desired to determine whether a shorter or longer duration might not offer a more utilitarian clinical means for discriminating cases with bad outcome from those that can be expected to do well. This is especially relevant because recent evidence suggests that our earlier definitions may be too conservative.[*] A total of 5903 cases were available for detailed study of this problem.

The decision sequence for arrest of dilatation requires documentation that the active phase is in progress.[†] The algorithm

just described provides this information and defines the time frame as well (from t_1 or t_1' to t_3 or t_2'). All rectified recordings within this time span are examined to determine if any two are identical. If equal values of dilatation are detected, the time data are examined to calculate the interval between them.

Graphing Descent Pattern by Computer

Similar data are obtainable from reconstruction of the fetal descent curves, based on serial recordings of station (recorded in centimeters above or below the plane of the ischial spines). The basic algorithm is equally applicable for calculation of the several derivative variables pertaining to descent. Despite the apparent simplicity of the concept, considerable effort was expended to evolve applicable standards for assessing valid fetal station data points and for tracing meaningful patterns.

From the outset, it was clear that not all station recordings would be usable because the active descent process through the birth canal related to clinical events of labor only after the dilatation process had already evolved well into the active phase. Therefore, all data on fetal station recorded prior to the end of the latent phase of dilatation had to be ignored. The exception was using such earlier station recordings to aid in establishing the station at which the active descent process began in those cases in which a later valid point was otherwise unavailable. Similarly, at the terminal end of the descent process just prior to delivery, sequences of frequent and sometimes widely divergent examinations yielded calculations of maximum slope of descent that were apparently unphysiologic (because they were so rapid that they were very unlikely to have actually occurred in nature, based on extensive preceding clinical experience and research.[*]) They were consi-

---

* Bottoms SF, Sokol RJ, Rosen MG: Short arrest of cervical dilatation: A risk for maternal/fetal/infant morbidity. *Am J Obstet Gynecol* 1981; 140:108.

† Friedman EA, Kroll BH: Computer analysis of labour progression. *J Obstet Gynaec Brit Comm* 1969; 76:1075; Friedman EA, Kroll BH: Computer analysis of labor progression: II. Diagnosis of secondary arrest of dilatation. *J Reprod Med* 1971; 7:176.

* Friedman EA, Sachtleben MR: Station of the fetal presenting part: I. Pattern of descent. *Am J Obstet Gynecol* 1965; 93:522; Friedman EA, Sachtleben MR: Station of the fetal presenting part: IV. Slope of descent. *Am J Obstet Gynecol* 1970; 107:1031.

dered unacceptable because one or more recordings upon which such calculations were based had to be in error.

Eventually, after introducing a series of operational testing mechanisms and cleansing procedures, we derived what we considered a good database from which subsequent analyses could be reliably developed. Briefly summarized, the descent program consisted of the following steps:

1. We computed the maximum slope of descent for every sequential pair of station-time recordings. This step demanded a minimum of two valid, properly timed, nonregressive (rectified) recordings of fetal station observed after the dilatation pattern had been documented to have entered the deceleration phase or second stage. In this regard we included the station recorded for all operative deliveries; alternatively, we assigned a value of station +4 for all spontaneous vaginal deliveries, designated at the time of delivery.

2. Maximum allowable maximum slope dimensions introduced limits for acceptance. If the calculated maximum slope exceeded these limits, then the station value with the earlier time value was deleted on the assumption it was probably in error (or at least more likely to be in error than the subsequent recording). After deletion, the first step was redone, again calculating the maximum slope for the remaining pairs of station-time recordings. The limits, as aforementioned, were established at first from clinical experience, but were later confirmed from distribution data showing the magnitude of outlying slope values.

3. Cases in which the numerator of the slope ratio (centimeters of station change over time in hours [cm/h]) used to compute maximum slope of descent was equal to 1 or less (that is, the station levels were no more than 1 cm apart) and the denominator greater than 1.5 (that is, the time interval between them was more than 1.5 hours), it was felt that a reliable slope could not be calculated. We did not consider the slope valid because the effect of the probable inherent error of the station recording was so great as to maximize the error it introduced into the maximum slope value computed by dividing the small difference between station estimates by the large interval difference in the time recordings.

4. A maximum slope of zero was considered abnormal by definition; these cases were to be dealt with specifically under the rubric of arrest of descent. These are the data manipulation mechanisms that resulted in reduction of the index population to the final residual figure of 14,357, all with certifiably reliable dilatation and descent variables for the more intensive detailed analysis to follow.

Graphing Incomplete Labor Patterns by Computer

A particularly knotty problem concerned patients delivered by cesarean section, usually undertaken before the dilatation and descent processes had fully evolved. Thus, the paradigms we had created for programmatic analyses of labor were seldom suitable to them. Both curves were constructed by computer algorithm on the basis of retrospective delineation of the active phase. Minimal criteria for case acceptability, as detailed above, had to be met to ensure that the labor pattern could be reconstructed reliably.

All but a small proportion of cesarean section cases failed to meet these criteria (especially those pertaining to the need for two defined active phase observations of dilatation time at 2.5-6.0 cm and 6.0-9.0 cm, respectively). Among the 3139 NCPP registrants (5.34%) who delivered by cesarean section, 95.5% failed these tests of acceptance. It was obvious to us that we had to recoup the critical information pertaining to these gravida by some special means. Various computer programming approaches were tried, all without success. Satisfactory selection and analyses were finally accomplished by manual techniques.

We first deleted twins, cases with unconfirmable recorded delivery time, and 1407 with no labor examinations (nearly all elective repeat cesarean sections and the remainder emergency sections prior to labor). This left 1345 sets of labor course records to be examined. All dilatation and station data with their pertinent time relationships (designated for convenience in retrograde intervals from the delivery time) were listed for each case, along with identification numbers and parity. Data for each case were also plotted graphically using ordinates of centimeters of cervical dilatation and fetal station against an abscissa of elapsed time from delivery (retrograde) in hours.

This latter graphic representation permitted us to examine the details of labor patterns of all gravidas for purposes of quantitating the range of relevant dilatation and descent variables (see above). It was feasible, for example, to measure maximum slope of dilatation in all cases in which the active phase had evolved (in many incompletely) before the cesarean section was done, even though the full set of criteria demanded by the computer algorithm could not be met. This approach allowed us to diagnose arrest of dilatation or arrest of descent visually and to provide data on both duration of arrest and the level of dilatation or station at which the arrest occurred. Tabular printout of the data, obtained simultaneously, provided greater degrees of accuracy for calculations of relevant durations and slopes than could be obtained from the graphic displays.

As expected, large numbers of aberrant labor patterns were encountered in this group of women who had been delivered by cesarean section. The data obtained from them were reincorporated into the index series for purposes of expanding our overview of the labor phenomena and to make it more representative of the gravid population with which we were dealing. The tedious manual manipulations were clearly beneficial in this regard; the derived information, which could readily be reintegrated into the mainstream of our index files, more than justified the time and effort expended.

CHAPTER 9

Labor Data Survey

Summary

The labor progression data derived from 17,056 index cases were analyzed in depth to provide a detailed quantitative description of the distribution of some of the relevant variables pertaining to patterns of cervical dilatation and fetal descent. Stratification by race, maternal age, and parity yielded additional data on labor course as affected by these factors, showing that parity alone could account for almost all the variations encountered. An attempt was made to produce linear transformation so as to facilitate logical division of the scale range of each variable into useful incremental groups. Cut points were established on this basis.

There were 17,056 cases in which the computer algorithm was fully capable of reconstructing the dilation and/or descent patterns from recorded NCPP data. From these reconstructed tracings, calculations of all definable measures of the labor progression (derivative variables) were done. In addition to quantitation of the durations of first and second stage, the durations of latent, active, and decelerations phases were obtained. The maximum slopes of both dilatation and descent were also computed.

Standard statistical descriptors of the distributions of each of these variables were formulated, including mean (numerical average), median (50th percentile value), modal (value with maximum frequency of occurrence), standard deviation, and standard error of the mean, as well as measurements (moment coefficients) of skewness and kurtosis. Minimum and maximum values, range, and variance were available also. Furthermore, we developed the actual frequency distributions of the data in terms of numerical incidence, percentiles, cumulative frequencies, and cumulative percentage tables for the entire series.

For completeness, we examined durations of deceleration phase and second stage by two different approaches according to whether the time designation for onset of deceleration phase and second stage (t_2 and t_3, Figure 8-1) were actual recordings or were instead derived by projection. This was done to ascertain the degree of inconsistency that might have been introduced by the pattern reconstruction paradigm; they were found to be essentially identical.

The labor data, thus displayed, were stratified in a series of different ways. Institutional distributions were examined to uncover any possible distinctive characteristics of the several patient populations or perhaps differences in the manner by which observations from the field units were obtained and recorded. Fractionation by race, maternal age, and parity was also done in the interest of determining from the outset whether or not we would of necessity have to maintain separate parallel study channels for one or more groups of distinctively different gravidas. We recognized, for example, that nulliparous labor differed quite characteristically from multiparous labor, requiring that we keep nulliparas separate from multiparas at all times. Our concern was to ensure there were no other,

less obvious but nonetheless important distinguishing characteristics that would mandate additional special considerations.

Overall Summary Data

The operational program produced summary data to describe the labor progression pattern for the entire index population of 17,056 gravidas, as shown in Table 9-1. On average, without regard for parity, the latent phase duration was 5.5 hours and active phase, 3.5 hours; this yielded a mean first stage duration of 9.0 hours. When the mean second stage of 0.6 hours was added, total duration of labor averaged 9.6 hours. Note that the median values of each variable fell on the low side, indicating skewed distributions toward the high end of the scale (see below), as might be expected. This confirmed previous findings.*

The degree of skewness was found to be moderately large, causing us concern about applicability and usefulness of the array of standard tests of statistical significance which are intended for data that have a normal (gaussian) distribution. Because of these concerns, we felt it necessary to undertake explorations into methods for effecting linear transformation (see below) or utilizing nonparametric analytic techniques (see chapter 8).

---

*Friedman EA, Kroll BH: Computer analysis of labour progression. *J Obstet Gynaecol Brit Comm* 1969; 76:1075.

Table 9-1
Overall Labor Progression Data

Variable	Mean	Median	Standard Deviation	Standard Error of Mean
Latent phase, hr.	5.52	5.1	5.44	0.042
Maximum dilatation slope, cm./hr.	5.06	3.0	9.37	0.072
Active phase, hr.	3.47	2.7	2.97	0.026
Deceleration phase, hr. (measured)	0.69	0.50	0.67	0.005
Deceleration phase, hr. (derived)	0.77	0.50	1.59	0.014
Maximum descent slope, cm./hr.	6.39	5.8	3.71	0.042
Second stage, hr. (measured)	0.62	0.35	2.57	0.020
Second stage, hr. (derived)	0.68	0.37	1.94	0.017

Racial Characteristics

Examination of these data stratified by race (Table 9-2) suggested that ethnicity affects labor. Second stage duration, for example, appeared to be significantly longer in white gravidas and those designated "other" (that is, other than black or white) than in black gravidas. Active phase durations followed a similar pattern in white cases, but they were shorter than expected for "other" races. The inconsistency of these trends raised questions about the possibility of a confounding factor at play. If each of the racial groups were not equivalently composed of the same parity admixture among its members, for example, then it may have been the parity effect we were seeing here rather than the influence exerted by race per se.

When the racial groups were stratified by parity (Table 9-3), it became clear that they were not comparable. There were proportionally (and significantly) more nulliparas (46.2% versus 40.5%) among white gravidas than among black. Similarly, there was almost twice the frequency of grand multiparas (para 5 or higher, 11.1% versus 6.5%) in the black population. The mean parity (before delivery) for the index population was 1.43 ± 0.013; for black women, parity averaged 1.58 ± 0.020 and for white gravidas, 1.36 ± 0.017, a very significant difference ($t = 8.38$, $p < .001$).

These data strongly suggested that some, if not all, the difference in labor course encountered between the black and the white groups may have been accounted for on the basis of the difference in parity make-up. As we subsequently learned, when corrected for parity effect, the labor course data did become nearly identical. Although racial, cultural, and economic fac-

Table 9-2
Labor Data by Race[a]

Variable	White	Black	Other
No.	7,906	7,066	1,702
Latent phase, hr.	$5.53\pm0.055(4.3)$	$5.38\pm0.070(3.9)$	$6.06\pm0.142(4.7)$[b]
Maximum dilatation slope, cm./hr.	$5.17\pm0.117(3.0)$	$4.98\pm0.104(3.0)$	$5.08\pm0.177(3.3)$
Active phase, hr.	$3.57\pm0.037(2.8)$[b]	$3.41\pm0.043(2.7)$	$3.04\pm0.066(2.3)$[b]
Deceleration phase, hr.	$0.68\pm0.007(0.50)$	$0.70\pm0.008(0.50)$	$0.59\pm0.012(0.45)$[b]
Maximum descent slope, cm./hr.	$6.42\pm0.070(5.8)$	$6.32\pm0.080(5.7)$	$6.47\pm0.110(5.9)$
Second stage, hr.	$0.80\pm0.030(0.39)$[b]	$0.40\pm0.028(0.16)$	$0.62\pm0.064(0.18)$[b]

[a] Data presented as mean ± standard error of mean; median value in parentheses.
[b] Statistically significant difference from referent black gravida group, $p < 0.01$.

Table 9-3
Parity Distribution by Race*

Parity	White		Black	
	No.	%	No.	%
Nullipara	3,644	46.2	2,857	40.5
Para 1-4	3,734	47.3	3,420	48.5
Para 5+	516	6.5	781	11.1

* Distribution statistically significant by chi-square analysis, $p < 0.001$.

tors may play a role in infant outcome results, at this point it was apparent that we did not need to maintain two or more parallel series of data according to race, at least insofar as the labor data were concerned.

Maternal Age Characteristics

The material on labor progression was next stratified by maternal age (Table 9-4). For each variable studied, there was clear evidence of a trend with advancing age. Since this ran counter to prior published observations,* it raised the suspicion that it may have been spurious. All duration measurements were longer in younger gravidas

---

*Friedman EA, Sachtleben MR: Relation of maternal age to the course of labor. *Am J Obstet Gynecol* 1965; 91:915; Cohen WR, Newman L, Friedman EA: Risk of labor abnormalities with advancing age. *Obstet Gynecol* 1980; 55:414.

and all slopes lower; the older the woman, the more rapid the labor. Intuitively, this suggested a parity effect, especially since older gravidas are obviously more likely to be multiparas.

As expected, teenagers were almost exclusively nulliparas (Table 9-5). Whereas the absolute numbers of parturients fell after age 30 years, there was still a relatively high proportion of nulliparas among them. Nonetheless, a counterbalancing increase in grand multiparas was seen; the frequency of grand multiparas in the over-30 group was more than three times that of the 20- to 29-year-old population. The average parity increased from essentially zero in those aged under 20 years to 1.47 ± 0.014 in the middle range and 1.73 ± 0.039 in those 30 years old or over. Looking at these data another way revealed the average age of nulliparas to be 22.77 ± 0.059 years old;

Table 9-4
Labor Data by Maternal Age

Variable	< 20 yr.	20–29 yr.	30–34 yr.	≥ 35 yr.
No.	4,614	9,461	1,594	1,005
Latent phase, hr.	6.05±0.088(4.6)*	5.37±0.054(4.1)	4.97±0.118(3.8)*	5.30±0.174(4.0)
Maximum dilatation, cm./hr.	3.90±0.090(2.5)*	5.28±0.103(3.1)	6.37±0.292(3.7)*	6.70±0.377(3.8)*
Active phase, hr.	4.09±0.053(3.3)*	3.30±0.033(2.6)	2.64±0.070(2.0)*	2.84±0.100(2.0)*
Deceleration phase, hr.	0.80±0.011(0.60)*	0.65±0.006(0.48)	0.57±0.015(0.40)*	0.58±0.018(0.39)*
Maximum descent slope, cm./hr.	4.02±0.092(3.0)*	5.34±0.068(3.4)	5.96±0.106(4.1)*	6.91±0.102(4.8)*
Second stage, hr.	0.86±0.038(0.54)*	0.59±0.028(0.34)	0.25±0.049(0.24)*	0.35±0.057(0.30)*

* Significantly different from 20–29 yr. group, $p < 0.01$.

Table 9-5
Parity Distribution by Maternal Age*

Parity	< 20 yr. No.	< 20 yr. %	20–29 yr. No.	20–29 yr. %	≥ 30 yr. No.	≥ 30 yr. %
Nullipara	4,611	99.9	3,459	36.6	1,167	44.9
Para 1–4	3	0.1	5,439	57.6	965	37.1
Para 5+	0	0.0	547	5.8	467	18.0

* Statistically significant, $p < 0.001$.

para 1-4 group, 26.50 ± 0.045 years old; and para 5+, 29.61 ± 0.157 years old.

Both sets of data showed statistically significant differences, reflecting the expected trends for parity to increase with age and for age to increase with parity. As before (with regard to race), the variations in labor progression patterns associated with advancing maternal age appeared to be entirely related to the changing parity composition of the gravid population. Thus, we realized that the age factor need not be retained as an ongoing discriminating variable for purposes of pursuing parallel data analyses, although it was to be studied later for its possible impact on the fetus and infant nonetheless.

Parity Characteristics

The relationship of parity to labor course is well recognized, of course, in that multiparous labor is generally shorter than nulliparous labor. What is not so apparent is the specific effect of multiparity on the different component parts of the labor pattern. Examination of the labor course in 7121 nulliparas (Table 9-6) showed how they differed from a like group of 9440 multiparas. On average, both latent and active phase durations were about 2 hours shorter in

multiparas (1.87 and 2.12 hours, respectively). The deceleration phase was 21 minutes (0.35 hour) shorter on average and the second stage, 42 minutes (0.70 hour) shorter. Thus, total mean multiparous labor was 4.69 hours briefer than mean labor in nulliparas. Of greater importance, the average rates of dilatation and descent were more than twice as fast in multiparas (by a factor of 2.02 for dilatation and 2.26 for descent).

It was interesting to note in passing that there were some substantive differences in these parity data from those obtained in the past by means of less sophisticated hand plotting and measurement.* As shown in Table 9-6, current latent phase durations were shorter than had previously been encountered, especially in nulliparas. Durations of the later phases of labor and second stage were also somewhat briefer, although not to the same degree.

The slopes of dilatation and descent were also more steeply inclined. It was, of course, very improbable that women had changed intrinsically in regard to their expected labor progression pattern. It was far more

*Friedman EA: Primigravid labor: A graphicostatistical analysis. *Obstet Gynecol* 1955; 6:567; Friedman EA: Labor in multiparas: A graphicostatistical analysis. *Obstet Gynecol* 1956; 8:691.

Table 9-6
Labor Data for Nulliparas and Multiparas

Variable	Current Study		Prior Study*	
	Nulliparas	Multiparas	Nulliparas	Multiparas
No.	7,212	9,440	500	500
Latent phase, hr.	6.58±0.072(5.3)	4.71±0.077(3.6)	8.6±0.272(7.5)	5.3±0.190(4.5)
Maximum dilatation slope, cm./hr.	3.21±0.058(2.2)	6.50±0.090(3.9)	3.0±0.085(2.7)	5.7±0.161(5.2)
Active phase, hr.	4.55±0.044(3.4)	2.43±0.046(2.1)	4.9±0.15(4.0)	2.2±0.080(1.5)
Deceleration phase, hr.	0.88±0.009(0.58)	0.53±0.008(0.29)	0.90±0.054(0.8)	0.23±0.015(0.2)
Maximum descent slope, cm./hr.	3.73±0.032(3.4)	8.42±0.060(7.6)	3.3±0.103(3.0)	6.6±0.179(5.8)
Second stage, hr.	1.04±0.019(0.60)	0.34±0.011(0.32)	0.95±0.036(0.8)	0.24±0.013(0.2)

* From Friedman, E.A.: Obstet. Gynecol. 6:567, 1955 and 8:691, 1956; Friedman, E.A.: Labor: Clinical Evaluation and Management, 2nd ed., New York: Appleton-Century-Crofts, 1978.

likely that we were seeing the effect of changing obstetrical practices, particularly as regards less use of agents that may inhibit progress, such as heavy narcotic analgesics, and/or more use of uterotonic agents for enhancing labor. Our data appeared to mirror almost exactly the pattern of labors that have been characterized as "ideal," namely those free of potentially dystocic problems of any kinds and unhampered by exogenous interference.*

Within parity subgroups, further insights could be obtained as to changing labor patterns with advancing parity (Table 9-7). Contrary to expectations, there seemed to be very little additional foreshortening of the several phase and stage durations or speeding of the rates of dilatation and descent beyond para 1 and 2. Whereas the maximum slopes of dilatation increased sharply from para 0 to para 1 and then again to para 2, the rates leveled off at higher parities. The same was seen with slopes of descent, and these trends were reflected somewhat by equivalent foreshortening of the related active phase and second stage durations. These trends are illustrated in Figure 9-1. In prior studies,* findings had suggested enhancement with high parity, but this could not be confirmed here.

A tangential issue was addressed at this time by an investigation to determine if prior nonviable pregnancy might have any discernible effect on the subsequent labor course. This was based on the clinical impression that nulliparas behaved differently according to whether or not they had had an earlier spontaneous or induced abortion. Therefore, nulliparas were stratified into 6723 primigravidas (para 0, gravida 1 only) and 489 multigravidas (para 0, gravida 2 or more). Their respective labor courses (Table 9-8) were found to be almost identical except for some minimal, albeit significant, foreshortening of the second stage in

multigravid nulliparas (6.6 minutes average difference, $t = 2.46$, p = .015) associated with a somewhat increased rate of descent (difference not statistically significant).

Linear Transformation

Having thus shown that only parity required stratification insofar as labor data distributions were concerned, we next undertook exploratory analyses of the derived labor variables. Our initial approach was to try to fit the data to a normal (gaussian) probability plot. The objective here was to provide a means for developing a straight line plot for the purpose of extracting the maximum information from these labor variables so that both parametric and graphical analytic techniques could be utilized along with tabular analyses. Given successful linear transformation, we felt we would be able to divide the scale range of a variable into logical and meaningful groupings.* Discrete groups thus created would offer subpopulations with outcome rates that could then be subjected to statistical testing, for example, by odds ratio relative to a designated modal referent group.

On a parametric scale, furthermore, we felt we could simultaneously proceed with logistic regression analysis of outcomes (each outcome dichotomized into normal and abnormal). At a later date, logistic regression would be done with the full data set, reincorporating the large number of cases temporarily tabled at this point because they failed to meet the minimal acceptance criteria of requisite labor data (see chapter 8). From the results of the logistic function, we expected to be able to plot the specific level of stated risk according to the value of the given derived labor variable. In this way, we felt we would be able to show the value of the variable at which the clinical pattern was demonstrated to expose the fetus to risk. This in

*Friedman EA: Primigravid labor: A graphicostatistical analysis. *Obstet Gynecol* 1955; 6:567; Friedman EA: Labor in multiparas: A graphicostatistical analysis. *Obstet Gynecol* 1956; 8:691.

*Cox DR: Some procedures connected with logistic qualitative response curve, in David FN (ed.): *Research Papers in Statistics*, London, John Wiley & Sons, 1966.

Table 9-7
Labor Data by Parity

Variable	Para 0	Para 1	Para 2	Para 3	Para 4	Para 5+
No.	7,212	3,412	2,183	1,464	955	1,426
Latent phase, hr.	6.58±0.072(5.3)	4.88±0.084(3.7)	4.70±0.090(3.7)	4.42±0.123(3.4)	4.39±0.143(3.3)	4.81±0.168(3.5)
Maximum dilatation slope, cm./hr.	3.21±0.058(2.2)	5.68±0.174(3.6)	6.99±0.306(4.0)	6.52±0.248(4.0)	6.97±0.330(4.3)	7.40±0.347(4.2)
Active phase, hr.	4.55±0.044(3.4)	2.61±0.041(2.2)	2.34±0.050(2.0)	2.38±0.068(2.0)	2.24±0.074(2.0)	2.29±0.076(2.1)
Deceleration phase, hr.	0.88±0.009(0.58)	0.55±0.009(0.38)	0.51±0.010(0.26)	0.52±0.014(0.22)	0.50±0.017(0.20)	0.53±0.016(0.24)
Maximum descent slope, cm./hr.	3.73±0.032(3.4)	7.94±0.071(7.1)	8.50±0.102(7.9)	8.76±0.116(8.0)	8.70±0.120(7.7)	8.82±0.092(7.6)
Second stage, hr.	1.04±0.019(0.60)	0.44±0.064(0.36)	0.32±0.036(0.30)	0.27±0.026(0.28)	0.22±0.010(0.30)	0.26±0.30(0.28)

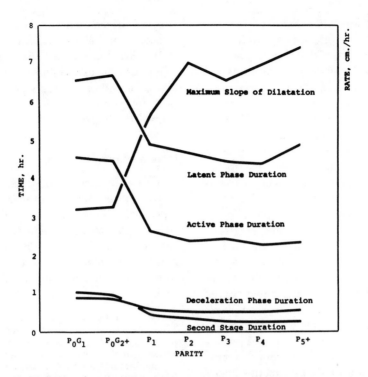

Figure **9-1.** Labor progression data by parity. Latent and active phase durations fall rapidly from nulliparity to primiparity, as does second stage duration and, to a lesser extent, deceleration phase duration. With further advanced parity, there is almost no additional trend seen, except as shown for latent phase (to para 4, but not beyond). Maximum slope of dilatation increases markedly from nulliparity to para 1 and further to para 2, without much further increment in higher parity groups.

Table 9-8
Labor Course in Nulliparas by Prior Obstetrical Experience

Variable	Primigravid Nulliparas	Multigravid Nulliparas
No.	6,723	489
Latent phase, hr.	6.57±0.07	6.68±0.24
Maximum dilatation slope, cm./hr.	3.20±0.09	3.27±0.19
Active phase, hr.	4.55±0.04	4.47±0.16
Deceleration phase, hr.	0.88±0.01	0.89±0.03
Maximum descent slope, cm./hr.	3.72±0.04	3.84±0.05
Second stage, hr.	1.05±0.02	0.94±0.04

turn would define abnormal labor on the basis of its adverse fetal and infant impact. We recognized that this operation was important because all the classical statistical machinery becomes applicable on the transform scale.

The distribution of each derived variable was, therefore, examined in detail. The skewed nature of the several distribution curves, as aforementioned, became apparent when plotted on a linear scale. Illustrative is the cumulative percent plot for maximum slope of dilatation values, presented here without regard for parity stratification (Figure 9-2); it shows the median value (50th percentile) at 3.0 cm/h and a large proportion of trailing tail values at the high end of the scale. Comparable curves were obtained for the other labor variables.

By the simple expediency of plotting the square root of the variable against a probability scale, we empirically modified several of the distribution curves by effecting linear transformation. The variables that were thus linearized were the durations of latent phase, second stage, and total labor (Table 9-9). Distribution data dealing with the maximum slopes and the durations of active and deceleration phases were made linear only by plotting the fourth root against probit* (Figure 9-3).

Incrementation Process

This transformation process permitted us to choose effective cut points for group intervals. To calculate the cut points, for any number of scale range divisions, given the mean x and the standard error of the mean s, we obtained: $c_i' = sc_i + \bar{x}$. The constants for c_i needed to obtain five cut points

---

*The probit scale reflects measurement of statistical probability based on deviations from the mean of a normal (gaussian) frequency distribution, expressed in the number and fraction of standard deviations above (+) or below (-) the mean for the distribution of a given data set.

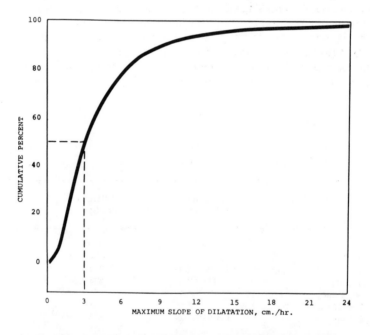

Figure 9-2. Distribution of data for maximum slope of dilatation plotted by cumulative frequency to show a markedly skewed pattern with principal concentration of values around the median (broken line) of 3.0 cm/h and an asymmetrically long tail of values extending far into the high range.

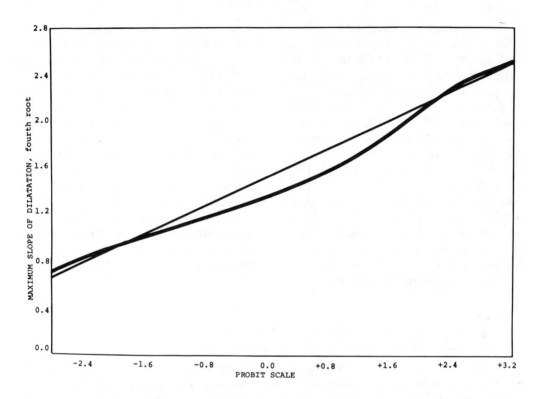

Figure **9-3.** Transformation of nonlinear data to linearity. Data for maximum slope of dilatation were linearized as shown by plotting the fourth root against the probit scale. The resulting transformation formed a distribution (heavy line) closely approximating linearity (thin line).

Table 9-9
Linear Transformation of Derived Labor Variables

Variable	Transformed Mean ± SD	Real Mean ± SD
Latent phase (square root)	2.178±0.940	4.744±5.62
Maximum dilatation slope (fourth root)	1.362±0.297	3.441±3.02
Active phase (fourth root)	1.297±0.241	2.676±9.40
Deceleration phase (fourth root)	0.845±0.171	0.510±0.720
Maximum descent slope (fourth root)	1.510±0.305	5.199±3.84
Second stage (square root)	0.524±0.449	0.274±0.920

(to yield six groupings) were -1.449, -0.660, 0.000, +0.660, and +1.449, as derived by Cox. The mean of the fourth root of the maximum slope of dilatation, for example, was 1.362 and its standard deviation 0.297; calculating the five cut points yielded 0.932, 1.166, 1.362, 1.558, and 1.792 in the fourth root scale. These translated to "real" values of 0.76, 1.84, 3.44, 5.89, and 10.31 cm/h on the original untransformed and skewed distribution.

Groups were constructed in this manner for all labor variables (Table 9-10) and outcomes studied within each group (see chapter 10). In due course, however, we determined that the logistic function was not an ideal model for deriving risk func-

tion. We found that risk factors did not follow a symmetrical sigmoid curve as specified by the logistic model. Instead, they tended to look more like the asymmetrical Gompertz function. Despite the great effort expended in pursuing this aspect of our studies, therefore, the results proved unsatisfactory. This led us ultimately to nonparametric analytic techniques, especially the Freeman-Tukey deviate type (see chapters 7 and 11). The latter approach proved much more effective in identifying values of the labor variables that were associated with bad outcomes, thereby helping define abnormal labor on the basis of such deleterious effects on offspring.

Table 9-10
Cut-Points for Labor Variables by Linear Transformation

Variable	Low Cut		Median Cut		High Cut
Latent phase duration					
Square root	0.809	1.554	2.178	2.802	3.547
Duration, hr.	0.654	2.415	4.744	7.851	12.581
Maximum slope of dilation					
Fourth root	0.932	1.166	1.362	1.558	1.792
Rate, cm./hr.	0.755	1.848	3.441	5.892	10.314
Active phase duration					
Fourth root	0.931	1.120	1.279	1.438	1.627
Duration, hr.	0.751	1.574	2.676	4.276	7.016
Deceleration phase					
Fourth root	0.698	0.833	0.945	1.058	1.193
Duration, hr.	0.237	0.481	0.797	1.253	2.026
Duration, min.	14.2	28.8	47.8	75.2	121.6
Maximum slope of descent					
Fourth root	1.068	1.309	1.510	1.711	1.952
Rate, cm./hr.	1.301	2.936	5.199	8.570	14.518
Second stage					
Square root	-	0.227	0.524	0.820	1.175
Duration, hr.	-	0.052	0.275	0.627	1.380
Duration, min.	-	3.1	16.5	40.3	82.8

CHAPTER 10

Labor Course and Outcome: Cut Point Strategy

Summary

The cut points derived earlier by linear transformation were used to assess the impact of given levels of the derived labor progression variables on fetal and infant outcome. Extreme values were associated with poor results, although not consistently across the range of the 35 outcome measures examined. In general, use of these cut points did not prove uniformly reliable or sufficiently sensitive, even though they served to demonstrate that the approach was feasible.

Several different statistical approaches, each successively more sophisticated, were utilized in our attempts to determine the impact of the labor course on the fetus and infant. We began merely by stratifying cases according to outcome, first having dichotomized specific outcomes (normal versus abnormal, including livebirth versus stillbirth or neonatal death, alert versus depressed by Apgar scoring, etc), and determining the mean of the derived labor variables for each of the resulting subgroups.

Next, we established cut points for the distribution data after appropriate linear transformation had been accomplished (chapter 9), thereby enabling us to subdivide cases according to labor pattern. Within each subset thus created, outcome results were tallied for comparison with a designated referent sample. Nonparametric techniques were then invoked for dealing with relative risk (chapters 7 and 11). The range scale of each derived labor variable was subdivided into predefined quanta. The expected number of abnormal results was generated for each quantum for comparison with the observed number. The deviation of each observed rate from its expected value was then assessed for statistical significance.

These techniques focused in sequence more closely on the several labor variables under surveillance, progressively clarifying the level at which fetal and infant risk could be objectively shown. Once defined, these risk limits allowed us to designate high-risk labors for comparison of results with those normal patterns. Combinations were also studied by establishing a "lexicon" of pattern groupings (chapter 12). This was done to ascertain how often abnormalities arose concurrently and also to help determine relative impact of such combinations on the offspring with regard to both enhancement or diminution of effect. These features were further investigated by discriminant function analysis and log linear modeling techniques for still better definition and quantitation of risk effects (chapter 14).

At-Risk Group Data

There were 128 stillborn infants (7.68/1000) and 132 neonatal deaths (7.92/1000) among the 16,667 index cases in which all of the relevant labor variables were derivable. The labor data for the gravidas who delivered these infants were collated (Table 10-1) and compared with data from the residual group of 16,407 women whose infants survived the newborn period, as a preliminary means for examining for gross differences. No statistically significant differences were encountered, perhaps because of the relatively small number of deaths.

By contrast, labors resulting in neonatal depression as measured by the low Apgar scores at both one and five minutes (2081 and 409 cases, respectively) showed important differences from labors yielding alert infants (Table 10-2). With the single exception of the maximum slope of dilatation as it pertained to five-minute Apgar scores, all labor variables showed verifiable differences among labors resulting in depressed infants. Lengthening of latent, active, and deceleration phases as well as of second stages was uniformly encountered, along with diminished mean rates of cervical dilatation and fetal descent. All trends were in the same direction, that is, toward longer labors with slower progression.

It should be noted in passing that no attempt was made to stratify these data by factors recognized to affect the labor

Table 10-1
Labor Data in Perinatal Death Groups

Variable	Stillbirth	Neonatal Death	Perinatal Death	Surviving Livebirth
No.	128	132	260	16,407
Latent phase duration, hr.	6.00±0.564	6.07±0.536	6.04±0.388	5.51±0.042
Maximum dilatation slope, cm./hr.	5.73±1.054	4.78±0.447	5.24±0.566	5.08±0.074
Active phase duration, hr.	3.96±0.515	3.59±0.344	3.76±0.298	3.44±0.026
Deceleration phase duration, hr.	0.75±0.074	0.72±0.060	0.73±0.048	0.68±0.014
Maximum descent slope, cm./hr.	6.49±0.902	6.61±0.510	6.55±0.412	6.39±0.042
Second stage duration, hr.	0.67±0.101	0.60±0.073	0.63±0.060	0.68±0.017

Table 10-2
Labor Data for Depressed Infants

Variable	1–Min. Apgar (<6)			5–Min. Apgar (<6)		
	Depressed	Normal	t	Depressed	Normal	t
No.	2,081	13,686		409	15,506	
Latent phase, hr.	6.07±0.136	5.42±0.044	4.55*	6.66±0.344	5.48±0.043	3.40*
Maximum dilatation slope, cm./hr.	4.49±0.171	5.19±0.083	3.68*	4.46±0.427	5.12±0.077	1.52
Active phase, hr.	3.99±0.083	3.35±0.027	7.33*	4.27±0.205	3.42±0.026	4.11*
Deceleration phase, hr.	0.79±0.017	0.66±0.005	7.34*	0.84±0.041	0.68±0.014	3.69*
Maximum descent slope, cm./hr.	5.40±0.134	6.54±0.093	6.99*	5.34±0.380	6.42±0.082	2.78*
Second stage, hr.	0.83±0.028	0.66±0.020	4.94*	0.92±0.071	0.67±0.018	3.41*

* $p < 0.01$.

course, such as maternal parity (chapter 9), for example. Thus, these findings could not yet be interpreted meaningfully. It was perhaps possible (if not likely) that what we encountered here was merely a reflection of an underlying difference in parity composition of the depressed versus the nondepressed infants. If the former resulted from proportionately more nulliparas, their labors would be expected to be longer and slower overall than a group containing a relatively greater fraction of multiparas. While the data were indeed suggestive, therefore, we were cautioned against concluding that prolonged labors are hazardous on this basis alone.

Nonetheless, these preliminary results—and comparable findings on a range of other adverse infant outcomes—encouraged us to believe that the basic premise of this project was not only feasible but actually thereby demonstrated. We were able to devise a workable system to examine the NCPP data file in detail, to select specified case material, to compile labor data and assess labor progression, to derive objective data for quantitating that progression, to group cases by outcome (and later by the magnitude of the derived labor variables, see below), to determine outcome results within designated groups, and finally, to compare the outcome data thus provided. Collectively, these enabling mechanisms placed us in a favorable

position to proceed to define abnormal labor on the basis of fetal and infant effects, and then to measure the degree of risk according to specific critical levels of those labor progression variables.

Incrementalized Labor Data

Logistic regression analysis was brought to bear at this point in order to focus more clearly on this issue. We expected it to provide us with some quantitation of risk according to scalar measurements of the derived labor course variables. The cut points described earlier (chapter 9) were applied for subdividing the range of each variable. The subpopulations formed in this way were then examined for the entire series of fetal and infant outcome results.

Neonatal death rates, for example, reflected the adverse impact of the extreme values of some of the labor variables (Table 10-3). Middle range (level 3) latent phase durations were associated with 5.05 deaths/1000. This contrasted rather sharply with a rate of 12.77/1000 at the high end of the scale (level 6, equivalent to latent phase durations in excess of 12.6 hours; see chapter 9, Table 9-10). The rate ratio here was 2.53—that is, the death rate in level 6 gravidas was more than 2½ times greater than in the level 3 groups, a highly significant difference (t = 2.36, p = .019).

Table 10-3
Impact of Labor Variables on Neonatal Death Rate

| Variable | Level of Variable [a] | | | | | |
	1 (Lowest)	2	3 (Referent)	4	5	6 (Highest)
Latent phase, No.	711	3564	4162	3291	2337	1331
NND per 1,000	4.22	8.70	5.05	6.99	6.42	12.77
Rate ratio	0.84	1.72	1.00	1.38	1.27	2.53
t	0.31	1.92	-	1.07	0.69	2.36[b]
Active phase, No.	963	3169	3611	3896	2499	1258
NND per 1,000	7.27	10.10	4.43	6.67	7.20	8.74
Rate ratio	1.64	2.28	1.00	1.51	1.63	1.97
t	0.96	2.71[b]	-	1.31	1.37	1.51
Maximum dilatation slope, No.	486	3441	3270	4620	2287	1287
NND per 1,000	2.06	7.56	5.80	6.32	10.49	8.55
Rate ratio	0.36	1.30	1.00	1.09	1.81	1.47
t	1.53	0.89	-	0.29	1.87	0.95
Deceleration phase, No.	1165	2850	4131	3542	2493	1215
NND per 1,000	7.73	11.58	5.08	5.93	6.02	9.05
Rate ratio	1.52	2.28	1.00	1.17	1.19	1.78
t	0.95	2.84[b]	-	0.50	0.49	1.35
Maximum descent slope, No.	509	3502	3750	3212	2190	1284
NND per 1,000	4.08	7.02	5.52	5.80	8.75	10.06
Rate ratio	0.74	1.27	1.00	1.05	1.59	1.92
t	0.37	0.99	-	0.34	1.54	1.75
Second stage, No.	-	4590	3871	3471	2065	1453
NND per 1,000	-	8.06	7.07	6.05	6.78	7.57
Rate ratio	-	1.33	1.17	1.00	1.12	1.25
t	-	1.08	0.54	-	0.33	0.58

[a] Range of each variable divided into 6 subgroups by means of cut-points chosen by method of Cox (see text).

[b] $p < 0.05$.

At the lower end of the latent phase range, inconsistent results were seen. Whereas extremely short latent phase durations (less than 0.65 hour) did not appear to be associated with increased neonatal death rates, short durations in level 2 (0.65 to 2.42 hours) were, to a degree that approached statistical significance. The rate of 8.70/1000 in this group represented a rate ratio of 1.72 or a 72% increase over the referent rate of 5.05/1000 for the referent group at level 3 (t = 1.92, p = .056). Thus, there was substantive evidence of an adverse relationship with long latent phase durations and suggestive evidence of a similar effect with short latent phases.

For active phase durations, deaths in level 2 (0.75 to 1.57 hours) were significantly increased to 10.10/1000, for a rate ratio of 2.28 over the referent value of 4.43/1000 in level 3 (t = 2.71, P = .008). In level 1, the rate ratio of 1.64, while impressive, was not statistically significant (t = 0.96). Similarly, at the high end of the active phase range, rate ratios of 1.63 and 1.97 (for levels 5 and 6, respectively, corresponding to durations greater than 4.28 and 7.02 hours) were also found to be insignificant when tested statistically.

High maximum slopes of dilatation were associated with increased neonatal death rates (rate ratios 1.81 and 1.47 in levels 5 and 6, which reflected rates of active-phase dilatation in excess of 5.89 and 10.31 cm/h), but they were not verifiable by statistical analysis. This provided only a suggestion, therefore, that excessively rapid rates of dilatation may be deleterious. Essentially the same relationships were encountered for high maximum slopes of descent, rate ratios of 1.59 and 1.92 being found in levels 5 and 6 (corresponding to 8.57 and 14.52 cm/h), but neither was statistically significant, however.

Increased death rates occurred at both extremes of the deceleration phase duration range, achieving statistical significance only in level 2. The rate ratio here was 2.28

for a neonatal death rate of 11.58/1000 compared with the referent rate of 5.08 (t = 2.84, p = .005). Second stage duration data were divided into five groups instead of six because the total number was reduced by those cases with no second stage. These latter consisted of women who had been delivered by cesarean section plus those whose second stage duration could not be accurately measured. Analysis showed only moderate increases in death rates at both extremes, but these were not meaningful in statistical terms.

Data were developed to assess the impact of the several labor variables on the frequency of neonatal depression as measured by the incidence of low Apgar scores (less than 6) at one and five minutes after birth (Table 10-4). More impressive results than those just reviewed for neonatal

Table 10-4
Labor Impact on Neonatal Depression (Low Apgar Score)[a]

Variable	12 (Lowest)		Level of Variable 345 (Referent)			6 (Highest)
Latent phase duration						
1-min. Apgar	0.52[b]	1.96[b]	1.00(10.90)	1.20[b]	1.35[b]	1.62[b]
5-min. Apgar	0.83	0.93	1.00(1.79)	1.37	1.51[b]	2.23[b]
Maximum dilatation slope						
1-min. Apgar	1.44[b]	1.36[b]	1.00(10.79)	1.11	0.92	0.94
5-min. Apgar	2.18[b]	1.39[b]	1.00(1.87)	1.13	1.09	1.08
Active phase duration						
1-min. Apgar	0.91	1.04	1.00(9.95)	1.23[b]	1.50[b]	1.82[b]
5-min. Apgar	1.24	1.19	1.00(1.73)	1.06	1.60[b]	2.39[b]
Decelertion phase duration						
1-min. Apgar	1.02	1.00	1.00(10.25)	1.25[b]	1.35[b]	1.67[b]
5-min. Apgar	1.15	1.16	1.00(1.78)	1.26	1.35	2.07[b]
Maximum descent slope						
1-min. Apgar	1.70[b]	1.54[b]	1.00(10.02)	1.01	0.97	1.41[b]
5-min. Apgar	2.16[b]	1.43[b]	1.00(1.90)	1.06	1.09	1.12
Second stage duration						
1-min. Apgar	-	0.91	0.85[b]	1.00(11.81)	1.20[b]	1.51[b]
5-min. Apgar	-	1.26	1.08	1.00(1.73)	1.73[b]	1.92[b]

a   Data are expressed as rate ratios relative to referent values shown in parentheses.

b   p < 0.05.

69

deaths were found. Long latent phase durations were associated with unexpectedly high frequencies of depressed infants (rate ratios 1.62 at one minute and 2.23 at five minutes for level 6 latent phases over 12.6 hours, yielding t values of 5.69 and 3.76, both with p less than .0002). Long active phases also appeared to have a similar effect, those in level 6 (over 7.02 hours) being associated with rate ratios of 1.82 at one minute and 2.39 at five minutes (t of 6.68 and 3.94, p less than .0001). Parallel trends were seen with long deceleration phase and second stage durations as well.

Not unexpectedly, excessively slow rates of dilatation and descent were also associated with high frequencies of depressed infants (Table 10-4). Levels 1 and 2 of the maximum dilatation slope range (less than 0.76 cm/h and 0.76 - 1.85 cm/h) showed significantly increased rate ratios, as did levels 1 and 2 of the maximum descent slope distribution (less than 1.30 and 1.30 - 2.94 cm/h).

For neonatal depression, therefore, we have uncovered a consistent relationship over the entire range of these labor variables. It should be noted, however, that we have not as yet been able to pinpoint the precise level beyond which any given labor variable can be said to impact unfavorably (to a statistically verifiable degree) on the fetus or infant. Although we have shown that extremes of duration and rates of progression are potentially harmful, we have not actually addressed the level at which that harm may actually be exerted.

Effect on Full Range of Outcomes

In our further efforts to delineate the fetal and infant effects of these derived variables, we examined each of them seriatim across the spectrum of outcomes. The outcome variables we concentrated upon here totalled 35 in all, including a series of both short- and long-term results, such as:

Stillbirth, neonatal death, and perinatal mortality

Neonatal depression at one and five minutes (Apgar scores 0-5)

Bayley developmental scale mental score at 8 months below 56 (definitely abnormal) and below 74 (suspect plus definite)

Bayley developmental scale motor score at 8 months at or below 19 (definitely abnormal) and below 26 (suspect plus definite)

Neurologic examination at 1 year abnormal and combined suspect plus definite

Communication disorder at age 3 years based on a battery of speech, language, and hearing tests of performance in language reception, language expression, hearing, speech mechanism, speech production, and global scoring, all evaluated as abnormal and combined suspect plus definite

Intelligence quotient summary scores at 4 and 7 years, stratified into six groups (below 70, 70-79, 80-89, 110-119, 120-139, and 140+) for comparison with average IQ levels (90-109)

Some of the resulting data are presented in Tables 10-5 through 10-10, each of which provides a summary of the detailed outcome material evolved for a different labor variable. In Table 10-5, for example, we offer a variety of outcome results for the latent phase duration groupings. The neonatal death and depression data were reviewed earlier (see above). Newly presented are 8-month to 7-year follow-up figures. They show a persistent residual adverse result in surviving infants associated with foreshortened latent phase durations in levels 1 and 2 (less than 0.65 hour and 0.65 - 2.42 hours), but no apparent comparable effect in the upper reaches of the range.

Maximum slope of dilatation data (Table 10-6) failed to follow suit except for statistically insignificant increases of abnormal 8-month results in the Bayley developmental scales and 3-year communication tests in

Table 10-5
Impact of Latent Phase Duration on Fetus and Infant[a]

| Outcome Variable | Level of Latent Phase Duration | | | | | |
	1 (Lowest)	2	3 (Referent)	4	5	6 (Highest)
Neonatal death	0.84	1.72	1.00(0.51)	1.38	1.27	2.53[b]
1-Min. Apgar score < 6	0.52[b]	1.96[b]	1.00(10.90)	1.20[b]	1.35[b]	1.62[b]
5-Min. Apgar score < 6	0.83	0.93	1.00(1.79)	1.37	1.51[b]	2.23[b]
8-Mo. Bayley mental score < 56	2.84[b]	1.02	1.00(0.61)	0.75	0.80	0.46
8-Mo. Bayley mental score < 74	1.81[b]	1.21[b]	1.00(6.47)	0.99	0.91	0.86
8-Mo. Bayley motor score < 19	2.33	1.24	1.00(0.49)	1.12	1.08	0.76
8-Mo. Bayley motor score < 26	2.32[b]	1.28[b]	1.00(4.47)	1.11	0.95	0.80
8-Mo. global abnormality	4.21[b]	1.64[b]	1.00(0.98)	1.08	1.69	1.37
1-Yr. neurological abnormality	1.98[b]	1.12	1.00(1.43)	1.07	0.91	0.91
3-Yr. communication disorder	2.01[b]	1.34	1.00(5.92)	1.12	0.98	0.82
4-Yr. intelligence quotient < 70	1.63[b]	0.96	1.00(3.83)	1.22	1.33	1.10
7-Yr. intelligence quotient < 70	1.46[b]	1.11	1.00(4.12)	1.05	1.16	1.12

[a] Rate ratios relative to referent values (%) in parentheses.
[b] $p < 0.05$.

Table 10-6
Maximum Slope of Dilatation and Outcome[a]

| Outcome Variable | Level of Maximum Dilatation Slope | | | | | |
	1 (Lowest)	2	3 (Referent)	4	5	6 (Highest)
Neonatal death	0.36	1.30	1.00(0.58)	1.09	1.81	1.47
1-Min. Apgar score < 6	1.44[b]	1.36[b]	1.00(10.79)	1.11	0.92	0.94
5-Min. Apgar score < 6	2.18[b]	1.39[b]	1.00(1.87)	1.13	1.09	1.08
8-Mo. Bayley mental score < 56	2.26	0.79	1.00(0.46)	1.08	2.20[b]	1.14
8-Mo. Bayley motor score < 19	1.49	0.82	1.00(0.52)	1.03	1.27	1.54
8-Mo. global abnormality	1.08	0.81	1.00(1.49)	1.15	1.35	1.44
1-Yr. neurological abnormality	0.68	0.97	1.00(1.46)	1.31	1.11	1.45
3-Yr. communication disorder	1.40	1.12	1.00(5.90)	1.10	1.49	1.60
4-Yr. intelligence quotient < 70	0.83	1.17	1.00(4.90)	1.00	1.15	0.84
7-Yr. intelligence quotient < 70	1.06	1.18	1.00(4.12)	1.06	1.24	1.22

[a] Rate ratios relative to referent values (%) in parentheses.
[b] $p < 0.05$.

level 1 offspring. In addition, there were suggestive increases at the high end of the range in tests of long-term neurologic and developmental disorders. Active phase duration (Table 10-7) mirrored these tenuous trends and added statistically significant findings at level 6 (greater than 7.02 hours) for 8-month global abnormalities and 3-year communication skill disorders. Deceleration phase duration (Table 10-8) showed possible adverse effects at the low end for all outcomes, none achieving statistical significance except low 8-month Bayley mental scores in level 2 (0.24 to 0.48 hour).

Data for maximum slope of descent (Table 10-9) were rather consistent throughout in terms of the previously encountered association of poor neonatal results, specifically depression, with both excessively rapid and very slow rates of progression. Abnormal 8-month mental and motor scale results were significantly

71

Table 10-7
Active Phase Duration and Outcome[a]

Outcome Variable	Level of Active Phase Duration					
	1 (Lowest)	2	3 (Referent)	4	5	6 (Highest)
Neonatal death	1.64	2.28[b]	1.00(0.44)	1.51	1.63	1.97
1-Min. Apgar score < 6	0.91	1.04	1.00(9.95)	1.23[b]	1.50[b]	1.82[b]
5-Min. Apgar score < 6	1.24	1.19	1.00(1.73)	1.06	1.60[b]	2.39[b]
8-Mo. Bayley mental score < 56	1.31	2.43[b]	1.00(0.42)	1.00	1.10	1.69
8-Mo. Bayley mental score < 74	1.33	1.16	1.00(6.42)	1.03	1.00	1.05
8-Mo. Bayley motor score < 19	1.49	1.60	1.00(0.45)	1.29	0.78	1.53
8-Mo. Bayley motor score < 26	1.37	1.44	1.00(4.44)	1.30	1.46	1.60[b]
8-Mo. global abnormality	1.17	1.40	1.00(1.55)	1.02	0.74	0.79
1-Yr. neurological abnormality	1.22	1.08	1.00(1.67)	1.03	0.72	0.96
3-Yr. communication disorder	1.34	1.12	1.00(6.12)	1.05	1.36	1.58[b]
4-Yr. intelligence quotient < 70	1.06	0.77	1.00(4.27)	1.15	1.15	1.09
7-Yr. intelligence quotient < 70	1.16	1.10	1.00(4.20)	1.18	1.26	1.24

[a] Rate ratios relative to referent values (%) in parentheses.
[b] $p < 0.05$.

Table 10-8
Deceleration Phase Duration and Outcome[a]

Outcome Variable	Level of Deceleration Phase Duration					
	1 (Lowest)	2	3 (Referent)	4	5	6 (Highest)
Neonatal death	1.52	2.28[b]	1.00(0.51)	1.17	1.19	1.78
1-Min. Apgar score < 6	1.02	1.00	1.00(10.25)	1.25[b]	1.35[b]	1.67[b]
5-Min. Apgar score < 6	1.15	1.16	1.00(1.78)	1.26	1.35	2.07[b]
8-Mo. Bayley mental score < 56	1.51	2.17[b]	1.00(0.46)	1.11	0.55	1.80
8-Mo. Bayley motor score < 19	1.30	1.37	1.00(0.52)	1.04	0.77	1.17
8-Mo. global abnormality	1.50	1.41	1.00(1.43)	1.16	0.91	0.88
1-Yr. neurological abnormality	1.37	1.18	1.00(1.47)	1.33	1.12	0.56
3-Yr. communication disorder	1.45	1.16	1.00(5.52)	1.10	1.14	0.98
4-Yr. intelligence quotient < 70	1.32	0.85	1.00(4.00)	1.18	1.27	1.24
7-Yr. intelligence quotient < 70	1.40	1.12	1.00(4.16)	1.16	1.26	1.12

[a] Rate ratios relative to referent values (%) in parentheses.
[b] $p < 0.05$.

increased in level 1 (less than 1.30 cm/h). Poor results in level 1 persisted into later testing activities, but not at significant levels. At the high end of the range of descent rates, similar adverse outcomes were encountered, none statistically significant. Second stage duration (Table 10-10) showed especially bad results at lowest levels (less than 0.05 hour), achieving statistical significance in several testing vehicles.

Interestingly, we encountered an apparent "protective" effect in some of the level 5 (0.63 - 1.38 hours) second stage results—that is, a significantly low rate ratio when compared with the referent value. This was seen, for example, in 8-month global abnormalities for levels 5 and 6 (0.63 - 1.38 hours and greater than 1.38 hours). While this may have resulted from an unwise choice of referent group or may merely have been a specious chance finding, it deserved special notation so that it might be subjected to closer scrutiny in the future. The latter applies especially because it arose paradoxically in a background of significant adverse neonatal effects.

Table 10-9
Maximum Slope of Descent and Outcome[a]

Outcome Variable	Level of Maximum Descent Slope					
	1 (Lowest)	2	3 (Referent)	4	5	6 (Highest)
Neonatal death	0.74	1.27	1.00(0.55)	1.05	1.59	1.92
1-Min. Apgar score < 6	1.70[b]	1.54[b]	1.00(10.02)	1.01	0.97	1.41[b]
5-Min. Apgar score < 6	2.16[b]	1.43[b]	1.00(1.90)	1.06	1.09	1.12
8-Mo. Bayley mental score < 56	2.02[b]	1.40	1.00(0.50)	1.10	1.42	1.55
8-Mo. Bayley motor score < 19	1.80[b]	0.90	1.00(0.54)	1.12	1.30	1.60
8-Mo. global abnormality	1.40	1.06	1.00(1.55)	1.20	1.42	1.56
1-Yr. neurological abnormality	1.10	0.92	1.00(1.52)	1.30	1.20	1.46
3-Yr. communication disorder	1.51	1.16	1.00(5.46)	1.12	1.50	1.62
4-Yr. intelligence quotient < 70	1.32	1.20	1.00(4.62)	1.02	1.10	1.28
7-Yr. intelligence quotient < 70	1.28	1.17	1.00(4.30)	1.05	1.12	1.16

a Rate ratios relative to referent values (%) in parentheses.
b $p < 0.05$.

Table 10-10
Second Stage Duration and Outcome[a]

Outcome Variable	Level of Second Stage Duration				
	2 (Lowest)	3	4 (Referent)	5	6 (Highest)
Neonatal death	1.33	1.17	1.00(0.61)	1.12	1.25
1-Min. Apgar score < 6	0.91	0.85[b]	1.00(11.81)	1.20[b]	1.51[b]
5-Min. Apgar score < 6	1.26	1.08	1.00(1.73)	1.73[b]	1.92[b]
8-Mo. Bayley mental score < 56	1.49	1.32	1.00(0.54)	2.10[b]	1.38
8-Mo. Bayley motor score < 19	1.41[b]	1.09	1.00(0.63)	0.74[b]	0.79
8-Mo. global abnormality	1.44[b]	1.06	1.00(1.58)	0.47[b]	0.45[b]
1-Yr. neurological abnormality	1.06	1.02	1.00(1.73)	0.72	0.66
3-Yr. communication disorder	1.45[b]	1.16	1.00(6.02)	0.94	1.06
4-Yr. intelligence quotient < 70	1.08	0.81	1.00(4.62)	0.83	0.76
7-Yr. intelligence quotient < 70	1.19	1.09	1.00(4.08)	1.02	0.90

a Rate ratios relative to referent values (%) in parentheses.
b $p < 0.05$.

CHAPTER **11**

Labor Course and Outcome: Logistic and Nonparametric Analysis

Summary

Because the logistic function did not yield a linear plot of risk effect, it was deemed to be an inadequate model for measuring risk. Nonparametric analytical approaches were, therefore, explored. Use of the Freeman-Tukey deviate proved especially valuable. By this method, it was found possible to demonstrate levels (durations and slopes) of labor progression variables beyond which there was a high probability of a bad result. Objective definitions of labor course disorders could then be developed on the basis of the expected adverse outcome.

Quantitation of the level of a given variable at which adverse impact existed was attacked preliminarily by logistic regression analysis (chapter 9). As previously described, we transformed the skewed distribution curves for each of the derived labor variables into an approximation of a straight line. This was necessary to enable us to bring standard parametric statistical testing techniques to bear. Insofar as logistic regression applications were concerned, we felt they would perhaps provide a means for describing the risk value for the range of levels of any given labor variable. If this were to prove feasible, we could thereby define abnormal labor with a degree of precision not previously available. That precision would not result from an assessment of statistical variation from the norm in terms of maternal factors, the method used in the past for identifying aberrant labor as one in which the course of progression fell outside acceptable limits of duration or rate. Instead, the precision would derive from outcome effects as encountered in the fetus and infant.

Nonlinearity of Transform Function

Logistic regression analysis was accomplished with the database pertaining to labor variables so as to display the relationship between the levels of each variable (linearly transformed) and outcome. Solving the logistic growth curve equation for latent phase (square root of the duration) as related to neonatal depression measured by low five-minute Apgar scores, for example, yielded a regression coefficient of 4.169 ± 0.142 (standard error) for the constant and -0.169 ± 0.056 for adverse Apgar score impact. The curvilinear relationship proved to be quite significant ($t = 5.65$, $p < .0001$).

When plotted to show estimated risk against square root of latent phase (Figure 11-1), the expected linear pattern failed to develop. Covariance analysis confirmed the unacceptable departure from linearity. This signified that logistic curve fitting was improper—that is, the criteria and basic assumptions of the logistic model had not been properly fulfilled. In order for logistic regression analysis to be correctly applicable, it is necessary for the risk factors to be distributed along the scale of the independent variable (square root of latent phase duration in this case) in a symmetrical sigmoid curve, the classical logistic growth law pattern described by the equation

$$y = \frac{a}{1 + bc^x}$$

The curvilinear relationship uncovered here appears to represent an asymmetric Gompertz-type function of the variety designated generically by

$$y = a + bc^x$$

To further emphasize the inappropriateness of the logistic model for our study needs, we can appreciate that the risk correlates with a broad range of transformed latent phase values in Figure 11-1. However, the portion of the range that is clinically relevant is very limited. It extends only to about 6.0 (equivalent to untransformed, real latent phase durations of up to 36 hours), which accounts for no more than 19% of the cumulated risk of neonatal depression attributable to the latent phase variable.

Other outcomes were examined in the same way for the latent phase variable, with much the same results. The risk impact was not distributed along a symmetrical logistic sigmoid curve. In each case, it caused the logistic regression analysis to yield a nonlinear plot of risk effect. This in turn meant that we had utilized an unacceptable assessment of risk. Furthermore, it meant we would be unable to quantitate that level of the latent phase duration at which fetal and infant risk might be considered excessive.

Similar data were evolved for all the other derived labor variables and outcomes. While some came closer to the symmetry needed for a valid logistic function than others, none was sufficiently congruent to be acceptable for deriving the risk function correctly. We even stratified our material by parity, maternal age, and race to ensure that a meaningful relationship was not somehow clouded over by possible confounding factors, but to no avail. We were, therefore, drawn to the inevitable conclusion that the logistic function was a poor mathematical model for our purposes in terms of risk measurement at this stage of the investigation.

Nonparametric Analysis

Recognizing belatedly that such parametric techniques could not be applied profitably here, we proceeded to explore nonparametric analytic approaches. We have detailed the underlying conceptual

75

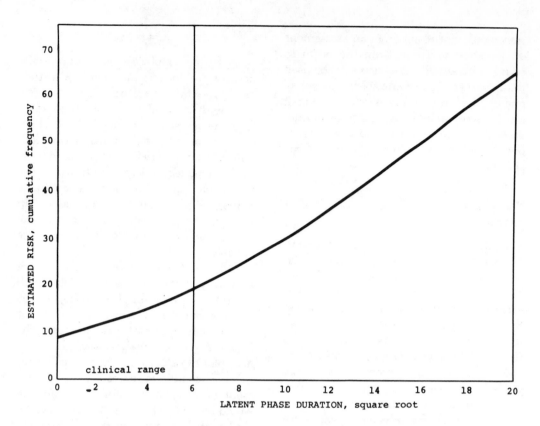

Figure 11-1. Latent phase duration and risk of neonatal depression (low five-minute Apgar score) as determined by logistic regression of transformed latent phase data. The relationship shown is very significant statistically, but has negligible practical meaning because it was nonlinear, as shown, and related to a spectrum of values falling far outside the clinical range of expected latent phase durations (6 here refers to 36 hours, latent phase duration being represented as the square root).

model in chapter 7. In practical terms, the Freeman-Tukey deviate (FTD) allowed us to determine those specific incremental levels of a given continuous variable that were associated with high risk for the fetus and infant. To accomplish this objective, each of the seven derived labor variables was separately stratified by increments of duration or rate. Then each matrix thus produced was studied for the frequency of bad outcomes (all of those previously listed) within each component cell.

The magnitude of this task can be appreciated by recognizing the possible impact of each of the seven labor variables on some of the outcome variables, making it necessary to take into account 2^7 or 128 different possible combinations. One of these will

include cases with entirely normal labor progression as a comparison standard for the other 127 groups. Enumerating 35 abnormal fetal and infant outcome results for all 127 abnormal labor combination groups yielded 4445 two-by-two tables. These were to be used for estimating the relative risk and the attributable risk of each labor progression abnormality taken individually and in all possible combinations, utilizing the normal labor group as the common referent.

Application to Neonatal Outcome

For illustrative purposes, we have tabulated the distribution of abnormally low

76

five-minute Apgar scores (0-5) in 8562 multiparas by latent phase duration (Table 11-1). The overall frequency of depressed infants was 2.24% (192 neonates). The rate for each incremental group ranged widely from 1.21% to 13.51%. Among the 57 women whose latent phase duration was between 14.0 and 14.9 hours, for example, there were five or 8.77% depressed infants. Based on the overall rate, however, only 1.28 should have been expected (2.24% of 57). The Freeman-Tukey deviate (FTD) for the number actually observed was 2.213. Based on the normal (gaussian) distribution of these deviates, it could have occurred by chance 1.3% of the time (p = .013). This suggested an adverse impact from latent phases of this duration, a finding that gathered considerable support from the fact that adjacent cells followed suit—that is, latent phases of 13.0 to 13.9 hours duration yielded a high rate of depressed neonates (five infants or 6.9%, when only 1.65 were expected), a frequency that resulted in a significant FTD of 1.955 (p = .025). Those

of 12.0 to 12.9 hours duration had more than three times the expected incidence (two or 7.69% when 0.60 was expected), although not quite statistically significant (FTD = 1.321, p = .093). Incremental groups beyond 16.0 hours duration comprised progressively smaller case numbers, but they showed further magnification of the adverse effect nonetheless. Collapsing all these cases of 20 hours or more left one tail group of 74 cases with ten depressed infants or 13.51%; only 1.70 such infants were expected, for an impressively high FTD of 3.764 (p = .00008). Thus, the analysis showed a zone of clear-cut adverse neonatal effect in the upper range of latent phase values, statistically verifiable from 13.0 hours upward and rather suggestive at 11.0 or 12.0 hours.

An interesting contrast appeared in the low-middle range between 2.0 and 5.9 hours, indicating a cluster of "protection." In the 4.0 to 4.9 hours increment group, there were 12 or 1.29% depressed infants, while 21.40 were expected; the large nega-

Table 11-1
Freeman-Tukey Deviates for Neonatal Depression
by Latent Phase Durations in Multiparas*

Duration hr.	Apgar Score (No.) 0-5	6-10	Depressed %	Expected No.	Freeman-Tukey Deviate	p
< 1.0	9	738	1.205	17.14	-2.084	0.019
1.0-1.9	32	1,172	2.658	27.62	0.961	
2.0-2.9	23	1,274	1.811	29.13	-1.025	
3.0-3.9	27	1,136	2.322	26.68	0.225	
4.0-4.9	12	921	1.286	21.40	-2.133	0.016
5.0-5.9	14	713	1.926	16.68	-0.522	
6.0-6.9	11	398	2.689	9.38	0.642	
7.0-7.9	11	412	2.600	9.70	0.540	
8.0-8.9	7	225	3.017	5.32	0.804	
9.0-9.9	7	271	2.518	6.38	0.381	
10.0-10.9	5	128	3.759	3.05	1.090	
11.0-11.9	4	76	5.000	1.86	1.377	0.084
12.0-12.9	2	24	7.692	0.60	1.321	0.093
13.0-13.9	5	67	6.944	1.65	1.955	0.025
14.0-14.9	5	52	8.772	1.31	2.213	0.013
15.0-15.9	2	15	11.765	0.39	1.557	0.060
16.0-19.9	6	41	12.766	1.08	2.811	0.002
20.0+	10	64	13.514	1.70	3.764	0.00008
Total	192	8,370	2.294			

* Based on the frequency of low 5-minute Apgar scores (0-5).

77

tive FTD of -2.133 was statistically significant (p = .016). A somewhat smaller (and statistically insignificant) negative deviate appeared in the adjacent groups based on the unexpectedly low frequencies of neonatal depression. Collapsing the zone of apparent protection between 2.0 and 5.9 hours resulted in an accumulation of 76 low Apgar scores in 4120 babies or 1.84% (94.51 expected, FTD = -1.757, p = .040). This range of latent phase durations yielded a significantly diminished frequency of poor results.

The contrasting adverse and protective zones that these data suggested are summarized in Table 11-2 in which the rate ratios are also presented. Relative to the zone representing both lowest risk and highest population density, namely those with latent phase durations between 2.0 and 5.9 hours, neonatal depression rates were significantly increased to nearly fourfold (rate ratio = 3.70, χ^2 = 26.61, p = 2.5 × 10^{-7}) in the 10.0 - 14.9 hours group and more than sevenfold (rate ratio = 7.09, χ^2 = 77.74, p < 1 × 10^{-10}) in those of 15.0 hours or more. Further collapsing the entire upper range from 10.0 hours produced a group of 373 gravidas with 34 or 9.12% depressed neonates. Since only 8.56 such infants were expected, the FTD was 5.88 (p = 2.1 × 10^{-9}) and rate ratio 4.96 (χ^2 = 76.02, p < 1 × 10^{-10}).

The "natural" sequestration of the latent phase data according to the level of fetal-infant impact, both good and bad, was thus shown to be clearly demonstrable by this approach. On this basis, we felt we could quantitate the effect of all of the derived labor variables, thereby forming the foundation for definitive descriptions of the limits of labor progression patterns that can be expected to affect the fetus and infant unfavorably.

Expansion to Other Outcomes

Latent Phase Duration

The other outcome variables fell into a similar pattern insofar as latent phase impact in multiparas was concerned (Table 11-3). While not all the results in both extreme value ("tail") groups could be determined to be statistically significant, the trends for long latent phase durations (of 10.0 hours or more) to be associated with relatively adverse outcomes showed rather good consistency over the range of the selected variables shown here, as well as in others not listed in the interest of avoiding unnecessary duplication.

Having thus developed a workable paradigm, we proceeded to examine all of the other derived labor variables, separately for multiparas and nulliparas, to determine the critical levels of durations and slopes that were associated with bad effects.

For latent phase duration in nulliparas, a parallel analysis was done with similar results. With regard to neonatal depression at age five minutes (Table 11-4), for example, affected cases were unevenly distributed. Compared to the overall rate of 3.64%, the frequency varied from a homogeneously low zone of 2.80% (in 2782 off-

Table 11-2
Neonatal Depression for Latent Phase Groups in Multiparas

Duration hr.	No.	Apgar 0-5 No.	%	Freeman-Tukey Deviate	p	Rate Ratio RR	p
< 2.0	1,910	41	2.15	-0.243		1.17	
2.0-5.9	4,120	76	1.84	-1.757	0.040	1.00*	
6.0-9.9	1,342	36	2.68	1.066		1.46	0.059
10.0-14.9	235	16	6.81	3.424	0.0003	3.70	<0.00001
15.0+	138	18	13.04	4.944	<0.00001	7.90	<0.00001

* Referent (1.84% rate)

Table 11-3
Outcome Results According to Latent Phase Duration in Multiparas[a]

Outcome Variable[b]	Latent Phase Duration, hr.				
	< 2.0	2.0–5.9	6.0–9.9	10.0–14.9	15.0+
SB	1.27	1.00(0.77)	0.88	2.43[c]	5.55[c]
NND	1.20	1.00(0.76)	1.48	4.40[c]	12.82[c]
PMR	1.13	1.00(1.57)	0.98	3.93[c]	8.20[c]
APG1	1.13	1.00(4.80)	1.43	3.07[c]	6.96[c]
APG5	1.17	1.00(1.84)	1.46	3.70[c]	7.09[c]
MENT8	1.34[c]	1.00(7.49)	1.08	0.99	1.99[c]
MOT8	1.22[c]	1.00(7.13)	0.94	1.16	2.00[c]
GLOB8	1.21[c]	1.00(12.05)	0.90	1.00	1.66[c]
NEUR1	1.04	1.00(8.72)	0.96	1.14	1.71[c]
SLH3	1.07	1.00(12.85)	0.91	0.91	1.28[c]
IQ4	1.13	1.00(1.98)	1.13	2.13[c]	1.18
IQ7	1.01	1.00(2.85)	0.85	1.26	1.27

a   Data presented as rate ratios relative to referent rate in 2.0–5.9 hr. group for each outcome variable under surveillance; referent rate shown in parentheses.

b   SB, stillbirth; NND, neonatal death rate; PMR, perinatal mortality rate; APG1 and APG5, Apgar score 0–5 at 1 and 5 minutes; MENT8, MOT8, and GLOB8, abnormal Bayley mental, motor, and global assessments at 8 months; NEUR1, abnormal neurological findings at age 1 year; SLH3, abnormal speech, language and hearing test results at 3 years; IQ4 and IQ7, abnormal score on IQ testing at 4 and 7 years (using race-sex specific cut-points).

c $p < 0.05$.

spring of women whose latent phase durations were 3.0 to 7.9 hours) to progressively higher zones culminating in a rate of 16.46% in the uppermost range (18.0+ hours). The incremental group data fell naturally into five segments based on stepwise increases in the frequency of neonatal depression. A block of negative FTD values identified the "protective" zone between 3.0 and 7.9 hours in which the rate of adverse effects was at its nadir. The next higher segment from 8.0 to 11.9 hours was likewise consistent in the somewhat greater frequency of depression (3.22%, rate ratio 1.15, not statistically significant). Next in order was the 12.0 to 17.9 hours group with a significantly increased adverse result (5.88%, rate ratio 2.10, $\chi^2 = 11.42$, p = .0007). The tail group from 18.0 hours upward was even more impressive in this regard (16.46%, rate ratio 6.43, $\chi^2 = 59.98$, p < 1 × 10^{-10}).

A similar relationship was encountered for neonatal death rates (Table 11-5), significantly increased mortality being found in the group with latent phase durations of 18.0 hours or more (24.84/1000 versus 5.52/1000 in the referent group, for a rate ratio of 4.50, $\chi^2 = 8.77$, p = .003). While similar enhancement of the stillbirth rate was seen in the upper ranges, it did not quite achieve statistical significance (18.63/1000 versus 6.21 in the referent group, rate ratio 3.00, $\chi^2 = 3.45$, p = .063). At age eight months, summary global abnormalities were also concentrated somewhat in the upper ranges of the distribution of latent phase durations; the rate was 38% greater than that seen in the referent group and could be shown to be statistically significant (rate ratio 1.38, $\chi^2 = 4.15$, p = .042). A residual adverse effect from long latent phase durations was also seen in other long-range results up to seven years.

79

Table 11-4
Neonatal Depression by Latent Phase Duration in Nulliparas

Duration hr.	No.	5-min Apgar 0-5 No.	%	Freeman-Tukey Deviate	p	Rate Ratio RR	p
< 3.0	1,446	49	3.39	0.481		1.32	
3.0-5.9	1,844	54	2.93	-0.573		1.14	
6.0-7.9	938	24	2.56	-1.063		1.00*	
8.0-9.9	508	16	3.15	0.028		1.23	
10.0-11.9	464	16	3.45	0.381		1.35	
12.0-13.9	276	14	5.07	1.610	0.054	1.98	0.035
14.0-17.9	157	12	7.64	2.493	0.006	2.98	0.001
18.0+	158	26	16.46	5.705	<0.00001	6.43	<0.00001

* Referent (rate 2.56%)

Table 11-5
Outcome Results by Latent Phase in Nulliparas[a]

Outcome Variable	Latent Phase Duration, hr. < 3.0	3.0-7.9	8.0-11.9	12.0-17.9	18.0+
SB	1.43	1.00(0.62)	1.89	1.74	3.00
NND	1.86	1.00(0.55)	1.42	1.95	4.50[b]
PMR	1.63	1.00(1.17)	1.67	1.84	3.71[b]
APG1	1.24	1.00(4.69)	1.16	2.00[b]	4.16[b]
APG5	1.19	1.00(2.80)	1.15	2.10[b]	5.76[b]
MENT8	1.20	1.00(5.74)	0.83	1.28	1.90[b]
MOT8	1.09	1.00(3.68)	0.92	1.56	2.16
GLOB8	1.12	1.00(8.53)	0.89	0.99	1.38[b]
NEUR1	1.10	1.00(6.65)	0.91	1.36[b]	1.50[b]
SLH3	1.10	1.00(16.42)	1.00	1.30[b]	1.32[b]
IQ4	1.12	1.00(2.95)	0.85	1.17	1.19
IQ7	0.73	1.00(2.89)	0.77	1.00	1.34[b]

[a] Data in rate ratios relative to rate in 3.0-7.9 hr. group for each outcome, shown in parentheses.

[b] $p < 0.05$.

Active Phase Duration

For active phase duration in multiparas (Table 11-6), the markedly skewed distribution of the data into the low end of the scale clustered half (49.0%) the cases—although not an equivalently proportional number of adverse effects—in the incremental groups under 2.0 hours. Thus, it was not feasible to isolate a critical low-end value for this variable. At the high end, it was clear that long active phases—5.0 hours or more and especially 8.0 hours or greater—impacted ad-

versely on the infant as evidenced by statistically significant increases in perinatal death and neonatal depression rates. Later in life, significant residual effects were seen mostly in the very prolonged active phase group (8.0+ hours) with only suggestions of persistent effect in the one-year neurological examination and seven-year IQ results in the 5.0-7.9 hours group.

Active phase duration limits for nulliparas were more obvious at both extremes, especially in the immediate deleterious effect on perinatal death rates (Table 11-7). Although low-end effect (under 2.0 hours duration) diminished with time, highly significant residual effect did persist into later years. It is of interest in passing to note an unexpected zone of apparent "protection" encountered in the speech, language, and hearing results at age three years. There was a significantly diminished frequency of bad results in the 6.0 to 9.9 hr. group. Although unexplained, it may have been a specious finding or suggest that the original choice of referent group cut points was incorrect.

Maximum Slope of Dilatation

The maximum slope of dilatation was examined in the same way by increments of 0.2 cm/h (in contrast to the other labor variables which heretofore were incremented by time intervals of 15 minutes or 0.25 hour). For multiparas, the data fell naturally into five strata (Table 11-8). The best outcome results were seen between slopes of 3.0 and 7.9 cm/h. The worst occurred below 1.5 cm/h and at 12.0 cm/h or more. They proved statistically significant for a variety of outcome variables. Neonatal depression, for example, showed impressive bimodal effects: At the low end, the rate ratio for low Apgar score frequency in this cell was 1.97 (x^2 = 13.82, p = .0002), based on a frequency of 4.12% versus the 2.09% referent rate). At the high end of the range, the

Table 11-6
Outcome by Active Phase in Multiparas

| Outcome Variable | Active Phase Duration, hr. | | | |
	< 1.0	1.0–4.9	5.0–7.9	8.0+
PMR	1.09	1.00(1.80)	1.72*	5.54*
APG5	1.01	1.00(2.08)	1.88*	6.81*
GLOB8	0.95	1.00(12.42)	1.10	1.83*
NEUR1	1.01	1.00(8.70)	1.36*	1.79*
SLH3	0.99	1.00(18.82)	0.98	1.47*
IQ4	0.75	1.00(2.32)	1.01	1.42*
IQ7	1.06	1.00(2.69)	1.40*	1.74*

* p < 0.05.

Table 11-7
Outcome by Active Phase in Nulliparas

| Outcome Variable | Active Phase Duration, hr. | | | |
	< 2.0	2.0–5.9	6.0–9.9	10.0+
PMR	3.99[a]	1.00(0.95)	1.64	3.94[a]
APG5	1.27	1.00(2.64)	1.67[a]	3.77[a]
GLOB8	1.02	1.00(7.50)	1.04	1.45[a]
NEUR1	0.86	1.00(6.12)	1.10	1.62[a]
SLH3	1.19[a]	1.00(16.51)	0.81[b]	1.47[a]
IQ4	0.85	1.00(3.15)	0.86	1.10
IQ7	1.33[a]	1.00(2.38)	1.11	1.46[a]

[a] p < 0.05.

[b] Apparent "protective" effect, p < 0.05.

rate ratio was 1.67 (χ^2 = 4.60, p = .032) with a frequency of 3.50% depressed infants. Longer-term follow-up data showed persistent effects associated with extreme values of the maximum slope variable. This effect was present at both high and low slope values, but was particularly significant at the upper end of the scale of dilatation rates, emphasizing the especially pervasive risk of precipitate labors.

The same relationships were also found for maximum dilatation rates in nulliparas (Table 11-9). Optimal outcomes were associated with active phase dilatation rates of 3.0 to 4.9 cm/h. Below 1.2 cm/h, a value that has previously been identified as being below clinical expectations on the basis of

maternal effects,* the offspring were found to be at some increased risk of death or depression. Permanent neurologic and developmental damage could not be clearly demonstrated, however, at this end of the range. Rates of 5.0 cm/h or more were likewise associated with poor immediate outcomes; there was an overall rate ratio for perinatal deaths of 3.29 (45.99/1000 versus 13.98 expected, χ^2 = 19.77, p = 8.7 x 10^{-6}) for all cases with dilatation slopes of 5.0 cm/h or greater and a startling rate ratio of 6.59 (χ^2 = 25.04, p = 5.6 x 10^{-7}) for slopes of 10.0+

*Friedman EA, Sachtleben MR: Dysfunctional labor: II. Protracted active phase dilatation in nulliparas. *Obstet Gynecol* 1961; 17:566.

Table 11-8
Outcome by Maximum Slope of Dilatation in Multiparas

| Outcome Variable | Maximum Dilatation Slope, cm./hr. | | | | |
	< 1.5	1.5–2.9	3.0–7.9	8.0–11.9	12.0+
PMR	1.77*	1.06	1.00(1.70)	1.43	1.50
APG5	1.97*	1.33	1.00(2.09)	1.44	1.67*
GLOB8	1.18	1.12	1.00(11.83)	0.99	1.33*
NEUR1	1.41*	0.95	1.00(8.93)	0.91	0.92
SLH3	1.10	1.09	1.00(17.90)	1.10	1.18*
IQ4	1.22*	0.97	1.00(2.37)	0.87	1.26*
IQ7	1.10	1.16	1.00(2.50)	0.88	1.72*

* p < 0.05.

Table 11-9
Outcome by Maximum Slope of Dilatation in Nulliparas

| Outcome Variable | Maximum Dilatation Slope, cm./hr. | | | | |
	< 1.2	1.2–2.9	3.0–4.9	5.0–9.9	10.0+
PMR	1.57	0.65	1.00(1.40)	2.87a	6.59a
APG5	1.94a	1.30	1.00(2.73)	1.55	4.28a
GLOB8	1.00	0.94	1.00(8.62)	0.87	1.67a
NEUR1	1.04	0.87	1.00(7.27)	1.09	1.18
SLH3	0.83	0.88	1.00(19.42)	1.13	1.79a
IQ4	1.01	0.83b	1.00(3.39)	1.17	1.98a
IQ7	0.88	0.79b	1.00(2.95)	1.22	1.62a

a p < 0.05.

b Apparently "protective," p < 0.05.

cm/h. The significantly deleterious impact of the upper extreme values was seen in the long-term follow-up data through seven years. This was almost exactly parallel to the effect just seen in multiparas, again pointing to precipitate dilatation as especially harmful.

Deceleration Phase Duration

Deceleration phase durations were markedly skewed to the low end of the range of values in both nulliparas and multiparas, 63.5% and 76.4% of cases falling under 1.0 hour duration, respectively. Moreover, short durations were associated with the best fetal and infant outcomes, especially those under 1 hour in nulliparas

and under 30 minutes in multiparas. Utilizing the outcome data from these cells as referents, therefore, we were able to recognize increasingly poor results with longer deceleration phases (Tables 11-10 and 11-11).

Perinatal death rates in multiparas rose abruptly in cases with deceleration phases of 1 hour or more. Residual late adverse impact existed in those with durations of 2.0 hours and greater, as indicated especially by the frequencies of neonatal depression, global scoring at eight months, three-year communications testing results, and IQ scores at four and seven years. High frequencies of speech, language, and hearing abnormalities were also seen in signifi-

Table 11-10
Outcome by Deceleration Phase in Multiparas

| Outcome Variable | < 0.50 | Deceleration Phase Duration, hr. | | |
		0.50–0.99	1.00–1.99	2.00+
PMR	1.00(1.61)	1.09	1.87*	5.26*
APG5	1.00(1.98)	1.05	1.31	2.98*
GLOB8	1.00(11.83)	1.09	1.10	1.53*
NEUR1	1.00(8.48)	0.98	1.17	1.30
SLH3	1.00(21.08)	1.05	1.18*	1.23*
IQ4	1.00(2.22)	1.04	0.85	1.60*
IQ7	1.00(2.81)	0.99	1.06	1.57*

* $p < 0.05$.

Table 11-11
Outcome by Deceleration Phase in Nulliparas

| Outcome Variable | < 1.0 | Deceleration Phase Duration, hr. | | |
		1.0–1.9	2.0–2.9	3.0+
PMR	1.00(1.43)	0.86	1.27	2.24[a]
APG5	1.00(2.75)	1.33	1.49	2.88[a]
GLOB8	1.00(8.07)	1.02	1.25	1.84
NEUR1	1.00(6.43)	1.06	1.35	0.95
SLH3	1.00(22.56)	0.98	0.77[b]	1.03
IQ4	1.00(3.03)	0.93	0.76	1.46[a]
IQ7	1.00(2.70)	0.84	0.84	1.17

[a] $p < 0.05$.

[b] Apparent "protection," $p < 0.05$.

cantly excess numbers in children born after labors with only moderate prolongation of this labor variable, namely those of 1.0 hour duration or more.

In nulliparas (Table 11-11), neonatal depression by frequency of low five-minute Apgar scores (as well as one-minute scores, not shown here) was especially enhanced by deceleration phase durations greater than 3.0 hours, and there was some effect (not significant) even with deceleration phases of as short a duration as 1.0 hour. Perinatal deaths, moreover, were likewise significantly increased beyond 3.0 hours. The long-term data only suggested a permanent impact from deceleration phases of 3.0 hours or more, especially the eight-month Bayley scale results (which were not statistically significant) and the four-year IQ scores (which were).

Maximum Slope of Descent

Maximum slopes of descent could be stratified into five well-demarcated zones of effect in both multiparas and nulliparas (Tables 11-12 and 11-13). In multiparas, rates of descent less than 2.0 cm/h were associated with particularly poor perinatal results. The effect persisted at a significant level through the eight-month examinations and continued thereafter, but to a lesser (and insignificant) extent. Perhaps because of the larger numbers of cases in the cells, significantly adverse impact was found for slopes of a somewhat greater magnitude, specifically 2.0-3.9 cm/h, for the results at eight months and four years. In the upper range of values, solid consistency

Table 11-12
Outcome by Maximum Slope of Descent in Multiparas

| Outcome Variable | Maximum Descent Slope, cm./hr. | | | | |
	< 2.0	2.0–3.9	4.0–5.9	6.0–9.9	10.0+
PMR	2.20*	1.06	1.00(1.61)	0.84	1.49*
APG5	2.04*	1.35	1.00(2.30)	0.73	1.86*
GLOB8	1.42*	1.25*	1.00(13.21)	0.88	1.22*
NEUR1	1.34	1.13	1.00(9.27)	0.95	1.29*
SLH3	1.18	1.06	1.00(28.91)	1.06	1.11
IQ4	1.11	1.38*	1.00(1.98)	1.16	1.44*
IQ7	1.16	1.09	1.00(2.85)	0.87	1.35*

* $p < 0.05$.

Table 11-13
Outcome by Maximum Slope of Descent in Nulliparas

| Outcome Variable | Maximum Descent Slope, cm./hr. | | | | |
	< 1.0	1.0–2.4	2.5–4.4	4.5–5.9	6.0+
PMR	1.74	1.10	1.00(1.01)	2.14*	2.49*
APG5	2.79*	1.14	1.00(2.33)	0.98	1.62*
GLOB8	1.55*	1.02	1.00(8.05)	1.12	1.26
NEUR1	1.92*	0.99	1.00(6.64)	0.83	1.17
SLH3	1.05	1.06	1.00(29.53)	1.11	1.27*
IQ4	1.18	1.27	1.00(2.78)	1.44*	1.65*
IQ7	2.25*	1.07	1.00(2.60)	1.10	1.37*

* $p < 0.05$.

was encountered across almost all testing vehicles (with the single exception of the speech, language, and hearing results) for descent slopes of 10.0 cm/h or more. Even at 6.0-9.9 cm/h, moreover, poor outcomes were found in both four-year and seven-year IQ scores.

For nulliparas (Table 11-13), similar findings existed below 1.0 cm/h descent rates and at or above 6.0 cm/h. The homogeneity of effect over a range of test results was fairly good at both ends of the scale. Additional effect was also apparent in the 4.5-5.9 cm/h incremental group especially for perinatal death. Except for the four-year IQ data, no residual effect was seen in other test results for this group.

Second Stage Duration

Tightly clustered second stage durations were skewed to the far left (lowest range). This made it impossible to define a group of multiparas with excessively foreshortened second stage, analogous to our experience with deceleration phase durations (see above). There were 83.7% multiparas with second stages of less than 30 minutes duration. Although studied in 15-minute increments, no discriminating risk characteristics could be uncovered in multiparas at the low end of the scale by this approach. At the high end, however, second stage durations of 1.0 hour or more were apparently associated with increased

perinatal death and neonatal depression (Table 11-14). The harmful impact was even more impressive with second stage durations of 2.0 hours or more.

Special note was taken of this latter observation in light of recent determinations that a prolonged second stage duration does not necessarily cause harm by itself; it may instead merely serve as a signal of an inherent obstetrical problem that warrants close attention and atraumatic delivery considerations.* Of more than passing interest, therefore, was the rather good long-term follow-up data for surviving infants, indicating no recognizable residual effect. The seven-year IQ data were especially gratifying in this regard.

In nulliparas, analysis of second stage data was able to isolate extremes of duration at both ends of the scale (Table 11-15). Those less than 30 minutes long (0.50 hour) were associated with significantly increased frequencies of perinatal death and neonatal depression plus some significant enhancement of other late bad outcomes as well. Durations of 2.0 hours or more also had increased rates of perinatal death, but not of any late adverse results; those 3.0 hours or greater, moreover, yielded a significantly increased incidence of dead and depressed

---

*Cohen WR: Influence of the duration of second stage labor on perinatal outcome and puerperal morbidity. *Obstet Gynecol* 1977; 49:266.

Table 11-14
Outcome by Second Stage in Multiparas

| Outcome Variable | Second Stage Duration, hr. | | | |
	< 0.50	0.50–0.99	1.00–1.99	2.00+
PMR	1.00(1.63)	0.60	2.02*	10.51*
APG5	1.00(1.96)	1.24	2.03*	7.60*
GLOB8	1.00(12.33)	1.15	0.98	1.53
NEUR1	1.00(8.80)	0.88	0.95	1.89
SLH3	1.00(19.52)	0.97	0.92	1.21
IQ4	1.00(2.29)	0.83	0.89	1.28
IQ7	1.00(2.93)	0.77	0.76	1.07

* $p < 0.05$.

85

babies. There were augmented rates of neurologic abnormalities at one year in association with long second stages, and this effect was still apparent in the data at four years.

Defining Limits of Normal

Our efforts to this stage have yielded the long-sought objective definitions of the levels of each of the labor course variables which are associated with—and perhaps causative of—untoward outcomes to fetus and infant. When these levels are encountered, one can anticipate poor results based on statistical probability and, of course, on the assumption that past experience (as determined empirically from preceding data collection) can be projected into the future for prognostication purposes.

The cut points for each of the derived labor variables are presented in Table 11-16. They are derived from the series of analyses detailed above. Note the absence of low-end cut points for active and deceleration phase durations in both nulliparas and multiparas as well as for second stage duration in multiparas. Our analytical approaches have not been able to provide us with meaningful values to aid us in discovering where these missing cut points may lie. Nonetheless, we are rather confident about the reliability of all the other designated values.

Table 11-15
Outcome by Second Stage in Nulliparas

Outcome Variable	Second Stage Duration, hr.			
	< 0.50	0.50–1.99	2.00–2.99	3.00+
PMR	2.95[a]	1.00(0.78)	2.49[a]	3.14[a]
APG5	1.44[a]	1.00(2.60)	1.40	2.35[a]
GLOB8	1.01	1.00(8.15)	1.03	1.14
NEUR1	0.98	1.00(6.49)	1.09	1.72[a]
SLH3	1.15[a]	1.00(18.03)	0.84	1.06
IQ4	1.07	1.00(2.99)	0.65[b]	1.34[a]
IQ7	1.41[a]	1.00(2.24)	0.83[b]	1.19

[a] $p < 0.05$.

[b] Apparent "protective" effect, $p < 0.05$.

Table 11-16
Selected Cut-Points for Defining Abnormal Labor Progression from Adverse Results to Offspring

Derived Labor Variable	Limits			
	Nulliparas		Multiparas	
	Low	High	Low	High
Latent phase, hr.	3.0	18.0	2.0	10.0
Active phase, hr.	-	6.0	-	5.0
Maximum dilatation slope, cm./hr.	1.2	5.0	1.5	12.0
Deceleration phase, hr.	-	2.0	-	1.0
Maximum descent slope, cm./hr.	1.0	4.5	2.0	10.0
Second stage, hr.	0.5	2.0	-	1.0

It should be noted that some of these cut points vary to a degree from levels heretofore considered to represent the abnormal state based on maternal prognosis for delivery.* In nulliparas, for example, latent phase duration of 20.1 hours or more was deemed abnormal instead of the 18.0-hour cut point now disclosed; in multiparas, a 13.6-hour limit for latent phase is now reduced to 10.0 hours. Limits of active phase duration are curtailed from 11.7 and 5.2 hours for nulliparas and multiparas, respectively, to 6.0 and 5.0 hours. Whereas the low-end cut points for maximum slope of dilatation are exactly the same as in the past, the upper limits are down to 5.0 and 12.0 cm/h from 6.8 and 14.7 cm/h. Similarly, the low end of the normal range for maximum slope of descent remains about as before, but the high end comes down from 6.4 and 14.0 cm/h to 4.5 and 10.0 cm/h. Deceleration phase duration is now limited to 2.0 hours for nulliparas instead of 2.7 hours, but increases to a very small degree (by an average of 8.4 minutes from 0.86 to 1.0 hour) for multiparas; this is the only instance in which the new limit was more conservative than the old. Second stage length is reduced from 2.0 and 1.1 hours to 2.0 and 1.0 hours.

---

*Friedman EA: *Labor: Clinical Evaluation and Management,* ed 2. New York, Appleton-Century-Crofts, 1978, p 49.

CHAPTER 12

Labor Course and Outcome: Lexicon Approach

Summary

The labor course and its disorders, as previously defined by nonparametric methods, were codified into a lexicon term for each of 42,972 gravidas. Six labor progression variables were incorporated to produce a term consisting of six characters with four possible code designations. Assessment of outcomes by lexicon groupings showed that concentrations of poor results were limited to a relatively small number. Simplification to eliminate redundancy reduced the code term to four characters and the number of possible codes to a more manageable size. Hierarchical patterns were also developed to study generic groupings and thereby assess the impact of code components and combinations of components. Specific patterns were thus identified as contributing greatly to adverse outcomes.

Having defined a number of variables that describe labor progression quantitatively and then having determined the level of those variables beyond which adverse fetal and infant effects can be expected to be encountered, we proceeded to study their interrelationships. Toward this end, we wished to assess the impact of combinations of concurrent labor disorders. The analytical approach we used was one by which we felt we could not only determine the relative influence of the various types of disorders under surveillance, but perhaps uncover synergistic or counterbalancing effects as well.

Codification

Our first step was to codify all case material, nulliparas and multiparas considered separately, according to the presence or absence of each of the disorders previously defined (chapter 11). For this purpose, we exposed the entire NCPP data set of 59,391 gravidas after first excluding those whose parity status was unknown. The resulting index population of 54,697 women encompassed 16,322 nulliparas and 38,375 multiparas. Because labor data or follow-up infant results were incomplete in some cases, the final study sample for this operation totalled 42,972, or 14,597 nulliparas and 28,375 multiparas in all.

A six-character code was established for every patient. Each character in sequence represented one of the derived labor progression variables. Reading from left to right, they were:

1. Latent phase
2. Active phase
3. Deceleration phase
4. Second stage
5. Maximum slope of dilatation
6. Maximum slope of descent

The code for a given character stipulated one of four possible options according to the condition of the labor variable it represented:

A, absent because it was unknown, not calculated or unrecorded
D, down range, that is, below the lower limit of normal cut point as previously determined, abnormally low
M, middle range, between the upper and lower cut point extreme limits of normal, within the normal range
U, up range, above the upper limit of normal, abnormally high

In order to familiarize the reader with this kind of codified designation, a few examples are in order at this point:

MMMMMM denotes a case in which all six variables are known and all fall within the normal limits.
MAMMAM is a situation in which all variables are normal except for unknown active phase duration and maximum slope of dilatation (second and fifth characters).
MUUMDD shows prolonged active and deceleration phases (second and third digits) with abnormally slow rates of dilatation and descent (last two characters).
AMMDMU unknown latent phase, foreshortened second stage with excessively rapid descent.

Permutations

A lexicon of six-character "terms" was thus devised, comprising one term for each of the 42,972 women being studied. There were in theory 1296 possible combinations of the six variables (6^4 = 1296). Taking parity into account might yield as many as 2592 such groupings (2 times 1296). Contrary to expectations, however, there were only 576 lexicon groups encountered (including normal), 295 for nulliparas and 281 for multiparas. These 576 constituted only 22.2% of the 2592 combinations that were possible. Nonetheless, they were so numerous as to make detailed analysis at best costly and at worst unprofitable (within the constraints of time and resources available for this project) and perhaps even meaningless in terms of practical usefulness.

This was verified by the finding that, aside from the normal pattern, only 47 groups (Table 12-1) among the 280 multiparous patterns encountered contained as few as 50 cases, and only 22 of the 294 nulliparous groups (Table 12-2) contained that minimum number. The operation thus fractionated the case material so that only 12.0% of the codified pattern sets were suf-

89

Table 12-1
Common Lexicon Patterns in Multiparas

Lexicon Code	No.	Lexicon Code	No.
MMMMMU*	1,429	MDDDUU	112
MAMAMA*	939	MDMMMM*	112
MAMAMU*	658	MMUMDU	111
MDMMMU*	527	MADAUU	97
MMMDMU*	458	UAMAMU	94
MMMMMA*	431	DAMAMU	90
MDMMUU*	307	UMMMMM	85
MAMAMM*	266	MUUMDU*	82
MAUADA*	245	MDMMUM	74
MDMDMU	239	MADAUA	72
MAMAMM	213	MUUMDM*	69
MMMDMA	211	DMMMMM*	67
DMMMMU*	192	MDMMUA	66
MMMUMU*	191	DMMDMU	66
UAMAMA	170	DMMMMA	64
MMMUMM*	160	MAUADU	64
MDMDUU	159	UAMAMM	58
UMMMMU	156	MUUMDA*	58
MAMAUU	152	DDMMMU	57
DAMAMA	147	MDMDUA	54
MDMDMA*	145	UMMMMA	54
MDDMUU	145	UAUADA	51
MAMAUA	145	UMMDMU	51
MMUMDA	144	MAUADM	50

* Frequently occurring pattern shared in common with nulliparas.

Table 12-2
Common Lexicon Labor Patterns in Nulliparas

Lexicon Code	No.	Lexicon Code	No.
MMMMMU*	1,554	DMMMMM*	125
DMMMMU*	310	MMMUMU*	120
MAMAMU*	248	MMMMDU	105
MMMDMU*	216	MUMMMU	96
MDMMMU*	187	MUUMDA*	81
MAMAMA*	179	MUUMDM*	80
MDMMUU*	175	MAUADA*	71
MAMAMM*	173	MDMMMM*	70
MUUMDU*	173	MMMUMM*	66
MDDMUU*	151	MDDMUM	60
MMMMMA*	125	MUMMDU	54

* Frequently occurring pattern shared in common with multiparas.

ficiently sizable to provide utilitarian rates of adverse outcomes (69 of the 574 groups that were actually found to exist). Moreover, these 69 groups accounted for only 14,007 patients or 32.6% of the 42,972 index population base from which they were drawn (9588 or 33.8% of multiparas and 4419 or 30.3% of nulliparas), leaving the majority of cases sequestered into cells containing too few cases to be rationally analyzable. Of passing interest, both nulliparas and multiparas shared these 69 populous pattern groups in common, although their relative positions when arranged according to descending order of frequency were somewhat dissimilar.

To demonstrate feasibility and to test validity of our basic thesis, however, we did pursue this approach anyway, completing an investigation of outcome results for all 576 groups. We selected a few representative outcome measures for this purpose, limiting ourselves to (1) stillbirth, (2) neonatal death, (3) low five-minute Apgar score, (4,5) abnormal eight-month Bayley mental and motor score, (6) three-year speech, language, and hearing disorder, and (7) abnormal four-year IQ score. Every subset of data produced in this manner was subjected to Freeman-Tukey analysis (chapter 7) to ascertain if it deviated significantly from the mean result for the population at large as well as from the mean of the normal labor group.

Sequencing by Score

Groupings were "scored" for purposes of identification, sequencing, and aligning them in an orderly and logical arrangement.

The score involved a four-integer sequence made up of:

1. Number of U (up range) designations in the coded term
2. Number of M (middle range) designations
3. Number of D (down range) designations
4. Number of A (absent) designations

Cases with no labor data (AAAAAA), for example, would be coded 0006 (no U, no M, no D, but six A codes). Normal labors with a full data set (MMMMMM) were coded 0600 (all M codes). A fairly common group, MAMAMU characterized by precipitate descent, was scored 1302 (one U, three M, zero D, and two A codes).

Compilation of Outcome Data

A sample page (Table 12-3) illustrates the extensive compilation of results obtained. A consecutive sequence, by score, of 54 lexicon patterns of labor are shown for multiparas, with stillbirth data for each. Freeman-Tukey deviates (FTD) are given

Table 12-3
Sample Page of Lexicon Labor Patterns in Multiparas Showing Stillbirths

Code Score	Lexicon Pattern	Total No.	Observed Stillborn No.	FTD_m[a]	FTD_n[a]
1023	DAUADA	34	1	0.461	0.986
1032	DAUADD	1		-0.041	-0.015
1041	DDDDUA	2		-0.080	-0.030
1113	DAMAUA	22		-0.680	-0.294
1113	DAUAMA	1		-0.041	-0.015
1113	MAAADU	2		-0.080	-0.030
1113	MADAUA	72	2	0.508	1.357
1113	MAUADA	245	3	-0.881	0.817
1122	DADAUM	1		-0.041	-0.015
1122	DAUADM	6		-0.223	-0.088
1122	MADAUD	1		-0.041	-0.015
1122	MAUADD	5		-0.189	-0.074
1131	DDDMUA	6		-0.223	-0.088
1131	DDMDUA	4		-0.154	-0.059
1131	DMUDDA	3		-0.117	-0.044
1131	MDDDUA	32	1	0.504	1.008
1140	DDDDUM	2		-0.080	-0.030
1203	MAMAUA	145		-2.606[b]	-1.332
1203	MAUAMA	1		-0.041	-0.015
1203	UAMAMA	170	3	-0.150	1.242

				FTD$_m$	FTD$_n$
1203	MAUAMA	1		-0.041	-0.015
1203	UAMAMA	170	3	-0.150	1.242
1212	DAMAMU	90		-1.907[b]	-0.937
1212	DAMAUM	6		-0.223	-0.088
1212	MADAUM	25		-0.752	-0.329
1212	MAUADM	50	1	0.148	0.824
1212	UAMAMD	1		-0.041	-0.015
1221	DDMMUA	7	2	1.890[b]	2.044[b]
1221	DMUDMA	1		-0.041	-0.015
1221	DMUMDA	23		-0.704	-0.305
1221	MDAMDU	3		-0.117	-0.044
1221	MDDMUA	31	2	1.258	1.750[b]
1221	MDMDUA	54	3	1.393	2.104[b]
1221	MMADDU	2		-0.080	-0.030
1221	MMDDUA	1		-0.041	-0.015
1221	MMUDDA	49		-1.248	-0.581
1221	UDMDMA	16	1	0.890	1.194
1230	DDDMUM	4		-0.154	-0.059
1230	DDMDMU	33		-0.932	-0.418
1230	MDDDUM	3		-0.117	-0.044
1302	MAMAMU	658		-6.447[b]	-3.597[b]
1302	MAMAUM	41		-1.096	-0.501
1302	MAUAMM	4		-0.154	-0.059
1302	UAMAMM	58	1	0.006	0.749
1311	DMMUMA	1		-0.041	-0.015
1311	DMUMMA	2		-0.080	-0.030
1311	DUMMMA	1	1	1.374	1.399
1311	MDMMUA	66	4	1.694[b]	2.499[b]
1311	MDMUMA	1	1	1.374	1.399
1311	MMAMDU	8		-0.289	-0.116
1311	MMAUDM	2		-0.080	-0.030
1311	MMDMUA	2		-0.080	-0.030
1311	MMUDMA	2		-0.080	-0.030
1311	MMUMDA	144		-2.594[b]	-1.324
1311	UDMMMA	15	1	0.917	1.206
1311	UMMDMA	21	2	1.492	1.864[b]

[a] FTD$_m$, Freeman-Tukey deviate based on comparison with overall series mean rate; FTD$_n$, deviate relative to mean rate for normal labor pattern, MMMMMM.

[b] Statistically significant FTD, p < 0.05.

with relation to both the overall stillbirth rate for the entire population and the rate for just the normal labor group (MMMMMM, 7.65/1000). Significant FTD values (1.645 or greater, p < .05) among these 54 groups occurred with patterns DDMMUA, MDDMUA, MDMDUA, MDMMUA, and UMMDMA when contrasted with the normal labor group, indicating an adverse effect; "protection" appeared to apply with pattern MAMAMU because of the large negative FTD, reflecting no mortality in 658 cases. In addition, comparison with the overall mean rate yielded significant FTD values for three more patterns, all on the "protective" side (MAMAUA, DAMAMU, and MMUMDA). Because the overall rate was higher than the normal labor rate, no new adverse patterns were uncovered by this exercise.

Deviant Patterns

A listing of all such deviant patterns for stillbirths in multiparas is presented in Table 12-4 along with each subset sample size and its associated stillbirth rate. Among the 281 multiparous labor pattern sets, stillbirths occurred in 48, ranging in number from one to 14. The largest number of deaths was found in the group designated MAMAMA, consisting of 14 in 939 cases or

Table 12-4
Labor Patterns Significantly* Associated with Stillbirth in Multiparas

Lexicon Pattern	No.	Stillbirth rate, per 1,000	FTD	p
Adverse Impact				
UDMMUA	6	500.00	2.644	0.004
DDMMUA	7	285.71	2.044	0.020
DUUMDA	10	200.00	2.004	0.023
MMMUMA	12	166.67	1.977	0.024
MUUUDA	12	166.67	1.977	0.024
UMMDMA	21	95.24	1.865	0.031
UAUADA	51	78.43	2.636	0.004
MDDMUA	31	64.52	1.750	0.040
MDMMUA	66	60.61	2.499	0.006
DMMDMA	36	55.56	1.697	0.044
MDMDUA	54	55.56	2.104	0.018
DAMAMA	147	47.62	3.130	0.0009
MDMMMA	213	28.17	2.354	0.009
MMMMMA	431	16.24	1.708	0.044
MAMAMA	939	14.91	2.163	0.015
Protective Effect				
MAMAMU	668	0.00	-3.597	0.0002
MDMDMU	239	0.00	-1.883	0.030
MMMDMU	458	0.00	-2.874	0.002
MDMMUU	311	0.00	-2.224	0.013
MMMMMU	1,429	1.40	-3.541	0.0002
MDMMMU	532	1.90	-1.724	0.042

* Based on Freeman-Tukey deviate (FTD) greater than 1.645, $p < 0.05$, relative to the death rate associated with normal labor pattern (MMMMMM), arranged in order of the magnitude of effect.

14.91/1000. The highest frequency, by contrast, was in group UDMMUA with three deaths among six offspring. Of the 48 groups in which a fetus had died, the stillbirth rate proved significantly increased only in the 15 shown here.

In terms of the kinds of abnormal labors represented by these patterns, little intergroup consistency was apparent when the pattern designations were compared, except for the inexplicable absence of second stage duration data throughout (A, the final or sixth character of the code). Low stillbirth rates—found to be statistically significant in those sets made up of large number of cases with few or no deaths—were encountered in six protective pattern groups (Table 12-2). Normal latent and deceleration phase durations occurred in all (M, the first and third characters), as did

excessively rapid rates of descent (U, the final character).

Neonatal deaths in multiparas appeared in significantly high frequencies, when compared with the referent rate in the normal labor group, in 18 pattern sets (Table 12-5) among the 68 sets in which any such deaths were found. No protective groups were detected for this outcome variable utilizing the normal labor group for reference. Examining the codes failed to disclose any consistency in the patterns thus designated as high risk for neonatal deaths. Moreover, little correlation was found between these codes and those with stillbirth risk (see above), perhaps related to the fragmentation of the groups into so many descriptors. The only two patterns identified as having similar results for both variables were DAMAMA (short latent phase,

Table 12-5
Patterns Significantly* Associated with Neonatal Death in Multiparas

Lexicon Pattern	No.	Neonatal Death Rate, per 1,000	FTD	p
Adverse Impact				
UMUMDM	5	400.00	2.109	0.018
UUMMMU	11	181.82	2.065	0.020
DDMMMA	33	60.61	1.919	0.028
MMUMDM	41	48.78	1.870	0.031
UMMUMU	49	40.82	1.823	0.034
UAUADA	51	39.22	1.823	0.034
UMMDMU	53	37.74	1.799	0.036
MMMUMM	165	36.36	3.216	0.0007
UAMAMM	59	33.90	1.766	0.039
MAUADA	249	28.11	3.278	0.0005
DAMAMA	147	27.21	2.444	0.007
UMMMMU	157	25.48	2.389	0.008
MDMDUU	163	24.54	2.364	0.009
MAMAMM	271	18.45	2.417	0.016
DMMMMU	195	15.38	1.734	0.042
MAMAMU	668	14.97	3.124	0.0009
MDMMUU	311	12.86	1.833	0.033
MDMMMU	532	11.28	2.067	0.019
Protective Effect				
None				

* See footnote, Table 12-4.

and unknown active phase, second stage, and rate of descent) and UAUADA (long latent and deceleration phases, slow dilatation rate, and the same missing data).

Paradoxical comparative findings were of special interest as pertaining to differential (indeed opposite) effects of certain labor abnormalities. Excessively rapid descent, for example, seemed to be protective insofar as stillbirth rates were concerned, but some of the same patterns (MAMAMU, MDMMUU, and MDMMMU) yielded significantly high frequencies of neonatal deaths. This could be explained intuitively by the recognized traumatic effect of precipitate delivery on the newborn infant, representing the adverse impact of the type of injury resulting from excessive contractility and descent at the very end of the labor process, that clearly does not usually apply to the fetus earlier in labor.

All other outcomes were studied in like manner by lexicon pattern. The kind of findings that were uncovered were similar to those just described. Patterns of different varieties were determined to be related to an assortment of poor outcomes. Only moderate degrees of consistency could be shown, however. The data in general, while interesting and suggestive in places (as indicated above, for example), appeared to be too finely tuned to permit us to grasp all the nuances of interaction that we sought. Accordingly, we modified our attack for purposes of diminishing the fragmentation of our data, that is, reducing the number of possible labor pattern combinations. Of course, we wished to accomplish this without losing important information.

Recoding to Eliminate Redundancies

We recognized certain redundancies that could be eliminated. Prolonged active phase was essentially synonymous with low maximum slope of dilatation in the active phase; similarly, short active phases resulted from rapid dilatation rates. Correlation between them proved to be very good, as expected. Indeed, it was exceedingly rare to find any case in which such correlation did not exist. Therefore, these two variables (active phase duration and maximum slope of dilatation) could be joined. Further, latent phase disorders appeared to have almost no discernible effect on the fetus, at least in relative terms when compared with the much greater effects of other aspects of the labor course. Thus, we rationalized that when a latent phase aberration occurred in conjunction with another abnormality of the derived labor variable, it could be ignored (that is, suppressed); if it occurred alone, it was to be retained. Finally, the duration of second stage reflected the maximum slope of descent (short if descent was rapid, long if descent was slow), allowing us to collapse these two variables into one as well.

This reduction operation offered the economy of a four-character code for labor patterns instead of the previous six. From left to right, the four-character condensed code included the following designations:

1. Latent phase
2. Deceleration phase
3. Maximum slope of dilatation (incorporating active phase)
4. Maximum slope of descent (incorporating second stage)

Still further in our efforts to simplify, we collapsed the aforementioned designation for A (absent or unknown) into M (median or normal range of variable) on the assumption that most labors in which a given segment could not be reconstructed were probably normal. Those labors in which no labor progression variable could be derived at all were still excluded, however. We also substituted the symbol X for all designations (D, M, and U) attributed to the latent phase variable when the pattern was associated with any other abnormality in deceleration, dilatation, or descent.

On the basis of this formulation, we postulated that no more than 29 labor patterns were possible for both nulliparas and multiparas, excluding patterns that were unreconstructable in any way (AAAA). These 29 patterns consisted of a normal labor pattern (MMMM), two latent phase disorders (DMMM and UMMM), and 26 other combinations of the three remaining variables. We actually found 16 such patterns in nulliparas and 19 in multiparas among NCPP gravidas. Notable by their absence were nine identical patterns in both nulliparas and multiparas, plus three additional ones in nulliparas only (Table 12-6).

The rare or absent pattern groups proved worthy of interest. Deceleration phase disorders, for example, never occurred in isolation in nulliparas and only rarely in multiparas. There were 27 XUMM cases, all multiparas, in 38,378 gravidas or 1:1412 (0.070%) and no XDMM representatives at all. In every case in which the deceleration phase was foreshortened in nulliparas, the maximum slope of dilatation was abnormally rapid (XDUM, XDUD, and XDUU, 438 cases). Similarly, every time the deceleration phase was prolonged (XUDM, XUDD, and XUDU, 788 cases), the dilatation slope was protracted. In multiparas, there were also no exceptions to the association between short deceleration phase duration and rapid dilatation (680 cases), but there were some patients with long deceleration phases who had normal dilatation rates (1602 had low dilatation slopes, only 49 had normal slopes, and none had increased slopes).

It was rather clear that the parity distinction we had heretofore maintained was superfluous because the pattern groupings that were identified were very similar in both nulliparas and multiparas, both with regard to their existence and their relative frequencies of occurrence. For purposes of further examination of the distribution of the various combinations of labor abnormalities, nonetheless, we continued to

95

Table 12-6
Composite Lexicon Patterns of Labor Abnormalities

Nulliparas		Multiparas	
Pattern	No.	Pattern	No.
XMMU	2,659	XMMU	3,780
XMUU	627	XMUU	2,024
XMDU	436	XUDM	816
XUDM	393	XMUM	807
XUDU	366	XUDU	618
XDUU	291	XDUU	470
XMUM	269	UMMM	365
XMDM	245	DMMM	307
DMMM	212	XMMD	260
XDUM	141	XDUM	206
XMMD	98	XUDD	168
XMMM	48	XMDU	83
XUDD	29	XMUD	33
XMDD	29	XMDM	28
XMUD	12	XUMM	27
XDUD	6	XMDD	22
		XUMU	15
		XDUD	4
		XUMD	4
Nonexistent patterns			
XDMM		XDMM	
XDMU		XDMU	
XDMD		XDMD	
XDDM		XDDM	
XDDU		XDDU	
XDDD		XDDD	
XUUM		XUUM	
XUUD		XUUD	
XUUU		XUUU	
XUMM			
XUMU			
XUMD			

examine the two populations as separate sets of data.

Hierarchical Patterns

We next sought to devise and examine hierarchical patterns. Hierarchical patterns differ from those just described in being more generically (rather than specifically) oriented. Thus, to form a group containing all gravidas presenting labor patterns characterized by protracted dilatation (abnormally slow maximum slope of dilatation in the active phase), we included every case with the designation D as the third code character (actual patterns XMDU, XUDM, XUDU, XMDM, XUDD, and XMDD). In hierarchical terms, the code for this group was XXDX. Based on the data for the actual patterns that made up this hierarchical group shown in Table 12-6, it was composed of 1498 nulliparas and 1735 multiparas, representing 10.3% and 6.1% of their representive parity groups. Similarly, precipitate dilatation patterns (XXUX) hierarchically encompassed all those actual patterns with the appropriate third character code (XMUU, XDUU, XMUM, XDUM, XMUD, and XDUD). They totalled 1346 nulliparas and 3627 multiparas or 9.2% and 12.8% of their respective base populations.

Table 12-7 displays the distributions of the hierarchical pattern groups derived in this way. The data for the latent phase

Table 12-7
Distribution of Hierarchical Composite Labor Patterns in Nulliparas

Lexicon Pattern	Nulliparas %	Multiparas %	Description
MXXX	91.8	92.6	Normal latent phase
DXXX	6.9	3.2	Foreshortened latent phase
UXXX	1.3	4.2	Prolonged latent phase
XXMX	80.5	81.1	Normal maximum dilatation slope
XXDX	10.3	6.1	Protracted dilatation
XXUX	9.2	12.8	Precipitate dilatation
XXXM	79.0	73.7	Normal maximum descent slope
XXXD	1.2	1.7	Protracted descent
XXXU	19.8	24.6	Precipitate decent
XXDM	4.4	3.0	Protracted dilatation, normal descent
XXDD	0.4	0.7	Protracted dilatation and descent
XXDU	5.5	2.5	Protracted dilatation, precipitate descent
XXUM	2.8	3.6	Precipitate dilatation, normal descent
XXUD	0.1	0.1	Precipitate dilatation, protracted descent
XXUU	6.3	1.7	Precipitate dilatation and descent
XXMD	0.7	0.9	Normal dilatation, protracted descent
XXMU	8.0	13.4	Normal dilatation, precipitate descent
XMXX	91.6	91.9	Normal deceleration
XDUX	3.0	2.4	Short deceleration, rapid dilatation
XUDX	5.4	5.7	Prolonged deceleration, slow dilatation

groups were dissimilar from those shown earlier because they now included those cases heretofore "suppressed" by the procedure we had used before to effectively ignore abnormally long or short latent phases when they were associated with other labor aberrations. The data now shown give the true incidence figures.

Outcome Analysis by Lexicon Pattern

Outcome data for each of the newly formed compressed lexicon patterns were developed in the same manner as described before for the fuller lexicon pattern groups, utilizing Freeman-Tukey deviate analysis. Stillbirth rates within each group were compared with the expected mortality rate for the overall group and, more pertinently, for the normal labor group (MMMM), as shown for nulliparas in Table 12-8 arrayed in descending order of adverse impact. Rate

ratios were also derived for purposes of developing impressions of relative risk. In regard to stillbirths, significant associations were disclosed for patterns XMUM, XDUM, and XUDD, which translate to precipitate dilatation in the first two and the combination of protracted dilatation and protracted descent in the last. Relative protection appeared to exist in the presence of patterns XMMU, XMUU, XMDU, XDUU, and XUDU, all associated with precipitate descent.

This analysis was expanded to include other outcome variables available to us for investigation. A sampling of the results for nulliparas are summarized in Table 12-9 as they pertain to the stillbirth data just detailed plus neonatal death rates, low five-minute Apgar score frequency, rates of low Bayley mental and motor scale assessments at eight months, and abnormal speech, language, and hearing at three years. Only the observed frequencies of each abnormality

Table 12-8
Stillbirths by Compressed Labor Patterns in Nulliparas

Lexicon Pattern	No.	Stillbirth No.	per 1,000	Freeman–Tukey Deviate	Rate Ratio
MMMM	1,101	13	11.81	–	1.000
XUDD	32	3	93.75	2.14[a]	7.938[a]
XDUM	146	7	47.95	2.66[a]	4.060[a]
XMUM	278	10	35.97	2.72[a]	3.046[a]
XMDM	249	6	24.10	1.52	2.041
XUDM	398	6	15.08	0.64	1.277
DMMM	213	2	9.39	0.18	0.795
XMUU	620	3	4.86	-1.77[b]	0.412
XMDU	433	1	2.31	-2.22[b]	0.196
XMMU	2,651	2	0.75	-8.09[b]	0.064[b]
UMMM	47	0	0.00	-0.79	0.000
XMMD	98	0	0.00	-1.39	0.000
XMDD	29	0	0.00	-0.54	0.000
XMUD	12	0	0.00	-0.25	0.000
XDUU	287	0	0.00	-2.82[b]	0.000[b]
XDUD	5	0	0.00	-0.11	0.000
XUDU	366	0	0.00	-3.28[b]	0.000[b]

[a] Significantly increased relative to referent rate in MMMM group, $p < 0.05$.

[b] Significantly decreased rate, $p < 0.05$.

associated with the labor pattern are presented here, together with the rate ratio that pertains. We have flagged those relationships that are statistically significant by the techniques previously described.

The negligibly adverse impact of isolated latent phase disorders (DMMM and UMMM) was verified throughout, except for the suggestive (but not statistically significant) effect on neonatal deaths (rate ratios 1.03 and 4.55 in foreshortened and prolonged latent phase cases, respectively). Long-term follow-up of these babies failed to show any residual effect; indeed, there was an apparent protective aspect to short latent phase durations encountered in the three-year communications testing results.

Abnormally protracted dilatation (XMDM) appeared to yield high frequencies of bad outcomes, but no result achieved statistical significance in this aspect of our study. Similarly, excessively rapid dilatation (XMUM) showed an initial impressively adverse impact on the stillbirth rate and some residual (statistically insignificant) effect on eight-month Bayley motor scores

only.

Better consistency was seen across the spectrum of outcomes for the pattern XMMU (rapid descent) with protective effects noted for many of the outcome variables. The single counterbalancing exception of the bad eight-month Bayley motor scores stood alone in this regard. Slow descent (XMMD) similarly showed some protective impact (although the data were not statistically significant); again there was only one exception in that the rate of neonatal depression was significantly increased, as shown by the frequency of low Apgar scores.

The more complex patterns, representing combinations of aberrations, provided additional important information. When both precipitate dilation and precipitate descent coexisted in the same labor, a common combination, neonatal deaths occurred in very high numbers (3½ times the frequency expected, a statistically significant increase). As previously noted, stillbirth rates were unaffected, however, except perhaps for some protective influ-

Table 12-9
Selected Outcome Results by Lexicon Labor Pattern in Nulliparas

Lexicon Pattern	No.	Stillbirth		Neonatal Death		Low 5-minute Apgar Score		Low 8-month Bayley Mental		Low 8-month Bayley Motor		Abnormal 3-year Communication	
		%	RR	%	RR	%	RR	%	RR	%	RR	%	RR
MMMM	1,101	1.18	1.00	0.46	1.00	3.00	1.00	0.23	1.00	0.22	1.00	8.16	1.00
DMMM	213	0.94	0.80	0.47	1.03	2.96	0.98	0.60	2.60	0.58	2.60	1.37	0.17[b]
UMMM	47	0.00	0.00	2.08	4.55	4.35	1.45	0.00	0.00	0.00	0.00	-	-[c]
XMDM	249	2.41	2.04	0.82	1.78	2.94	0.98	0.00	0.00	0.52	2.34	11.27	1.38
XMUM	278	3.60	3.05[a]	0.37	0.81	1.95	0.65	0.00	0.00	0.44	1.99	8.33	1.02
XMMD	98	0.00	0.00	0.00	0.00	8.51	2.83[a]	0.00	0.00	0.00	0.00	6.06	0.74
XMMU	2,651	0.08	0.06[b]	0.38	0.82	2.23	0.74[b]	0.37	1.64	0.41	1.86[a]	6.05	0.74[b]
XDUM	146	4.80	4.06[a]	1.42	3.10	2.94	0.98	0.96	4.21	0.94	4.24	3.85	0.47
XUDM	398	1.51	1.28	0.25	0.56	5.72	1.90[a]	0.67	2.93	0.97	4.36[a]	10.77	1.32
XMUU	620	0.49	0.41[b]	1.59	3.49[a]	2.92	0.97	0.60	2.63	0.39	1.76	8.44	1.03
XMDD	29	0.00	0.00	0.00	0.00	7.14	2.38	0.00	0.00	0.00	0.00	-	-
XMDU	433	0.23	0.20[b]	0.92	2.01	3.50	1.17	0.55	2.39	0.54	2.42	3.82	0.47[b]
XMUD	12	-	-[c]	-	-	-	-	-	-	-	-	-	-
XDUU	287	0.00	0.00[b]	1.03	2.26	3.52	1.17	0.00	0.00	0.00	0.00	7.84	0.96
XDUD	5	-	-	-	-	-	-	-	-	-	-	-	-
XUDD	32	9.38	7.94[a]	0.00	0.00	0.00	0.00	0.00	0.00	0.00	0.00	-	-
XUDU	366	0.00	0.00[b]	1.35	2.95[a]	5.18	1.72[a]	0.96	4.19[a]	0.31	1.40	5.13	0.63

a Significantly increased rate ratio, p < 0.05.
b Significantly decreased rate ratio, p < 0.05.
c Rates based on small sample size (less than 20) have been omitted.

ence. Rapid descent following protracted dilatation (XMDU) had a very similar effect with increased neonatal deaths (although not statistically significant) and diminished fetal deaths. Follow-up data on surviving infants showed only poor eight-month results (not significant).

Patterns of still greater complexity offered essentially the same results. Rapid dilatation and descent with a short deceleration phase (XDUU) provided effects parallel to those of rapid dilatation and descent associated with normal deceleration (XMUU), namely low stillbirth and high neonatal death rates. Rapid descent and protracted dilatation had comparable effects whether accompanied by a normal deceleration phase (XMDU) or a long one (XUDU). In this last group, bad early results (significantly high neonatal death rates and poor five-minute Apgar and eight-month Bayley mental scores) were counterbalanced somewhat by good late results (few low three-year communications problems) in surviving infants. The combination of slow dilatation, slow descent, and prolonged deceleration (XUDD) was an especially deleterious one with regard to stillbirth rates, nearly eight times the expected number having been encountered. Survivors did well, nonetheless.

Results for multiparas were examined in the same way (Table 12-10). Shortened latent phases (DMMM) provided unexpectedly bad short-term results with significantly elevated stillbirth, neonatal death, and neonatal depression rates, but no apparent permanent impact on survivors. Prolonged latent phase durations (UMMM) had a similar effect in terms of increased risks of death or depression, but only the Apgar score results were statistically significant.

Both protracted (XMDM) and precipitate dilatation (XMUM) showed bad short-term effects, but only the slow dilatation group yielded any apparent residual effect on surviving children as evidenced by high frequencies of poor results at the eight-month testing. Protracted descent (XMMD) did not affect the stillbirth rate, but it had a particularly adverse influence on neonatal death and depression and eight-month abnormality rates; subsequent results showed no residual effect. Precipitate descent (XMMU), by contrast, showed either no effect or a protective effect in both immediate and long-term outcome variables.

Deceleration phase effects tended to enhance those of the dilatation or descent abnormality with which they were associated. A short deceleration phase accompanying precipitate dilatation (XDUM) showed the same bad results as with precipitate dilatation alone (XMUM), especially augumenting neonatal death and depression rates (the latter achieving statistical significance). Prolonged deceleration phase with protracted dilatation (XUDM) parallelled the early effects of protracted dilatation in isolation (XMDM) in a like manner.

Combinations of protracted dilatation and descent (XMDD) yielded frequent (but not statistically significant) neonatal deaths. This was especially apparent because of the larger numbers of cases involved when accompanied by prolonged deceleration phase (XUDD), impacting unfavorably on stillbirth and neonatal deaths as well as neonatal depression rates (the last two significantly so). Precipitate dilatation and descent combinations (XMUU and XDUU) showed a suggestion of negative effect on the neonate but some apparent protective effect on the fetus.

In general, there was good concordance between the results to offspring of nulliparas and those of multiparas. The adverse effects of short latent phase duration in multiparas were not seen in nulliparas, although prolonged latent phase had comparable impact. Protracted and precipitate dilatation correlated almost exactly, as did protracted and precipitate descent. The complementary influence of the deceleration phase was seen in both parity groups. Minor discrepancies seen in the lexicon patterns representing combinations of disorders might have been accounted for on

Table 12-10
Outcome Results by Labor Pattern in Multiparas

Lexicon Pattern	No.	Stillbirth		Neonatal Death		Low 5-minute Apgar Score		Low 8-month Bayley Mental		Low 8-month Bayley Motor		Abnormal 3-year Communication	
		%	RR	%	RR	%	RR	%	RR	%	RR	%	RR
MMMM	2,159	1.20	1.00	0.84	1.00	2.03	1.00	0.99	1.00	1.29	1.00	7.82	1.00
DMMM	310	2.90	2.41a	1.95	2.34a	3.85	1.90a	0.93	0.94	0.90	0.70	6.84	0.87
UMMM	367	1.91	1.58	1.37	1.64	3.50	1.73a	0.00	0.00b	0.36	0.28	9.38	1.20
XMDM	28	3.57	2.97	3.57	4.27	3.57	1.76	5.00	5.07	4.55	3.52	-	-c
XMUM	816	1.96	1.63a	0.87	1.04	2.71	1.34	0.63	0.64	0.63	0.48	6.86	0.88
XMMD	257	1.17	0.97	2.31	2.76	3.75	1.85a	1.96	1.99	1.93	1.50	5.68	0.73
XMMU	3,760	0.48	0.40b	1.01	1.20	2.08	1.03	0.55	0.56	0.90	0.70b	5.88	0.75b
XDUM	207	1.93	1.60	1.46	1.74	4.62	2.28a	1.32	1.34	1.27	0.98	4.65	0.59
XUDM	810	1.60	1.33	2.33	2.78a	3.79	1.87a	0.95	0.97	1.10	0.86	4.64	0.59b
XMUU	2,007	0.30	0.25b	1.14	1.36	1.83	0.91	1.02	1.03	0.76	0.59b	6.93	0.89
XMDD	21	0.00	0.00	4.55	5.43	0.00	0.00	-	-	-	-	-	-
XMDU	80	1.25	1.04	4.82	5.76	8.54	4.21a	1.75	1.78	3.57	2.77	5.00	0.64
XMUD	34	5.88	4.88a	3.03	3.62	0.00	0.00	0.00	0.00	0.00	0.00	-	-
XDUU	468	0.21	0.18b	0.64	0.76	1.11	0.55	0.84	0.85	1.10	0.86	6.63	0.85
XDUD	4	-	-c	-	-	-	-	-	-	-	-	-	-
XUDD	167	2.40	1.99	2.98	3.56a	5.13	2.53a	0.00	0.00	0.00	0.00v	10.20	1.31
XUDU	618	0.32	0.27b	0.32	0.39	1.16	0.57	0.20	0.21b	0.80	0.62	2.45	0.31b

a Significantly increased rate ratio, p < 0.05.
b Significantly decreased rate ratio, p < 0.05.
c Rates based on small sample size (less than 20) have been omitted.

the basis of instability of the frequency data due to small sample size. Despite this problem, we were favorably impressed with the degree of consistency we had been able to achieve thus far.

Hierarchical Results Summarized

The aforementioned hierarchical groupings gave us further insights into the effects of labor disorders, whether alone or in combination, by allowing us to examine possible effects in perspective. All cases with protracted dilatation patterns (XXDX), for example, could be studied. Their results to offspring could be compared with an especially relevant referent group, namely those with normal dilatation rates (XXMX) rather than an overall normal labor population.

The data derived in this manner (Tables 12-11 and 12-12) showed some interesting facets.

The adverse effects of foreshortened latent phase in multiparas (DXXX), seen in the specific pattern groups, were repeated here. No comparable effect was found in nulliparas, except perhaps for the eighth-month Bayley scores. Prolonged latent phase (UXXX), however, showed bad effects in both nulliparas and multiparas, analogous to the earlier findings. The deleterious effects of protracted dilatation (XXDX) were also confirmed. By contrast, protracted descent (XXXD) had demonstrably adverse impact in multiparas, but not nulliparas. Precipitate dilatation (XXUX) was accompanied by poor infant outcomes in nulliparas, but not in multiparas. Precipitate

Table 12-11
Outcomes for Hierarchical Labor Pattern Groups in Nulliparas[a]

Pattern	Stillbirth	Neonatal Death	Low 5-min. Apgar Score	Abnormal 8-mo. Mental Score	Abnormal 8-mo. Motor Score	Abnormal 3-yr. Communications
MXXX	1.00	1.00	1.00	1.00	1.00	1.00
DXXX	0.80	1.03	1.02	2.60[b]	2.60[b]	0.17[b]
UXXX	0.00[b]	4.55[b]	1.45[b]	0.00[b]	0.00[b]	0.00[b]
XXMX	1.00	1.00	1.00	1.00	1.00	1.00
XXDX	2.57[b]	1.14	1.67[b]	2.14[b]	1.58[b]	1.12
XXUX	3.59[b]	2.33[b]	1.10	1.13	1.03	1.24[b]
XXXM	1.00	1.00	1.00	1.00	1.00	1.00
XXXD	0.93	1.06	2.01[b]	0.00	0.00	0.68[b]
XXXU	0.75[b]	1.35[b]	0.84[b]	1.42[b]	0.84	0.80[b]
XXMM	1.00	1.00	1.00	1.00	1.00	1.00
XXDM	1.68[b]	0.91	1.52[b]	0.00[b]	2.96[b]	1.58[b]
XXDD	4.46[b]	0.00	1.24	0.00	0.00	0.00
XXDU	1.06	2.40[b]	1.41[b]	2.65[b]	2.13[b]	0.64
XXUM	3.64[b]	1.42[b]	0.75[b]	1.11	2.23[b]	1.02
XXUD	0.00	10.74[b]	1.93[b]	0.00	0.00	1.61
XXUU	0.30[b]	2.74[b]	1.03	1.49[b]	0.99	1.20[b]
XXMD	0.00	0.00	2.80[b]	0.00	0.00	0.88
XXMU	0.69[b]	0.73[b]	0.73[b]	1.35[b]	1.53[b]	0.88[b]
XMXX	1.00	1.00	1.00	1.00	1.00	1.00
XDUX	2.48[b]	2.31[b]	1.29[b]	0.86[b]	0.71[b]	1.04
XUDX	1.75[b]	1.27[b]	1.93[b]	2.26[b]	1.51[b]	1.16

a Expressed in rate ratios relative to rate in the normal hierarchical pattern for the subgroup.

b $p < 0.05$.

102

Table 12-12
Outcomes for Hierarchical Labor Pattern Groups in Multiparas[a]

Pattern	Stillbirth	Neonatal Death	Low 5-min. Apgar Score	Abnormal 8-mo. Mental Score	Abnormal 8-mo. Motor Score	Abnormal 3-yr. Communications
MXXX	1.00	1.00	1.00	1.00	1.00	1.00
DXXX	2.41[b]	2.34[b]	1.11	0.94	0.70[b]	0.87[b]
UXXX	1.58[b]	1.64[b]	1.73	0.00[b]	0.28[b]	1.20[b]
XXMX	1.00	1.00	1.00	1.00	1.00	1.00
XXDX	1.31[b]	1.74[b]	1.38[b]	0.81[b]	1.12	0.64[b]
XXUX	0.88[b]	0.99	0.91	1.10	0.76[b]	1.00
XXXM	1.00	1.00	1.00	1.00	1.00	1.00
XXXD	1.13	2.69[b]	1.34[b]	1.02	0.97	0.88
XXXU	0.25[b]	1.02	0.69[b]	0.91	0.82[b]	0.86[b]
XXMM	1.00	1.00	1.00	1.00	1.00	1.00
XXDM	1.12	2.33[b]	1.57[b]	1.28[b]	1.05	0.58[b]
XXDD	1.42[b]	3.10[b]	1.88[b]	0.00	0.00	1.16
XXDU	0.29[b]	0.84[b]	0.85[b]	0.43[b]	0.92	0.34[b]
XXUM	1.30[b]	0.97	1.28[b]	0.90	0.64[b]	0.81[b]
XXUD	3.50[b]	2.66[b]	0.00	0.00	0.00	0.00
XXUU	0.19[b]	1.02	0.70	1.17[b]	0.70[b]	0.88
XXMD	0.77	2.23[b]	1.53[b]	2.29[b]	1.63[b]	0.71[b]
XXMU	0.32[b]	0.98	0.87[b]	0.87	0.77[b]	0.74[b]
XMXX	1.00	1.00	1.00	1.00	1.00	1.00
XDUX	0.81[b]	0.79[b]	0.99	1.13	1.19[b]	0.89
XUDX	1.32[b]	1.46[b]	1.16[b]	0.64[b]	0.91[b]	0.64[b]

a   Expressed in rate ratios relative to rate in the normal hierarchical pattern for the subgroup.

b $p < 0.05$.

descent (XXXU) also yielded poor results only in nulliparas.

Among hierarchical combinations of labor aberrations, several stood out because of their impact. In nulliparas, protracted dilatation yielded high rates of bad infant results when followed by normal or precipitate descent (XXDM and XXDU), but paradoxically not when followed by protracted descent (XXDD). We could conceive of the possibility that the delivery practices under the latter circumstances would be more likely to lead to cesarean section, thereby perhaps averting some of the potential damage of an operative vaginal delivery, but this remained to be ascertained.

Precipitate dilatation behaved differently as shown by the bad outcomes associated with all variants, including those followed by normal (XXUM), protracted (XXUD), and precipitate descent (XXUU). Among these, long-term effects were especially untoward in cases with both precipitate dilatation and precipitate descent (XXUU). Cases of precipitate descent yielded adverse effects if preceded by either protracted or precipitate dilatation (XXDU or XXUU), but not a normal rate of dilatation (XXMU).

The influence of deceleration phase disorders was equivalently bad whether prolonged (XUDX) or foreshortened (XDUX). The effects seen with deceleration phase patterns appeared to mirror those encountered in cases with dilatation aberrations; specifically, prolonged deceleration, which always accompanied protracted dilatation,

103

showed the same results as protracted dilatation; and foreshortened deceleration showed the same effects as the precipitate dilatation pattern with which it was in such constant association.

The results of these analyses provided us with an overall gestalt for subsequent investigation in still greater depth of detail.

Except for the matter of arrest disorders, we were in a position, at this point, to proceed to determine relative risk of these various labor disorders, thereby to designate which of them could be expected to yield poor outcomes and, further, to quantitate those risks.

CHAPTER 13

Labor Course and Outcome: Arrest Disorders

Summary

Arrest of dilatation and descent was studied in a 14,357-case sample and in the remaining 44,449 NCPP population. Frequency and duration of arrest were found related to degree of dilatation or level of station at which it occurred. Outcome results varied with duration. Objective definition of cut points was possible for clinical diagnostic purposes. The interrelationships that existed between degree of dilatation and duration of arrest were determined to affect outcome as well.

The foregoing analyses of labor data dealt exclusively with quantitation of the several identifiable component phases and slopes of the labor patterns among patients who followed the characteristic sigmoid and hyperbolic curves of dilation and descent, respectively. Our next objective was to study arrest of labor progression. To embark upon this investigation we needed to assess the labor progression data as related to both dilatation and descent for purposes of providing a meaningful computer-definable and clinically compatible diagnosis of arrest disorders.

In this regard, a computer program capable of offering such useful information was designed, written, and implemented (chapter 8). In brief, we utilized all sequences of dilatation and descent data that fulfilled the minimum requirements for valid, properly timed, nonregressive (rectified) recordings of the sequence necessary to define the course of labor. Given this information, any sequence of two or more identical values of cervical dilatation or fetal station was identified as an arrest of progression. The maximum time during which the arrest phenomenon was observed to exist was measured.

Study Populations

We defined arrest of dilatation in the context of the ongoing active phase of dilatation. Arrest of descent was similarly defined as limited to the time interval from the beginning of the deceleration phase of dilatation to delivery. The analysis dealt seriatim with three defined populations. First, we examined that portion of our index population (here designated "sample" population) with adequate data for reconstructing the labor patterns completely; second were cases in which the labor pattern could be partially reconstructed from available data principally by hand operations (called formally the "index" group); and third, the full NCPP data set was studied in depth.

Arrest in Sample Population

Based on the sample population of 14,357 gravidas with reliable dilatation and descent labor variables under our surveillance, we were able to identify 1777 with documented arrest sequences, or 12.4%. These constituted 833 nulliparas from a total of 7932 nulliparas or 10.5%; and 945 multiparas from a total of 6425 multiparas or 14.7%.

The duration of arrest of dilatation in nulliparas averaged 0.97 hour (SD 1.02 hours), with a median value of 0.67 hour and a range up to 8.23 hours (Table 13-1). For multiparas, the arrest lasted on average 0.48 hour (SD 0.68 hour), median 0.26 hour and maximum 9.50 hours. The data were markedly skewed in their distribution. From this, it was clear that the major component of the population with failure to progress as herein defined was probably constituted of essentially normal variants.

Rather than representing a true pathologic arrest process, the apparent cessation of progress was perhaps the result of a sequence of examinations made in close approximation one to the other. In consideration of the inherent error of such estimates of dilatation and station, it was felt plausible to consider that one would have been unable to detect normally occurring changes when examinations were made in rapid sequence.

The distribution of the arrest of dilatation data (Table 13-2 and Figure 13-1) showed that the greatest proportion of cases had very short durations of arrest, confirming the above contention. It followed, therefore, that it was necessary for us to examine these arrest data according to increments of duration so as to ascertain the impact, if any, of more prolonged arrest on outcome as contrasted with relatively short durations of arrest. In this way, we felt we might be able to determine the specific cut point at which a diagnosis of pathological arrest could be made meaningfully. By this we intended to determine a clinically applicable definition in terms of the potential impact of arrest of labor on the fetus or infant.

Arrest of descent was documented in 2216 patients in the sample population of 14,357 gravidas, or 15.4%. These included 1535 nulliparas (19.4%) and 681 multiparas (10.6%). The duration of arrest in nulliparas averaged 0.55 hour (SD 0.68 hour), with a median value of 0.34 hour and a range up to maximum of 8.00 hours (Table 13-3). For multiparas, arrest of descent averaged 0.24 hour in duration (SD 0.34 hour), median 0.34 hour and maximum 4.76 hours. As with the arrest of dilatation data, the distribution of the descent durations was skewed. This indicated that most of the population affected with arrest of descent probably constituted normal variants. As before, we reasoned the phenomenon was likely to have been caused by examinations done in close proximity rather than by a true pathological arrest process. The

Table 13-1
Distribution of Arrest of Dilatation Data in Sample Population

	Nulliparas	Multiparas
No.	7,932	6,425
Arrest, No.	833	945
%	10.50	14.71
Mean duration, hr.	0.97	0.48
Standard deviation, hr.	1.02	0.68
Skewness (moment coefficient)	2.60	5.43
Kurtosis (moment coefficient)	9.27	48.39
Quantiles: 5%	0.05	0.03
10%	0.16	0.06
25%	0.33	0.13
50% median	0.67	0.26
75%	1.20	0.58
90%	2.08	1.13
95%	3.01	1.50
Maximum	8.23	9.50
Modal	0.50	0.25

Table 13-2
Distribution of Duration of Arrest of Labor Progress by Type of Arrest and Parity

Duration, hr.	Arrest of Descent				Arrest of Dilatation			
	Nulliparas		Multiparas		Nulliparas		Multiparas	
	No.	Cum%	No.	Cum%	No.	Cum%	No.	Cum%
0.00-0.24	490	31.9	468	68.7	119	14.3	401	42.4
0.25-0.49	519	65.7	152	91.0	167	34.3	245	68.4
0.50-0.74	203	79.0	26	94.9	164	54.0	135	82.6
0.75-0.99	102	85.6	12	96.6	99	65.9	51	88.0
1.00-1.24	63	89.7	10	98.1	81	75.6	34	91.6
1.25-1.49	36	92.1	4	98.7	43	80.8	25	94.3
1.50-1.74	32	94.1	4	99.3	33	84.8	15	95.9
1.75-1.99	29	96.0	1	99.4	28	88.1	9	96.8
2.00-2.24	18	97.2	1	99.6	24	91.0	8	97.7
2.25-2.49	13	98.0	1	99.7	15	92.8	6	98.3
2.50-2.74	5	98.4	1	99.9	5	93.4	4	98.7
2.75-2.99	10	99.0	0	99.9	11	94.7	2	98.9
3.00-3.24	3	99.2	0	99.9	4	95.2	3	99.3
3.25-3.49	1	99.3	0	99.9	8	96.2	0	99.3
3.50-3.74	3	99.5	0	99.9	4	96.6	1	99.4
3.75-3.99	0	99.5	0	99.9	6	97.4	0	99.4
4.00+	8	100.0	1	100.0	21	100.0	6	100.0
Total	1,535		681		833		945	

markedly skewed distribution (Table 13-2) is shown in the cumulative curves illustrated in Figure 13-2.

Arrest by Degree of Dilatation

Before embarking on our assessment of the impact of arrest of dilatation and de-scent on the fetus or infant, we sought to examine the arrest data according to the level of progress that had been achieved by the time the arrest occurred. Cases identified as showing arrest of dilatation, for example, were stratified according to the cervical dilatation that had been reached. They were grouped by increments of 0.5

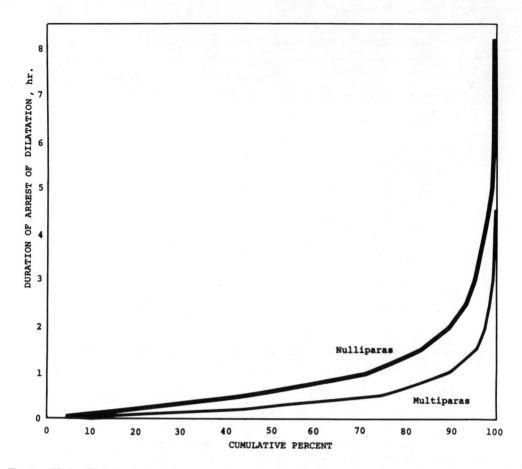

Figure **13-1.** Distribution of duration of arrest of dilatation by parity, plotted by cumulative frequency to show the intense concentration at the low end of the scale, especially in multiparas. Arrest was less than 2.0 hours long in 88% of nulliparas and 97% of multiparas.

cm. The distribution of the duration of arrest was determined within each group thus formed.

The distribution data derived in this way (Table 13-4) showed a preponderance of cases arresting at large cervical dilatation levels in both nulliparas and multiparas. Less than one-third of the cases of arrest occurred at dilatation of less than 8.0 cm (28.9% in nulliparas and 30.5% in multiparas); arrest at 9.0 cm or greater occurred in 45.2% of nulliparas with arrest of dilatation and 40.8% of multiparas who arrested.

Arrest by Level of Station

We also examined arrest of descent according to the station at which the arrest had occurred. The distribution data for fetal station (Table 13-5) showed a comparable cluster of cases at the most caudad stations in both nulliparas and multiparas. There were 81.8% arrests at stations +3 and +4 in nulliparas and 67.7% at these stations in multiparas. In addition, there were greater relative frequencies of arrest at high stations in multiparas than in nulliparas, 7.8% versus 2.2% at station +1 or more cephalad.

Duration of Arrest

Among the nulliparas, we encountered a subtle trend toward shorter durations of arrest when arrest cases were studied by the level of dilatation at which that arrest occurred (Table 13-6). This suggestion of a

108

Table 13-3
Distribution of Arrest of Descent Data in Index Population

		Nulliparas	Multiparas
No.		7,932	6,425
Arrest, No.		1,535	681
%		19.35	10.60
Mean duration, hr.		0.55	0.24
Standard deviation, hr.		0.68	0.34
Standard error, hr.		0.017	0.013
Skewness (moment coefficent)		4.06	5.85
Kurtosis (moment coefficient)		27.14	56.44
Quantiles:	5%	0.04	0.02
	10%	0.08	0.02
	25%	0.20	0.07
	50% Median	0.34	0.15
	75%	0.63	0.27
	90%	1.25	0.46
	95%	1.83	0.75
Maximum	8.00	4.76	
Modal	0.25	0.15	

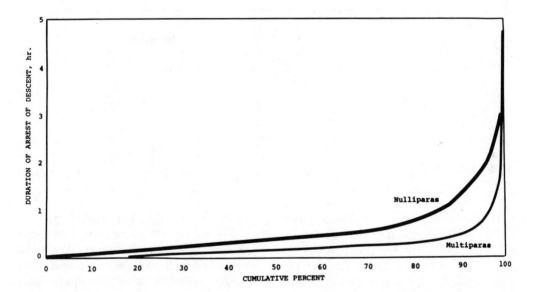

Figure **13-2.** Distribution of duration of arrest of descent by parity, showing skewed concentration at short durations. Arrest lasted less than 1.0 hour in 86% of nulliparas and 97% of multiparas.

trend toward somewhat shorter durations with advancing dilatation in nulliparas took the form of the regression equation

$$y = 1.388 - 0.060x$$

The standard error of the regression coefficient for the slope of this line (-0.060 ± 0.056) showed that the trend was not statistically significant ($t = 1.07$). By contrast, shorter durations of arrest were clearly associated with greater degrees of cervical dilatation at the time of arrest. The regression equation for this relationship in multiparas was

$$y = 1.218 - 0.096x$$

109

Table 13-4
Distribution of Arrest of Dilatation by Degree of Dilatation Achieved

Cervical Dilatation at Arrest, cm.	Nulliparas			Multiparas		
	No.	%	Cum%	No.	%	Cum%
5.0	18	2.2	2.2	13	1.4	1.4
5.5	8	1.0	3.2	4	0.4	1.8
6.0	70	8.5	11.7	47	5.0	6.8
6.5	14	1.7	13.4	26	2.8	9.6
7.0	118	14.4	27.8	164	17.4	27.0
7.5	9	1.1	28.9	33	3.5	30.5
8.0	196	23.8	52.7	254	27.0	57.5
8.5	17	2.1	54.8	16	1.7	59.2
9.0	223	27.1	81.9	242	25.7	84.9
9.5	149	18.1	100.0	142	15.1	100.0
Total	822	100.0		941	100.0	

Table 13-5
Distribution of Arrest of Descent by Station Achieved

Fetal Station at Arrest	Nulliparas			Multiparas		
	No.	%	Cum%	No.	%	Cum%
-2	0	0.0	0.0	1	0.1	0.1
-1	0	0.0	0.0	1	0.1	0.2
0	6	0.4	0.4	12	1.8	2.0
+1	27	1.8	2.2	38	5.6	7.6
+2	246	16.0	18.2	168	24.7	32.3
+3	590	38.4	56.6	193	28.3	60.6
+4	666	43.4	100.0	268	39.4	100.0
Total	1,535	100.0		681	100.0	

The slope proved to be rather steeply inclined relative to its standard error (-0.096 ± 0.033), making the trend statistically significant (t = 2.91, p = .0054). This relative foreshortening of the average duration of arrest with advancing cervical dilatation, particularly in multiparas, suggested the possibility that obstetrical personnel became more alert in detecting this problem late in labor. Moreover, they were perhaps more aggressive in intervening either with uterotonic stimulation or surgical delivery. It is obvious that if these observations proved to be correct, such interventive factors may have had major impact on the results to the offspring. It remained to be seen, however, whether or not any trend existed with regard to outcome impact.

The more serious nature of arrests of descent occurring at higher station was suggested by their longer durations as contrasted with the relatively shorter durations of arrests occurring at lower stations in the pelvis (Table 13-7). Arrests in nulliparas at station +2, for example, averaged nearly four times the duration of arrests at station +4 (1.07 ± 1.22 hours versus 0.29 ± 0.23 hour). Comparable differences were seen in multiparas who arrested at station +1 (mean duration 0.46 ± 0.64 hour) versus those arrested at station +4 (duration 0.13 ± 0.16 hour), a 3.5-fold increment.

That these trends are real is shown in Figure 13-3, which demonstrates the actual

Table 13-6
Duration of Arrest of Dilatation by Degree of Dilatation at the Arrest

Cervical Dilatation at Arrest, cm.	Nulliparas		Multiparas	
	Duration[a]	Median	Duration[ab]	Median
5.0	0.76±0.39	0.63	0.61±0.62	0.42
5.5	1.14±1.73	0.50	0.96±0.70	1.17
6.0	1.16±1.04	0.91	0.54±0.50	0.50
6.5	1.40±0.82	1.34	0.44±0.41	0.34
7.0	1.09±1.06	0.75	0.70±1.04	0.42
7.5	0.62±0.95	0.17	0.52±0.56	0.50
8.0	0.94±1.06	0.67	0.49±0.70	0.25
8.5	0.59±0.31	0.58	0.25±0.24	0.20
9.0	0.87±0.88	0.59	0.39±0.43	0.25
9.5	0.94±1.16	0.55	0.34±0.57	0.17

[a] Mean ± standard deviation, expressed in hours.

[b] Statistically significant trend, p = 0.005.

Table 13-7
Duration of Arrest of Descent by Level of Station at the Arrest

Fetal Station at Arrest	Nulliparas		Multiparas	
	Duration[a]	Median	Duration[ab]	Median
0	0.69±0.70	0.51	0.33±0.47	0.16
+1	0.93±0.62	0.88	0.46±0.64	0.18
+2	1.07±1.22	0.64	0.33±0.46	0.21
+3	0.61±0.54	0.43	0.24±0.21	0.20
+4	0.29±0.23	0.25	0.13±0.16	0.10

[a] Mean ± standard deviation, expressed in hours.

[b] Statistically significant trend, p = 0.03.

cumulative distribution curves for each subset of data in nulliparas by the fetal station at which the arrest occurred. There is clear evidence presented that very few arrests at low stations persisted (or were permitted to persist) for longer that 1.0 hour, yet this was not uncommon at higher stations of arrest. In this regard, there were less than 2% of arrests lasting more than 1.0 hour in duration at station +4 as contrasted with 34% at either station +1 or +2.

The trend for shorter arrests of descent to occur at progressively lower stations is shown in the regression equations for nulliparas and multiparas:

$$y = 0.942 - 0.112x \qquad y = 4.22 - 0.062x$$

In these relationships, the standard errors of the regression coefficients for the slopes were 0.089 and 0.027, respectively. On this latter basis, only the regression line for multiparas proved statistically significant (t = 2.30, p = .026). It is possible that these trends were specious in that lower stations of arrest may have made feasible the management option for effecting vaginal delivery by forceps instrumentation. Whether or not this approach was appropriate is not

111

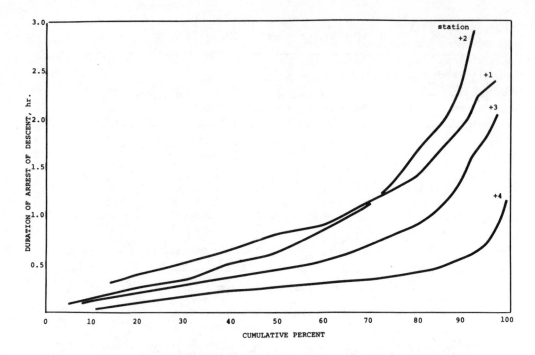

Figure **13-3.** Distribution of duration of arrest of descent by the fetal station at which the arrest occurred. The lower the station of arrest, the shorter its duration. This suggests more expeditious recognition, evaluation, and intervention when arrest took place at low stations.

relevant to this discussion.

Still to be ascertained is whether or not forceps intervention in some of these cases may have artificially shortened the arrest duration. The trend we encountered, therefore, was perhaps a reflection of intervention rather than a characteristic of the arrest process per se. We expected in due course to determine if the delivery procedure, that is, the intervention technique, affects outcome. This was an obvious concern both for our investigational objectives and for obstetrical practice in general.

Intuitively, it was felt that many, if not most, of the cases with arrest of dilatation or arrest of descent may have represented variations of normal in which the duration of arrest was very short and perhaps even artifactual. If specious, such arrest of progression would perforce have little relevance to the patient, to her labor, or to fetal and infant outcome. In order to resolve this issue pertaining to how long an arrest had to persist before it could be considered

meaningful in terms of its potential impact on the offspring, we studied the range of outcome variables for all infants delivered of women with arrest disorders according to the duration of the arrest.

Outcome by Duration

Patients were stratified by the duration of both forms of arrest in 15-minute increments. The subsets of cases thus created were examined for each of the outcomes. Relative rates of adverse outcomes were calculated for such important measures of result as stillbirth, neonatal death, perinatal mortality, low Apgar score at one and five minutes, abnormal eight-month Bayley mental, motor, and global scores, abnormal one-year neurologic examination, abnormalities of speech, language, and hearing at age three years, and low IQ scores (race-sex specific) at four and seven years. As before, offspring of nulliparas were analyzed separately from those of multiparas.

Results based on the index population were tabulated and subjected to Freeman-Tukey analysis (chapter 7). Illustrative are the data produced for neonatal depression, reflecting the frequency of low five-minute Apgar scores, according to the increasingly prolonged durations of arrest of descent (Table 13-8). It was found that, in general, the longer the duration of arrest, the greater the adverse effect. This was not unexpected, of course, but the data permitted us to ascertain a practical cut point for purposes of defining the best criterion for diagnosing a clinically significant arrest disorder. Clinical significance in this context, representing a major objective of this series of investigations, refers to the adverse impact on the fetus and infant as documentable here.

The data in Table 13-8 show a relatively homogeneous low frequency of neonatal depression for durations of arrest of descent in nulliparas under 0.75 hour (collectively 2.52% among the 1192 cases). A sharp rise in poor results is seen among cases with longer durations of arrest, all but one incremental group yielding a uniform zone of positive Freeman-Tukey deviates, distinctive from the negative deviates forming the "protective" zone with arrests of less than 0.75 hour.

Rate ratios were studied for each of the incremental groups as well and subjected to statistical verification. When compared with the arbitrarily chosen referent group with durations of arrest of less than 0.25 hour, several subsets achieved statistical significance, showing clear-cut adverse impact from arrests of descent that lasted a relatively long period of time.

Beyond 2.0 hours duration, the number of cases in each incremental group became too small to provide stability in the observed relationships. To offset this instability resulting from small sample sizes, the groups were variously collapsed at the upper end of the range of durations. For example, there were 61 cases with durations of arrest of 2.0 hours or greater in the material displayed in Table 13-8. These yielded 6.56% depressed infants for a Freeman-Tukey deviate of 1.278 and rate ratio of 2.66 (not quite statistically significant, $p = .074$).

When this approach was expanded to other outcome variables, relative uniformity of impact could be demonstrated (Table 13-9). This uniformity helped serve the aforementioned purpose of defining a meaningful cut point for arrest of descent.

Table 13-8
Neonatal Depression by Duration of Arrest of Descent in Nulliparas

Duration of Arrest, hr.	No.	Apgar Score < 6 No.	%	Freeman-Tukey Deviate	Rate Ratio
0.00-0.24	485	12	2.47	-0.844	1.00 Referent
0.25-0.49	509	13	2.55	-0.757	1.03
0.50-0.74	198	5	2.53	-0.429	1.02
0.75-0.99	100	7	7.00	1.772*	2.83*
1.00-1.24	62	4	6.45	1.256	2.61*
1.25-1.49	36	1	2.75	0.053	1.12
1.50-1.74	31	1	3.23	0.192	1.30
1.75-1.99	29	1	3.45	0.250	1.39
2.00-2.24	18	1	5.56	0.601	2.25
2.25-2.49	13	0	0.00	-0.628	0.00
2.50-2.74	5	1	20.00	1.135	8.10*
2.75-2.99	10	1	10.00	0.907	4.05
3.00+	15	1	6.67	0.710	2.70

* $p < 0.05$.

Across the range of outcomes that were studied, for example, it became apparent that arrest of descent exceeding 1.0 hour in duration was associated with adverse results. This was more strongly shown in short-and medium-term outcome assessments (such as death, neonatal depression, eight-month and one-year abnormalities) than in long-term testing (low four-year and seven-year IQ scores), but it was nonetheless present in all outcomes studied.

Cut-Point Options

To demonstrate the effect of cut-point selection, data for neonatal deaths were compiled (Table 13-10) for all cases with arrest of descent dichotomized at a 1.0-hour trial cut point. This manipulation yielded distinctively different neonatal death rates. There were more than four times the frequency of deaths associated with arrests lasting 1.0 hour or more as compared with those of shorter duration.

Other cut points also yielded higher mortality rates in association with longer arrest durations, but the rate ratios failed to achieve comparable statistical significance (Table 13-11). Nearly identical relationships were encountered for the frequency of neurologic abnormalities at one year of age. Neonatal depression, by contrast, showed

Table 13-9
Selected Outcomes by Duration of Arrest of Descent in Nulliparas[a]

Duration of Arrest, hr.	Neonatal Death	Low 5-min. Apgar Score	1-yr. Neurological Abnormality	Low 4-yr. IQ	Low 7-yr. IQ
0.00-0.24	1.00	1.00	1.00	1.00	1.00
0.25-0.49	1.45	1.03	1.17	0.79	1.17
0.50-0.74	-	1.02	1.05	1.17	1.01
0.75-0.99	-	2.83[b]	-	1.54[b]	1.14
1.00-1.24	3.97[b]	2.61[b]	6.26[b]	1.21	1.20
1.25-1.49	-	1.12	-	1.02	1.10
1.50-1.74	-	1.30	-	1.65[b]	1.76[b]
1.75-1.99	-	1.39	-	0.95	2.17[b]
2.00+	4.92[b]	2.25	2.00[b]	1.34[b]	1.18

a   Data expressed as rate ratios relative to referent rate for cases with arrest durations less than 0.25 hr.

b   p < 0.01.

Table 13-10
Neonatal Death as a Function of the Duration of Arrest of Descent in Nulliparas

Outcome	Duration of Arrest, hr.	
	< 1.00	1.00+
Liveborn survivor, No.	1,309	217
Neonatal death, No.	5	4
Neonatal death rate, per 1,000	3.81	18.10
Rate ratio	1.00	4.75*

*   p = 0.029.

significant differences at cut points even as low as 0.5 hour. Nonetheless, the 1.0-hour cut point for arrest of descent appeared to be most applicable across the range of outcomes.

The same approach was taken with regard to data derived from multiparas as distinct from nulliparas. This was done to ascertain whether the cut point of 1.0 hour duration of arrest of descent shown to apply for nulliparas was also appropriate for multiparas. Parity did not appear to influence the choice of cut point for defining a clinically significant arrest of descent. The data for multiparas were found to be essentially identical with those for nulliparas in regard to the impact that the duration of arrest had on offspring. Thus, we felt we were on very firm ground in designating the 1.0-hour cut point as a utilitarian measure of the duration of an arrest of descent process that can be expected to yield an adverse outcome.

The data for arrest of dilatation were studied in the same way. The trends we encountered were comparable in general terms, that is, the longer the arrest, the greater the frequency of adverse effects. However, there was much less consistency encountered across outcome measures. The frequency of neurologic abnormality at age one year, for example, correlated well with increasing durations of arrest of dilatation in multiparas (Table 13-12), but perinatal mortality did not. Moreover, there was considerably less uniformity as to cut point options than had been encountered with arrest of descent (Table 13-13).

Defining Arrest

In clinical practice, we have heretofore utilized a definition of arrest of dilatation that considered failure to progress in the active phase exceeding 2.0 hours to be abnormal. This has proved reasonably reliable for practical case-finding purposes. Our current analysis did not find the 2.0-hour cut point to be as meaningful a predictor of bad outcome as the 1.0-hour cut point had for arrest of descent. The only other cut point option that appeared to be any more effective for purposes of prognostication with regard to duration of arrest of dilatation was 1.0 hour, which did seem to hold more or less consistently across the range of outcomes.

For both convenience and statistical pur-

Table 13-11
Cut-Point Selection Options for Arrest of Descent
Duration in Nulliparas Based on Outcome

Outcome	Cut at 0.50 hr.		Cut at 0.75 hr.		Cut at 1.00 hr.	
	Below	At/above	Below	At/above	Below	At/above
Neonatal death						
Rate, per 1,000	4.98	7.53	4.14	12.20	3.81	18.10
Rate ratio	1.00	1.51	1.00	2.94	1.00	4.75*
p-value		0.53		0.090		0.010
Neonatal depression (Low 5-min. Apgar)						
Rate, %	2.50	4.49	2.52	5.64	2.88	4.87
Ratio ratio	1.00	1.79*	1.00	2.24*	1.00	1.69
p-value		0.037		0.005		0.12
Neurological abnormality (1 yr.)						
Rate, %	1.33	1.96	1.31	2.36	1.23	3.33
Rate ratio	1.00	1.47	1.00	1.80	1.00	2.70*
p-value		0.40		0.22		0.034

* Statistically significant, $p < 0.05$.

Table 13-12
Neurological Abnormality at 1 Year as a Function of the
Duration of Arrest of Dilatation in Multiparas

Outcome	Duration of Arrest, hr.	
	< 1.00	1.00+
Neurologically normal	443	136
Neurologically abnormal	8	7
Abnormality rate, %	1.77	4.90
Rate ratio	1.00	2.76*

*   p = 0.001.

Table 13-13
Cut-Point Selection Options for Arrest of Dilatation
Duration in Multiparas Based on Outcomes

Outcome	Cut at 0.50 hr.		Cut at 0.75 hr.		Cut at 1.00 hr.	
	Below	At/above	Below	At/above	Below	At/above
Neonatal death						
Rate, per 1,000	7.74	16.72	11.52	7.46	10.82	12.05
Rate ratio	1.00	2.16	1.00	0.65	1.00	1.11
Neonatal depression (Low 5-min. Apgar)						
Rate, %	1.74	2.65	1.83	3.08	1.72	4.94
Rate ratio	1.00	1.53	1.00	1.69	1.00	2.88*
Global abnormality (8 mo.)						
Rate, %	0.58	1.98	0.65	3.00	0.92	1.72
Rate ratio	1.00	3.41	1.00	4.61*	1.00	1.88
Neurological abnormality (1 yr.)						
Rate, %	1.60	2.21	1.79	2.80	1.77	4.90
Rate ratio	1.00	1.38	1.00	1.56	1.00	2.76*

*   Statistically significant, p < 0.05.

poses, therefore, we felt it appropriate to use a 1.0-hour cut point throughout for all arrest disorders in both nulliparas and multiparas on a preliminary basis. Introduction of this definition yielded diagnoses of arrest of dilatation in 283 nulliparas and 113 multiparas from the limited index sample population. These constituted 34.0% of nulliparas and 12.0% of multiparas with documentable arrest of dilatation. They totaled 2.76% of the 14,357 NCPP gravidas with plottable cervical dilatation patterns sufficient to reconstruct their labor courses (3.57% and 1.76% of nulliparas and multipa-

ras, respectively). Arrest of descent was diagnosed in 221 nulliparas and 23 multiparas, representing 14.4% and 3.4% of cases with some cessation of progressive descent. These 244 women constituted 1.70% of the index sample population of gravidas with definable labor patterns (2.79% of nulliparas and 0.36% of multiparas).

Expanding the Data Base

The next step in pursuing this aspect of our investigations was to incorporate cases of arrest disorders derived by extensive hand-screening operations from among those which our computer selection program had excluded by virtue of incomplete labor data, but which were considered likely candidates for arrest disorders. These operations specifically concentrated on patients who had been delivered by cesarean section during a labor that had not evolved completely to full cervical dilatation. The survey yielded a total of arrest cases that exceeded 6200. Several hundred had to be deleted because parity was not designated; since all our data were required to be stratified into nulliparas versus multiparas for substantive and overriding reasons (chapter 9), this step was necessary in order to ensure that this stratifying factor would be maintained. As a result, we were left with 5903 arrest cases. It should be noted in passing that this was by far the largest accumulated series of this type of case on record, being at least 25 times larger than the greatest published series to date.

Stratified by parity, there were 2642 nulliparas and 3261 multiparas, including all who had any arrest of dilatation or descent, regardless of duration. Specifically addressing ourselves to arrest of dilatation, we sought to determine the level of cervical dilatation that had been achieved at the time the arrest occurred. This averaged 6.48 cm in nulliparas (SD 1.76, SE 0.03, modal value 4.0 cm) and 6.60 cm in multiparas (SD 1.70, SE 0.03, modal value 8.0 cm).

Distribution by Degree of Dilatation

The distribution of these data according to the level of dilatation at the time of arrest was examined in some detail. We noted that estimates of dilatation were recorded exclusively in 0.5-cm steps as a discrete, noncontinuous variable. Not unexpectedly, we encountered clustering of cases into zero end-digit dilatation values. Zero end-digit pooling is a well-recognized phenomenon in which excessive concentrations of scalar readings ending in zero are commonly encountered. Rounding of measurements

to the zero end-digit value, while a common practice, makes such data difficult to handle statistically.*

Thus, we found (Table 13-14) relatively large numbers of cases in which arrest occurred at 4.0 cm, 5.0 cm, and so forth up to 9.0 cm and relatively few at 4.5 cm, 5.5 cm, and further to 9.5 cm. In view of this saw-toothed distribution (Figure 13-4), we felt it appropriate to enlarge the interval of dilatation for grouping purposes and thereby reduce the number of divisions for future consideration. This was done by coalescing the group achieving 4.0 cm dilatation together with those arresting at 4.5 cm. Thereafter, we dealt with 1.0-cm increments rather than 0.5-cm divisions. The newly created distribution is shown in the "envelope" of the bar graph included in Figure 13-4.

In this way, we could recognize that arrest of dilatation prior to 4.0 cm was a rarity, totalling 192 cases or 1.06% of the index population and 3.25% of all documented arrest cases. Beyond this point, moreover, the frequency remained at a rather constant level regardless of the degree of dilatation at which the arrest occurred, averaging 15.2% for each centimeter increment subgroup from 4.0 to 9.0 cm.

The distribution of levels of dilatation at which arrest occurred is shown in Table 13-15, stratified by parity. In general terms, multiparas arrested labor at more advanced cervical dilatation than nulliparas, but the range was broad in both groups.

Of greater interest was the duration of arrest according to the level of dilatation achieved (Tables 13-16 and 13-17). These data dealing with cases of arrest of dilatation can be compared with those from the sample population satisfying all necessary criteria for reconstructing the labor course (Table 13-1). One can see that we have apparently succeeded in including a large number of cases with more prolonged dura-

---

*Yule GU: On reading a scale. *J R Stat Soc* 1927; 90:570.

Table 13-14
Distribution of the Degree of Dilatation Achieved at Time of
Arrest of Dilatation

Cervical Dilatation at Arrest, cm.	Nulliparas			Multiparas		
	No.	%	Cum%	No.	%	Cum%
< 2.0	2	0.1	0.1	1	0.03	0.03
2.5	3	0.1	0.2	7	0.2	0.2
3.0	48	1.8	2.0	76	2.3	2.6
3.5	25	1.0	2.9	31	1.0	3.5
4.0	252	9.5	12.5	216	6.6	10.2
4.5	63	2.4	14.8	63	1.9	12.1
5.0	441	16.7	31.5	456	14.0	26.1
5.5	71	2.7	34.2	83	2.6	28.6
6.0	408	15.4	49.7	533	16.3	45.0
6.5	55	2.1	51.7	102	3.1	48.1
7.0	307	11.6	63.4	428	13.1	61.2
7.5	61	2.3	65.7	85	2.6	63.8
8.0	396	15.0	80.7	612	18.8	82.6
8.5	51	1.9	82.6	44	1.4	83.9
9.0	330	12.5	95.1	374	11.5	95.4
9.5	131	5.0	100.0	151	4.6	100.0
Total	2,642	100.0		3,261	100.0	

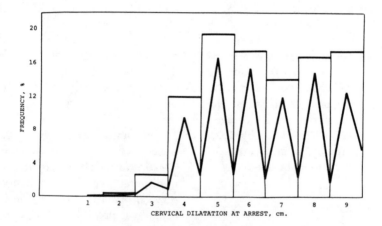

Figure 13-4. Degree of cervical dilatation achieved in nulliparas with arrest of dilatation, showing zero end-digit clustering at full integers to produce a saw-toothed distribution curve (heavy line). Envelope illustrates incrementation used for meaningful analysis (thin line).

tions of arrest, ostensibly more serious disorders of labor with worse prognosis for the fetus and infant. This is evidenced by the relatively larger overall mean durations for nulliparas (1.57 ± 0.34 hours versus 0.97 ± 1.02 hours in the sample group pre-viously studied) and multiparas (0.93 ± 0.55 hour versus 0.48 ± 0.68 hour).

Similarly, the duration of arrest according to the degree of cervical dilatation at which the arrest occurred may be compared here with the data earlier derived from the

118

Table 13-15
Arrest of Dilatation by Parity in Incremental Groupings

Cervical Dilatation at Arrest, cm.	Nulliparas		Multiparas	
	No.	%	No.	%
< 3.0	5	0.11	8	0.21
3.0-3.5	73	2.76	107	3.28
4.0-4.5	315	11.92	279	8.56
5.0-5.5	512	19.38	539	16.53
6.0-6.5	463	17.52	635	19.47
7.0-7.5	368	13.93	513	15.73
8.0-8.5	447	16.92	656	20.12
9.0-9.5	461	17.41	525	16.07
Total	2,642	100.00	3,261	100.00

Table 13-16
Duration of Arrest of Dilatation by Dilatation Achieved in Nulliparas

Cervical Dilatation at Arrest, cm.	No.	Mean Duration, hr.	Standard Deviation	Standard Error
3.0-3.5	73	3.02	4.23	0.50
4.0-4.5	315	2.04	2.81	0.16
5.0-5.5	512	1.53	2.13	0.10
6.0-6.5	463	1.55	1.81	0.09
7.0-7.5	368	1.49	1.82	0.10
8.0-8.5	447	1.52	1.51	0.07
9.0-9.5	461	1.17	1.15	0.05
Total	2,642	1.57	0.34	0.01

Table 13-17
Duration of Arrest of Dilatation by Dilatation Achieved in Multiparas

Cervical Dilatation at Arrest, cm.	No.	Mean Duration, hr.	Standard Deviation	Standard Error
3.0-3.5	107	3.71	5.94	0.57
4.0-4.5	279	1.41	2.20	0.13
5.0-5.5	539	0.89	1.45	0.06
6.0-6.5	635	0.84	0.87	0.04
7.0-7.5	513	0.81	0.88	0.04
8.0-8.5	656	0.78	1.15	0.05
9.0-9.5	525	0.57	0.70	0.03
Total	3,261	0.93	0.55	0.01

sample population (Table 13-5). Without exception, the mean durations of arrest in the large index population arrest group were consistently greater than in the original sample group for each increment of dilatation level reached.

In addition, there were clear-cut trends for arrest durations to be shorter when arrest occurred at more advanced degrees of cervical dilatation. These trends were expressed by the regression equations

$$y = 3.181 - 0.237x \qquad y = 3.593 - 0.384x$$

in nulliparas and multiparas, respectively. The standard errors of the coefficient for the regression slopes, -0.237 ± 0.069 and -0.384 ± 0.149, indicated that both trends were statistically significant (for nulliparas t = 3.43, p = .0012, and for multiparas, t = 2.58, p = .013).

Expanding the Data Base Maximally

The full NCPP data bank was ultimately utilized in an effort to verify the previous findings with regard to the relationship between outcome and the duration of arrest. Whereas earlier we had limited ourselves strictly to those sample and index cases in which the labor progress pattern could be reconstructed either entirely by computer programming methods or partially by hand operations, we now examined all NCPP cases so as to determine whether any arrest of progression beyond a critical limit of duration had comparable adverse effects. We studied the bulk of project cases that had not been included within the sample or index populations, specifically concentrating on the 44,449 case records that had been excluded from the index population (total NCPP series 58,806 women less 14,357 index cases).

It seemed logical to us that many of their labors had been excluded from consideration because the full dilatation and descent processes had not evolved sufficiently to satisfy the minimum criteria for inclusion (chapter 8). Indeed, we were convinced that

the very abnormalities under surveillance (arrest of dilatation and of descent) made it likely that such criteria would not be fulfilled. Further, we recognized from foregoing studies that these cases represented an especially adverse group in terms of fetal and infant outcome. Therefore, we persisted in the extreme.

Beginning with 13 magnetic tape reels of basic data files from the gravid population encompassing 5.7 million punch cards of data, we were able to identify 9882 cases with available parity status information in which there was indisputable arrest of progress recorded. This number exceeded by a factor of 67.4% even our own record number of arrest cases (see above).

Outcome Results

Having already recognized the adverse impact of arrested labor on the fetus and infant, we proceeded to determine the range of outcomes for offspring of women who had had arrest of progression in labor (Table 13-18). Even though these cases admittedly included many in which the arrest was very short in duration (and therefore probably specious), the deleterious effect was nonetheless apparent in some of the outcome variables. This was seen particularly in the neonatal and perinatal death rates among multiparas and the frequency of low Apgar scores in nulliparas. It was of passing interest to note that the overall stillbirth rate did not appear to have been affected by the existence of an arrest disorder. If such an effect did exist (see below), it was perhaps diluted by the presence of so many cases of inconsequential arrest durations.

Outcome By Degree of Dilatation

Stratifying by the level of cervical dilatation that was achieved at the time of the arrest demonstrated an interesting, albeit inconsistent, trend (Table 13-19). We have already seen that the neonatal death rate was increased in association with arrest of dilatation. By examining the material

Table 13-18
Outcomes for Arrest of Dilatation in Full Data Set

| Outcome | Nulliparas with Arrest | | Multiparas with Arrest | |
	No.	%	No.	%
Total	4,442		5,440	
Stillbirth	29	0.653	40	0.735
Neonatal death	38	0.855	58	1.066*
Perinatal mortality	67	1.508	98	1.801*
Low 5-min. Apgar	171	3.850*	143	2.629
Abnormal 8-mo. mental	15	0.338	35	0.643
Abnormal 8-mo. motor	16	0.360	33	0.607
Abnormal 1-yr. neurological	52	1.171	74	1.360
Abnormal 3-yr. communications	132	2.972	121	2.224
Low 4-yr. IQ	79	1.178	70	1.287
Low 7-yr. IQ	62	1.396	88	1.618

* Statistically significant, p < 0.01.

Table 13-19
Neonatal Death Rates by Degree of Dilatation
Achieved at Time of Arrest of Dilatation

| Cervical Dilatation at Arrest, cm. | Nulliparas | | Multiparas | |
	Rate per 1,000	Rate Ratio	Rate per 1,000	Rate Ratio
3.0–3.5	27.40	3.62*	46.73	6.17*
4.0–4.5	6.35	0.84	14.34	1.89
5.0–5.5	25.49	3.37*	24.12	3.19*
6.0–6.5	10.80	1.43	4.72	0.62
7.0–7.5	10.87	1.44	19.49	2.57
8.0–8.5	2.24	0.30*	9.15	1.21
9.0–9.5	4.35	0.57*	7.63	1.01

* Statistically significant, p < 0.01.

according to the degree of dilatation, we could now ascertain that the mortality rates were not uniformly distributed across the range of the divisions of dilatation level.

Instead, the deaths were concentrated in the 3.0–7.0 cm level groups. In fact, it appeared as if there was some degree of protection against the infant dying among nulliparas if an arrest occurred at or beyond 8.0 cm cervical dilatation. Although the frequency of neonatal deaths in multiparas diminished with increasing cervical dilatation, there was no such comparable protec-

tion encountered. We conjectured that earlier recognition and more aggressive intervention may have had a beneficial effect in these cases. As previously stated, this was a particularly interesting observation that deserved to be explored. Similar results, although not quite so impressive, were found with other outcomes as well.

Outcome by Duration of Arrest

When cases of arrest of dilatation were stratified by the duration of arrest, for example, we were able to confirm the particularly deleterious effects of arrest lasting 2.0 hours or more in both nulliparas (Table 13-20) and multiparas (Table 13-21). In addition, these data suggested that there may have been some adverse effect from arrest of dilatation of shorter duration, especially at 1.25 and 1.50 hours or more.

As to arrest of descent, the most impressive negative impact on the fetus and infant was seen with durations of at least 2.0 hours in length, but shorter durations affected offspring unfavorably as well, especially in multiparas (Table 13-22 and 13-23). Durations of 1.0 hour or greater yielded rather poor outcomes as shown by perinatal mortality, neonatal depression, and abnormal global scoring at eight months of age, with some residual effect still apparent up to age seven years. Arrest of descent lasting more than 1.5 hours showed very impressive long-term results, apparently reflecting the permanent damaging effects of this labor disorder on surviving children in multiparas. There was little doubt that these data accurately reflected the insult to the fetus and infant of this labor process.

Table 13-20
Outcome by Duration of Arrest of Dilatation in Nulliparas[a]

Duration of Arrest, hr.	No.	Perinatal Mortality	Low 5-min. Apgar	Abnormal 8-mo. Global	Abnormal 3-yr. Communications	Low 4-yr. IQ	Low 7-yr. IQ
0.00-0.24	207	0.96	0.61	1.28	0.64	0.92	1.07
0.25-0.49	432	0.77	1.08	0.64	0.93	0.73	1.07
0.50-0.74	485	0.68	0.78	0.57	0.99	1.08	0.73
0.75-0.99	405	0.82	0.44b	1.63	1.11	1.42	0.75
1.00-1.24	424	0.47	0.66	0.64	1.07	1.12	0.88
1.25-1.49	333	1.19	1.08	-	0.59	0.94	0.87
1.50-1.74	319	2.29b	1.32	-	1.15	1.52b	1.47b
1.75-1.99	230	1.16	0.77	-	0.87	0.88	1.02
2.00+	1,607	1.53b	1.38b	2.21b	2.31b	1.24	1.03

a   Data for 4,442 cases represented as rate ratios relative to rate for offspring of cases without arrest.

b $p < 0.05$.

Table 13-21
Outcome by Duration of Arrest of Dilatation in Multiparas[a]

Duration of Arrest, hr.	No.	Perinatal Mortality	Low 5-min. Apgar	Abnormal 8-mo. Global	Abnormal 3-yr. Communications	Low 4-yr. IQ	Low 7-yr. IQ
0.00–0.24	541	0.99	0.80	0.82	1.62[b]	1.11	0.98
0.25–0.49	1,143	0.63[b]	0.87	0.82	0.93	1.16	1.30
0.50–0.74	884	0.69	0.71	1.23	0.96	1.38	1.03
0.75–0.99	567	0.59	0.73	1.18	0.63	0.89	0.77
1.00–1.24	464	0.72	1.17	0.99	0.86	1.12	0.96
1.25–1.49	330	1.01	1.39[b]	1.26	1.29	1.29	1.11
1.50–1.74	260	1.28	1.02	0.70	1.44[b]	1.24	1.26
1.75–1.99	195	2.84[b]	0.81	0.69	0.80	1.69[b]	1.58[b]
2.00+	1,056	2.37[b]	1.77[b]	2.14[b]	1.42[b]	1.60[b]	1.51[b]

a   Data for 5,440 cases represented as rate ratios relative to rate for offspring of cases without arrest.

b $p < 0.05$.

124

Table 13-22
Outcome by Duration of Arrest of Descent in Nulliparas[a]

Duration of Arrest, hr.	No.	Perinatal Mortality	Low 5-min. Apgar	Abnormal 8-mo. Global	Abnormal 3-yr. Communications	Low 4-yr. IQ	Low 7-yr. IQ
0.00–0.24	227	1.72[b]	0.75	0.69	1.14	0.96	0.97
0.25–0.49	628	1.09	0.96	1.01	1.03	1.28	1.44[b]
0.50–0.74	526	0.56	0.70	1.25	0.86	1.14	1.01
0.75–0.99	367	1.33	0.77	0.44	0.75	1.19	1.09
1.00–1.24	253	0.77	1.10	0.67	1.79[b]	0.81	1.20
1.25–1.49	152	0.64	0.99	2.10	0.89	1.16	1.10
1.50–1.74	129	–	1.49	0.00	1.04	1.21	1.76[b]
1.75–1.99	77	–	1.13	1.86	1.11	2.41[b]	2.17[b]
2.00+	378	5.75[b]	2.41[b]	8.08[b]	1.73[b]	1.04	1.18

[a] Data for 2,737 cases expressed as rate ratios relative to rate for offspring of cases without arrest.

[b] $p < 0.05$.

125

Table 13-23
Outcome by Duration of Arrest of Descent in Multiparas[a]

Duration of Arrest, hr.	No.	Perinatal Mortality	Low 5-min. Apgar	Abnormal 8-mo. Global	Abnormal 3-yr. Communications	Low 4-yr. IQ	Low 7-yr. IQ
0.00-0.24	503	0.98	0.72	0.86	1.12	0.93	0.99
0.25-0.49	682	0.91	0.86	1.01	0.98	0.97	1.29
0.50-0.74	236	1.05	0.46	1.23	0.99	1.15	1.04
0.75-0.99	93	-	0.79	1.09	0.87	0.74	1.12
1.00-1.24	64	0.96	1.74	0.75	0.84	0.93	1.28
1.25-1.49	41	1.51	2.86b	1.19	1.26	1.07	1.58b
1.50-1.74	21	2.94b	3.62b	1.34b	0.67	1.03	3.51b
1.75-1.99	16	7.72b	2.29b	0.83	-	1.40b	1.63b
2.00+	68	10.29b	8.29b	3.16b	3.37b	1.33b	1.46b

a   Data for 1,724 cases expressed as rate ratios relative to rate for offspring of cases without arrest.

b $p < 0.05$.

126

CHAPTER 14

Labor Course: Designation of Risk Variables

Summary

A series of analyses was carried out to identify those labor progression variables significantly associated with poor fetal and infant results and to quantitate their risk effects. The factors determined to be related to bad outcomes by bivariate analysis were screened by cluster analysis for redundancy of informational content. Remaining variables were then subjected to logistic regression analysis to determine the impact of each while all others were being considered simultaneously. Investigation was limited to cases without serious congenital anomalies within the birth weight range of 2500–4000 g and outcomes were consolidated to reduce analytical complexities. Only eight of the original 22 labor progression variables were flagged as being especially relevant adverse influences on offspring.

All preliminary exploratory analyses of the labor progression data having been completed, we next undertook a series of investigations to assess which of the defined variables were significantly associated with fetal/infant risk and to quantitate the degree of relative risk. Moreover, it was now feasible to pursue the several lines of study outlined in chapter 7 pertaining to the application of a sequence of methods for designating risk variables. Beginning with a nonparametric technique, such as the Freeman-Tukey deviate (see p 40), we could specify those labor progression variables significantly related to a variety of specified adverse outcomes. Relative risk statistics, derived simultaneously to indicate the level of potential effect, could also be weighed for relevance by significance testing, as by the Mantel-Haenszel chi-square test or similar methods.

Design of Analytical Sequence

These examinations were expected to highlight those bivariate risk variables worthy of further study in depth. It was felt that the number might be diminished somewhat by means of cluster analysis (chapter 7) to identify risk variables with similar or nearly identical informational content in regard to poor outcomes. Tightly clustered variables are informationally highly interrelated. Selecting one variable from such a group of clustered variables allows one to reduce the number of variables to be studied without losing important information. The reduced set of risk variables is then tested by successive multivariate analytic techniques. For our purposes, logistic regression proved especially valuable for studying all relevant variables simultaneously so as to help distinguish those with unique or independent adverse impact from those whose effect was likely to reflect the influence of some other concurrent factor with which it was associated.

Using information from the foregoing exploratory analyses, we chose the cut points for designating abnormal states of labor progression (see Table 11-16) and for arrest disorders (chapter 13). This yielded a series of 22 variables, all dealing with labor progression, for study (Table 14-1). We thus satisfied our desire to make continuous variables discontinuous by grouping, thereby to enable us to examine incremental data by a sensitive and reliable nonparametric testing vehicle. Before proceeding with the definitive Freeman-Tukey analysis, however, we had to define both the population to be examined and the type or types of outcomes which could be considered relevant.

Table 14-1
Labor Progression Variables Defined

Variable Code	Definition	Cut-Point	
		Nulliparas	Multiparas
LAT1	Normal latent phase duration		
LAT2	Foreshortened latent phase	< 3.0 hr.	< 2.0 hr.
LAT3	Prolonged latent phase	>18.0 hr.	>10.0 hr.
ACT1	Normal active phase duration		
ACT2	Foreshortened active phase	< 2.0 hr.	< 1.5 hr.
ACT3	Prolonged active phase	> 6.0 hr.	> 5.0 hr.
DEC1	Normal deceleration phase duration		
DEC2	Foreshortened deceleration phase	< 0.2 hr.	< 0.1 hr.
DEC3	Prolonged deceleration phase	>2.0 hr.	> 1.0 hr.
SEC1	Normal second stage duration		
SEC2	Foreshortened second stage	< 0.5 hr.	< 0.1 hr.
SEC3	Prolonged second stage	>2.0 hr.	> 1.0 hr.
MAXS1	Normal maximum slope of dilatation		
MAXS2	Protracted dilatation	< 1.2 cm./hr.	< 1.5 cm./hr.
MAXS3	Precipitate dilatation	> 5.0 cm./hr.	>12.0 cm./hr.
DESC1	Normal maximum slope of descent		
DESC2	Protracted descent	<1.0 cm./hr.	< 2.0 cm./hr.
DESC3	Precipitate descent	>4.5 cm./hr.	>10.0 cm./hr.
ARRD1	No arrest of dilatation		
ARRD3	Arrest of dilatation	>2.0 hr.	> 2.0 hr.
ARRS1	No arrest of descent		
ARRS3	Arrest of descent	>1.0 hr.	> 1.0 hr.

Limiting Index Population

To this point, we had imposed stratification of our data by parity alone, having demonstrated little impact from other demographic factors. It was clear that the results of all antecedent exploratory analyses were not necessarily applicable to all subpopulations, although the assumption was implicit (albeit aknowledged to be suspect). For the purposes of the critical examinations about to be undertaken, however, this assumption could not be permitted to go unchallenged. Most actuarial and demographic characteristics were to be examined both in isolation (as bivariate factors) and collectively in multivariate analyses of the risks associated with intrinsic variables (chapter 21). Nonetheless, some few were recognized in advance to be so powerful as predictors of bad outcome that prior corrections were warranted for them. Two were singled out at this juncture, namely major anomalies incompatible with survival or with normal development and low birth weight.

A total of 18 specified diagnostic anomalous entities were identified. The data files were exhaustively searched and 198 relevant cases were identified with 237 diagnoses (Table 14-2). It was obvious that these conditions were unrelated in any way to the labor-delivery events under surveillance and that the expected poor outcomes for them could not be ascribed to or accounted for by factors relating to parturition. It was appropriate, therefore, to delete all 198 cases from further consideration in this portion of the investigation. This would ensure that such cases would not somehow implicate an otherwise innocuous variable if by chance they were associated.

The same concept was felt to apply to the adverse effects on infant survival and development recognized to occur in response to premature birth. Correcting for this factor suggested that cases be stratified by gestational age at delivery. However, the errors inherent in gestational age, as calculated from the last menstrual period, are well-documented. Moreover, a cutoff by gestational age would not permit such errors to

Table 14-2
Congenital Disorders Unrelated to Labor-Delivery Factors

Diagnosis*	No.	Incidence per 10,000
Down syndrome	49	28.3
Hydrocephaly	40	23.1
Anencephaly	39	22.5
Meningomyelocele	33	19.1
Microcephaly	12	6.9
Encephalocele	12	6.9
Post-rubella syndrome	11	6.4
Inborn error of metabolism	11	6.4
Craniosynostosis	10	5.8
Microphthalmia	9	5.2
Robin syndrome	4	2.3
Hydrancephaly	3	1.7
Dandy-Walker syndrome	1	0.6
Potter's syndrome	1	0.6
Congenital retardation	1	0.6
Chorioretinitis	1	0.6
Total diagnoses	237	
Total cases	198	114.5

* From NCPP data file 1408 based on PED8 forms for 17,925 cases.

129

be taken into account. Use of birth weight for stratification was considered to be more acceptable because it was clearly more accurate than gestational age. It failed to deal with the problem of intrauterine growth retardation, but this can be remedied by including small-for-gestational-age as an important intrinsic variable in a subsequent phase of the analysis. At the upper end of the birth weight spectrum, very large babies are also at risk because they tend to develop in women who have underlying or overt diabetes mellitus. Moreover, they may be subjected to the trauma of delivery if cephalopelvic disproportion is unrecognized, difficult forceps delivery is attempted, or shoulder dystocia should occur. Accordingly, the index population was trimmed to include only those who delivered infants weighing between 2500 and 4000 g. Low and high birth weight cases were set aside for study at a later time, if warranted.

Redefining Outcomes

The next step was to define outcomes more precisely and succinctly than heretofore. Given the complexity of the definitive analyses about to be undertaken and their cost in terms of effort and computer time, it was prudent to try to diminish the large number of outcome variables to a more economical and workable number. To this end, we consolidated the number of existing outcomes into three logical time frames, namely perinatal, infancy, and childhood. Perinatal outcomes included stillbirth, neonatal and perinatal death, as well as neonatal depression based on low five-minute Apgar scores (definite or severe 0-3, suspect or moderate 4-7). Infancy outcomes included the results of neurologic and psychological examinations at 8 months and 1 year (definite and suspect abnormalities considered separately). Childhood outcomes reflected the scores achieved on the 3-year speech, language, and hearing battery and the IQ examinations at 4 and 7 years (also divided into definite and sus-

pect). Parity distinctions were maintained as before (nulliparas versus multiparas).

As analytical results from this reduced number of outcomes were obtained, it became increasingly clear that there were variable degrees of consistency across the three time frames. Therefore, a single "union" variable was derived as a composite of the aforementioned outcomes. It consisted of any definite adverse result occurring at any time to a given individual. Use of this union variable simplified the final thrust of our investigational sequences, considerably reducing the prior necessary duplication and redundancy.

Screening Analysis

The aforementioned stratifications for major anomalies and extremes of birth weight yielded an index group containing 6688 nulliparas and 8481 multiparas with reliable labor progression and infant outcome data for our purposes. Freeman-Tukey bivariate analyses were conducted to ascertain the potential effect of each of the defined labor progression variables on the fetus and infant. The Freeman-Tukey deviate (FTD) derived by this approach provided a means for designating those items significantly associated with adverse or beneficial outcomes. The rate ratio (RR) of the observed frequency of the outcome relative to the expected rate gave the magnitude of the effect.

An example of the data generated is shown in Table 14-3 for offspring of the subset of nulliparas with protracted active phase dilatation patterns (code MAXS2, see Table 14-1). The outcome designated "definite perinatal" refers to either death (stillbirth or neonatal death) or severe asphyxia (Apgar score 0-3 at five minutes of age). In all, there were 41 of these results among 1233 cases or 3.3%; 2.4% occurred in the total nulliparous population from which these cases were derived, for a rate ratio of 1.39, representing a 38.6% excess occurrence rate. The FTD was 2.125, equivalent to a two-sided p value of .0335, indicating a low probability that this was a chance event. The results for "suspect perinatal" outcome (moderate neonatal depression, Apgar score 4-7 at five minutes) were even more impressive with RR 1.41 and FTD 3.807, p = .00014. These data supported the preliminary observation that the variable MAXS2 was probably a significant contributor to poor perinatal outcome. Later infant outcome results were relatively good. The only suggestion of a problem occurred in the "suspect infancy" subgroup (RR 1.14, FTD 1.882), but it failed to achieve more than a marginal level of statistical significance (p = .060).

This approach demonstrated the utilitarian value of the screening technique used here. Accordingly, it was expanded to provide the full panoply of rate ratios and Freeman-Tukey deviates for all the 22 labor progression variables for both nulliparas (Table 14-4) and multiparas (Table 14-5). Among nulliparas, significantly adverse perinatal outcomes were identified for:

ACT2, foreshortened active phase duration
ACT3, prolonged active phase duration

DEC2, foreshortened deceleration phase duration (suspect only)
DEC3, prolonged deceleration phase duration
SEC2, foreshortened second stage duration
SEC3, prolonged second stage duration
MAXS2, protracted dilatation pattern
DESC2, protracted descent pattern
ARRD3, arrest of dilatation (suspect only)
ARRS3, arrest of descent

Significant protective perinatal factors included:

ACT1, normal active phase duration
DEC1, normal deceleration phase duration (suspect only)
SEC1, normal second stage duration (suspect only)
MAXS3, precipitate dilatation (suspect only)
DESC1, normal maximum slope of descent (suspect only)
ARRD1, no arrest of dilatation (suspect only)

Table 14-3
Outcomes for Cases with Protracted Dilatation[a]

Adverse Outcome	No.	Observed Rate, %	Expected Rate, %	RR	z-Statistic	p-Value
Perinatal						
Definite	1233	3.33	2.40	1.39[b]	2.125[b]	0.034
Suspect	1305	8.66	6.13	1.41[b]	3.807[b]	0.00014
Infancy						
Definite	972	2.34	2.61	0.90	-0.467	0.64
Suspect	1123	15.49	13.57	1.14	1.882	0.060
Childhood						
Definite	346	19.36	17.70	1.09	0.811	0.42
Suspect	537	48.04	46.22	1.04	0.847	0.40

a Based on 6,688 nulliparous deliveries resulting in birth of infants weighing 2500-4000 g. following labor characterized by abnormally low maximum slope of dilatation (less than 1.2 cm./hr.), code MAXS2.

b Statistically significant, p<0.05.

Table 14-4
Outcomes by Labor Progression Variables in Nulliparas*

Variable	Perinatal				Infancy				Childhood			
	Definite		Suspect		Definite		Suspect		Definite		Suspect	
	RR	p	RR	p	RR	p	RR	p	RR	p	RR	p
LAT1	0.96		0.95		0.93		1.00		1.01		0.98	
LAT2	1.11		1.10		1.31	0.092	1.06		1.02		1.09	0.047
LAT3	1.26		1.40		0.46		0.61	0.038	0.81		0.77	0.053
ACT1	0.71	0.0051	0.89	0.74	0.96		1.01		0.95		0.98	
ACT2	1.40	0.034	0.85		1.10		0.92		1.07		1.04	
ACT3	1.65	0.0012	1.58	0.000001	1.04		1.04		1.09		1.02	
DEC1	0.86		0.86	0.014	1.04		0.99		0.98		0.98	
DEC2	1.48	0.063	1.48	0.0014	1.02		0.99		1.02		1.11	
DEC3	1.43	0.051	1.41	0.0023	0.77		1.05		1.13		1.04	
SEC1	0.83	0.077	0.82	0.0020	0.99		0.96		0.95		0.96	
SEC2	1.34	0.039	1.31	0.0015	1.00		1.06		1.14		1.12	0.0036
SEC3	1.67	0.058	1.86	0.000039	1.06		1.14		1.01		0.94	
MAXS1	0.89		0.93		0.97		0.97		0.97		0.99	
MAXS2	1.39	0.034	1.41	0.00014	0.90		1.14	0.060	1.09		1.04	
MAXS3	0.95		0.70	0.032	1.25		0.91		0.99		1.00	
DESC1	0.93		0.87	0.027	0.91		0.99		1.02		0.98	
DESC2	1.85	0.00052	2.02	10^{-6}	1.46	0.075	1.21	0.029	1.16		1.03	
DESC3	0.77		0.85		1.03		0.87		0.79		1.08	
ARRD1	0.93		0.87	0.016	1.06		1.03		0.99		1.01	
ARRD3	1.28		1.54	10^{-6}	0.76		0.87	0.097	1.05		1.17	
ARRS1	0.93		0.92		0.97		1.00		0.99		1.00	
ARRS3	1.53	0.028	1.55	0.00010	1.21		0.96		1.07		1.04	

* Data for Freeman-Tukey screening analyses from midrange birthweight offspring of 6,688 nulliparas; p-values above 0.10 suppressed.

Similar adverse infancy outcomes were found in:

MAXS2, protracted dilatation pattern (suspect only)
DESC2, protracted descent pattern (suspect only)

Comparable childhood outcomes occurred in:

LAT2, foreshortened latent phase duration (suspect only)
SEC2, foreshortened second stage duration (suspect only)

Infancy protection was found only in LAT3, prolonged latent phase duration, and limited to the suspect subset.

Outcome Results Summarized
The outcome results are summarized in Table 14-6, along with those derived by the same method for multiparas. It is clear that perinatal outcomes are the most sensitive indicators of adverse results because, with few exceptions, all bad late outcome variables were already signalled by poor early outcome data. The same held true for good results as well. The reverse was seldom the case—that is, perinatal outcome data indicated several variables to be potentially harmful, even though later results were not necessarily consistent in this regard. Both parity groups showed largely similar findings, lending weight to the validity of these observations.

It is tempting to examine the results from the viewpoint of the relative quantitative impact of the labor progression variables being surveyed here. This can be done using these data in anticipation of the more sophisticated multivariate analytic techniques, bearing in mind that the screening

Table 14-5
Outcomes by Labor Progression Variables in Multiparas*

Variable	Perinatal Definite RR	Perinatal Definite p	Perinatal Suspect RR	Perinatal Suspect p	Infancy Definite RR	Infancy Definite p	Infancy Suspect RR	Infancy Suspect p	Childhood Definite RR	Childhood Definite p	Childhood Suspect RR	Childhood Suspect p
LAT1	0.75	0.0043	0.95		1.02		1.01		0.97		0.99	
LAT2	1.65	0.00048	1.13		0.95		1.12		1.10		1.05	
LAT3	1.79	0.00072	1.18		0.94		0.75		1.11		0.98	
ACT1	0.80	0.047	0.98		0.96		0.99		0.98		1.01	
ACT2	1.13		0.98		1.09		0.99		0.99		0.97	
ACT3	2.11	0.00052	1.40		0.75		1.21	0.055	1.34		1.13	
DEC1	0.81	0.023	0.95		0.97		0.97		0.94		0.98	
DEC2	1.91	0.00010	1.35	0.051	1.48	0.013	1.12		1.34	0.031	1.05	
DEC3	1.51	0.019	1.04		0.75		1.14	0.064	1.14		1.12	0.035
SEC1	0.85		0.92		0.90		0.93	0.051	0.85	0.044	0.96	
SEC2	1.08		1.02		1.11		1.07	0.069	1.13	0.066	1.03	
SEC3	2.38	0.0042	2.10	0.0026	0.64		1.06		1.06		0.96	
MAXS1	0.86		1.00		0.95		0.96		1.00		1.00	
MAXS2	1.88	2.0×10^{-5}	1.32	0.047	0.87		1.20	0.0046	1.11		1.13	0.011
MAXS3	0.89		0.93		1.25	0.058	1.02		0.95		0.93	0.089
DESC1	0.79	0.038	0.96		1.03		1.04		1.02		1.01	
DESC2	3.29	10^{-6}	2.17	10^{-6}	1.40	0.051	1.23	0.0064	1.01		0.98	
DESC3	0.75	0.043	0.77	0.015	0.86		0.88	0.0060	0.97		0.99	
ARRD1	0.93		0.98		0.98		0.99		1.01		1.00	
ARRD3	1.68	0.049	1.23		1.17		1.05		0.93		1.04	
ARRS1	0.95		0.98		1.02		1.00		1.00		1.00	
ARRS3	4.02	1.0×10^{-6}	2.44	0.0018	0.00	0.045	1.14		1.03		0.74	

* Data based on 8,481 multiparas delivered of infants weighing 2500-4000 g.; p-values above 0.10 suppressed.

method examined each variable in isolation without consideration for any possible concurrent or interactional effects from other variables with which it may have been associated. Given this constraint, we may note that the most consistent and strongest adverse relationships were disclosed in nulliparas for:

ACT3, prolonged active phase
DESC2, protracted descent

To a lesser extent, poor results followed:

ACT2, foreshortened active phase
DEC3, prolonged deceleration phase
SEC2, foreshortened second stage
SEC3, prolonged second stage
MAXS2, protracted dilatation
ARRS3, arrest of descent

In multiparas, strong relationships were found for:

LAT2, foreshortened latent phase
LAT3, prolonged latent phase
DEC2, foreshortened deceleration phase
MAXS2, protracted dilatation
DESC2, protracted descent
ARRS3, arrest of descent

Lesser associations were disclosed in multiparas for:

ACT3, prolonged active phase
DEC3, prolonged deceleration phase
SEC3, prolonged second stage
ARRD3, arrest of dilatation

In descending rank order by rate ratio for both parity series, the greatest impact was shown from:

DESC2, protracted descent
ARRS3, arrest of descent
ACT3, prolonged active phase

133

SEC3, prolonged second stage
MAXS2, protracted dilatation
DEC3, prolonged deceleration phase

Protection was less consistently or definitively encountered, but it was found in:

ACT1, normal active phase
DEC1, normal deceleration phase
SEC1, normal second stage
DESC1, normal slope of descent

This undoubtedly reflected the fact that normalcy (the absence of abnormality) in these labor variables protected against the adverse effects of the specific abnormality.

All six disorders thus identified as having strong adverse effects referred to dysfunctional labors, that is, slow or arrested progress. Rapid or precipitate patterns also resulted in adverse outcomes, especially DEC2, SEC2, LAT2, and ACT2, but the magnitude of effect appeared to be somewhat smaller and there was less homogeneity of effect across parity and outcome groupings. Intergroup consistency across parity groups was greatest in all the aforementioned seven dysfunctional patterns and the four dysfunctional subsets with minor variations in rank order only. Inconsistencies were apparent in some, either as a result of the disclosure of opposite effects— that is, protection in one parity group and deleterious result in the other—or because the significant findings in one were unsupported by comparably significant effect in the same outcome variables of the other. The former inconsistency included LAT3 and MAXS3; the latter, included all eight of the remaining labor progression variables.

Table 14-6
Significant Labor Progression Variables as Identified
by Screening Analysis[a]

Variable	Nulliparas			Multiparas		
	Perinatal	Infancy	Childhood	Perinatal	Infancy	Childhood
LAT1				0.75c		
LAT2		1.31	1.09A[b]	1.65E		
LAT3		0.61a[b]	0.77a[b]	1.79D		
ACT1	0.71c			0.80a		
ACT2	1.41A					
ACT3	1.65D			2.11C	1.21a[b]	
DEC1	0.86b[b]			0.81a		
DEC2	1.48D[b]			1.91F		1.34A
DEC3	1.43A			1.51B	1.14[b]	1.12A[b]
SEC1	0.82c[b]				0.93a[b]	0.85a
SEC2	1.34A		1.12C[b]		1.07[b]	1.13
SEC3	1.67A			2.38C		
MAXS2	1.39A	1.14[b]		1.88F	1.20C[b]	1.13B[b]
MAXS3	0.70a[b]				1.25	0.93[b]
DESC1	0.87a[b]			0.79a[b]		
DESC2	1.85E	1.21A[b]		3.29F	1.40A	
DESC3				0.75a	0.88c[b]	
ARRD1	0.87b[b]					
ARRD3	1.54F[b]			1.68C		
ARRS3	1.53A			4.02F	0.00a	

[a] Data presented in the form of relative risk; the significance coding for p-values is as follows:

    Adverse: A 0.05, B 0.01, C 0.005, D 0.001, E 0.0005, F 0.0001 or less.
    Protective: a 0.05, b 0.01, c 0.005, d 0.001, e 0.0005, f 0.0001 or less.

[b] Association is relevant for "suspect" outcome only.

Assessment by Composite Outcome Variables

It was clear that the analytical approach was thus far ineffective for demonstrating which of these factors could be discounted as relevant to outcome. Although we had derived information by this screening method showing qualitative relationships suggesting an impact, we were not as yet able to determine with precision what the relative effects were in objective quantitative terms, except of course for those variables in which clear-cut consistency existed. While it is unlikely that the latter factors were important, it was neither certain that they were all meaningful nor apparent that the others were not.

Therefore, we proceeded to introduce a composite outcome variable (see p 130) at this point in an attempt to determine the overall effect of the labor progression vari-

ables on the fetus and surviving infant. The objective here was to reduce all definitely adverse outcomes to a single marker so that every affected infant would be designated, whether the effect occurred in the perinatal period or subsequently during infancy or childhood as reflected in the results of long-term evaluations.

The bivariate screening analysis carried out using the single composite outcome variable yielded much utilitarian information about the influence of the labor progression patterns (Table 14-7). Of greatest significance was the finding of major adverse effects associated with protracted descent (DESC2) pattern in both nulliparas and multiparas. The rate ratios indicated more than ten and 13 times the rate of deleterious outcomes, respectively, highly significant observations in statistical terms. No other labor progression variable demon-

Table 14-7
Composite Variable[a] as an Index of Outcome Effect of Labor
Progression Factors

Variable	Nulliparas				Multiparas			
	Rate	RR[b]	FTD	p	Rate	RR[b]	FTD	p
LAT1	7.60	0.97	-0.62	0.54	7.96	0.94	-1.33	0.18
LAT2	8.79	1.12	1.33	0.18	9.43	1.12	1.32	0.19
LAT3	7.11	0.91	-0.40	0.69	10.28	1.22	1.96	0.050
ACT1	6.94	0.89	-2.16	0.031	7.97	0.95	-1.15	0.24
ACT2	9.44	1.21	2.13	0.033	8.91	1.06	0.99	0.32
ACT3	9.36	1.20	1.93	0.054	9.78	1.16	1.04	0.29
DEC1	7.58	0.97	-0.66	0.51	7.89	0.94	-1.58	0.11
DEC2	8.80	1.12	0.94	0.34	12.20	1.45	3.95	0.000077
DEC3	8.49	1.08	0.74	0.46	8.80	1.04	0.44	0.66
SEC1	7.37	0.94	-1.18	0.24	7.36	0.87	-2.42	0.015
SEC2	9.04	1.16	1.87	0.062	9.38	1.11	2.23	0.025
SEC3	8.02	1.02	0.13	0.89	9.13	1.08	0.37	0.71
MAXS1	7.41	0.95	-1.06	0.29	8.06	0.96	-1.01	0.31
MAXS2	8.70	1.11	1.20	0.23	9.56	1.13	1.35	0.18
MAXS3	8.66	1.11	0.89	0.37	8.91	1.06	0.72	0.47
DESC1	7.85	1.00	0.04	0.96	8.14	0.97	-0.69	0.49
DESC2	10.59	1.35	2.90	0.0037	13.21	1.57	4.84	0.0000012
DESC3	5.96	0.76	-2.44	0.014	7.62	0.90	-1.62	0.11
ARRD1	7.77	0.99	-0.18	0.86	8.29	0.98	-0.45	0.65
ARRD3	8.10	1.03	0.36	0.72	9.81	1.16	1.40	0.16
ARRS1	7.72	0.99	-0.32	0.75	8.38	0.99	-0.18	0.86
ARRS3	8.66	1.11	0.86	0.39	11.68	1.39	1.37	0.17

a   Composite variable constructed as a union of all identified adverse results of a definite nature affecting the offspring from birth to age 7 years.

b   Risk ratio relative to referent rate of 7.83% for nulliparas or 8.43% for multiparas.

135

strated a comparable influence insofar as magnitude or consistency were concerned.

Nonetheless, some surfaced as possibly important as factors affecting outcome. Excessively rapid labors—shown by patterns of foreshortened second stage (SEC2), active phase (ACT2), and deceleration phase (DEC2), and precipitate descent (DESC3)—were all more or less associated with bad outcomes, but either weakly (as with SEC2) or inconsistently (in one parity group but not in the other). The only dysfunctional pattern of comparable interest was prolonged latent phase (LAT3) which showed adverse effects in offspring of multiparas only. Protective effects, also not consistent, were identified for normal active phase (ACT1) and second stage (SEC1).

This phase of the analysis confirmed that DESC2, which headed the list of adverse factors when examined in relation to subgroups of outcome variables, remained as the strongest contender when those outcomes were collapsed into a single composite variable. Some labor progression variables were no longer shown to be meaningful (for example, DEC3, SEC3, MAXS2, ARRD3, ARRS3, and LAT2), while the effect of others was somewhat enhanced (for example, SEC2, DEC2, and DEC3). Those eight factors having been shown to be clearly associated with (but not necessarily causative of) either adverse or beneficial outcome were now subjected to more in-depth surveillance for purposes of elucidating their relative effects in quantitative terms.

Cluster Analysis

The reduced sequence of labor progression variables was studied by the aggregative hierarchical clustering technique described in chapter 7. A Pearson product-moment correlation matrix was computed to identify those variables containing very similar informational content dealing with the outcome of offspring. As previously stated, those variables found to offer much

the same information could be considered redundant. By studying just one member of such a tightly interrelated set of variables, we would in effect be studying them all. In other words, no substantive information would be lost if only one were retained for future study and, in complementary fashion, nothing would be gained by keeping the others. Logic and the economics of investigative cost and effort dictated the appropriateness of this approach.

The factors under study were the labor progression variables previously derived by bivariate screening (see above) documented to be significantly associated with adverse or beneficial outcomes (definite only). We first deleted those variables that were clearly superfluous, such as ACT1, DEC1, SEC1, and DESC1 in nulliparas and LAT1, DEC1, and SEC1, in multiparas. By contrast, it was felt inappropriate to delete ACT1 in multiparas because the rule concerning mutual exclusivity did not apply since only ACT3 (and not ACT2) was included as a significantly adverse variable for future consideration. Deletion of these redundant variables was done because it was quite clear that they merely represented the mutually exclusive residual case data counterbalancing relevant adverse variables, all of which were included among the list of variables to be studied.

Had they been left in, they would obviously have been shown to cluster tightly with their opposite member—that is, ACT1 would of necessity have clustered with ACT2 and ACT3, since it has a high negative correlation with those two variables and reflects the counterbalancing "goodness" left after the "badness" associated with the other two variables had been accounted for. Leaving these superfluous variables in place would not only have unnecessarily increased the complexity of the cluster analysis but, more importantly, it might have prevented other, more subtle interrelationships from being disclosed. The final list of variables that were to be studied, therefore, totaled nine for nulliparas and 13 for multiparas.

This aspect of the study proceeded by attempting to quantify the similarity between pairs of variables. Once such similarity is known, the variables can be aggregated into subgroups according to their similarity. The similarity between a pair of variables is defined as the absolute value of their product-moment correlation. The aggregative hierarchical clustering method yielded the desired series or heirarchy of different clusterings of the variables under study. They begin with trivial clusterings and proceed in stepwise fashion to merge pairs of clusters successively (again on the basis of similarities between the larger subgroupings) until all variables have been merged. The result of this process can be represented graphically in the form of a tree, each twig representing an individual variable and each branching point representing the junction of pairs of clusters into larger clusters of variables.

Cluster Results

The results of this analytic operation are shown in Figures 14-1 and 14-2. The output tree is depicted with its root or main trunk on the right and the branches on the left. The clustering process moves from left to right on the page. The horizontal scale in the tree diagram is important. The position of each branching or junction point on the page is proportional to the value of the mean intercluster similarity of the two subclusters joined at that point. The further the junction is from the right margin of the tree, the greater the value of the mean intercluster similarity and the higher and more significant the correlation coefficient. The position, therefore, offers a measure of the compactness or relative intensity of the similarity of the cluster.

The cluster analysis for nulliparas (Figure 14-1) showed little compactness. The correlation coefficients (r) between vari-

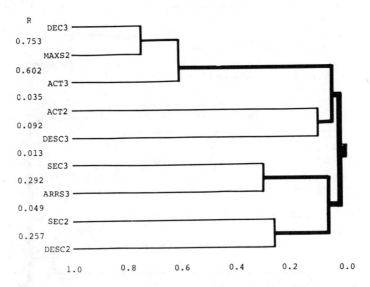

Figure 14-1. Cluster analysis of labor progression variables in nulliparas showing clustering of variables with the greatest intercluster similarity. Horizontal location of the branch junction is proportional to the degree of intercluster similarity of the subclusters joining at that point. The strongly compact cluster of DEC3 with MAXS2 (and somewhat less with ACT3) demonstrates that they contain similar information pertaining to outcome. Horizontal axis is correlation of coefficient (R) between variables and subclusters.

137

ables were uniformly low except for the cluster of DEC3 with MAXS2 ($r = .753$) and to a lesser extent, the subcluster of these two variables with ACT3 ($r = .602$). No other interrelationship even approached these levels of significance. This can be interpreted to mean that the degree of similarity between all but the three variables mentioned was so small that each contained information about outcome which warranted retaining them as potentially important variables for future study in greater depth. As to the significantly clustered items, it was intuitively apparent that they represented comparable kinds of labor progression problems, namely protracted dilatation, prolonged deceleration, and prolonged active phase. Indeed, it is probably that they frequently occurred in the very same cases and, therefore, the adverse

outcomes they reflected were perhaps those of the same infants.

Given the strong correlation between DEC3 and MAXS2 in both cluster analysis and clinical observation, it was felt quite acceptable to delete one. Accordingly, MAXS2 was retained as representative of this two-variable cluster and DEC3 was suppressed. Whereas we might have done likewise with ACT3, it was nonetheless retained because the statistical correlation was a bit weaker (although the clinical correlation was felt to be stronger). Moreover, we felt it preferable here to err on the side of conservatism rather than to risk losing data of possible relevance to the overall study.

For multiparas, the 13 preselected labor progression variables yielded a cluster (Figure 14-2) that was almost identical to that

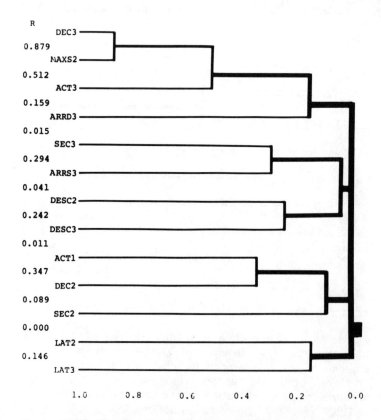

Figure 14-2. Results of cluster analysis of labor progression variables in multiparas, showing findings comparable to those disclosed in nulliparas (compare Figure 14-1).

138

obtained for nulliparas. The index of similarity between DEC3 and MAXS2 was even greater ($r = .879$), but it was smaller when clustered with ACT3 ($r = .512$). This supported the validity of deleting DEC3 and retaining ACT3 as had been done with the nulliparas. Again, there were no other significant subclusters, indicating the need to retain all the designated variables as possible or even probable risk factors.

The cluster analyses thus reduced our list of labor progression variables to eight and 12 for nulliparas and multiparas, respectively, Whereas it did not greatly reduce the effort that will be required for the multivariate analysis to follow, it did point out one or possibly two redundancies in each parity group. It also showed quite a strong degree of consistency between the parity groups. In addition, it suggested that each of the variables under study was acting independently of the others or, if they themselves were not responsible for the deleterious result, they were reflecting diverse intermediary or associated factors. Their relevance to the primary goal of this investigation was thereby confirmed.

Logistic Regression Analysis

As discussed in chapter 7, logistic regression analysis was preferred over linear discriminant function because it circumvented problems related to the validity of inferences about the multivariate indicators. It will be recalled that linear discriminant function requires the data for each category of the outcome variable to be distributed normally, that is, to show relatively uniform and symmetrical gaussian distributions. This must apply to both normal and abnormal outcomes. It should be obvious that at least one outcome does not fulfill this basic requirement, namely Apgar scores. They have a markedly skewed distribution concentrated almost exclusively near the upper end of the scale range, falling into a more typical Poisson distribution. Examination of our outcome data in this regard showed positive zero-order correla-

tion coefficients, confirming objectively what had been felt likely on an intuitive basis, namely that linear discriminant function was not optimally applicable here and, if applied, would risk producing analytic results which might be either specious or difficult to interpret.[*]

Logistic regression analysis, by contrast, offered no such constraints and was felt to be appropriate for our needs. Its only real drawback was the great intensity of computation time and expense it required. The burdens it imposed increased geometrically with the number of variables that were to be studied. Logistic regression analysis offered a means for estimating the effects of each indicator variable while simultaneously controlling for the effects of all others in the composite model. This estimate of effect, controlled for all other risk factors, represented the relative risk. The odds ratio was used to estimate the relative risk, especially for situations in which the rate of adverse effect was small, as it was in most of the outcomes currently under investigation. The odds ratio for any given variable was derived from the logistic regression coefficient.

The logistic regression program was first invoked to examine all labor progression variables simultaneously. Subsequently, a step-up analysis was to be undertaken. The latter was an iterative logistic regression process begun with the core or base model of only significant variables. Those variables not previously found to be significant in the first analysis were then to be added back seriatim to verify whether or not they might prove significant in the absence of the other nonsignificant variables. The aim here was to identify all variables of possibly significant relevance by ensuring that marginal items or highly intercorrelated variables would not be missed. Recall that we had taken care not to miss the highly intercorrelated variables because we had identified them in the aforementioned cluster

---

[*]Moore DH: Evaluation of five discriminating procedures for binary variables. *J Am Stat Assoc* 1973; 68:342.

analysis.

Logistic Regression Results

The results of the primary logistic regression analyses are shown in Tables 14-8 and 14-9 for nulliparas and multiparas, respectively. The relative impact of each of the variables was studied as it applied to the composite outcome variables—that is, definite adverse outcome, as opposed to definite plus "suspect," in one or more of the series of perinatal outcomes or tests of neurologic and developmental status. As stated, the estimate of relative risk was derived from the logistic regression coefficient; its statistical significance was defined by the

Table 14-8
Logistic Regression Analysis of Labor Progression Variables
in Nulliparas for Composite Outcome

Variable	Regression Coefficient	Standard Error	Ratio[a]	Relative Risk	p–Value
Constant	-2.599	0.072	-36.12		
ACT2	0.322	0.118	2.74	1.38[b]	0.0085
ACT3	0.309	0.150	2.06	1.36[b]	0.044
SEC2	0.146	0.108	1.36	1.16	
SEC3	-0.002	0.208	-0.01	1.00	
MAXS2	-0.077	0.139	-0.56	0.93	
DESC2	0.194	0.140	1.39	1.21	
DESC3	-0.329	0.133	-2.47	0.72[b]	0.017
ARRS3	0.106	0.147	0.72	1.11	

[a] Relation of regression coefficient to standard error, based on data for 6,688 nulliparas. This represents an index of t-statistic or z-score from which to derive the p-value for probability of chance occurrence.

[b] Statistically significant, $p < 0.05$.

Table 14-9
Logistic Regression Analysis of Labor Progression Variables in Multiparas
for Composite Outcome

Variable	Regression Coefficient	Standard Error	Ratio[a]	Relative Risk	p–Value
Constant	-2.577	0.097	-26.58		
LAT2	0.075	0.110	0.68	1.08	
LAT3	0.196	0.124	1.58	1.22	
ACT1	0.002	0.092	-0.02	1.00	
ACT3	0.172	0.209	0.82	1.19	
DEC2	0.290	0.139	2.09	1.34[b]	0.042
SEC2	0.193	0.082	2.34	1.21[b]	0.023
SEC3	0.084	0.263	0.32	1.09	
MAXS2	-0.093	0.139	-0.67	0.91	
DESC2	0.351	0.134	2.62	1.42[b]	0.012
DESC3	-0.088	0.088	-1.00	0.92	
ARRD3	0.625	0.133	0.47	1.06	
ARRS3	0.259	0.292	0.89	1.30	

[a] Relation of regression coefficient to standard error, based on data for 8,481 multiparas.

[b] Statistically significant, $p < 0.05$.

relationship of the regression coefficient to its standard error. Labor progression factors determined to be most significant under this form of close surveillance were:

ACT2, foreshortened active phase
ACT3, prolonged active phase
DESC3, precipitate descent (protective)

For multiparas, the list included:

DEC2, foreshortened deceleration phase
SEC2, foreshortened second stage
DESC2, protracted descent

The analysis was also applied to the examination of the same series of labor progression variables as related to perinatal outcome or severe depression. This was done to recheck that no variable might be lost as a consequence of the use of the composite outcome variable. The results are detailed in Tables 14-10 and 14-11. From these, we learned that the same adverse effects still accrued to ACT2 and ACT3 in nulliparas, but the ostensibly protective effects of DESC3 were no longer present. Rather unexpected findings developed in the data from multiparas. Only DESC2 (protracted descent) retained its primacy as

an index of bad outcome and actually demonstrated an even stronger impact. Neither DESC2 nor SEC2 were significant any longer, whereas LAT2 and LAT3 achieved statistical significance now even though they had not done so before.

Step-Up Analysis

A step-up form of logistic regression analysis was also undertaken to provide additional elucidation. The most critical labor progression variables were examined as a block. They consisted of the aforementioned eight variables identified for nulliparas (ACT2, ACT3, SEC2, SEC3, MAXS2, DESC2, DESC3, and ARRS3) and 12 for multiparas (the same as those for nulliparas without ACT2, but with the addition of LAT2, LAT3, ACT1, DEC2, and ARRD3).

The preliminary or initial model for the composite outcome variables in nulliparas was preselected to include only those three labor progression variables yielding the greatest collective significance as determined by the logistic regression process (namely ACT2, ACT3, and DESC3). When these were examined in isolation, the logistic regression analysis yielded regression coefficients and standard errors as before to provide relevant rate ratios for quantitation of effects and t values as indices of statistical

Table 14-10
Logistic Regression Analysis of Labor Progression Variables in Nulliparas for Perinatal Outcome

Variable	Regression Coefficient	Standard Error	Ratio[a]	Relative Risk	p-Value
Constant	-4.197	0.145	-28.86		
ACT2	0.652	0.212	3.08	1.92[b]	0.0034
ACT3	0.752	0.257	2.92	2.12[b]	0.0052
SEC2	0.334	0.195	1.71	1.40	0.088
SEC3	0.471	0.325	1.45	1.60	
MAXS2	-0.071	0.240	-0.30	0.93	
DESC2	0.377	0.238	1.59	1.46	
DESC3	-0.240	0.242	-0.99	0.79	
ARRS3	0.347	0.247	1.40	1.41	

[a] Relation of regression coefficient to standard error, based on data for 6,086 nulliparas.

[b] Statistically significant, $p < 0.05$.

141

significance. These are shown in Table 14-12.

The results of this analysis differed from the earlier logistic regression for the same data (compare Table 14-8) because all the preliminarily screened variables had been included before, but only those of documented significance were to be considered at this point. It will be noted that the apparent impact of ACT2 was greater than previously observed both in magnitude (RR increased from 1.38 to 1.44) and statistical confidence (p value fell from .0085 to .0025). The protective effect of DESC3 increased comparably (RR 0.72 to 0.69 and p .017 to .0071). The influence of ACT3 remained the same (RR 1.36).

All the remaining variables were surveyed by testing all combinations of four-variable models to ascertain if any retained significance under these circumstances. Only DESC2 and SEC2 surfaced as possible candidates for inclusion in such a step-up model (at probability levels of .074 and .091, respectively). To determine the impact of including them, the variable DESC2 was added first because its associated p-value was smaller. Logistic regression analysis of this first step-up model produced the data shown in Table 14-12. Adding this fourth variable changed the relative associations to a limited extent, but the previously encoun-

Table 14-11
Logistic Regression Analysis of Labor Progression Variables in Multiparas for Perinatal Outcome

Variable	Regression Coefficient	Standard Error	Ratio[a]	Relative Risk	p–Value
Constant	-4.137	0.197	-21.01		
LAT2	0.487	0.198	2.43	1.62[b]	0.019
LAT3	0.692	0.216	3.10	2.00[b]	0.0024
ACT1	-0.205	0.187	-1.10	0.81	
ACT3	0.281	0.330	0.85	1.32	
DEC2	0.023	0.267	0.08	1.02	
SEC2	-0.050	0.169	-0.30	0.95	
SEC3	0.399	0.399	1.00	1.49	
MAXS2	0.119	0.231	0.52	1.13	
DESC2	0.934	0.391	2.39	2.55[b]	0.021
DESC3	0.099	0.233	0.42	1.10	
ARRD3	-0.0014	0.188	-0.01	1.00	
ARRS3	1.208	0.221	5.48	3.35[b]	1.4×10^{-6}

[a] Relation of regression coefficient to standard error, based on data for 7,847 multiparas.

[b] Statistically significant, p<0.05.

Table 14-12
Step-Up Logistic Regression Modeling of Labor Progression Variables for Composite Outcome in Nulliparas

Variable	Initial Model			Step-Up Model		
	RR	t	p	RR	t	p
ACT2	1.44	3.18	0.0025	1.38	2.74	0.0085
ACT3	1.36	2.64	0.011	1.33	2.38	0.021
DESC3	0.69	-2.18	0.0071	0.72	-2.44	0.018
DESC2				1.27	1.82	0.072

tered qualitative relationships remained essentially the same. A further survey of all remaining variables failed to disclose any that even approached statistical significance (even at the 10% probability level) in terms of its possible relationship to the composite outcome. Therefore, no significant models remained to be evaluated. It was clear from this that the four labor progression variables thus identified carried the brunt of the effect of the outcome in this subpopulation.

Similar step-up logistic regression modeling was done in multiparas for the composite outcome variable. Once again, the three significant variables disclosed by the original logistic regression assessment of all prescreened variables (see Table 14-9) were incorporated into the initial model. These included DEC2, SEC2, and DESC2. The analysis revealed some enhancement of the effect of DESC2 on outcome (RR increased from 1.42 to 1.53, p fell from .012 to .0012), but diminished the relationship for DEC2 (RR 1.34 to 1.31, p .043 to .034); SEC2 remained about the same (RR 1.21 to 1.20, p .023 to .028). In this instance, all the tests of each of the remaining variables as possible candidates for inclusion in a four-factor model yielded none capable of achieving statistical significance. Thus, no step-up model was feasible. The three variables thus identified provided all the information available on the relationship to composite outcome.

Perinatal outcome, having previously been shown to be somewhat more sensitive than the composite variable as an indicator of adverse effect, was also utilized as an outcome variable in this form of step-up logistic regression analysis. For nulliparas, three labor progression variables were flagged as having significant associations with this outcome at the outset to form the initial model. These variables included two that had previously been identified by logistic regression (see Table 14-10), namely ACT2 and ACT3, plus one other (SEC2) that had failed to reach a level of statistical significance earlier (Table 14-13). This preliminary procedure of designating the initial model components had effectively enhanced the relative impact of one variable (ACT3, RR 2.12 to 2.31, p .0052 to .00014) and the significance of another (SEC2, RR 1.40 to 1.41, p .093 to .058), leaving the third essentially unchanged (ACT2, RR 1.92 to 1.91, p .0034 to .0026).

Testing for four-factor models revealed three possible contenders for inclusion, namely DESC2 (p = .032), SEC3 (p = .034), and ARRS3 (p = .041). DESC2 was added to the original initial model first because it was associated with the smallest p value. As shown in Table 14-13, the newly formed model altered the relative impacts of the prior variables somewhat. As expected, the newly added variable DESC2 was significantly related to adverse perinatal outcome (RR = 1.65, p = .030). The relative effects of all others, however, were correspondingly reduced; the reduction actually caused the variable SEC2 to become nonsignificant in regard to its relation to outcome (RR = 1.26, p = .24).

Table 14-13
Step-Up Logistic Regression Modeling of Labor Progression Variables for Perinatal Outcome in Nulliparas

Variable	Initial Model			Step-Up Model 1			Step-Up Model 2		
	RR	t	p	RR	t	p	RR	t	p
ACT2	1.91	3.17	0.0026	1.77	2.74	0.0085	1.83	2.87	0.0060
ACT3	2.31	4.13	0.00014	2.20	3.86	0.00033	2.15	3.75	0.00046
SEC2	1.41	1.94	0.058	1.26	1.20	0.24	1.36	1.58	0.12
DESC2				1.65	2.23	0.030	1.55	1.93	0.056
SEC3							1.84	1.97	0.050

Further testing for five-factor models showed both SEC3 (p = .066) and ARRS3 (p = .068) still within range. An expanded step-up model with the addition of SEC3 (Table 14-13) showed that this new factor did have a significant relationship to perinatal outcome (RR = 1.84, p = .050). The other four variables remained more or less consistent in terms of magnitude of effect and significance. Additional testing of six-factor models yielded no residual effects even for ARRS3, which had previously surfaced as potentially relevant. Thus, no other significant models were disclosed and no other variables achieved significance.

For multiparas (Table 14-14), the perinatal outcome variable yielded an initial base model for logistic regression analysis containing four variables: LAT2, LAT3, ARRS3, and DESC2. All had increased their levels of effect, most especially ARRS3 (RR 2.55 to 3.33, p .021 to .00082) and DESC2 (RR 3.35 to 3.66, p 1.4×10^{-6} to 1.9×10^{-9}).

Survey of five-factor models showed ACT3 (p = .074) and ACT1 (p = .096) as possible entrants for consideration at the next step up. The addition of ACT3 (Table 14-14) showed that this variable fell somewhat short of statistical significance at the 5% level (RR = 1.62, p = .064). Inclusion of this fifth factor did not meaningfully alter the standings of three of the other factors insofar as magnitude or significance of effect was concerned. Only ARRS3 was softened in its relation to perinatal outcome (RR 3.33 to 2.88, p .00082 to .0038), although its effect remained quite strong

with relative impact second in magnitude only to DESC2.

Testing of six-factor models did not disclose any other labor progression variable that might contribute in any noteworthy way. None of the remaining variables approached statistical significance even at the 10% probability level, including ACT1 which had previously surfaced as a potentially protective candidate for inclusion in the model.

Summary of Risk Variables for Labor Progression

A summary of the findings from the several logistic regression analyses is presented in Table 14-15, indicating the significant variables and their levels of significance stratified by parity. This listing indicates those labor progression variables determined to be verifiably related to adverse outcomes for fetus and infant. They have been studied collectively in relation to one another by this foregoing set of analyses. They have thus been clearly identified as relevant to outcome when all other labor progression variables were considered simultaneously.

Having come this far, we have concluded the first major phase of the investigative program dealing with the task of defining labor progression, reducing that progression to quantifiable terms, designating cut points for defining abnormalities, and determining the relative impact of those defined disorders in isolation and in relation

Table 14-14
Step-Up Logistic Regression Modeling of Labor Progression Variables for Perinatal Outcome in Multiparas

Variable	Initial Model			Step-Up Model		
	RR	t	p	RR	t	p
LAT2	1.73	2.90	0.0055	1.66	2.68	0.0099
LAT3	2.08	3.47	0.0011	2.06	3.43	0.0012
ARRS3	3.33	3.56	0.00082	2.88	3.04	0.0038
DESC2	3.66	7.32	1.9×10^{-9}	3.64	7.28	3.5×10^{-9}
ACT3				1.62	1.87	0.064

Table 14-15
Summary of Significant Labor Progression Variables by Logistic Regression*

Variable	Full Model				Initial Model				Step-Up Model			
	Composite		Perinatal		Composite		Perinatal		Composite		Perinatal	
	N	M	N	M	N	M	N	M	N	M	N	M
LAT2				B				C				B
LAT3				C				D				D
ACT2	B		E		C		C		B		C	
ACT3	A		E		B		F		A		E	A
DEC2		A				A						
SEC2		A				A		A				
SEC3									A			
DESC2		B		F		D		F		A		F
DESC3	a				b				a			
ARRS3			A				D				C	

* Significance code: A 0.05, B 0.01, C 0.005, D 0.001, E 0.0005, F 0.0001 or less. Lower case code for protective effects.

N nulliparas, M multiparas.

to each other. Similar studies will now be undertaken to do the same for adjunctive drugs in labor, for intrinsic obstetric factors, and for delivery-related events. After the relevant constellation of significant variables has been defined and studied for each of these subsequent phases, we will be in a position to reassess the entire series which will then comprise four sets of variables determined to be significant on the basis of the results of four parallel series of investigations such as the one just described. The final assessment (see chapter 25) will repeat the sequence of statistical analyses for purposes of examining each of the flagged variables for its impact on offspring while all others are being simultaneously considered.

145

CHAPTER 15

Adjunctive Pharmacologic Agents

Summary

Drugs and anesthetics administered to parturients were studied extensively to ascertain the spectrum of usage, route, dosage levels, and schedules, and when in labor they were given. In all, 168 specific agents and anesthetics were identified for study. Those invoked most frequently could be examined according to drug dosage regimen and the time in labor they were ordered. Conduction anesthetic techniques were stratified by the local anesthetic drug used to achieve the block; inhalation and intravenous anesthetics were likewise divided by agent. A valuable data resource was thus produced.

The second group of variables pertinent to these investigations was the array of drugs administered to the parturient. These encompassed a large number of agents given for a variety of purposes, including, most commonly, sedatives, tranquilizers, analgesics, anesthetics, belladonna alkaloids, and uterotonic agents for induction or stimulation of labor; less often, various other drugs were given, including antibiotics, diuretics, magnesium sulfate, cardiotropic drugs, and numerous others. Our purpose, of course, was to identify any effects these drugs might have on the fetus and infant within the context of this series of analyses. We sought to study the possible effects of the pharmacologic agents used in and around labor by examining outcomes for the offspring of women grouped according to whether or not they had beengiven a drug, ultimately taking into account other associated risk factors that may have been acting simultaneously.

Survey of Labor Drug Usage

The NCPP data bank was first surveyed in depth to determine drug usage. This was intended to provide information on the kinds of agents actually administered to Project patients and the frequency of their administration. Further, we felt it worthwhile to ascertain the distribution of drug dosages individually and in broad generic categories. Such details were expected to help assess the feasibility of pursuing a meaningful analysis of this material. If it were learned, for example, that a given agent was actually seldom utilized in labor, pursuing an analysis of its effects on outcome could be expected to yield little by way of useful data, unless of course the impact was of major magnitude.

In addition to general interest in the kind of drugs given to laboring gravidas and how often they were given, we felt it important to specify when in the course of labor they had been administered. This latter aspect of study had relevance insofar as possible intercalary effects on the labor itself were concerned. That is to say, if adverse fetal or infant effects were found to be associated with an agent, knowledge about the interposed effect of that agent on the labor process, perhaps manifested by the development of a noxious labor disorder, would offer insights into the mechanism by which that effect was produced.

Moreover, information about the timing of drug administration, particularly with reference to the duration prior to delivery, might help address issues of direct drug-mediated effects. We appreciated, for instance, the time-related depressive effects of narcotic analgesics on the newborn infant. Their greatest negative impact was expected to be encountered if birth occurred in the time interval when the drug levels were at their maximum in mother and fetus. It seemed obvious, therefore, that the time of administration of drugs

with reference to delivery could offer potentially useful information for our purposes.

Finally and perhaps most relevant, we desired data on dosage and route of administration. Lacking blood drug levels, we felt such data would prove an acceptable substitute, particularly since one of our prime objectives was to evaluate obstetrical practices as actually carried out in the clinical field. Drug levels would, of course, have afforded us greater precision here, but they could only have served as indirect indicators of the impact of specific drug-use practices.

This consideration applied especially to anesthetic agents. The local anesthetic drugs, for example, were known to have markedly different effects according to the route, site, and technique of administration, with drug dosage contributing in only a relatively minor way. A specific dose of lidocaine given locally into the perineum for episiotomy, for example, has a far different maternal effect (and perhaps fetal effect as well) from that of the same or smaller dose given intrathecally for spinal anesthesia.

Insofar as these several considerations were concerned (type of drug, dosage regimen, route of administration, and timing in regard to the labor process), we recognized that stratification of our case material into large numbers of finely detailed subsets would probably yield very few data cells containing a sample size sufficient for valid analysis. In order to satisfy our aims, therefore, it was a foregone conclusion that we would have to introduce methodologic compromises. The most obvious of these was that stratification along several dimensions simultaneously was not likely to be feasible, expect perhaps for those agents or classes of drugs that had been given most frequently.

Combining Data Sources

A major preliminary problem confronting us in our attempt to compile a comprehensive data file on drug utilization among NCPP patients was the need to combine dissimilar data derived from multiple sources. The main source of drug information was the ADM-51 form (Labor and Delivery Drugs), which contained entries pertaining to all agents given during the course of labor and at the time of delivery. This form provided extensive codified information on every agent received by a patient along with the date and time it was given, the dosage, and the route. For intravenous (IV) infusions, the time discontinued was also noted. Drugs were identified by a four-digit code encompassing 1330 individually identified generic and proprietary products.

In addition, form OB-57 (Anesthetic Agents) provided similar information on gaseous, IV, and conduction anesthetic agents, along with the time started and stopped (the latter where relevant), dosages, routes, depth or level of anesthesia attained before the cord was clamped, and any resulting patient reactions or complications. Codes for anesthesia encompassed 36 agents in all.

For uterotonic agents, additional information was provided on forms OB-34 (Obstetrician's Summary of Labor and Delivery) and OB-55 (Delivery Report). These files detailed the use of oxytocin or other uterine-stimulating agents, whether used for induction or augmentation, when it was given in the course of labor (by actually phase of dilatation pattern), method and dosage, as well as indication and reaction, if any.

Much effort was expended in compiling a utilitarian data resource encompassing use of the full gamut of pharmacologic agents in labor. The extensive experience of the Boston University Drug Epidemiology Unit had been brought to bear earlier for evolving an updated and edited computer tape summary of drug exposure during pregnancy for all NCPP gravidas.* The primary thrust of that program was determining the

effects of early pregnancy exposures on the fetus. Codification of agents under that program required reorganization of the drug data so as to identify each compound by generic components. Standard nomenclature was assigned and all agents were then classified appropriately according to pharmacologic conventions, drug indications, and frequency of usage.

We had the advantage of this foregoing classification system and the wisdom of its creators. However, we did not have a complete and uniformly coded data tape on drugs given in labor comparable to the tape that the Drug Epidemiology Unit had produced for drugs in pregnancy (their material based on data from form OB-15, Drugs in Pregnancy). For reference purposes, the main groupings of their classification are presented here (Table 15-1).

Survey Results

Our first task, after assembling the available drug information from the several sources described above, was to reproduce an analogous listing for labor drugs given to NCPP parturients and then to embellish that enumeration of drug usage by expanding the data according to dosage patterns. Because the latter would perforce require substantive numbers of cases to be meaningful, we limited our attention to those groups of drugs which had been administered relatively often in labor. Indeed, we determined that while the number of agents given during the course of labor was moderately large, totaling 123 in all, most of them had been invoked in a negligible number of patients (less than 20). Exclusive of anesthetic agents which will be dealt with separately (see below), this left only those 37 specifically designated drugs shown in Table 15-2 for our investigative analytical purposes.

Among general categories of pharmacologic agents, sedatives and tranquilizers led the list in order of frequency with 6317 cases exposed. Analgesics and antipyretics followed with 4946, mostly in the narcotic

---

*Heinonen OP, Slone D, Shapiro S: *Birth Defects and Drugs in Pregnancy.* Littleton, Mass, Publishing Sciences Group, 1977.

Table 15-1
Drug Exposure in NCPP Pregnancies*

Group	Agent	No.	%
Analgesics and antipyretics		33,841	67.30
	Non-addicting	32,856	65.34
	Narcotic analgesics	6,754	13.41
Antimicrobial and antiparasitic		17,538	34.88
	Antibiotics	9,560	19.01
	Sulfonamides	5,689	11.31
	Systemic antimicrobials	3,185	6.33
	Topical antimicrobials	4,792	9.53
Immunizing agents		22,707	45.16
Antinauseants, antihistamines, and phenothiazines		14,641	29.12
	Antihistamines and antinauseants	12,678	25.21
	Phenothiazines	3,675	7.31
Sedatives, tranqilizers, and antidepressants		14,278	28.40
	Barbiturates	12,639	25.14
	Tranquilizers and nonbarbiturate sedatives	3,231	6.43
	Antidepressants	152	0.30
Autonomic nervous system drugs		12,502	24.86
	Sympathomimetic	9,719	19.33
	Parasympatholytic	5,623	11.18
	Parasympathomimetic	44	0.09
Anesthetics, anticonvulsants, etc.		6,990	13.90
	Local anesthetics	5,703	11.34
	General anesthetics and oxygen	492	0.98
	Anticonvulsants (nonbarbiturate)	425	0.85
	CNS stimulants	228	0.45
	Muscle relaxants	266	0.53
	Smooth muscle stimulants	196	0.39
Caffeine and other xanthines		13,509	26.87
Diuretics and cardiovascular drugs		15,887	31.60
	Diuretics	15,671	31.17
	Antihypertensives	525	1.04
	Vasodilators	129	0.26
	Digitalis glycosides	129	0.26
Cough medicines		7,941	15.79
	Expectorants	6,277	12.48
	Antitussives	867	1.72
Gastrointestinal agents		806	1.60
Hormones		3,506	6.97
	Progestational	1,399	2.78
	Estrogenic	761	1.51
	Thyroid	825	1.64
	Corticosteroids	275	0.55
	Antidiabetic	234	0.47
	Other	1,246	2.48
Inorganic compounds		10,116	20.12

* From Heinonen, O.P. et al.: Birth Defects and Drugs in Pregnancy. Littleton, Massachusetts: Publishing Sciences Group, 1977.

subcategory. Anesthetics (3417), uterotonic agents (3216), and drugs affecting the
autonomic nervous system (2781) trailed,
but they were still far ahead of the much
less often used antimicrobials, diuretics, and
cardiovascular drugs. The most frequently
administered single agent was meperidine
(Demerol), which was recorded as having
been given to 3589 women in labor or
9.38% of the index population. Only hyoscine (scopolamine), synthetic oxytocin
(Syntocinon), and promazine (Sparine)

even approached it in the number of times
administered (2402, 2335, and 2129 cases,
respectively). Nearly all other agents were
encountered in much smaller numbers,
except secobarbital (1408), promethazine
(Phenergan, 1174), and alphaprodine
(Nisentil, 1015).

Temporal Considerations

The common usage of meperidine gave
us the opportunity to stratify the data per-

Table 15-2
Pharmacological Agents Administered in Labor[a]

Group	Agent	No.	%
Analgesics and antipyretics		4,946	12.92
Nonaddicting analgesics		40	0.10
	Aspirin	23	0.06
	All others	17	0.04
Narcotic analgesics		4,906	12.82
	Meperidine	3,589	9.38
	Alphaprodine	1,015	2.65
	Phenazocine	132	0.34
	Lorfan	74	0.19
	Morphine sulfate	71	0.19
	All others	25	0.07
Antimicrobials		325	0.85
	Achromycin	112	0.29
	Penicillin	98	0.26
	Streptomycin	53	0.14
	Chloramphenicol	25	0.07
	Gantrisin	20	0.05
	All others	17	0.04
Sedatives and tranquilizers		6,317	16.51
	Barbiturates	2,198	5.74
	Secobarbital	1,408	3.68
	Pentobarbital	530	1.38
	Phenobarbital	246	0.64
	All others	14	0.04
Tranquilizers		4,119	10.76
	Promazine	2,129	5.56
	Promethazine	1,174	3.07
	Hydroxyzine pamoate	294	0.77
	Propiomazine	215	0.56
	Triflupromazine	180	0.47
	Perphenazine	28	0.07
	Mepromazine	28	0.07
	Prochlorperazine	21	0.05
	All others	50	0.13
Autonomic nervous system drugs		2,781	7.27
	Hyoscine	2,402	6.28
	Atropine	324	0.85
	Ephedrine	28	0.07
	All others	27	0.07
Anesthetics			
	Gaseous	1,813	4.74
	Intravenous	29	0.08
	Conduction	3,417	8.93

150

Diuretics and cardiovascular agents	254	0.66
Reserpine	57	0.15
Apresoline	42	0.11
Methoxamine	32	0.08
Hydrochlorothiazide	30	0.08
Acetazolamide	30	0.08
Chlorothiazide	19	0.05
All others	44	0.11
Uterotonic agents	3,216	8.40
Syntocinon	2,335	6.10
Oxytocin	539	1.41
Sparteine	99	0.26
All others	9	0.02
Miscellaneous agents	792	2.07
Magnesium sulfate	262	0.68
Vitamin K	318	0.83
Deladumone	46	0.12
All others	166	0.43
Total parturients given drugs	18,651[b]	48.74

[a] All agents administered to 20 patients or more are listed by generic name.

[b] Because more than one drug may have been given to a patient, the number of patients is necessarily smaller than the total number of drugs administered as represented by the column total.

taining to this agent not only by dosage but also by patterns of administration in terms of five definable time periods relating to labor and delivery: (1) those in which the drug was given at or before the onset of labor, (2) those given the drug during the latent phase, (3) during the active phase, (4) in the second stage, and (5) for completeness, just at or after the delivery.

Enumeration of drug dosage and administration time in labor yielded a matrix of data such as shown in Table 15-3. Among the 3589 patients to whom it was given, most received it in the active phase of the first stage (68.7%); an additional 25.4% were given it during the latent phase. Meperidine was administered to a small proportion at or before labor (3.7%) and to even fewer in the second stage (2.0%). Administered doses per patient ranged from 5 to 200 mg, with clusters expectedly found at 25, 50, 75 and 100 mg. As can be seen, the 50-mg dosage was most popular (57.59%), concentrated especially in the active phase (40.26% of the entire drug use experience with meperidine and 69.91% of this dosage level usage).

Comparable distributions of doses and timing were evolved for each of the other

drugs and the general classes of drugs as aforementioned. Table 15-4 displays the relative distributions over the course of labor of those agents that had been given in reasonable numbers (that is, to at least 100 gravidas). As expected, all narcotic analgesics showed consistent concentration in the active phase, as shown above for meperidine. Tranquilizers, which were commonly used in conjunction with narcotic analgesics to potentiate their pain-relieving effects, were similarly distributed, as were both atropine and hyoscine. Barbiturates in labor were given somewhat more equally in latent and active phases, although most of the phenobarbital appeared to have been given at or before the onset of labor. Uterotonic agents were about evenly divided between onset, latent phase and active phase time groups.

In general, drugs were seldom used in the second stage. Relative to the total use of any drug, the only apparent exceptions were atropine, Syntocinon, magnesium sulfate, and phenazocine (Prinadol). However, among them, only Syntocinon was actually given in second stage to sizable numbers of patients (147 in all). Even meperidine was used only in 72, and hyoscine and proma-

Table 15-3
Meperidine Administration by Dose and Time in Labor

Dosage, mg.	At or before onset	Latent phase	Active phase	Second stage	Post partum	Total
< 25	0	1	8	0	0	9
25–49	9	89	320	23	3	444
50–74	53	527	1,445	37	5	2,067
75–99	24	128	339	4	0	495
100–149	45	167	351	6	1	570
150+	0	1	3	0	0	4
Total	131	913	2,466	70	9	3,589

Table 15-4
Distribution of Principal Pharmacological Agents*
Administered in the Course of Labor

Agent	No.	At or before onset %	Latent phase %	Active phase %	Second phase %
Analgesics					
Meperidine	3,589	3.7(0.7)	25.4(4.9)	68.7(13.2)	2.0(0.4)
Alphaprodine	1,015	0.8(0.0)	25.0(1.4)	71.6(3.9)	2.5(0.1)
Phenazocine	132	0.0(0.0)	33.3(0.2)	62.1(0.4)	4.6(0.0)
Barbiturates					
Secobarbital	1,408	18.9(1.4)	43.2(3.3)	37.3(2.8)	0.6(0.1)
Pentobarbital	530	10.9(0.3)	39.3(1.1)	49.3(1.4)	0.6(0.0)
Phenobarbital	246	66.3(0.9)	13.4(0.2)	18.7(0.3)	1.2(0.0)
Tranquilizers					
Promazine	2,129	3.8(0.4)	31.5(3.6)	61.2(7.0)	3.3(0.4)
Promethazine	1,174	2.5(0.2)	28.9(1.8)	66.9(4.2)	1.4(0.1)
Hydroxyzine	294	5.1(0.1)	31.3(0.5)	62.6(6.0)	1.0(0.0)
Propiomazine	215	1.9(0.0)	30.7(0.4)	66.1(0.8)	0.9(0.0)
Triflupromazine	180	2.2(0.0)	32.8(0.3)	64.4(0.6)	0.6(0.0)
Autonomic drugs					
Hyoscine	2,402	2.8(0.4)	27.8(3.6)	65.8(8.5)	3.3(0.4)
Atropine	324	4.0(0.1)	14.8(0.3)	68.8(1.2)	10.8(0.2)
Uterotonic agents					
Syntocinon	2,335	25.1(3.1)	38.3(4.8)	29.3(3.7)	6.3(0.8)
Oxytocin	539	38.0(1.1)	24.0(1.0)	24.7(0.7)	2.8(0.1)
Other					
Magnesium sulfate	262	11.8(0.2)	31.7(0.4)	50.4(0.7)	5.7(0.1)
Vitamin K	318	26.1(0.4)	50.9(0.9)	22.6(0.4)	0.3(0.0)

* Includes all drugs administered in at least 100 cases. Row percentages do not add to 100% because postpartum use is omitted; parentheses enclose percentages of the total population of patients given drugs in labor.

zine in only 70 cases each.

Utilization of oxytocin, dealt with separately here in its natural and synthetic forms, was further complicated by considerations of induction versus augmentation or both (Table 15-5). As shown, induction with oxytocin was done 485 times in this series (21.8%). Only 55 of these inductions were unassociated with continued use of the agent into labor for further augmentation purposes.

To put oxytocin usage into temporal perspective, we established a grid (Table 15-6) to show when oxytocin was initiated and how long it was continued in the course of labor. This exercise was limited, of course, to those cases in which the labor progression pattern could be adequately reconstructed for purposes of determining the specific labor phases in which the oxytocin was started and stopped. In most cases, it was begun in the active phase (66.2%), and in most of these, it was also concluded in the

active phase (85.1% of those begun in the active phase and 56.4% of all cases in which oxytocin was used).

Anesthetic Agents and Techniques

Our survey of anesthetic agents (Table 15-7) was similarly complicated by a time factor, but since gaseous and IV agents had been given almost exclusively in the terminal moments of the labor process for purposes of delivery support only, temporal considerations were given low priority interest in regard to our analysis of their effects. Conduction anesthesia, by contrast, not only had a time factor that needed to be taken into account, but it also presented the much more compelling issues of dosage, route, and technique to lend a complexity of serious proportions to these investigations. Stratification in just two dimensions by agent and by method (Table 15-8), for

Table 15-5
Distribution of Uterotonic Agents by Induction Versus Augmentation

	Induction only No. (%)	Augmentation only No. (%)	Both No. (%)	Total No. (%)
Oxytocin	15 (0.7)	294 (13.2)	72 (3.2)	381 (17.1)
Syntocinon	37 (1.7)	1,427 (64.1)	340 (15.3)	1,804 (81.0)
Both	3 (0.1)	21 (0.9)	18 (0.8)	42 (1.9)
Total	55 (2.5)	1,742 (78.22)	430 (19.3)	2,227 (100.0)

Table 15-6
Oxytocin Use by Phase of Labor

Labor phase begun in	Drug continued to be used through			
	Latent phase No. (%)	Active phase No. (%)	Second stage No. (%)	Total No. (%)
Latent phase	58 (5.6)	86 (8.2)	86 (8.2)	230 (22.0)
Active phase		589 (56.4)	103 (9.9)	692 (66.2)
Second stage			123 (11.8)	123 (11.8)
Total	58 (5.6)	675 (64.6)	312 (29.9)	1,045 (100.0)

153

Table 15-7
Distribution of Anesthetic Agents

Group	Agent	No.	%
Gaseous			
	Nitrous oxide	1,071	20.4
	Cyclopropane	285	5.4
	Ether	106	2.0
	Trilene	216	4.1
	Ethylene	2	0.0
	Halothane	13	0.3
	Fluoromar	2	0.0
	Chloroform	22	0.4
	Gas-oxygen-ether	76	1.5
	Penthrane	20	0.4
	Total	1,813	34.5
Intravenous			
	Surital sodium	9	0.2
	Pentothal sodium	20	0.4
	Total	29	0.6
Conduction			
	Cyclaine	393	7.5
	Metycaine	62	1.2
	Nesacaine	53	1.0
	Nupercaine	185	3.5
	Pontocaine	712	13.5
	Novocaine	139	2.6
	Xylocaine	1,292	24.6
	Carbocaine	580	11.0
	Cytamest	1	0.0
	Total	3,417	65.0

Table 15-8
Conduction Anesthesia by Drug Type and Route of Administration

Agent	Spinal No. (%)	Caudal No. (%)	Epidural No. (%)	Local No. (%)	Pudendal No. (%)	Paracervical No. (%)
Cyclaine	377(11.0)	–	–	1(0.0)	14(0.4)	1(0.0)
Metycaine	1(0.0)	38(1.1)	4(0.1)	4(0.1)	14(0.4)	1(0.0)
Nesacaine	2(0.1)	42(1.2)	6(0.2)	2(0.1)	–	–
Nupercaine	185(5.4)	–	–	–	–	–
Pontocaine	700(20.5)	–	–	–	–	–
Novocaine	38(1.1)	–	–	54(1.6)	42(1.2)	3(0.1)
Xylocaine	577(16.9)	10(0.3)	67(2.0)	209(6.1)	396(11.6)	33(1.0)
Carbocaine	–	38(1.1)	35(1.0)	99(2.9)	270(7.9)	138(4.0)
Cytamest	–	–	–	–	1(0.0)	–
Total	1,880(55.0)	128(3.7)	112(3.3)	369(10.8)	737(21.6)	176(5.2)

example, illustrated that few subset populations would be large enough to support analysis in depth. Therefore, further stratification by additional factors was felt to be neither warranted nor practicable at this time.

The considerable effort that had been expended in preparing this material was felt to be warranted, despite the apparent limitations based on sample size considerations, in order to allow us to assess the impact of these agents on the fetus and infant. We felt we were now in a position to proceed with that assessment at least in regard to those agents that had been administered to NCPP parturients in relatively large numbers. We realized that the analysis of drug effects, based on the paradigms previously evolved in this series of investigations, would offer little by way of problems compared to the difficulties we had had in compiling this resource on drug exposure in labor.

CHAPTER **16**

Adjunctive Drugs and Outcome

Summary

Exploratory nonparametric analyses were done to isolate agents likely to have an effect on the fetus or infant. Outcomes for various classes of agents and specific agents were surveyed. Rates of adverse results were compared with rates encountered among cases in which the specific drug was not given as well as cases in which no drugs at all had been administered. The value of using two types of controls was supported by indications that confounding effects were probably present.

Having thus detailed the drug experiences of our study population, we were in a position to embark upon the analytical phase of this portion of the investigational program. Specifically, we were prepared to relate pharmacologic agents to fetal and infant outcomes. These relationships were to be assessed both by the broad brushstroke approach of determining if any labor usage of a drug correlated at all with adverse results found in the offspring and the more delicate examination of possible effects according to the phase of labor in which the drug was given. The latter will be dealt with separately (chapter 17).

Designation of Control Group

The same nonparametric techniques were invoked as those that had been previously developed for the analysis of labor effects because they had proved so useful for our needs. Beginning with an analysis of drug use independent of the time factor, we grouped cases simply according to whether a drug had been given or not, for direct comparison. While inherently logical, use of the drug-not-used group as a control was recognized to lack a critical component in that other drugs may have been given to these patients. If so, it would make them possibly suboptimal as a valid control. A more meaningful control group was developed for this purpose, therefore; it consisted of cases in which no drug at all had been administered in labor from the entire list of drugs under surveillance. Each subset thus formed (drug X used, drug X not used, and no drug used) was examined in detail for the entire gamut of fetal and infant outcome variables as detailed earlier.

Narcotic Analgesic Agents

An illustration of the kind of data provided by the overview analysis (Table 16-1) gives us some insight into the possible effects of drugs on the infant. Low IQ scores at age four years appeared to be much more common in multiparas (RR 1.66) after Demerol use than in those not so exposed, but no more frequent than those receiving no drugs at all in labor (RR 0.95); the former proved very significant on statistical testing (p < .0001), the latter not significant at all. These apparently paradox-

ical findings confirmed the intuitive logic that militated use of two different kinds of controls. It also stressed the need, in further explorations, to bear in mind the possibility that confounding factors were at play. High cut points of IQ score at 90 were chosen arbitrarily here for illustrative purposes only. In the data to follow, the more critical cut points for IQ were those designated on the basis of race- and sex- specific distributions (see chapter 5).

Analyses of the range of outcomes yielded data such as summarized in Table 16-2. The aforementioned trends in four-year IQ data were encountered in nulliparas, but they were not duplicated in multiparas. The association was less apparent at seven years, except for some persistent effect in multiparas when compared to the Demerol-not-used group. Additionally, neonatal depression was significantly increased, as might have been expected on the basis of the recognized depressant effect of this agent in neonates. Stillbirth rates were clearly unaffected, but neonatal mortality may have been, especially in multiparas (albeit not statistically significant).

Surveying the narcotic analgesic agents in general use, separately for nulliparas and multiparas (Table 16-3), we noted similar kinds of effects on both Apgar and IQ scores, when compared with no-drug-use groups, for morphine, levallorphan (Lor-

Table 16-1
Meperidine Use in Labor as Related to 4-Year IQ Scores
in Offspring of Multiparas

	Demerol Used in Labor	Demerol Not Used	No Drugs Used	Total
IQ < 90	250* 30.23%	89 18.20%	1,045 31.71%	1,446 31.00%
IQ 90+	577 69.77%	400 81.80%	2,250 68.29%	3,218 69.00%
Total	827	489	3,295	4,664

* Frequency of low IQ relative to rate in Demerol-Not-Used group, rate ratio 1.66, χ^2 = 23.25, p = 1.42 x 10^{-6}. Low IQ relative to No-Drug-Used group, rate ratio 0.95, not significant.

157

fan), and phenazocine (Prinadol). They were also replicated, but less impressively, in nulliparas exposed to meperidine (Demerol) in labor. Contrastingly, alphaprodine (Nisentil) showed apparent protective effects for both early and late outcome variables, suggesting a selection bias in patients to whom this agent may have been given. This was an alternative and more plausible explanation for this finding than the inference that the drug somehow actually protected the fetus; while it was conceivably correct, one would need much more evidence to rely upon it as proven fact. This finding emphasized one of the pitfalls of simple associations and confirmed the

Table 16-2
Fetal and Infant Outcome by Meperidine Use in Labor[a]

Outcome	Nulliparas		Multiparas	
	RR_1	RR_2	RR_1	RR_2
Stillbirth	0.98	1.01	0.99	0.85
Neonatal death	1.09	1.68	1.81	1.81
Low 5-min. Apgar	1.53[b]	2.01[b]	1.29	1.49
Abnormal 8-mo. mental	1.67	0.80	1.10	0.39
Abnormal 8-mo. motor	1.46	1.20	1.68	0.79
Abnormal 3-yr. communications	0.92	0.97	1.10	3.94[b]
Low 4-yr. IQ	1.14[b]	1.17[b]	0.89	0.96
Low 7-yr. IQ	0.97	1.10	1.04	1.15[b]

[a] Data expressed in rate ratios: RR_1, relative to no-drug-use group; RR_2, relative to this drug nonuse.

[b] $p < 0.05$.

Table 16-3
Outcomes Associated with Narcotic Usage in Labor by Parity[a]

Agent	Parity	No.	SB	NND	APG5	MENT8	MOT8	SLH3	IQ4	IQ7
Meperidine										
	Nulliparas	1,395	0.98	1.09	1.53[b]	1.67	1.46	0.92	1.14[b]	0.97
	Multiparas	1,210	0.99	1.81	1.29	1.10	1.68	1.10	0.89	1.04
Nisentil										
	Nulliparas	321	0.43	0.39	0.57	1.77	1.16	0.13[b]	0.61[b]	0.38[b]
	Multiparas	392	0.49	0.53	0.54	0.99	0.94	0.11[b]	0.59[b]	0.45[b]
Morphine										
	Nulliparas	23	0.00	5.49[b]	0.00	0.00	0.00	0.00	1.28	1.42
	Multiparas	42	4.04	0.00	2.92[b]	12.76[b]	8.54[b]	0.00	4.54[b]	2.02
Lorfan										
	Nulliparas	40	0.00	0.00	3.27[b]	0.00	0.00	2.44[b]	0.00	0.00
	Multiparas	28	0.00	6.30[b]	2.55[b]	0.00	0.00	0.00	3.63[b]	3.78[b]
Prinadol										
	Nulliparas	39	0.00	3.24	3.27	0.00	0.00	0.00	2.67	1.46
	Multiparas	33	5.14	0.00	1.19	0.00	0.00	0.00	1.33	1.15

[a] Data expressed in rate ratio relative to no-drug-use group. SB, stillbirth; NND, neonatal death; APG5, low 5-min. Apgar score; MENT8, mental score deficit at 8 mo.; MOT8, motor deficit at 8 mo.; SLH3, abnormal speech, language, hearing at 3 yr.; IQ4, IQ score below 70 at 4 yr.; IQ7, IQ score below 70 at 7 yr.

[b] $p < 0.05$

need for simultaneous considerations of sample make-up (to ensure comparability of populations) and confounding factors.

When these data groupings were collapsed as as to omit consideration of parity differences (Table 16-4), the pattern of overt effects changed somewhat. For meperidine, only neonatal depression persisted in significant frequencies, although other outcomes showed comparably high, but statistically insignificant, rate ratios (such as with abnormal eight-month Bayley scores and neonatal deaths). Nisentil yielded the same overall good results as seen before, with very significantly diminished rates of low three-year communications abnormalities and four- and seven-year IQ scores. Morphine demonstrated rather consistent adverse effects for most of the outcome variables. Lorfan continued to demonstrate adverse effects on Apgar scores at five minutes and IQ scores at four and seven years, but it no longer had a significant impact on neonatal deaths or three-year speech, language, and hearing results. Prinadol showed a deleterious influence on four-year IQ scores.

Consideration of all narcotic analgesics collectively without regard for specific drug type, dose, route or timing of administration, or for parity either (Table 16-4), was accomplished by coalescing all the aforementioned data on 3536 women to whom

any form of these agents had been given in labor. This was done to give us an overview of effect on the fetus and infant. Taken altogether, these cases documented rather clearly that the only adverse effect that could be deemed consistent (even allowing for the exception of the Nisentil data) was neonatal depression as reflected in the high frequency of low five-minute Apgar scores. This was not unexpected, of course. Contrariwise, the incidence of low IQ scores at four and seven years was correspondingly decreased, supporting a tentative conclusion that use of narcotic analgesics in labor had no apparent lasting effect on the offspring.

Tranquilizers

Similar data were generated for all other pharmacologic agents administered in reasonable numbers to laboring patients. The accompanying tables reduce these analyses to a quickly digestible form by flagging the statistically significant rate ratios for each specific drug, thereby designating the adverse or protective fetal and infant results that were disclosed.

Among the tranquilizers (Table 16-5), for example, promazine (Sparine) was largely protective (significantly so in the neonatal deaths and four-year IQ results for offspring of multiparas). In nulliparas, there

Table 16-4
Outcome by Narcotic Usage in Labor[a]

Agent	No.	SB	NND	APG5	MENT8	MOT8	SLH3	IQ4	IQ7
Meperidine	2,605	0.98	1.34	1.39[b]	1.47	1.49	1.03	1.02	1.00
Nisentil	735	0.41	0.50	0.55	1.36	0.99	0.12[b]	0.60[b]	0.42[b]
Morphine	65	2.34	2.28	2.50	3.76	3.57	0.00	3.39[b]	1.81[b]
Lorfan	68	0.00	2.11	2.88[b]	0.00	0.00	1.42	1.49[b]	1.56[b]
Prinadol	72	2.11	2.04	2.16	0.00	0.00	0.00	2.06[b]	1.32
All narcotics	3,536	0.89	1.19	1.28[b]	1.43	1.29	0.84	1.01	0.91[b]
No drug used (referent)	11,064	0.669%	0.687%	2.11%	0.475%	0.490%	6.21%	2.20%	2.81%

a   Data for this table and those following are rate ratios (except percentage referent rates for no-drug-used group) for specific and general drug usage without regard for parity classes.

b $p < 0.05$.

Table 16-5
Outcome by Use of Tranquilizers in Labor

Agent Parity	No.	SB	NND	APG5	MENT8	MOT8	SLH3	IQ4	IQ7
Promazine									
Nulliparas	451	1.22	0.84	1.51	0.00	0.00	1.93	0.90	0.97
Multiparas	561	1.51	0.33[a]	0.82	0.76	0.71	0.68	0.64[a]	0.74
Promethazine									
Nulliparas	517	0.80	0.73	1.56	2.73[a]	1.54	0.35[a]	1.47[a]	0.74
Multiparas	482	0.71	1.52	1.33	0.91	0.83	0.96	0.92	1.00
Hydroxyzine									
Nulliparas	122	1.12	1.03	1.49	1.72	1.56	0.52	1.62[a]	1.69[a]
Multiparas	116	0.00	1.58	1.61	3.67	3.31	0.98	1.47[a]	2.07[a]
Propriomazine									
Nulliparas	102	0.00	1.24	2.42	0.00	0.00	1.24	0.86	1.21
Multiparas	86	0.00	0.00	0.86	0.00	0.00	0.39	0.72	0.72
Triflupromazine									
Nulliparas	68	0.00	0.00	0.00	0.00	0.00	0.00	1.97[a]	2.62[a]
Multiparas	74	0.00	4.94[a]	2.57[a]	0.00	10.14[a]	0.96	1.60[a]	1.84[a]
Others[b]									
Nulliparas	45	0.00	0.00	1.48	5.20	5.09	0.00	1.68	1.57
Multiparas	48	0.00	0.00	1.54	8.84[a]	7.37[a]	0.87	0.58	0.86

[a] $p < 0.05$.

[b]   Includes 28 cases of perphenazine (Trilafon), 28 mepromazine, 21 prochlorperazine (Compazine), 12 meprobamate (Equanil, Miltown), 1 chlordiazepoxide (Librium), 18 chlorpromazine (Thorazine), 3 dimenhydrinate (Dramamine), 3 trimethobenzamine (Tigan), 3 thiethylperazine (Torecan), 1 chlorpheniramine (Chlor-Trimeton), 8 diphenhydramine (Benadryl), and 1 trimepramine (Temaril).

was a counterbalancing increase in abnormal three-year communications testing results (nearly twofold, but not statistically significant). The protective nature of the effect with promazine is to be noted in view of its similarity to that of alphaprodine (Nisentil) because both agents were often used concurrently. We have already suggested that this might represent preferential patient selection rather than true drug effect (see above).

No comparable effect was found for the other tranquilizers studied. Indeed, some of them—particularly hydroxyzine (Vistaril) and triflupromazine (Vesprin)—appeared to have especially adverse effects extending uniformly to the long-term outcome variables of four- and seven-year IQs. Promethazine showed similar results for nulliparas only and with less consistency. Neither beneficial nor adverse effect was seen for propriomazine. Pooled data from all other tranquilizers showed rather impressively

bad eight-month results. The correlations with poor outcome were felt to be important because they were expected to serve as flags to direct more in-depth analysis in the future.

Discounting parity distinctions (Table 16-6), as we had done earlier for the narcotic analgesic agents, we found promazine still associated with significantly decreased rates of neonatal deaths and low four-year IQ scores. Promethazine yielded high frequencies of neonatal depression and eight-month mental score abnormalities. The frequencies of abnormal three-year communications and four-year intelligence testing results were no longer statistically significant. Hydroxyzine and triflupromazine retained their adverse association with four- and seven-year IQ scores. Propriomazine data remained as before without clearcut trends in outcome variables. Adverse eight-month motor and mental scores associated with other tranquilizers persisted

160

here.

The overall effects of tranquilizers was examined as before by collapsing all the data into a single population base of 2668 patients to whom one or more of these drugs had been given in the course of labor (Table 16-6). All the effects just detailed vanished as a consequence of this manipulation, except that related to low five-minute Apgar scores. Persistent neonatal depression was thus demonstrated to be rather clearly associated with use of tranquilizers in labor. While this was not intended to imply that the relationship was one of cause and effect, the observation did suggest either that tranquilizers themselves caused depression or that a factor commonly associated with the use of tranquilizers did. Since narcotic analgesics were so very commonly given in conjunction with ataractic agents, it was felt the latter was perhaps the more likely explanation. The data further suggested that exposure to tranquilizers in labor had no discernible lasting effect on offspring.

Barbiturates

Use of barbiturates, as expected, resulted in some increase in neonatal depression, but this achieved statistical significance only with phenobarbital in multiparas (Table 16-7). Phenobarbital, moreover, showed rather impressively bad outcome results overall, most apparent in multiparas. This was an unanticipated finding without obvious explanation in terms of possible drug effect. We conjectured that the drug was perhaps being administered to patients who were specially selected by virtue of a

Table 16-6
Outcome by Tranquilizer Usage in Labor

Agent	No.	SB	NND	APG5	MENT8	MOT8	SLH3	IQ4	IQ7
Promazine	1,012	1.33	0.58*	1.12	0.26	0.26	1.20	0.76*	0.84
Promethazine	999	0.75	1.02	1.51*	2.13*	1.30	0.70	1.20	0.87
Hydroxyzine	238	0.63	1.22	1.56	2.24	2.05	0.81	1.55*	1.88*
Propriomazine	188	0.00	0.78	1.53	0.00	0.00	0.81	1.78*	0.99
Triflupromazine	142	0.00	2.05*	1.38	0.00	3.46	0.49	1.78*	2.21*
Others	93	0.00	0.00	1.50	6.01*	5.83*	0.60	1.11	1.20
All tranquilizers	2,668	0.84	0.87	1.37*	1.31	1.16	0.78	1.07	1.04

* $p < 0.05$.

Table 16-7
Outcome by Use of Barbiturates in Labor

Agent	Parity	No.	SB	NND	APG5	MENT8	MOT8	SLH3	IQ4	IQ7
Secobarbital										
	Nulliparas	580	1.42	0.87	1.50	2.14	2.16	0.48	0.64*	0.73*
	Multiparas	585	1.45	0.41	1.05	2.12	0.65	0.46*	1.01	1.12
Pentobarbital										
	Nulliparas	196	0.69	1.29	1.29	1.09	0.00	0.73	1.17	1.21
	Multiparas	257	1.32	0.71	1.21	1.63	3.12	1.04	1.16	0.88
Phenobarbital										
	Nulliparas	60	0.00	2.10	2.05	3.23	3.29	0.75	1.12	1.26
	Multiparas	110	3.09	3.22	3.11*	11.74*	10.94*	2.51*	1.46*	2.74*

* $p < 0.05$.

161

disease process—such as pregnancy-induced hypertension—that itself yielded poor outcomes. Thus, the drug might have served merely as a marker of the disorder for which it was used (analogous to insulin serving as a marker for diabetes mellitus).

This suspicion was partially supported by the observation that secobarbital, which was used routinely in early labor in otherwise normal gravidas for its hypnotic effects, had no parallel adverse impact on the fetus and infant. In fact, secobarbital appeared to have some protective effects, especially in the long-term follow-up data for three-year speech, language, and hearing and four- and seven-year IQ results (the latter in nulliparas only). Pentobarbital (given commonly as Carbrital in a proprietary combination of pentobarbital sodium and carbromal, a nonbarbiturate brominated monoureide) showed no comparable protective or deleterious effects.

We discounted parity as we had done for other agents in order to obtain a broader perspective (Table 16-8). The good three-year communications and four-year IQ effects of secobarbital were the same as before, but the bad eight-month motor results were now significantly increased. Pentobarbital again showed no meaningful effects at all. Phenobarbital yielded particularly poor results across the entire range of outcomes, and these data were statistically significant for all observations from five minutes to seven years. Collapsing all these data into a single all-encompassing barbiturate-use group (Table 16-8) produced evidence of deleterious early effects

up to eight months and paradoxically beneficial ones at three years.

Antibiotics

The marker effect was even more obvious in regard to outcomes of offspring whose mother was exposed to antibiotics in labor (Table 16-9). The results we encountered were rather devastating with very significantly increased rates of fetal and neonatal deaths as well as long-term damage to surviving infants. The effect, however, was not necessarily permanent as shown by the apparently acceptable four- and seven-year IQ findings. Whereas some fetal risks from antibiotics are recognized to exist—such as the ototoxicity of streptomycin or the rare marrow depression of chloramphenicol—nothing of this magnitude has been described. The more likely explanation, therefore, is that we were seeing the effect of the infectious processes for which the antibiotics were being administered in the course of labor, particularly the documented hazards relating to amnionitis.

Hypotensive Agents

The outcomes associated with use of magnesium sulfate mirrored the kind of poor results expected of the fetus and infant of a gravida with severe enough pregnancy-induced hypertension to require use of this powerful agent (Table 16-9). Similarly, reserpine and hydralazine hydrochloride (Apresoline), both given only to women with severe hypertension, fol-

Table 16-8
Outcome by Barbiturate Usage in Labor

Agent	No.	SB	NND	APG5	MENT8	MOT8	SLH3	IQ4	IQ7
Secobarbital	1,165	1.44	0.75	1.26	2.12*	1.53	0.47*	0.83*	0.93
Pentobarbital	453	0.99	0.97	1.23	1.17	1.13	0.99	1.16	1.02
Phenobarbital	170	1.77	2.57	3.05*	6.10*	5.96*	2.41*	1.34*	2.22*
All barbiturates	1,788	1.34	0.98	1.46*	2.20*	1.85*	0.76*	0.96	1.08

*   p < 0.05.

162

Table 16-9
Outcome by Use of Miscellaneous Agents in Labor

Agent Parity	No.	SB	NND	APG5	MENT8	MOT8	SLH3	IQ4	IQ7
Antibiotics[a]									
Nulliparas	89	6.16[b]	2.90	4.32[b]	4.96[b]	5.09[b]	3.46[b]	0.99	1.02
Multiparas	102	1.67	3.58[b]	2.18[b]	12.46[b]	3.91	0.50	1.10	1.06
Atropine									
Nulliparas	139	2.96[b]	0.92	2.16	3.04	1.46	1.56	1.07	1.01
Multiparas	146	1.16	0.00	2.09[b]	0.00	0.00	0.87	1.28	0.91
Hyoscine									
Nulliparas	740	0.93	0.34	0.95	1.14	0.85	0.98	0.74[b]	0.90
Multiparas	627	0.54	0.58	0.91	1.43	0.65	0.75	0.97	0.91
Magnesium sulfate									
Nulliparas	53	0.00	0.00	1.16	4.36	0.00	1.70	1.51[b]	1.26
Multiparas	114	1.49	1.60	0.99	7.41[b]	6.55[b]	1.27	1.82[b]	1.69[b]
Reserpine									
Nulliparas	10	0.00	0.00	0.00	16.13[b]	0.00	0.00	1.62	1.40
Multiparas	32	0.00	5.71[b]	3.58[b]	0.00	0.00	0.00	8.35[b]	5.09[b]
Apresoline									
Nulliparas	7	0.00	0.00	0.00	0.00	0.00	0.00	1.58	1.32
Multiparas	20	0.00	18.27[b]	7.79[b]	0.00	0.00	1.55	1.60	1.38

a   Includes 98 cases of penicillin and all its derivatives, 53 streptomycin, 112 tetracycline and related agents, 25 chloramphenicol, and 37 sulfonamide congeners.

b $p < 0.05$.

lowed a parallel trend pattern. The effect was so strong in fact that the results were statistically significant despite the relatively small numbers of cases represented here. The bad outcomes seen were undoubtedly the results one should expect as a consequence of the maternal hypertensive diathesis.

Belladonna Alkaloids

Neither atropine nor scopolamine showed this effect, except for the high frequency of neonatal depression with atropine use, perhaps more reflective of concomitant use of depressing narcotic analgesics. The apparently protective four-year IQ effect of scopolamine in nulliparas (with good seven-year outcome data as well, although not statistically significant) could also have represented a selection bias that required closer scrutiny. This was felt to be the case because use of scopolamine during the years of the NCPP data collection was a common practice, especially among private physicians who dealt principally with relatively healthy women. The apparent fetal and infant protection accompanying scopolamine use occurred here despite the fact that this agent has fallen into almost complete disuse because of its adverse maternal effects.

Uterotonic Agents

Rather paradoxical results were obtained from analysis of the data pertaining to offspring of gravidas receiving uterotonic stimulation in labor examined without consideration for the intent of the usage (that is, whether for induction or augmentation) or other aspects of dose schedule or timing (Table 16-10). Syntocinon, the synthetic hormone, was associated with very good four- and seven-year IQ results (statistically significant in multiparas), yet early outcomes appeared much less favorable, although not significantly so. Furthermore, use of oxytocin (Pitocin)—ostensibly the same substance pharmacologically, albeit

163

Table 16-10
Outcome by Use of Uterotonic Agents in Labor

Agent	Parity	No.	SB	NND	APG5	MENT8	MOT8	SLH3	IQ4	IQ7
Oxytocin										
	Nulliparas	117	2.34	1.09	1.61	0.00	0.00	2.98*	0.76	0.80
	Multiparas	68	7.49*	0.00	1.74	0.00	0.00	0.47	0.94	1.12
Syntocinon										
	Nulliparas	366	1.50	0.35	1.18	1.65	1.09	0.46	0.90	0.83
	Multiparas	348	1.47	2.10	1.51	2.42	1.12	0.77	0.71*	0.48*
Sparteine										
	Nulliparas	99	0.00	1.28	1.23	1.85	1.88	0.70	0.86	0.99
	Multiparas	61	5.57*	0.00	1.28	0.00	0.00	0.00	0.88	0.77

* $p < 0.05$.

naturally occurring—yielded particularly poor early results, especially stillbirths in multiparas (also increased in nulliparas, but not to a statistically significant degree) and three-year communications results in nulliparas; the good four- and seven-year IQ results contrastingly parallelled those of Syntocinon. Sparteine sulfate had no documentably adverse effect when used in nulliparas; however, in multiparas, it was associated with a high stillbirth rate, comparable to that of Pitocin, with no residual effect on surviving infants.

These data were coalesced (Table 16-11) to provide more generalized information on the effects of uterotonic stimulation (without regard for type, indication, technique, dose, route, or timing, and also without consideration of parity). When thus combined, the data reconfirmed a significantly adverse association between natural oxytocin and the stillbirth rate as well as the frequency of abnormal three-year speech, language, and hearing results. For Syntocinon, the beneficial impact on four-and seven-year IQ results was shown again as the only significant finding. Sparteine sulfate use yielded no data to suggest either a beneficial or deleterious effect. Collapsing all uterotonic agent usage into a single population sample (Table 16-11) for 1059 cases showed a significantly high stillbirth rate and a gratifying decrease in the rates of low four- and seven-year IQ scores.

To this point, the relationships between the drugs used in labor and outcome have been outlined both in general terms with regard to broad classes of agents and specifically vis-à-vis individual drugs. Dosage aspects, while examined superficially as part of these investigations, were not pursued in depth by virtue of the small numbers of cases that were found to compose any subset, except perhaps the very few agents utilized most prevalently (chapter 15). Our difficulties in this regard were compounded by the fact that, almost without exception, drug use practices were homogeneous in that a single dosage was usually prescribed for a given drug. Differentiating the effects of that common dosage from others given only infrequently was perforce not readily achievable. Remaining to be reported were the studies undertaken to review the modifying influence of the timing of drug administration in labor as such timing might alter the effects that those drugs appeared to have on the fetus and infant.

Table 16-11
Outcome by Uterotonic Agent Use in Labor

Agent	No.	SB	NND	APG5	MENT8	MOT8	SLH3	IQ4	IQ7
Oxytocin	185	4.15*	0.82	1.65	0.00	0.00	1.86*	0.83	0.92
Syntocinon	714	1.48	1.02	1.42	1.82	1.10	0.59	0.81*	0.66*
Sparteine	160	1.88	0.92	1.22	1.63	1.61	0.41	0.87	0.91
All uterotonics	1,059	1.99*	0.97	1.42	1.49	0.96	0.84	0.82*	0.74*

* $p < 0.05$.

CHAPTER 17

Adjunctive Drugs: Temporal Considerations

Summary

The outcome effects of a number of commonly administered agents were examined to determine if they were influenced by the time in labor when the drugs were given. Study was limited to those invoked often enough to permit meaningful stratification by time increments, such as narcotic analgesics, tranquilizers, barbiturates, belladonna alkaloids, and uterotonics. Especially interesting relationships were disclosed for Demerol and oxytocin.

Analyses followed that delved further into drugs effects, focusing upon the phase of labor in which the agents were administered. It has been generally accepted, for example, that narcotic analgesics given late in labor will have a greater adverse effect on the neonate, especially in terms of depression as measured by Apgar scores, than if given earlier. Potential interplay (whether synergistic, additive, or counterbalancing) between these drugs and labor progression disorders, particularly as regards diminishing or enhancing concurrent fetal effects, needed further elucidation as well. To study modifications of drug effects according to time of exposure, the material developed earlier for each relevant drug and drug group was stratified by labor phase. The matrix of subsets thus created was then examined for the spectrum of fetal and infant outcomes.

Neonatal Effects of Demerol by Time

An example of our systematic approach to this problem is shown in Table 17-1 for use of meperidine (Demerol) as it may have affected the five-minute Apgar score in the offspring of nulliparas. All patients who received Demerol were stratified according to the phase of labor in which the drug was given. Within each subgroup thus created, outcomes were assessed. The frequency of neonatal depression among those 920 infants whose mothers were given Demerol in the active phase only was 2.50%. This was to be compared with either the frequency of depression in those to whom no study drug had been administered (955 cases, 1.26% rate of neonatal depression) or that of cases given no drugs at all (6049 in all, 1.65% depression). Both referent groups were available, of course, and were actually utilized for our full analytical program; for our purposes here, however, we chose the latter as a better control groups for drug evaluations and more representative of the unaffected labor-delivery process.

Nonparametric techniques were brought to bear as in the past. Freeman-Tukey deviates (FTD) showed the clear significance of the adverse effect of Demerol on Apgar scores when it was given in the active phase (FTD 1.831, $p = .034$). Similarly, significantly increased rates of neonatal depression were seen when this drug was given to women in both active phase and second stage, even though the number of such cases was small (FTD 1.937, $p = .026$). A high frequency of depressed babies was encountered with Demerol use in both latent and active phases, but this was not quite statistically significant. Administration only in the latent phase failed to show any adverse effect on this outcome variable. Isolated second stage use was too infrequent (only 13 cases) to offer useful data. No other temporally isolated usage was associated with low Apgar scores.

When examined by timing of administration without consideration for use at other times in the same labor in a given patient (Table 17-2), these data were expected to provide further insights. As anticipated, for example, latent phase usage had no definable effect. We verified the very significant impact of active phase administration of Demerol; the frequency of neonatal depression was increased in this group nearly twofold overall (RR 1.72, $p = .0090$). This approach also provided additional information on second stage usage which had not been disclosed before. Even though the

Table 17-1
Neonatal Depression by Specific Time Frame of Demerol Usage in Nulliparas

Labor Phase	No.	Low 5-min. Apgar		Expected No.	Freeman-Tukey		Rate Ratio	
		No.	%		Deviate	p	RR	p
Onset only	30	0	0.00	0.50	-0.727		0.00	
Latent phase only	272	5	1.84	4.50	0.328		1.12	
Active phase only	920	23	2.50	15.21	1.831	0.034	1.52	0.068
Latent and active phases	98	4	4.08	1.62	1.501	0.067	2.47	0.064
Second stage only	13	0	0.00	0.22	-0.364		0.00	
Active phase and second stage	7	2	28.57	0.12	1.937	0.026	17.32	3.0×10^{-8}
Latent phase and second stage	1	0	0.00	0.02	-0.033		0.00	
Latent, active, and second stage	1	0	0.00	0.02	-0.033		0.00	
No Demerol usage	955	12	1.26	15.79	-0.940		0.76	
No drug use at all	6,049	100	1.65	100.00	-		1.00	

Table 17-2
Neonatal Depression by General Time Frame of Demerol Usage in Nulliparas

Labor Phase	No.	Low 5-min. Apgar No.	%	Expected No.	Freeman-Tukey Deviate	p	Rate Ratio RR	p
All latent phase usage	372	9	2.42	6.15	1.103		1.47	
All active phase usage	1,026	29	2.83	16.99	2.564	0.0050	1.72	0.0090
All second stage usage	22	2	9.09	0.36	1.579	0.057	5.51	0.0067
All Demerol usage	1,342	34	2.53	22.19	2.274	0.012	1.53	0.029

sample size was small (22 cases), the impact of drug use was so great as to satisfy statistical testing criteria for confirmation. The incidence of neonatal depression when Demerol was given in the second stage was more than five times the expected rate (RR 5.51, p = .0067) for offspring of gravidas given no drugs at all in labor and more than seven times the rate for those who had not been given Demerol at all (RR 7.23, p = .0016).

The sequence of evaluative analyses had thus been delicate enough to enable us to elucidate the effect of Demerol on the infant. Earlier, we showed that its use in labor was associated with neonatal depression. The current analysis was able to show that its effect on this outcome variable was most pronounced if it was given either in the active phase or in the second stage. Administration earlier did not appear to affect the infant in the same way. None of this was unexpected, of course, based on confirmatory clinical experience; nonetheless, it was gratifying to be able to test our basic premise and to demonstrate the functional capability of the analytical techniques that were applied.

Other Outcome Results for Demerol

These techniques were invoked for assessing other outcome variables as well. Demerol use had not previously been found to be related to any other adverse results. Our intention in pursuing such other outcomes was to ensure that no deleterious effects had been obscured by inundation with superimposed confounding information. For example, if the active phase and second stage usage impact on neonatal depression had not been so strong, it was conceivable that the nonimpacting latent phase usage could have hidden it. Under those circumstances, unless the cases were to be stratified temporally, it is not likely that the error (of omission) would ever have been discernible.

Having thus rationalized the need to examine even negative relationships in depth, we proceeded to do just that for Demerol (Table 17-3). As if to provide justification for this effort, we did find rate ratios for eight-month mental and motor score abnormalities to be quite high, but they were not statistically significant. Second stage use of this drug, even though cases were few in number, did yield significantly increased frequencies of eight-month abnormalities but not of abnormal three-year communications skills.

Neonatal deaths had been reported to be high (chapter 16), but not significantly so, in the overall data assessment for nulliparas (RR 1.34). Here we could appreciate their concentration in the group with exposure to Demerol at or before the onset of labor. This suggested that these women may have had some underlying disease process requiring pain relief or perhaps a condition (such as heart disease, especially with actual or marginally functional decompensation) which made the expected pain of the labor process medically unacceptable. If this proved to be correct, it would be logical to attribute the fetal or infant losses to the disease rather than to the drug; but this needed testing, of course.

The temporal overview of Demerol effect (Table 17-4) across a variety of outcomes showed no latent phase effects except the aforementioned increased rate ratios for stillbirths, neonatal deaths, and neonatal depression (none of which were statistically significant). No late effects were even suggested by these data, however. For active phase exposure, both neonatal depression and eight-month abnormalities were noted (only the former was significant); again, there was no late impact at all. Second stage administration yielded very high and very significant five-minute and eight-month effects. As before, late follow-up results were entirely satisfactory.

The same approach was applied to multiparas (Table 17-5). Neonatal depression, as reflected in low five-minute Apgar scores, was high when Demerol had been given at or before labor onset and in the rare cases in which it was given in all three time periods in labor. Here active phase use of this agent did not appear to have the same magnitude of depressing effect it had had in nulliparas—that is, although the frequency of depressed infants was higher than expected (RR 1.20 with active phase use only and 3.09 if given in both active phase and second stage), it did not reach statistical significance. Since the number of cases in the active phase subset should surely have been adequate for this form of analysis (760 patients), failure to achieve significance here could not be categorically discounted as specious.

As to other outcomes, stillbirth rates were unexpectedly high in conjunction

Table 17-3
Outcome by Specific Time Frame of Demerol Usage in Nulliparas

Labor Phase	No.	SB	NND	APG5	MENT8	MOT8	SLH3
Onset only	31	0.00	4.07	0.00	0.00	0.00	0.00
Latent phase only	279	1.47	1.37	1.12	0.78	0.00	1.40
Active phase only	956	0.72	0.79	1.52	1.94	1.88	0.89
Latent and active phases	107	2.56	2.36	2.47	0.00	0.00	0.40
Second stage only	13	0.00	0.00	0.00	16.13*	15.78*	0.00
Active phase and second stage	7	0.00	0.00	17.32*	0.00	0.00	0.00
No Demerol used	980	1.01	0.64	0.76	2.07*	1.22	0.94
No drugs used	6,313	0.714%	0.792%	1.65%	0.620%	0.634%	5.59%

* $p < 0.05$.

Table 17-4
Outcome by General Time Frame of Demerol Usage in Nulliparas

Labor Phase	No.	SB	NND	APG5	MENT8	MOT8	SLH
All latent phase usage	388	1.77	1.63	1.47	0.57	0.00	1.09
All active phase usage	1,071	0.90	0.94	1.72*	1.76	1.86	0.83
All second stage usage	22	0.00	0.00	5.57*	8.96*	8.77*	0.00
All Demerol usage	1,395	0.98	1.09	1.53*	1.67	1.12	0.92

* $p < 0.05$.

with use of Demerol in second stage (as well as active phase plus second stage). Since the subsets consisted of very small numbers of gravidas, we questioned whether or not this was meaningful. Moreover, if correct, it was conjectured that it might reflect liberal use of narcotizing agents for parturients who were about to deliver a fetus known to be dead. This was supported by the absence of a like effect on the neonatal death rates. Deaths among newborn infants were increased in association with the usage in latent and active phase but not second stage; in fact, no neonatal deaths occurred at all in the second stage subsets.

The questions raised by this detailed analysis were resolved by utilizing the more generalized paradigm for examining temporal effects (Table 17-6). Except for the stillbirth rates associated with second stage use (RR 7.07), no significant impact could be verified for any time period usage or any outcome variable. Some were rather suggestive, such as neonatal death rates with latent or active phase drug usage, neonatal depression with second stage usage, and eight-month motor abnormalities with active phase or second stage usage, but statistical testing failed to show that they were not likely to have occurred merely by chance.

Table 17-5
Outcome by Specific Time Frame of Demerol Usage in Multiparas

Labor Phase	No.	SB	NND	APG5	MENT8	MOT8	SLH3
Onset only	18	0.00	0.00	4.11*	0.00	0.00	6.98*
Latent phase only	195	0.00	2.81	1.35	2.05	0.00	1.14
Active phase only	760	1.12	1.92	1.20	1.21	2.21	1.07
Latent and active phases	191	0.00	0.96	1.01	0.00	0.00	0.90
Second stage only	10	16.98*	0.00	0.00	0.00	0.00	0.00
Active and second stage	26	6.53*	0.00	3.09	0.00	0.00	1.00
Latent phase and second stage	8	0.00	0.00	0.00	0.00	0.00	1.99
Latent, active, and second stage	4	0.00	0.00	12.34*	0.00	81.10*	0.00
No Demerol usage	731	1.16	1.00	0.88	2.84*	2.12	0.30
No drugs used	4,753	0.589%	0.547%	2.70%	0.290%	0.308%	7.16%

* p < 0.05.

Table 17-6
Outcome by by General Time Frame of Demerol Usage in Multiparas

Labor Phase	No.	SB	NND	APG5	MENT8	MOT8	SLH3
All latent phase usage	398	0.00	1.84	1.25	1.03	0.00	1.05
All active phase usage	981	1.04	1.66	1.24	0.92	2.10	1.03
All second stage usage	48	7.07*	0.00	2.58	0.00	9.83	1.03
All Demerol usage	1,212	0.99	1.81	1.24	1.09	1.68	1.10

* p < 0.05.

Nisentil Impact by Time

Although the use of alphaprodine (Nisentil) was much less frequent than that of meperidine in this series, it had been given in large enough numbers to permit a similar temporal analysis in some depth. As expected, some of the subsets contained so few cases (for example, the drug had been administered to only four nulliparas in the second stage) that the outcome data therein could not be considered valid. Where sample size proved adequate, the results to fetus and infant (Table 17-7) confirmed good long-term outcomes. Eight-month examination results showed the opposite effect, namely an apparently deleterious one. For multiparas exposed to this agent in both latent and active phases, the adverse

eight-month outcomes achieved statistical significance (more than five times the expected frequency of bad outcomes in these testing vehicles).

Coalescing these several Nisentil groups into logical time frames, as had been done for Demerol, revealed no new information. The protective nature of drug use, reflected in three-year communications test data for active phase usage, was confirmed here, but its deleterious aspect with regard to eight-month results was not. As before, second stage usage was too infrequent to allow for meaningful assessment of effect.

In regard to the unexpected protective influence that Nisentil appeared to show so uniformly in these analyses, it is essential to reemphasize that confounding factors (par-

Table 17-7
Outcome by Nisentil Usage Time Frames

Labor Phase	Parity	No.	SB	NND	APG5	MENT8	MOT8	SLH3
Latent phase only								
	Nulliparas	67	2.04	1.88	0.90	2.83	2.67	0.00
	Multiparas	55	0.00	0.00	0.00	0.00	0.00	0.00
Active phase only								
	Nulliparas	225	0.00	0.00	0.73	1.67	0.83	0.00
	Multiparas	264	0.64	0.69	0.42	0.00	0.00	0.15*
Latent and active phases								
	Nulliparas	23	0.00	0.00	2.63	0.00	0.00	0.00
	Multiparas	69	0.00	0.00	1.11	6.27*	5.49	0.00
Second stage only								
	Nulliparas	2	0.00	0.00	0.00	0.00	0.00	0.00
	Multiparas	8	0.00	4.63	0.00	0.00	0.00	0.00
All latent phase usage								
	Nulliparas	90	1.49	1.37	1.34	2.12	1.96	0.53
	Multiparas	129	0.00	0.00	0.58	3.22	2.92	0.00
All active phase usage								
	Nulliparas	250	0.00	0.00	0.48	1.52	0.74	0.00
	Multiparas	340	0.49	0.53	0.54	1.21	1.11	0.13*
All second stage usage								
	Nulliparas	4	0.00	0.00	0.00	0.00	0.00	0.00
	Multiparas	21	0.00	0.00	0.00	0.00	0.00	0.00
All Demerol usage								
	Nulliparas	321	0.43	0.39	0.57	1.77	1.16	0.13*
	Multiparas	412	0.41	0.44	0.54	0.99	0.93	0.11*

* p < 0.05.

ticularly as related to preselection of patients for drug administration) had not yet been taken into account. It was thus possible (indeed likely) that this ostensible protection may have been specious and have reflected instead the effects of hidden underlying influences. To put this into perspective by example, it is conceivable that Nisentil was preferentially administered to healthy women at term, systematically excluding those with any serious complication or those in premature labor. If true, this would account for the good results we found associated with the use of this narcotic analgesic, perhaps even counterbalancing and obscuring an adverse effect, if one existed.

Effects of Other Narcotics by Time

Other narcotic analgesics were also studied in the same way. None of the others, however, had been given to sufficient numbers of gravidas to allow us to derive outcome frequencies that could be considered even marginally worthwhile when fully stratified by labor phases. There were a few isolated subgroups that could be pooled sufficiently to satisfy our investigational needs. Active phase use of Lorfan, for example, could be examined in 25 nulliparas and 19 multiparas. A significantly increased frequency was encountered for low four-year IQ scores in nulliparas (RR 2.02, p = .005); low IQ scores were increased in multiparas also, but not significantly so (RR 1.70). Similarly, the frequencies of neonatal depression were increased (RR 2.63 in nulliparas and 1.95 in multiparas), but they did not prove statistically significant.

Morphine use, when stratified by labor phase, yielded unacceptably small subset sizes, the largest being 14 multiparas who had been given the drug in the latent phase. Among them, Apgar scores at five minutes were quite low (RR 6.17, p = .003). Prinadol, when examined in the same way according to the labor phase in which it was administered, was also used too infrequently except

for 23 nulliparas given it in the active phase. Their outcome results were characterized by significantly increased neonatal depression (RR 5.76, p = .005).

Tranquilizer Effects by Time

The modifying influences on outcome of the time frame of drug administration were examined for the tranquilizers as well. Promazine's protective effect, previously seen when we studied the overall impact without regard for the time in labor when it was given (chapter 16), was displayed (Table 17-8) in much greater detail. Generally good results were encountered with impressive consistency regardless of the labor phase exposed. Uncovered by this approach was an unexplained isolated discrepant finding of apparent adverse effect on three-year speech, language, and hearing results, especially significant in multiparas when the drug was given in the latent phase. Additionally, the stillbirth rate was unexpectedly high in the same subgroup.

The possible effects of promethazine (Table 17-9) were discordant. Little, if any, impact could be discerned from use of this agent in multiparas. In nulliparas, however, both adverse and beneficial effects were seen. Active phase exposure, for example, was associated with significantly poor five-minute Apgar and eight-month mental scores but equally significant good results in the stillbirth and three-year communications outcome variables. Because of problems relating to diminishing sample size in some subsets, data for second stage administration could not be evaluated meaningfully for this drug or other tranquilizers given even less often.

Hydroxyzine pamoate (Table 17-10) also failed to provide homogeneous data. Only administration in the active phase seemed to have some deleterious effects on short-term (neonatal death and low five-minute Apgar scores) and moderate-term (abnormal eight-month mental and motor scores) outcomes. While these trends were present in both parity groups, the rates proved sta-

Table 17-8
Outcome by Promazine Usage Time Frames

Labor Phase Parity	No.	SB	NND	APG5	MENT8	MOT8	SLH3
Latent phase only							
Nulliparas	80	1.71	1.58	1.57	0.00	0.00	1.49
Multiparas	71	4.78*	0.00	0.00*	0.00	0.00	2.99*
Active phase only							
Nulliparas	262	1.57	0.77	1.18	0.00	0.00	2.08
Multiparas	271	1.25	0.00*	0.70	0.00	0.00	0.00*
Latent and active phases							
Nulliparas	89	0.00	1.09	2.09	0.00	0.00	2.56
Multiparas	164	1.04	1.11	1.39	2.57	2.40	0.00
Second stage only							
Nulliparas	11	0.00	0.00	5.50	0.00	0.00	0.00
Multiparas	29	0.00	0.00	1.28	0.00	0.00	2.79
All latent phase usage							
Nulliparas	170	0.81	1.48	1.82	0.00	0.00	1.88
Multiparas	259	1.97	0.78	0.89	1.63	1.66	1.16
All active phase usage							
Nulliparas	358	1.15	0.71	1.55	0.00	0.00	2.07
Multiparas	478	1.07	0.42	0.96	0.89	0.91	0.22
All second stage usage							
Nulliparas	13	0.00	0.00	4.65	0.00	0.00	0.00
Multiparas	53	0.00	0.00	0.71	0.00	0.00	1.55
All promazine usage							
Nulliparas	451	1.22	0.84	1.51	0.00	0.00	1.93
Multiparas	559	1.51	0.33	0.82	0.76	0.70	0.68

* p < 0.05.

tistically significant only for eight-month data in multiparas. Results at three years and later did not mirror this earlier effect.

Propriomazine (Table 17-11) was almost without any discernible impact on the fetus based on these analyses. The only exception appeared in the frequency of neonatal depression in nulliparas given the drug in the latent phase (also perhaps reflected in the neonatal death rate for the same subset). Triflupromazine, which had previously been shown to have an apparently invidious effect across the range of outcomes (chapter 16), again showed that all adverse impact was limited exclusively to multiparous subgroups (Table 17-12). It was present with both latent and active phase administration. Nearly all subsets here, however, became so small that it was difficult to formulate acceptable conclusions from the analytical results. The data were, nonetheless, prepared for completeness with appropriate caveats as to their probable lack of validity.

The same constraints applied, only more so, to exposure to all other tranquilizers (Table 17-13). Among them, poor eight-month outcomes appeared to be associated with administration in either latent or active phase. In addition, latent phase exposure also enhanced neonatal depresssion in both nulliparas and multiparas, and active phase exposure augmented low eight-month mental and motor scores.

173

Table 17-9
Outcome by Promethazine Usage Time Frames

Labor Phase	Parity	No.	SB	NND	APG5	MENT8	MOT8	SLH3
Latent phase only								
	Nulliparas	121	1.13	1.04	0.00*	1.61	0.00	0.66
	Multiparas	122	0.00	1.50	1.56	0.00	0.00	0.51
Active phase only								
	Nulliparas	360	0.00*	0.70	1.90*	2.88*	1.68	0.22*
	Multiparas	301	1.13	1.21	1.38	1.51	1.36	1.17
Latent and active phases								
	Nulliparas	25	6.22	0.00	2.75	0.00	0.00	0.00
	Multiparas	43	0.00	0.00	0.00	0.00	0.00	0.00
All latent phase usage								
	Nulliparas	146	2.82	0.88	0.43	1.34	0.00	0.61
	Multiparas	166	0.00	1.07	1.11	0.00	0.00	0.44
All active phase usage								
	Nulliparas	385	0.72	0.66	1.95*	2.69*	1.57	0.25*
	Multiparas	349	0.98	1.05	1.19	1.30	1.18	1.07
All promethazine usage								
	Nulliparas	537	0.80	0.73	1.56	2.73*	1.54	0.35*
	Multiparas	482	0.71	1.52	1.41	0.90	0.83	0.96

* $p < 0.05$.

Table 17-10
Outcome by Hydroxyzine Usage Time Frames

Labor Phase	Parity	No.	SB	NND	APG5	MENT8	MOT8	SLH3
Latent phase only								
	Nulliparas	35	0.00	0.00	1.49	0.00	0.00	0.00
	Multiparas	31	0.00	0.00	1.19	0.00	0.00	1.99
Active phase only								
	Nulliparas	80	1.71	1.58	1.30	2.60	2.39	0.78
	Multiparas	64	0.00	2.86	2.35	6.76*	6.36*	0.72
All latent phase usage								
	Nulliparas	39	0.00	0.00	1.34	0.00	0.00	0.00
	Multiparas	46	0.00	0.00	0.80	0.00	0.00	1.50
All active phase usage								
	Nulliparas	84	1.63	1.52	1.24	2.52	2.32	0.76
	Multiparas	80	0.00	2.28	1.87	5.47	5.07	0.61
All hydroxyzine usage								
	Nulliparas	122	1.12	1.03	1.28	1.72	1.56	0.52
	Multiparas	116	0.00	2.15	1.61	3.67	3.31	0.98

* $p < 0.05$.

Table 17-11
Outcome by Propriomazine Usage Time Frames

Labor Phase	Parity	No.	SB	NND	APG5	MENT8	MOT8	SLH3
Latent phase only								
	Nulliparas	33	0.00	3.83	3.67*	0.00	0.00	1.38
	Multiparas	15	0.00	0.00	0.00	0.00	0.00	1.27
Active phase only								
	Nulliparas	64	0.00	0.00	1.92	0.00	0.00	1.28
	Multiparas	57	0.00	0.00	1.30	0.00	0.00	0.00
All latent phase usage								
	Nulliparas	36	0.00	3.41	3.36	0.00	0.00	1.19
	Multiparas	26	0.00	0.00	0.00	0.00	0.00	0.87
All active phase usage								
	Nulliparas	68	0.00	0.00	1.83	0.00	0.00	1.19
	Multiparas	68	0.00	0.00	1.09	0.00	0.00	0.00
All propriomazine usage								
	Nulliparas	102	0.00	1.24	2.42	0.00	0.00	1.25
	Multiparas	86	0.00	0.00	0.86	0.00	0.00	0.39

* $p < 0.05$.

Table 17-12
Outcome by Triflupromazine Usage Time Frames

Labor Phase	Parity	No.	SB	NND	APG5	MENT8	MOT8	SLH3
Latent phase only								
	Nulliparas	23	0.00	0.00	0.00	0.00	0.00	0.00
	Multiparas	15	0.00	0.00	2.47	0.00	21.63*	0.00
Active phase only								
	Nulliparas	38	0.00	0.00	0.00	0.00	0.00	0.00
	Multiparas	48	0.00	7.61*	2.41	0.00	8.54*	0.00
All latent phase usage								
	Nulliparas	29	0.00	0.00	0.00	0.00	0.00	0.00
	Multiparas	24	0.00	0.00	3.09	0.00	13.52*	0.00
All active phase usage								
	Nulliparas	44	0.00	0.00	0.00	0.00	0.00	0.00
	Multiparas	58	0.00	6.30*	2.64*	0.00	6.76*	0.00
All triflupromazine usage								
	Nulliparas	68	0.00	0.00	0.00	0.00	0.00	0.00
	Multiparas	72	0.00	4.94*	2.57*	0.00	10.14*	0.00

* $p < 0.05$.

Table 17-13
Outcome by Other Tranquilizer Usage Time Frames

Labor Phase Parity	No.	SB	NND	APG5	MENT8	MOT8	SLH3
Latent phase only							
Nulliparas	9	0.00	0.00	6.72*	0.00	0.00	0.00
Multiparas	12	0.00	0.00	3.09	0.00	40.55*	2.79
Active phase only							
Nulliparas	23	0.00	0.00	0.00	10.08*	9.18*	0.00
Multiparas	23	0.00	0.00	0.00	17.23*	0.00	0.00
All latent phase usage							
Nulliparas	13	0.00	0.00	4.65	0.00	0.00	0.00
Multiparas	19	0.00	0.00	3.90*	0.00	21.63*	2.33
All active phase usage							
Nulliparas	26	0.00	0.00	0.00	8.49*	7.80*	0.00
Multiparas	29	0.00	0.00	1.19	13.26	0.00	0.00
All other tranquilizer usage							
Nulliparas	45	0.00	0.00	1.48	5.20	5.04	0.00
Multiparas	48	0.00	0.00	1.54	8.84*	8.32*	0.87

* $p < 0.05$.

Barbiturate Effect by Time

Moving on to the barbiturates, we utilized this sharply focused paradigm for examining those agents administered with sufficient frequency to permit us to derive useful information. Specifically, this meant that secobarbital could be examined in most detail, but the others only somewhat sketchily according to available clusters of drug usage. When stratified by time in labor when the drug had been given, even secobarbital did not yield all subsets of adequate population size. For example, second stage usage was negligible (only eight cases in all).

The outcome data for secobarbital (Table 17-14) revealed apparent protection in the three-year communications testing vehicle when drug administration was either in latent or active phase, but the data failed to achieve statistical significance. In nulliparas, there was some increase in neonatal depression (not significantly so, however) if secobarbital had been given in the latent phase and, to a lesser extent, in the active phase as well. Significantly increased rates of eight-month abnormalities were disclosed among

those given this drug in the active phase; however, as just noted, the effect did not persist into the three-year tests. The possible causes of these apparently paradoxical effects remained to be elucidated.

Outcome data pertaining to pentobarbital usage (Table 17-15) mirrored those of secobarbital. They also showed some protective impact at three years (again not significant) in cases in which drug had been given in the active phase. There was some increased neonatal depression as well (not significant) associated with latent phase use in nulliparas. Latent phase administration in multiparas yielded poor eight-month results. When given in the active phase, contrary to expectations, effects were negligible except for an insignificant increase in abnormal eight-month results.

Phenobarbital, by contrast, was associated with poor outcomes in both short-term and long-term tests (Table 17-16). It must be emphasized, however, that the samples here had become very small. Caution must be exercised when interpreting such data because validity is dubious.

176

Table 17-14
Outcome by Secobarbital Usage Time Frames

Labor Phase	Parity	No.	SB	NND	APG5	MENT8	MOT8	SLH3
Latent phase only								
	Nulliparas	218	1.89	1.74	1.70	0.93	0.00	0.57
	Multiparas	274	1.23	0.67	0.97	2.93	0.00	0.44
Active phase only								
	Nulliparas	254	1.08	0.50	1.24	3.26*	4.20*	0.45
	Multiparas	188	1.81	0.00	1.03	2.27	2.11	0.20
Latent and active phases								
	Nulliparas	17	0.00	0.00	0.00	0.00	0.00	0.00
	Multiparas	37	0.00	0.00	1.03	0.00	0.00	0.93
All latent phase usage								
	Nulliparas	235	1.75	1.61	1.58	0.86	0.00	0.50
	Multiparas	314	1.08	0.58	0.97	2.59	0.00	0.50
All active phase usage								
	Nulliparas	271	1.01	0.47	1.17	3.03*	3.89*	0.40
	Multiparas	226	1.50	0.00	1.01	1.84	1.74	0.32
All secobarbital usage								
	Nulliparas	581	1.42	0.87	1.50	2.14	2.16	0.48
	Multiparas	585	1.45	0.63	1.04	2.12	0.65	0.46*

* $p < 0.05$.

Table 17-15
Outcome by Pentobarbital Usage Time Frames

Labor Phase	Parity	No.	SB	NND	APG5	MENT8	MOT8	SLH3
Latent phase only								
	Nulliparas	68	0.00	1.86	1.86	0.00	0.00	1.05
	Multiparas	100	1.70	0.00	1.16	4.25	7.82*	1.03
Active phase only								
	Nulliparas	103	0.00	1.23	0.62	1.88	0.00	0.75
	Multiparas	119	1.43	1.54	0.95	0.00	0.00	0.48
All latent phase usage								
	Nulliparas	70	0.00	1.80	2.71	0.00	0.00	1.05
	Multiparas	120	1.41	0.00	1.31	3.48	6.49*	1.69
All active phase usage								
	Nulliparas	105	0.00	1.20	1.22	1.85	0.00	0.75
	Multiparas	138	1.23	1.32	1.11	0.00	0.00	1.23
All phenobarbital usage								
	Nulliparas	196	0.51	1.29	1.29	1.09	0.00	0.73
	Multiparas	257	1.32	0.71	1.20	1.63	3.12	1.04

* $p < 0.05$.

Table 17-16
Outcome by Phenobarbital Usage Time Frames

Labor Phase Parity	No.	SB	NND	APG5	MENT8	MOT8	SLH3
Latent phase only							
Nulliparas	11	0.00	0.00	0.00	0.00	0.00	5.97*
Multiparas	20	0.00	9.14*	4.11*	21.54*	20.28*	2.33
Active phase only							
Nulliparas	12	0.00	0.00	0.00	0.00	0.00	0.00
Multiparas	30	0.00	0.00	4.94*	16.41*	14.75*	2.79
All latent phase usage							
Nulliparas	11	0.00	0.00	0.00	0.00	0.00	5.79*
Multiparas	23	7.72*	8.31*	5.55*	40.55*	38.17*	2.33
All active phase usage							
Nulliparas	12	0.00	0.00	0.00	0.00	0.00	0.00
Multiparas	33	5.14	0.00	5.79*	31.33*	28.21*	2.79
All phenobarbital usage							
Nulliparas	59	0.00	2.10	1.70	3.23	3.29	0.75
Multiparas	110	3.09	3.32	3.11*	11.75*	10.94*	2.51*

* $p < 0.05$.

Although the number of nulliparas to whom the drug had been given was relatively small, late results at three years were particularly bad, especially if the drug had been given in the latent phase. Similarly, in multiparas, significantly poor outcomes were encountered quite consistently for latent and active phase administration. Noteworthy were the adverse effects of increased neonatal death among those with drug given in the latent phase and still worse outcome results at eight months for both latent and active phase usage.

Again, the possible confounding effects of other factors deserved consideration here. As noted earlier, it was certainly conceivable, for example, that this agent was used preferentially in gravidas exhibiting preeclamptic diatheses; such hypertensive episodes have a documented adverse impact on infant well-being that cannot be directly attributable to the drug used to treat the hypertension. Coupled with the expected instability of the data based on small sample size, these observations make suspect any conclusion as to the possible effect this drug may have had on the offspring.

Antibiotic Effects by Time

The poor outcomes associated with antibiotic usage in labor, previously shown so graphically (chapter 16), were repeated when the data were divided according to the time in labor when these agents were given (Table 17-17). Equivalent effects were seen whether they were administered in the latent or the active phase of labor. Too few cases had second stage involvement (one nullipara and seven multiparas) to permit any form of study. The magnitude and pervasive nature of the adverse results strongly suggested the truth of our earlier conjecture concerning the likelihood that they reflected the effects of serious underlying disease rather than those of the drug itself.

Hypotensive Agent Effects by Time

Magnesium sulfate, studied in the same way (Table 17-18), yielded little new information. The data stratified by time frame, however, did show that active phase use

178

Table 17-17
Outcome by Antibiotic Usage Time Frames

Labor Phase	Parity	No.	SB	NND	APG5	MENT8	MOT8	SLH3
Latent phase only								
	Nulliparas	29	14.15*	0.00	7.56*	7.68*	7.89*	2.56
	Multiparas	20	0.00	9.14*	3.70*	20.27*	0.00	0.00
Active phase only								
	Nulliparas	25	0.00	5.05	5.04*	0.00	0.00	4.48*
	Multiparas	44	3.86	4.15	2.52	0.00	0.00	0.95
All latent phase usage								
	Nulliparas	31	13.27*	0.00	6.98*	7.01*	7.17*	2.24
	Multiparas	30	0.00	6.09*	3.70*	29.97*	14.75*	0.00
All active phase usage								
	Nulliparas	33	0.00	4.68	4.65*	0.00	0.00	3.64*
	Multiparas	53	3.14	3.38	2.74*	8.41*	7.54*	0.84
All antibiotic usage								
	Nulliparas	90	6.16*	2.90	4.32*	4.96*	5.09*	3.46*
	Multiparas	102	1.68	3.58	2.18*	12.46*	3.91	0.54

* p < 0.05.

Table 17-18
Outcome by Magnesium Sulfate Usage Time Frames

Labor Phase	Parity	No.	SB	NND	APG5	MENT8	MOT8	SLH3
Latent phase only								
	Nulliparas	21	0.00	0.00	0.00	0.00	0.00	0.00
	Multiparas	30	0.00	0.00	0.00	0.00	0.00	1.75
Active phase only								
	Nulliparas	26	0.00	0.00	2.33	0.00	0.00	2.98
	Multiparas	57	0.00	0.00	1.30	7.66*	6.62*	0.73
All latent phase usage								
	Nulliparas	23	0.00	0.00	0.00	10.08*	0.00	0.00
	Multiparas	40	0.00	0.00	0.00	0.00	0.00	1.55
All active phase usage								
	Nulliparas	28	0.00	0.00	2.16	8.49*	0.00	2.75
	Multiparas	71	0.00	0.00	1.07	5.94*	5.15	1.16
All magnesium sulfate usage								
	Nulliparas	53	0.00	0.00	1.16	4.36	0.00	1.70
	Multiparas	114	1.49	1.60	0.99	7.41*	6.55*	1.27

* p < 0.05.

Neither reserpine nor Apresoline had been given to enough patients in this project to provide a sufficiently ample database to satisfy the needs of this type of fragmentation analysis.

Belladonna Alkaloid Effects by Time

Hyoscine was administered to large numbers, as previously reported (chapter 15). The same applied, but to a lesser degree, to atropine as well. We had previously uncovered an apparently protective effect from scopolamine (chapter 16). Stratification of scopolamine outcome data by phase of labor (Table 17-19) showed this ostensible benefit to be concentrated among cases in which the drug had been given in the active phase. Indeed, a previously undetected adverse effect was disclosed for latent phase usage in several of the outcome variables we studied, including neonatal death and depression as well as abnormal eight-month and three-year test results (achieving statistical significance only in the last subset for nulliparas).

For atropine (Table 17-20), the high frequencies of neonatal depression seen before were replicated throughout the time frames examined, becoming increasingly noteworthy the later in labor it was given. Thus, giving atropine in the latent phase only increased the numbers of depressed newborn infants somewhat, but not significantly so and only in nulliparas. In the active

Table 17-19
Outcome by Scopolamine Usage Time Frames

Labor Phase	Parity	No.	SB	NND	APG5	MENT8	MOT8	SLH3
Latent phase only								
	Nulliparas	129	0.00	0.00	1.46	1.65	1.64	2.98*
	Multiparas	77	0.00	4.21	1.50	5.47	0.00	2.07
Active phase only								
	Nulliparas	493	1.39	0.52	0.65	1.28	0.86	0.63
	Multiparas	354	0.48	0.92	0.43	0.00	1.19	0.59
Latent and active phases								
	Nulliparas	87	0.00	0.00	2.19	0.00	0.00	0.00
	Multiparas	131	0.00	0.00	1.75	3.10	5.74*	0.00
Second stage only								
	Nulliparas	11	0.00	0.00	0.00	0.00	0.00	0.00
	Multiparas	13	0.00	0.00	2.85	0.00	0.00	0.00
All latent phase usage								
	Nulliparas	217	0.00	0.00	1.74	0.97	0.95	2.47
	Multiparas	229	0.74	1.42	1.68	3.53	3.31	1.12
All active phase usage								
	Nulliparas	580	1.17	0.43	0.88	1.07	0.71	0.61
	Multiparas	529	0.64	0.61	0.79	0.84	2.31	0.44
All second stage usage								
	Nulliparas	17	0.00	0.00	0.00	0.00	0.00	0.00
	Multiparas	60	2.83	0.00	1.28	0.00	0.00	0.00
All scopolamine usage								
	Nulliparas	735	0.93	0.34	0.95	1.14	0.85	0.98
	Multiparas	628	0.54	1.03	0.91	1.40	1.94	0.75

* $p < 0.05$.

Table 17-20
Outcome by Atropine Usage Time Frames

Labor Phase	Parity	No.	SB	NND	APG5	MENT8	MOT8	SLH3
Latent phase only								
	Nulliparas	24	0.00	5.26	2.52	0.00	0.00	7.16*
	Multiparas	14	0.00	0.00	0.00	0.00	0.00	0.00
Active phase only								
	Nulliparas	97	2.83	0.00	2.57*	4.42*	2.16	0.00
	Multiparas	103	1.65	0.00	2.18*	0.00	0.00	1.27
Second stage only								
	Nulliparas	9	0.00	0.00	13.44*	0.00	0.00	0.00
	Multiparas	18	0.00	0.00	1.76	0.00	0.00	0.00
All latent phase usage								
	Nulliparas	24	0.00	5.26	2.52	0.00	0.00	7.16*
	Multiparas	23	0.00	0.00	1.95	0.00	0.00	0.00
All active phase usage								
	Nulliparas	97	2.83	0.00	2.57*	4.42*	2.16	0.00
	Multiparas	112	1.52	0.00	2.67*	0.00	0.00	1.16
All second stage usage								
	Nulliparas	9	0.00	0.00	13.44*	0.00	0.00	0.00
	Multiparas	22	0.00	0.00	1.76	0.00	0.00	0.00
All atropine usage								
	Nulliparas	140	2.96*	0.92	3.11*	3.01	1.46	1.56
	Multiparas	146	1.16	0.00	2.09*	0.00	0.00	0.87

* $p < 0.05$.

phase, the increase was quite significant in both nulliparas and multiparas. The impact, reflected in the rate ratio, rose sharply (and proved very significant despite the very small sample size) when atropine was given in the second stage. Other scattered flags pertaining to high rates of stillbirths and abnormal eight-month and three-year outcomes did not appear to represent consistent effects related to atropine usage.

Uterotonic Effects by Time

Uterotonic stimulation was also fractionated temporally to try to clarify our prior paradoxical results (chapter 16). Syntocinon (Table 17-21) again appeared to have some late protective effect, but it was not significant and it appeared to be limited principally to late labor usage. That is to say, second stage exposure yielded no adverse three-year outcomes, whereas earlier usage in labor did not. By contrast, isolated untoward effects were found that had not previously been detected, such as the significantly increased neonatal death and depression rates in multiparas exposed in the active phase. The high neonatal mortality was repeated in the second stage subset for multiparas (but the rate ratio was not significant). These results deserved our special attention even though they might well have represented spurious observations.

Oxytocin (Pitocin) usage, when similarly stratified by time (Table 17-22), showed parallel results in general. There were relatively poor immediate outcomes, especially reflected in the frequency of low Apgar scores (none achieving statistical significance, however). The stillbirth data, cited earlier (chapter 16) for multiparas, was found to be strictly limited to latent phase

181

Table 17-21
Outcome by Syntocinon Usage Time Frames

Labor Phase	Parity	No.	SB	NND	APG5	MENT8	MOT8	SLH3
Latent phase only								
	Nulliparas	90	3.05	0.00	0.70	0.00	0.00	0.90
	Multiparas	79	2.15	0.00	1.42	5.56	0.00	0.78
Active phase only								
	Nulliparas	94	1.46	0.00	0.66	2.04	2.10	1.49
	Multiparas	116	1.49	4.73*	2.62*	0.00	3.23	1.12
Latent and active phases								
	Nulliparas	40	3.43	0.00	3.10	0.00	0.00	0.00
	Multiparas	52	0.00	0.00	1.45	8.21*	0.00	2.79
Second stage only								
	Nulliparas	40	0.00	0.00	0.00	4.74	4.51	0.00
	Multiparas	38	0.00	4.81	0.97	0.00	0.00	0.00
All latent phase usage								
	Nulliparas	133	3.09*	0.00	1.88	0.00	0.00	0.69
	Multiparas	145	1.17	0.00	1.29	5.94*	0.00	1.16
All active phase usage								
	Nulliparas	141	1.95	0.00	1.74	1.43	1.46	1.19
	Multiparas	190	0.89	2.86	1.97*	2.20	2.00	1.31
All second stage usage								
	Nulliparas	48	0.00	0.00	1.26	3.93	3.76	0.00
	Multiparas	67	0.00	2.69	0.54	0.00	0.00	0.00
All Syntocinon usage								
	Nulliparas	366	1.50	0.35	1.18	1.65	1.10	0.46
	Multiparas	346	1.47	2.10	1.51	2.42	1.12	0.77

* p < 0.05.

usage of this agent. This supported a contention that it was probably used for inducing or stimulating a labor with known intrauterine fetal death rather than that the drug somehow caused the death. Nonetheless, this could not readily explain the high (albeit insignificant) neonatal death rates in nulliparas (nor the analogous late findings of significantly increased three-year speech, language, and hearing abnormalities), unless one could conjecture that the oxytocin had been given preferentially to especially high-risk gravidas whose fetuses were in jeopardy by virtue of the concurrent maternal condition.

Despite the diminishing numbers of cases in the various subsets of the oxytocin data matrix, it was of interest to note that the analytical approach we used was capable of uncovering these potentially important relationships. Less encouragingly, the sample sizes became unacceptably small for sparteine use. Although the detailed analysis was done for this drug, it is not reported here because the results (all essentially negative in terms of the kinds of outcomes described above) could not be considered even remotely reliable.

Summary of Drug Effects by Time

To provide an overview of these rather detailed and perhaps confusing data, a summary listing is presented (Table 17-23). We feel constrained to reiterate that the drug

Table 17-22
Outcome by Oxytocin Usage Time Frames

Labor Phase	Parity	No.	SB	NND	APG5	MENT8	MOT8	SLH3
Latent phase only								
	Nulliparas	37	0.00	0.00	1.68	0.00	0.00	3.77*
	Multiparas	10	16.98*	0.00	0.00	0.00	0.00	0.00
Active phase only								
	Nulliparas	26	0.00	0.00	2.33	0.00	0.00	0.00
	Multiparas	25	0.00	0.00	1.48	0.00	0.00	0.00
All latent phase usage								
	Nulliparas	47	0.00	2.69	1.31	0.00	0.00	4.26*
	Multiparas	22	8.08*	0.00	1.85	0.00	0.00	0.00
All active phase usage								
	Nulliparas	36	0.00	3.51	1.68	0.00	0.00	1.79
	Multiparas	37	0.00	0.00	2.06	0.00	0.00	0.00
All Pitocin usage								
	Nulliparas	113	2.43	1.13	1.61	0.00	0.00	2.98*
	Multiparas	68	7.49*	0.00	1.74	0.00	0.00	0.47

* $p < 0.05$.

Table 17-23
Summary of Temporally Related Drug Effects*

| Agent | Time Frame of Drug Usage | | |
	Latent phase	Active phase	Second stage
Meperidine	Negligible	Moderately adverse	Adverse
Alphaprodine	Protective	Protective	-
Promazine	Mixed	Protective	Protective
Promethazine	Negligible	Mixed	-
Hydroxyzine	Negligible	Adverse	-
Propriomazine	Adverse	Negligible	-
Triflupromazine	Adverse	Adverse	-
Other tranquilizers	Adverse	Adverse	-
Secobarbital	Mixed	Mixed	-
Pentobarbital	Mixed	Negligible	-
Phenobarbital	Adverse	Adverse	-
Antibiotics	Adverse	Adverse	-
Magnesium sulfate	Negligible	Adverse	-
Hyoscine	Adverse	Protective	Protective
Atropine	Adverse	Adverse	Adverse
Syntocinon	Mixed	Adverse	Mixed
Oxytocin	Mixed	Adverse	-

* Stated effects here must be understood as not taking into account any confounding factors that could be expected to affect the fetus. Adverse, significantly poor results documented; Protective, significantly better outcome than expected; Mixed, inconsistent outcome results, some good and some bad; Negligible, no apparent outcome trend identified; blank, sample size inadequate.

effects must be considered to reflect an association rather than a cause-and-effect relationship. If is, of course, possible that some of the outcomes we found do represent the direct effects of the drugs acting on the fetus. Indeed, it is likely in some instances, such as the depressive effects of late labor administration of Demerol on the newborn infants. For others, however, we must not be tempted to jump prematurely to an inappropriate conclusion about the fetal impact of these agents until other relevant confounding factors are considered in perspective.

Our next undertaking in the pursuit of the goals of this endeavor was to try to discriminate, from among the various pharmacologic agents under study, those drugs that place the fetus and infant at greatest relative risk and to quantitate that risk. This was to be done while simultaneously taking into account concomitant use of other agents, a matter we have not heretofore dealt with at all except by way of commentary concerning the prescribing habit patterns of practicing obstetricians. We noted, for example, that tranquilizers were commonly used (not inappropriately) in conjunction with narcotic analgesics for their synergistic effects, making it rather difficult to separate the effect of one from that of the other (except perhaps intuitively). In addition, there was a demonstrated need for temporal consideration as herein described, bearing in mind the sometimes clear distinctions between the effects of a drug when given early in labor versus its effects when given late. The degree of analytical sophistication required for this increasing complex problem was apparent.

CHAPTER 18

Adjunctive Drugs: Designation of Risk Variables

Summary

The analytical sequence of bivariate, cluster, and logistic regression analyses was pursued to identify those pharmacologic agents and anesthesias significantly associated with poor results to offspring. The large numbers of drug-related variables were collapsed into a series of 45 items. Only cases yielding nonanomalous infants weighing 2500 to 4000 g were included for study. Outcomes were coalesced as well. Seventeen of the original adjunctive drug variables were determined to retain a statistically significant impact on results when the effects of all others were weighed concurrently.

The paradigm used to evaluate the labor progression variables, as detailed extensively in chapter 14, was invoked here for purposes of identifying those agents that were significantly related to adverse fetal/infant outcomes. Screening analyses were undertaken by the Freeman-Tukey nonparametric technique (chapter 7). Those variables identified by this approach were then scrutinized by cluster analysis (see p 42) to determine if any were interrelated and showed similarity of informational content. This was done to eliminate redundant variables and thereby reduce the number left to be examined by multivariate techniques. Logistic regression methods were then utilized to study the selected adjunctive drug variables simultaneously so as to assess which of them carried significant independent adverse effects.

The gamut of drugs administered to patients in labor was examined. These agents included all those reviewed in chapter 15, such as analgesics, anesthetics, and uterotonic agents. As will be recalled, there were 123 identified pharmacologic products, only 37 of which had been given often enough within the course of labor to permit meaningful analysis (see Table 15-2). To these were added oxytocin (Table 15-6) and anesthetic agents (Tables 15-7 and 15-8).

From the foregoing series of exploratory analyses, it had become increasingly clear that any adverse effects of the many different specific pharmacologic agents could not be studied in greater depth because the subsets dwindled to such small size as a consequence of the necessary stratifications. This was especially apparent in our attempts to assess effects of individual drugs (see chapter 16) in isolation and on the basis of temporal considerations, that is, in relation to the time in labor when the agent was administered (see chapter 17).

Accordingly, we tried to enhance our efforts by concentrating the data for related group variables, merging Pitocin use with Syntocinon use, for example. Similarly, all agents given for a different form of anesthetic block were collapsed into a single variable to address the possible impact of the anesthetic method rather than the anesthetic agent used to produce the block. Commonly used analgesics, tranquilizers, and antibiotics were left as single variables, but those used less often were pooled together. This operation created seven variables for uterotonic agents, 13 for anesthesias, and 25 for all other drugs, for a total of 45 codified items for study. These isolated and composite variables for the range of adjunctive drugs, including oxytocin and anesthesia, are defined in Table 18-1.

The population to be studied was made homogeneous by stratification according to parity (that is, nulliparas and multiparas), by deletion of those delivering infants with anomalies incompatible with survival or with normal neurologic development and growth (Table 14-2), and by restricting the investigation at this point to cases with infants of birth weights in the 2500 to 4000 g range. The rationale for this operation was the same as that presented in chapter 14. The residual index population consisted of 6688 nulliparas and 8481 multiparas, all with reliable information pertaining not only to the labor progression, but also to the adjunctive drugs used in labor and the infant outcomes.

The numerous outcome variables were collapsed as before into three collective outcomes, namely perinatal (death and severe neonatal depression), infant (8-month and 1-year neurologic and psychological abnormalities), and childhood (disorders or defects at ages 3, 4, and 7 years) adverse results. In addition, a single composite "union" outcome variable was constructed to flag any infant adversely affected at any time over the course of the project (definite abnormalities only).

Screening Analysis

The index populations thus derived were subjected to Freeman-Tukey nonparametric bivariate analysis to identify those variables most likely to affect the fetus and infant. The resultant Freeman-Tukey deviates (FTD) served to identify items of interest for further study, and the associated rate ratios (RR) provided a measure of the magnitude of the apparent effect on the offspring. We addressed the large number of drug-related variables in two phases, arbitrarily considering oxytocin and anesthetics first and all others subsequently. Later cluster and logistic regression analyses dealt with the entire range of drugs together.

Table 18-2 illustrates the kind of data output from this form of analysis. Infants delivered of mothers under paracervical block (code PARAC, see Table 18-1) were examined to verify the recognized adverse effects of this form of anesthesia. As expected, the analysis confirmed the

186

Table 18-1
Adjunctive Drugs and Anesthesias Defined

Variable Code	Definition
OXYT0	Oxytocin not used
OXYT1	Oxytocin induction of labor
OXYT2	Oxytocin augmentation of labor
ONSET1	Spontaneous onset of labor
ONSET2	Induced onset of labor
SPINAL	Spinal anesthesia (includes saddle block)
CAUDAL	Caudal block anesthesia
EPIDUR	Epidural block anesthesia
LOCAL	Local infiltration block anesthesia
PUDEND	Pudendal block anesthesia
PARAC	Paracervical block anesthesia
NOBLOCK	No regional anesthesia administered
NOGAS	No gaseous inhalation agent used for anesthesia
GAS1	Gaseous agent used intermittently
GAS2	Gaseous agent used continuously
GAS3	Gaseous agent used both intermittently and continuously
IVD0	No intravenous anesthetic agent used
IVD1	Intravenous anesthetic agent given
AGT1	Meperidine, Demerol, Pethadol
AGT2	Alphaprodine, Nisentil
AGT3	Prinadol, phenazocine
AGT4	Lorfan, levallorphan
AGT5	Morphine sulfate
AGT6	Achromycin
AGT7	Penicillin
AGT8	Streptomycin
AGT9	Chloramphenicol
AGT10	Sulfisoxazole, Gantrisin
AGT11	Secobarbital
AGT12	Pentobarbital sodium, Carbrital
AGT13	Phenobarbital
AGT14	Promazine, Sparine
AGT15	Phenergan, promethazine
AGT16	Hydroxyzine, Atarax, Vistaril
AGT17	Propiomazine, Largon
AGT18	Triflupromazine, Vesprin
AGT19	Hyoscine, scopolamine
AGT20	Atropine
AGT21	Reserpine
AGT22	Apresoline
AGT23	Syntocinon
AGT24	Oxytocin, Pitocin
AGT25	Sparteine sulfate
AGT26	Magnesium sulfate
AGT27	Other antibiotics
AGT28	Other ataractic agents

Table 18-2
Outcome for Cases Delivered under Paracervical Block[a]

Adverse Outcome	No.	Observed Rate, %	Expected Rate, %	RR	z-Statistic	p-Value
Perinatal						
Definite	298	4.36	2.40	1.82[b]	2.215[b]	0.027
Suspect	316	9.81	6.13	1.60[b]	2.726[b]	0.0064
Infancy						
Definite	249	2.01	2.61	0.77	-0.591	0.554
Suspect	274	10.94	13.57	0.81	-1.267	0.205
Childhood						
Definite	102	12.74	17.70	0.72	-1.311	0.190
Suspect	144	38.19	46.22	0.83	-1.932	0.053

[a] Based on 6,688 nulliparous deliveries resulting in infants weighing 2500–4000 g.

[b] Statistically significant, $p < 0.05$.

increased perinatal risk with FTD 2.215 for "definite" effects (death plus severe depression evidenced by five-minute Apgar scores 0-4) and FTD 2.726 for "suspect" effects (five-minute Apgar scores 5-7). Both were quite significant statistically with p values of .027 and .0064, respectively.

The rate ratios indicate that there were nearly twice the expected frequency of adverse perinatal effects. The rate ratio of 1.82 for definite adverse outcomes and rate ratio of 1.60 for suspect outcomes demonstrated that the increase or excess of effect was 81.7% and 60.0% greater than in the rest of the offspring of the general gravid population. It should be noted that the latter represented multiplier factors, not additive ones; this is to say, the observed 4.3% rate of perinatal death and depression was 81.7% times greater than the 2.4% expected rate.

The data shown in Table 18-2 indicate that the adverse impact of paracervical block, regardless of its apparent serious perinatal effect, does not seem to persist among surviving infants. Indeed, the late (childhood) suspect results fell just short of statistical significance as a protective variable (FTD = -1.932, p = .053). This might reflect that the intensity of effect was so great as to "cleanse" the surviving population of all infants who were deleteriously affected (by ensuring that few if any survived) or that other factors were confounding the results.

In this latter regard, it is possible, for example, that the paracervical block was utilized for delivery of gravidas who were essentially healthy with normal and uncomplicated pregnancy, labor, and delivery. If the infants of these women could be expected to do better than those of the general population, any residual effects of paracervical block on surviving infants may have been counterbalanced so that they would thereby no longer be apparent. This merely reemphasized the need for the multivariate analytic approach.

Bivariate screening was applied to the entire range of drug and anesthesia variables in both nulliparas and multiparas. The data for oxytocin and anesthesia are shown in Tables 18-3 and 18-4. The results for the rest of the drugs under investigation will be dealt with separately (see below). This division was arbitrary and done merely for

Table 18-3
Outcomes by Oxytocin and Anesthesia Use in Nulliparas*

Variable	Perinatal		Infancy		Childhood	
	Definite	Suspect	Definite	Suspect	Definite	Suspect
OXYT0	0.83	0.88a	0.96	0.98	0.98	1.00
OXYT1	0.00	1.63	0.00	0.76	1.07	0.69
OXYT2	1.57D	1.40F	0.95	0.92	0.90	1.02
OXYT3	0.91	1.15	2.03A	0.84	0.89	0.83
ONSET1	0.98	0.99	0.95	1.00	0.99	1.00
ONSET2	1.29	1.17	1.72A	0.87	1.23	0.98
SPINAL	0.64e	0.79d	0.91	1.00	1.01	1.03
CAUDAL	1.13	1.57A	1.06	1.04	1.27	1.17
EPIDUR	0.85	1.42	0.57	0.64a	1.04	1.09
LOCAL	1.03	1.15	0.76	1.01	0.77a	0.90a
PUDEND	1.33	1.24A	1.00	1.14	0.67d	0.79f
PARAC	1.82A	1.60B	0.77	0.80	0.72	0.83
NOBLOCK	1.88F	1.42D	1.58B	0.95	1.46C	1.17B
NOGAS	0.73c	0.86b	0.94	0.99	0.91	0.98
GAS1	0.99	0.71	1.20	1.10	0.95	1.02
GAS2	2.19F	1.74F	0.97	0.97	1.46D	1.09
GAS3	2.78E	1.67A	1.93	1.42	1.69A	1.08
IVD0	0.96	0.97	0.96	1.00	1.01	1.01
IVD1	5.61F	2.97E	1.78	0.50	0.35	0.62

* Data presented as rate ratios based on Freeman-Tukey screening analysis for midrange birthweight offspring of 6,688 nulliparas, coded for significant p-values:

Adverse relationships: A 0.05, B 0.01, C 0.005, D 0.001, E 0.0005, F 0.0001 or less.

Protective relationships: a 0.05, b 0.01, c 0.005, d 0.001, e 0.0005, f 0.0001 or less.

convenience. In nulliparas, significantly adverse perinatal results were associated with:

OXYT2, oxytocin augmentation of labor
CAUDAL, caudal block anesthesia
PUDEND, pudendal block anesthesia
PARAC, paracervical block anesthesia
NOBLOCK, no regional anesthesia administered
GAS2, continuously administered gaseous agent
GAS3, both intermittent and continuous gas given
IVD1, intravenous anesthetic agent given

These were confirmed or supplemented in nulliparas by infancy and childhood associa-

tions with the following variables:

OXYT3, combined induction and augmentation with oxytocin
ONSET2, induced labor (all forms)
NOBLOCK, no regional anesthesia used
GAS2, continuous gas anesthesia
GAS3, combined intermittent and continuous gas given

Verification or supplementation was provided in multiparas for infancy and childhood outcomes for:

OXYT1, oxytocin induction
OXYT2, oxytocin augmentation
EPIDUR, epidural anesthesia
NOBLOCK, no regional anesthesia
GAS1, intermittent gas anesthesia

Table 18-4
Outcomes by Oxytocin and Anesthesia Use in Multiparas*

Variable	Perinatal		Infancy		Childhood	
	Definite	Suspect	Definite	Suspect	Definite	Suspect
OXYT0	0.88	0.90	0.80c	0.93a	0.97	1.02
OXYT1	2.85D	1.73	1.18	1.69E	0.66	0.97
OXYT2	1.28	1.32A	1.18	0.86a	1.31A	0.99
OXYT3	1.77A	1.07	1.38	0.93	0.86	0.79b
ONSET1	0.93	0.97	0.98	0.98	1.00	1.00
ONSET2	1.68B	1.26	1.25	1.16	1.04	0.97
SPINAL	0.69a	1.01	0.69b	0.98	0.82	0.88d
CAUDAL	1.23	1.73A	1.05	0.95	0.65	0.81
EPIDUR	0.93	2.60D	2.47C	1.41A	0.95	0.93
LOCAL	0.92	1.26	1.44B	1.04	0.88	0.95
PUDEND	1.18	1.05	1.34C	1.01	1.10	0.96
PARAC	1.68	1.14	0.72	0.69a	1.03	1.00
NOBLOCK	1.07	0.86	0.91	0.99	1.08	1.11F
NOGAS	0.80a	0.94	1.04	1.02	0.93	0.93c
GAS1	1.01	0.87	0.87	1.02	1.04	1.06
GAS2	1.61D	1.24	1.07	1.01	1.19	1.13C
GAS3	1.42	1.31	0.69	0.71a	1.67A	1.34D
IVD0	0.99	0.98	1.01	1.00	1.01	1.00
IVD1	3.49B	2.75A	0.00	1.43	1.24	0.97

* Data and probability coding comparable to Table 18-3, for offspring of 8,481 multiparas.

GAS2, continuous gas anesthesia
GAS3, combined intermittent and continuous gas anesthesia

Protection appeared to be afforded in nulliparas by:

OXYT0, no exposure to oxytocin
SPINAL, spinal anesthesia
EPIDUR, epidural anesthesia (suspect outcomes only)
LOCAL, local infiltration anesthesia
NOGAS, no inhalation agent used

Similar protective effects were seen in nulliparas for:

SPINAL, spinal anesthesia
PARAC, paracervical block (suspect only)
NOGAS, no gas anesthesia used

Those variables demonstrating a clear relationship with definite adverse outcomes are tallied in Table 18-5 for clarification purposes. This list illustrates the areas of relatively consistent effect, such as for NOBLOCK (no regional block anesthesia), GAS2 and GAS3 (continuous administration of an inhalation agent with and without intermittent use), IVD1 (administration of an intravenous anesthetic agent). Consistency was also seen for the protective effects of SPINAL (spinal and saddle block anesthesia) and NOGAS (no exposure to inhalation anesthesia). Induction and augmentation of labor (OXYT1, OXYT2, OXYT3, and ONSET2) showed varying degrees of significantly adverse effects. Mixed results (both positive and negative outcomes) were encountered for LOCAL (local infiltration anesthesia) and PUDEND (pudendal block).

In view of the various degrees of homogeneity thus demonstrated, we proceeded to examine the data as related to the single composite outcome variable (see p 130). This was done to try to provide a means for identifying in a more consistent way those labor drug variables affecting the

190

population of fetuses and infants under surveillance. It was felt that reducing all definite adverse outcomes to a single index of bad outcome might serve this objective.

The screening analysis was repeated using the composite outcome variable to assess the overall impact of the oxytocin and anesthesia variables on the offspring. The data shown in Table 18-6 were derived. They documented the clear-cut risk asso-

Table 18-5
Significant Oxytocin and Anesthesia Variables by Screening Analysis*

| Variable | Nulliparas | | | Multiparas | | |
	Perinatal	Infancy	Childhood	Perinatal	Infancy	Childhood
OXYT0					0.80c	
OXYT1				2.85D		
OXYT2	1.57D					1.31A
OXYT3		2.03A		1.77A		
ONSET2		1.72A		1.68B		
SPINAL	0.64e			0.69a	0.69b	
EPIDUR					2.47C	
LOCAL			0.77a		1.44B	
PUDEND			0.67d		1.34C	
PARAC	1.82A					
NOBLOCK	1.88F	1.58B	1.46C			
NOGAS	0.73c			0.80a		
GAS2	2.19F		1.46D	1.61D		
GAS3	2.78E		1.69A			1.67A
IVD1	5.61F			3.49B		

* Probability code as in Table 18-3.

Table 18-6
Drug Effect for Oxytocin and Anesthesia as Reflected in Composite Outcome Variables

| Variable | Nulliparas | | | | Multiparas | | | |
	Rate	RR*	FTD	p	Rate	RR*	FTD	p
OXYT0	7.75	0.99	-0.19	0.84	7.93	0.94	-1.30	0.19
OXYT1	7.54	0.96	-0.08	0.94	11.85	1.41	1.43	0.15
OXYT2	7.27	0.93	-0.79	0.43	9.04	1.07	0.72	0.47
OXYT3	9.16	1.17	0.78	0.43	11.50	1.36	2.21	0.027
ONSET1	7.67	0.98	-0.48	0.63	8.22	0.98	-0.66	0.51
ONSET2	10.56	1.35	2.10	0.036	10.85	1.29	2.27	0.023
SPINAL	6.51	0.83	-3.09	0.0020	6.45	0.77	-3.32	0.00088
CAUDAL	9.68	1.24	1.08	0.28	8.24	0.98	-0.09	0.93
EPIDUR	8.70	1.11	0.53	0.59	12.96	1.54	1.69	0.090
LOCAL	7.91	1.01	0.07	0.94	10.07	1.19	1.82	0.069
PUDEND	8.2	1.05	0.47	0.64	10.58	1.26	3.46	0.00054
PARAC	8.98	1.15	0.78	0.44	10.57	1.25	1.16	0.24
NOBLOCK	11.11	1.42	3.82	0.00013	8.13	0.96	-0.64	0.52
NOGAS	6.84	0.87	-2.64	0.0082	8.08	0.96	-0.93	0.35
GAS1	8.84	1.13	0.76	0.44	9.04	1.07	0.79	0.43
GAS2	11.46	1.46	4.10	0.000041	9.52	1.13	1.52	0.13
GAS3	15.06	1.92	3.46	0.00053	7.94	0.94	-0.33	0.74
IVD0	7.74	0.99	-0.28	0.78	8.45	1.00	0.07	0.95
IVD1	14.52	1.85	1.96	0.050	11.63	1.38	0.75	0.45

* Risk ratio relative to referent rate of 7.83% for nulliparas and 8.43% for multiparas.

191

ciated with ONSET2 (all inductions), NOBLOCK (no regional block), GAS2 and GAS3 (continuous gas with and without intermittent use), and IVD1 (intravenous anesthesia) in nulliparas, plus ONSET2 and PUDEND (pudendal block) in multiparas. The protection from SPINAL (spinal anesthesia) and NOGAS (no exposure to gas anesthesia) was verified as well.

All the remaining 28 drug variables were assessed in the same manner by bivariate screening. The resulting data are shown in Table 18-7. Paradoxical results were encountered for narcotic analgesics. Demerol (AGT1) was associated with significantly adverse outcomes in nulliparas for both perinatal and composite variables; this was not duplicated in multiparas. In sharp contrast, the use of Nisentil in labor

(AGT2) appeared to be protective, significantly so in all subcategories of outcome except perinatal outcome in offspring of nulliparas. Phenazocine (AGT3) showed deleterious effects, but they did not reach statistical significance because the numbers of cases were not large. The effect of Lorfan (AGT4) was inconsistent, again because it was so seldom administered, achieving significance in nulliparas for perinatal outcome only.

Antibiotics were generally associated with poor results to the infant. Strong adverse effects were encountered for penicillin (AGT7), streptomycin (AGT8), and chloramphenicol (AGT9). Rather impressively bad outcomes occurred in multiparous cases given other antibiotics (AGT27). Deleterious effects were also seen after

Table 18-7
Outcome Results for Adjunctive Drugs by Parity*

| Variable | Perinatal | | Composite | |
	Nulliparas	Multiparas	Nulliparas	Multiparas
AGT1	1.37A	1.10	1.28B	1.03
AGT2	0.60	0.33a	0.59a	0.65a
AGT3	1.90	2.86	1.96	1.99
AGT4	3.33A	0.00	0.98	1.55
AGT5	2.78	0.00	1.77	0.00
AGT6	1.43	0.00	1.20	1.74
AGT7	3.47A	3.28A	1.96	1.65
AGT8	2.61	5.91C	2.02	2.13
AGT9	0.00	6.33A	4.25A	1.82
AGT10	0.00	0.00	2.13	3.19
AGT11	0.98	1.10	1.08	1.21
AGT12	1.06	0.56	1.08	0.73
AGT13	1.54	0.00	2.13D	1.13
AGT14	0.73	0.98	0.91	0.97
AGT15	1.16	0.75	1.20	0.94
AGT16	2.13A	0.47	1.96C	1.01
AGT17	0.61	1.64	1.06	1.19
AGT18	2.53A	0.00	1.82A	0.21a
AGT19	0.69	0.85	1.01	1.00
AGT20	2.03A	1.28	1.54A	1.14
AGT21	3.97A	0.00	1.53	1.28
AGT22	7.58D	0.00	2.74A	1.82
AGT23	1.09	0.78	1.04	0.68a
AGT24	3.27B	1.08	2.46D	1.54
AGT25	1.74	1.25	2.09B	1.19
AGT26	0.00	0.00	1.36	1.09
AGT27	0.00	14.77E	0.00	8.51E
AGT28	1.13	1.53	1.16	1.16

*   See Table 18-3 for probability code.

Achromycin, but they were not statistically significant. Use of sulfisoxazole (Gantrisin) (AGT10) did not appear to affect the perinatal results, but the composite outcome variable showed some degree (statistically insignificant) of long-term effect. It was not clear from these data whether the findings reflected the impact of the drug or, as is more likely, the influence of the infection for which the drug was used.

Barbiturates had negligible effects in general, especially secobarbital and pentobarbital (AGT11-12). However, there was some adverse effect related to phenobarbital use (AGT13) in nulliparas, but not multiparas; it reached significance for the composite outcome. Tranquilizers yielded mixed outcomes, most falling into the expected range. Only hydroxyzine (AGT16) and triflupromazine (AGT18) showed a significantly deleterious impact and this was limited exclusively to offspring of nulliparas; in both instances results for infants of exposed multiparas were quite good, significantly so in the composite outcome data for AGT18. Pooled ataractic data (AGT28) were poor in terms of outcome, but not at a significant level.

Scopolamine (AGT19) showed generally good results, whereas atropine (AGT20) yielded contrastingly bad ones, especially in nulliparas. Similarly, there were paradoxically good outcomes for Syntocinon (AGT23) and adverse results for Pitocin (AGT24); the former attained statistical significance in multiparas for composite outcome, the latter, in nulliparas for both outcome variables. Sparteine sulfate (AGT25) also showed bad results, significant only in nulliparas for the composite variable. Use of magnesium sulfate (AGT26) failed to demonstrate the effect expected from the condition of pregnancy-induced hypertension (PIH) for which it was given.

These findings supported the results of the preceding analyses to some extent, especially as regards the several variables thus shown to be consistently related to good and bad outcomes. In this manner we had arrived at the point at which these flagged variables could be studied in greater detail to determine possible confounding effects among them and to quantitate their relative impact on the fetus and infant.

Cluster Analysis

As had been done with the labor progression variables earlier (see chapter 14), cluster analysis was applied to those drug variables identified by bivariate screening to be associated with poor immediate or long-term outcomes for fetus and infant. The principles and technique were detailed in chapter 7 and the practical implementation and interpretation in chapter 14. Therefore, they need not be repeated here.

The results for the sequence of flagged adjunctive drug variables are shown in Figures 18-1 and 18-2 for nulliparas and multiparas, respectively, presenting 22 variables in nulliparas and 17 in multiparas. Clustering of adjunctive agents in nulliparas demonstrated no meaningful relationships at all in most cases. In some, the obvious and expected correlation was found between pairs of drugs and often given conjointly, such as penicillin and streptomycin (AGT7 and AGT8, $r = .634$), Demerol and atropine (AGT1 and AGT20, $r = .274$), and Nisentil and hydroxyzine (Vistaril) (AGT2 and AGT16, $r = .123$). Even among these pairs, however, the level of correlation was quite low.

The findings for oxytocin and anesthesia in multiparas can be dispensed with summarily. None of the variables examined showed any significant similarity to any other in regard to informational content. The only pair of variables even remotely related were SPINAL and PUDEND, but their intercorrelation was very low ($r = .309$), suggesting this was merely a chance occurrence. For nulliparas, a similar relationship (also statistically insignificant, $r = .500$), was disclosed for these two anesthesia variables insofar as their similarity of impact on the outcome was concerned.

A greater degree of similarity, this time

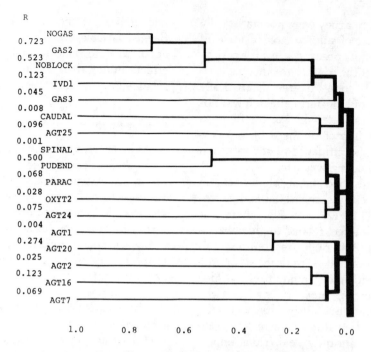

R

NOGAS	
0.723	
GAS2	
0.523	
NOBLOCK	
0.123	
IVD1	
0.045	
GAS3	
0.008	
CAUDAL	
0.096	
AGT25	
0.001	
SPINAL	
0.500	
PUDEND	
0.068	
PARAC	
0.028	
OXYT2	
0.075	
AGT24	
0.004	
AGT1	
0.274	
AGT20	
0.025	
AGT2	
0.123	
AGT16	
0.069	
AGT7	

```
1.0     0.8     0.6     0.4     0.2     0.0
```

Figure 18-1. Cluster analysis of adjunctive drug variables in nulliparas indicating the cluster of factors with greatest similarity of informational content as related to adverse outcome. Few items show any meaningful degree of intercluster correlation. The strongest relationship exists between AGT7 and AGT8 (penicillin and streptomycin). Position of branching on horizontal axis is proportional to correlation coefficient (R) between variables and cluster of variables.

verified as just achieving statistical significance (r = .723), was found between NOGAS and GAS2 (continuous administration of inhalation anesthesia). Given the intensity of apparent adverse association of GAS2, it seems logical that the protective aspects of NOGAS probably reflected the absence of the deleterious effects of the anesthesia. Thus, retaining the variable NOGAS could be considered somewhat superfluous or redundant in terms of some of its informational content. However, the level of similarity was not felt to be sufficiently high to warrant deletion of the variable at this time.

Despite our objective to reduce the number of variables for future consideration in the logistic regression model, we did not wish to omit consideration of any that might prove relevant, lest a potentially

important relationship to outcome be lost. As a consequence, all variables flagged by bivariate screening were passed through the cluster net to be evaluated by the multivariate techniques to follow. Each appeared to be acting independently of all others in regard to possible impact on outcome.

Logistic Regression Analysis

The details of the modelling technique have been reviewed in chapter 7 and its application to labor progression variables was shown in chapter 14. All oxytocin, anesthesia, and other drug variables were examined simultaneously to determine their relative impact as reflected in the composite outcome variable (all definite adverse outcomes collapsed into a single variable)

194

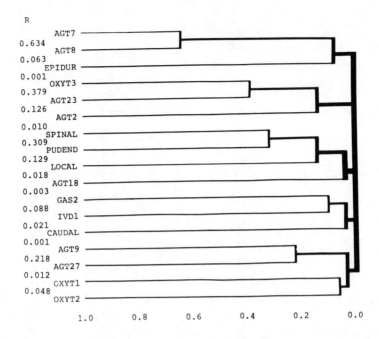

Figure 18-2. Cluster analysis tree for adjunctive drugs in multiparas. Close correlation is encountered for NOGAS and GAS2, and to a lesser extent for NOBLOCK. SPINAL and PUDEND are also correlated to a degree. AGT1 and AGT20 (Demerol and atropine) have similar informational content as well, but their correlation is not significant.

for offspring of nulliparas (Table 18-8) and of multiparas (Table 18-9).

The anesthesia variables determined to be particularly significant by this multivariate approach in nulliparas were SPINAL (significantly protective, RR = 0.77, p = .019), GAS2 and GAS3 (continuous and combined use, significantly adverse effects, RR 1.48 and 1.94, respectively, p .0043 and .0071). AGT16 (hydroxyzine) and AGT24 (oxytocin) were both associated with significantly bad effects (RR 1.96 and 2.45, p .037 and .021), whereas AGT2 (Nisentil) had a good effect (RR = 0.48, p = .014). For multiparas, the significant adverse variables were OXYT3 (combined induction and augmentation, RR = 1.86, p = .0012) and PUDEND (RR = 1.29, p = .0074). SPINAL was again significantly protective (RR = 0.75, p = .0087). OXYT1 (induction) fell short of statistical significance (RR = 1.62, p = .087), but AGT23 (Syntocinon) was quite protective (RR = 0.49, p = .019). AGT27

(antibiotics other than penicillin, streptomycin, and chloramphenicol) had very poor results (RR = 24.13, p = .026), probably reflecting the conditions for which they were given.

When assessed in the same manner for perinatal outcome (death or severe depression), other variables surfaced. For nulliparas (Table 18-10), SPINAL, GAS2, and GAS3 were found to be statistically significant. PARAC (paracervical block) fell just short of achieving statistical significance (RR = 1.93, p = .056). OXYT2 (augmentation use, RR = 1.93, p = .00085) and IVD1 (intravenous anesthesia, RR = 2.99, p = .017) also surfaced as important. No other drugs even approached significance except AGT22 (Apresoline) which did not quite reach the cut off level (RR = 8.41, p = .056).

For multiparas (Table 18-11), there were four significant variables. Only one was the same as before, OXYT3, although its magnitude of relative risk and statistical signifi-

Table 18-8
Logistic Regression Analysis of Drug Variables in
Nulliparas for Composite Outcome

Variable	Regression Coefficient	Standard Error	t-Statistic	Relative Risk	p-Value
Constant	-2.459	0.089	-27.77		
OXYT2	-0.091	0.114	-0.79	0.91	
SPINAL	-0.255	0.106	-2.41	0.77*	0.019
CAUDAL	0.041	0.249	0.17	1.04	
PUDEND	-0.218	0.177	-1.23	0.80	
PARAC	0.140	0.203	0.69	1.15	
NOBLOCK	-0.151	0.198	-0.76	0.86	
NOGAS	-0.163	0.187	-0.87	0.85	
GAS2	0.390	0.131	2.99	1.48*	0.0043
GAS3	0.663	0.236	2.81	1.94*	0.0071
IVD1	0.282	0.373	0.75	1.33	
AGT1	0.029	0.170	0.17	1.03	
AGT2	-0.732	0.293	-2.49	0.48*	0.014
AGT9	1.439	1.390	1.04	4.22	
AGT13	0.563	0.342	1.65	1.76	0.10
AGT16	0.674	0.314	2.14	1.96*	0.037
AGT18	0.504	0.402	1.25	1.66	
AGT20	0.016	0.308	0.05	1.02	
AGT22	0.574	0.772	0.74	1.78	
AGT24	0.894	0.374	2.39	2.45*	0.021
AGT25	0.643	0.391	1.64	1.90	0.10

* Statistically significant, $p < 0.05$.

Table 18-9
Logistic Regression Analysis of Drug Variables in
Multiparas for Composite Outcome

Variable	Regression Coefficient	Standard Error	t-Statistic	Relative Risk	p-Value
Constant	-2.401	0.058	-41.29		
OXYT1	0.480	0.278	1.73	1.62	0.087
OXYT2	0.136	0.116	1.17	1.15	
OXYT3	0.622	0.181	3.44	1.86*	0.0012
SPINAL	-0.289	0.106	-2.73	0.75*	0.0087
CAUDAL	-0.061	0.266	-0.23	0.94	
EPIDUR	0.436	0.294	1.48	1.55	
LOCAL	0.114	0.119	0.96	1.12	
PUDEND	0.255	0.092	2.79	1.29*	0.0074
GAS2	0.130	0.102	1.27	1.14	
IVD1	0.312	0.482	0.64	1.37	
AGT2	-0.270	0.301	-0.90	0.76	
AGT18	-1.538	0.922	-1.67	0.21	0.098
AGT23	-0.708	0.294	-2.41	0.49*	0.019
AGT27	3.183	1.388	2.29	24.13*	0.026

* Statistically significant, $p < 0.05$.

Table 18-10
Logistic Regression Analysis of Drug Variables in
Nulliparas for Perinatal Outcome

Variable	Regression Coefficient	Standard Error	t-Statistic	Relative Risk	p-Value
Constant	-3.923	0.177	-22.14		
OXYT2	0.655	0.191	3.44	1.93*	0.00085
SPINAL	-0.573	0.205	-2.62	0.58*	0.010
CAUDAL	-0.204	0.474	-0.43	0.82	
PUDEND	0.053	0.304	0.17	1.05	
PARAC	0.606	0.313	1.93	1.83	0.056
NOBLOCK	-0.104	0.339	-0.31	0.90	
NOGAS	-0.112	0.349	-0.32	0.89	
GAS2	0.775	0.226	3.43	2.17*	0.0012
GAS3	0.990	0.375	2.64	2.69*	0.0096
IVD1	1.100	0.442	2.48	2.99*	0.017
AGT1	0.332	0.311	1.07	1.39	
AGT4	1.281	0.805	1.59	3.60	
AGT7	0.980	1.131	0.87	2.66	
AGT16	0.529	0.561	0.94	1.70	
AGT18	0.361	0.675	0.54	1.43	
AGT20	0.457	0.509	0.90	1.58	
AGT21	1.215	0.952	1.28	3.37	
AGT22	2.129	1.104	1.93	8.41	0.056
AGT24	0.825	0.627	1.32	2.28	

* Statistically significant, $p < 0.05$.

Table 18-11
Logistic Regression Analysis of Drug Variables in Multiparas for
Perinatal Outcome

Variable	Regression Coefficient	Standard Error	t-Statistic	Relative Risk	p-Value
Constant	3.977	0.120	-33.16		
OXYT1	1.424	0.394	3.62	4.15*	0.00046
OXYT2	0.499	0.214	2.33	1.65*	0.022
OXYT3	1.141	0.307	3.71	3.13*	0.00034
SPINAL	-0.363	0.211	-1.72	0.70	0.087
CAUDAL	0.099	0.466	0.21	1.10	
EPIDUR	-0.113	0.730	-0.16	0.89	
LOCAL	-0.154	0.257	-0.60	0.86	
PUDEND	0.178	0.180	0.99	1.20	
GAS2	0.555	0.179	3.10	1.74*	0.0025
IVD1	0.905	0.624	1.45	2.47	
AGT2	-0.798	0.766	-1.04	0.45	
AGT7	-0.598	1.704	-0.35	0.55	
AGT8	2.437	1.715	1.42	11.43	
AGT9	0.874	1.396	0.63	2.40	
AGT27	2.893	1.555	1.86	18.05	0.066

* Statistically significant, $p < 0.05$.

cance were much greater in this analysis than earlier. The relative risk of OXYT3 increased from 1.86 to 3.13 (p .0012 to .00034). Neither SPINAL nor PUDEND, which had shown statistical significance in the composite outcome analysis, were verified to affect perinatal outcome in the same manner (although SPINAL retained a marginally insignificant protective impact, RR = 0.70, p = .087). OXYT1, which fell short of significance earlier, now demonstrated a strongly adverse influence on perinatal outcome (RR = 4.15, p = .00046). OXYT2, previously without apparent effect, now achieved significance as well (RR = 1.65, p = .022), as did GAS2 (RR = 1.74, p = .0025). The effect of IVD1 was suggestive only (at p = .10) and, therefore, worth exploring. Similarly, AGT27 (other antibiotics) repeated its adverse effect with a large, but insignificant relative risk (RR = 18.05, p = .066).

Step-Up Logistic Modelling

Step-up logistic regression analyses were also undertaken for these variables, as previously had been done for labor progression variables (see chapter 14). The significant oxytocin, anesthesia, and other drug variables were studied as a block to provide base data. Subsequent surveillance would then be undertaken to determine if other models, containing combinations which included more variables, would add more information pertaining to outcome.

The initial or base model for the composite outcome yielded the data shown in Table 18-12 for nulliparas. The eight variables previously identified as potentially significant on the basis of the prior findings shown in Table 18-8 were incorporated into the full logistic model. Examining these variables together in regard to their impact on offspring, but without reference to any other drug variables, did not change the magnitude of effect or its significance to any great extent, except for AGT13 (phenobarbital). Whereas it had previously yielded an insignificant relative risk of 1.76 (p = .10), it was now associated with a highly significant one of 2.47 (p = .015). There was no obvious explanation for this transformation.

The sequence of tests of each of the remaining variables for possible inclusion in a nine-factor model showed that none of them would be worthy contenders at a cutoff p value of .10 or less. Accordingly, no further step-up models could be constructed for the composite outcome in nulliparas.

The same step-up process in multiparas (Table 18-13) for the composite outcome produced a base model containing the seven variables previously identified: OXYT1, OXYT3, SPINAL, PUDEND, AGT18, AGT23, and AGT27. Their relative impact and statistical significance were almost precisely what they had previously been for the full model (Table 18-9). Tests for an eight-

Table 18-12
Step-Up Logistic Regression of Drug Variables
for Composite Outcome in Nulliparas

Variable	Initial Model		
	RR	t	p
SPINAL	0.79	-2.27	0.025
GAS2	1.49	3.10	0.0024
GAS3	1.96	2.90	0.0046
AGT2	0.56	-2.30	0.023
AGT13	2.08	2.47	0.015
AGT16	2.09	2.55	0.012
AGT24	2.50	2.62	0.010
AGT25	1.87	1.66	0.099

factor model failed to disclose any factor that could be added even at a 10% probability level. Only AGT5 (morphine) even approached this cut point (p = .106). No further step-up modelling was done, therefore.

The procedure was repeated in nulliparas for perinatal outcome data. Again, the same seven variables previously identified as carrying significant or potentially significant impact (Table 18-10) were incorporated into the initial logistic model. These included OXYT2, SPINAL, PARAC, GAS2, GAS3, IVD1, and AGT22. Only AGT22 showed any marked difference in effect from that seen earlier, the relative risk having increased from 8.41 to 9.58 (p .056 to .0067).

Surveillance of other factors to identify any of the remaining variables for inclusion

in an eight-variable model disclosed one that could qualify, namely AGT26 (magnesium sulfate). A step-up model was thus created, as shown in Table 18-14. The effect of the newly added item was negligible, although it further enhanced that of AGT22 (Apresoline), its relative risk rising still further to 10.64 (p = .0052). Further testing for a nine-factor model showed only AGT1 (Demerol) to be in contention (p = .0833). When it was added to the second step-up model, it failed to affect the relative impact of the other items to any great extent (Table 18-14). Only AGT22 responded by diminishing its relative risk all the way back to 8.06 (p = .013), about where it had been in the full logistic model.

A final step-up logistic regression operation involved perinatal outcome in offspring of multiparas. The six variables

Table 18-13
Step-Up Logistic Regression of Drug Variables
for Composite Outcome in Multiparas

| Variable | Initial Model | | |
	RR	t	p
OXYT1	1.59	1.68	0.096
OXYT3	1.84	3.50	0.00070
SPINAL	0.75	-2.83	0.0063
PUDEND	1.28	2.74	0.0073
AGT18	0.20	-1.74	0.085
AGT23	0.50	-2.49	0.014
AGT27	20.44	2.36	0.020

Table 18-14
Step-Up Logistic Regression of Drug Variables for
Perinatal Outcome in Nulliparas

| Variable | Initial Model | | | Step-Up Model 1 | | | Step-Up Model 2 | | |
	RR	t	p	RR	t	p	RR	t	p
OXYT2	1.89	3.49	0.00072	1.91	3.55	0.00059	1.93	3.61	0.00048
SPINAL	0.56	-2.89	0.0047	0.56	-2.90	0.0046	0.57	-2.83	0.0056
PARAC	1.83	1.99	0.048	1.84	2.01	0.047	1.83	1.98	0.049
GAS2	2.09	3.33	0.0012	2.09	3.33	0.0012	2.08	3.32	0.0014
GAS3	2.81	2.86	0.0052	2.79	2.83	0.0063	2.79	2.83	0.0063
IVD1	2.94	2.46	0.016	2.88	2.41	0.018	2.96	2.47	0.015
AGT22	9.58	2.77	0.0067	10.64	2.86	0.0052	8.06	2.48	0.013
AGT26				0.01	-1.08		0.01	-1.13	
AGT1							1.46	1.79	0.076

flagged earlier (Table 18-11) were incorporated into the initial model for the analysis. The results (Table 18-15) were almost identical with those seen before for three of the variables, OXYT2, SPINAL, and GAS2. Markedly reduced effects were seen with the rest, especially OXYT1 (RR 4.15 to 3.49) and OXYT3 (RR 3.13 to 2.28) with corresponding diminution in significance as well.

Testing for seven-factor models disclosed four variables of possible relevance, namely AGT2 (Nisentil, p = .0928), AGT8 (streptomycin, p = .0824), AGT18 (triflupromazine, p = .0769), and AGT23 (Syntocinon, p = .0635). As the drug with the lowest p value, AGT23 was incorporated into the first step-up model (Table 18-15) for perinatal outcome in multiparas. This operation enhanced all drug effects. Special augmentation appeared for OXYT1 (RR 3.49 to 3.81), OXYT3 (RR 2.28 to 2.80), and AGT27 (RR 11.25 to 12.20). AGT23 itself appeared protective here, albeit not significantly so (p = .093).

Additional testing of the remaining drug variables for possible inclusion in an eight-factor model flagged AGT8 (streptomycin, p = .0637). It was added to the second step-up model (Table 18-15), where it proved to have an impressively adverse effect (RR = 5.84, p = .027). It did not alter the other relationships, however, to any great extent. No other factors surfaced as relevant for purposes of continuing the analysis beyond the eight-factor model.

These observations are summarized in Table 18-16, which succinctly lists all variables demonstrated to be clearly significant by logistic regression analysis. They are shown separately for both parity groups and the two major outcome variables (composite and perinatal). These are the drug variables we have found to have the greatest impact on offspring whether acting alone or in concert with all other comparable drug variables. They will be incorporated into the final stages of this project (see chapter 25) to ascertain possible confounding effects from other concurrently acting variables related to labor progression, intrinsic characteristics, and delivery events.

Table 18-15
Step-Up Logistic Regression of Drug Variables for
Perinatal Outcome in Multiparas

Variable	Initial Model			Step-Up Model 1			Step-Up Model 2		
	RR	t	p	RR	t	p	RR	t	p
OXYT1	3.49	3.26	0.0015	3.81	3.46	0.00083	3.83	3.47	0.00077
OXYT2	1.52	2.00	0.048	1.61	2.25	0.027	1.60	2.22	0.029
OXYT3	2.28	2.92	0.0043	2.80	3.47	0.00082	2.67	3.27	0.0015
SPINAL	0.67	-1.99	0.048	0.69	-1.82	0.072	0.70	-1.76	0.081
GAS2	1.79	3.33	0.0012	1.80	3.37	0.0011	1.82	3.40	0.00097
AGT27	11.25	1.93	0.056	12.20	1.93	0.056	12.63	1.94	0.055
AGT23				0.44	-1.69	0.093	0.42	-1.78	0.078
AGT8							5.84	2.24	0.027

Table 18-16
Summary of Significant Drug Variables by Logistic Regression*

| Variable | Full Model | | | | Initial Model | | | | Step-Up Model | | | |
| | Composite | | Perinatal | | Composite | | Perinatal | | Composite | | Perinatal | |
	N	M	N	M	N	M	N	M	N	M	N	M
OXYT1				E				C				D
OXYT2			D	A			E	A			E	A
OXYT3		B		E		E		C				C
SPINAL	a	b	b		a	b	c	a			b	
PUDEND		B				B						
PARAC			A					A	A			
GAS2	C		D	C	C		C	C	C		D	
GAS3	B		B		C		C		B			
IVD1			A					A	A			
AGT2	a				a							
AGT8												A
AGT13					A							
AGT16	A				A							
AGT22			A				B				A	
AGT23		a				a						
AGT24	A				B							
AGT27		A				A						

* Significance code: A 0.05, B 0.01, C 0.005, D 0.001, E 0.0005, F 0.0001 or less. Protective relationships designated by lower case coding; adverse by capital letter coding.

CHAPTER 19

Intrinsic Maternal, Fetal, and Pelvic Factors

Summary

Potentially relevant prelabor conditions that might affect fetal and infant outcome were examined in detail, including the spectrum ranging from maternal demographic and socioeconomic traits to current and past medical disorders and obstetrical characteristics, for the 45,142 core cohort of gravidas under investigation. The survey yielded an important data resource for purposes of assessing the possible effects of these numerous factors on the offspring.

A wide variety of factors intrinsic to the patient and her pregnancy may affect the fetus. Needless to say, it is logical to take them all into account, if possible, whenever weighing risks to offspring. Publications on the subject of labor-delivery risk (including our own) have not heretofore dealt effectively with this issue, even though the hazards of some of the factors themselves are so widely recognized. Our aim in this segment, therefore, was to identify as many of these potentially relevant factors as feasible from the spectrum of variables known or suspected to impact unfavorably on the gravida, on her labor, on the delivery process, and most importantly, on her fetus. It was felt to be critical to assess such factors carefully because some (perhaps many) may serve as possible confounders of the outcome effects which we may ascribe to labor and delivery factors. This consideration was, of course, especially relevant to this series of investigations.

Spectrum of Variables

The first step was to determine which factors might be relevant insofar as possible direct impact on the fetus was concerned and which other factors might serve as markers of adverse outcome. Gestational age at delivery was an obvious example of the former and poor prior obstetrical history, of the latter. More remotely relevant variables were to be studied in addition, over a range of demographic, actuarial, socioeconomic, historical, medical, and obstetrical characteristics. Because of the thoroughness with which NCPP data had been collected, much of this information had already been sought after and, for the most part, was available for study. A partial list of the general topics examined here is shown in Table 19-1. Within each, subgroups of cases were to be collated for assessment of outcomes.

Combining Data Resources

Having decided upon the spectrum of variables to be investigated, we next proceeded with the difficult task of collecting diverse data from multiple sources within the NCPP data bank for purposes of compiling a workable data file for our purposes. This accomplished, we then isolated each of these factors as they pertained to intrinsic maternal, fetal, and pelvic conditions, and determined the frequency of occurrence of each of them among the Project gravidas.

For this purpose, we returned to the full database encompassing 58,806 cases, concentrating particularly on the 45,142 core cohort cases, there being no longer any rational justification to limit ourselves here just to those patients in whom all the necessary labor data were available for the other aspects of this investigation. This operation duplicated, in somewhat less detail and more limited scope, the extensive descriptive survey undertaken and

completed previously.* The published details need not be repeated here, of course, because that fine reference book is available as a resource work, but a few examples of the information made accessible for these analyses may put matters into better perspective.

Population Characteristics

Some reference to general population make-up was alluded to in chapter 4 where the data base was superficially characterized by the proportional distributions of age, race, parity, and gestational age at registration. As to actual numbers, study gravidas fell into age, marital status, race, and parity groupings as shown in Tables 19-2 through 19-5. Considerations concerning the limiting subset sizes were expected to apply to some of these subgroups. For example, the 31 women of age 45 years or older would probably prove insufficient in number to warrant separate analysis in depth. In general, however, the groupings were substantive, suggesting that meaningful information would indeed be forthcoming from the type of analytic approaches we were using.

Obstetrically Relevant Features

More critical to our needs was information pertaining to those variables with a greater likelihood of unfavorably affecting the fetus and infant than the above descriptors. Among them, gestational age at registration into the Project (that is, when they presented themselves for obstetrical care) and gestational age at delivery were surveyed (Tables 19-6 and 19-7). The unexpectedly high numbers of late registrants (14,290 at or after 28 weeks or 26.08% of NCPP patients) and premature

*Niswander, KR and Gordon, M: *The Collaborative Perinatal Study of the National Institute of Neurologic Diseases and Stroke: The Women and Their Pregnancies*. Philadelphia, WB Saunders Co, 1972.

Table 19-1
Selected Intrinsic Maternal, Fetal, and Pelvic Factors Under Surveillance

Institution	Gestational age at registration
Maternal age	Gestational age at delivery
Patient status	Multiple pregnancy
Marital status	Birth weight
Race	Fetal sex
Gravidity	Sterility investigation
Parity	Radiation
Prior abortion	Smoking
Prior premature	Abruptio placentae
Prior stillbirth	Placenta previa
Prior neonatal death	Cord prolapse
Maternal height	Incompetent cervix
Prepregnancy weight	Pregnancy-induced hypertension
Ponderal index	Hydramnios
Socioeconomic index	Uterine rupture
Weight gain	Pelvic adequacy
Prenatal visits	Fetal growth retardation
Walk-in (no prenatal care)	Fetal macrosomia
Vaginal bleeding	Uterine bleeding (by trimester)
Rh factor, sensitization	Leiomyomata uteri
Diabetes mellitus	Neuromuscular disease
Urinary tract infection	Seizure disorder
Anemia	Psychiatric disease
Sicklemia	Respiratory disease
Venereal disease	Cardiovascular disease

Table 19-2
Maternal Age Distribution

Age, yr.	No.	%
11-13	149	0.27
14-16	2,860	5.24
17-19	9,813	17.99
20-24	19,980	36.64
25-29	11,666	21.39
30-34	6,268	11.49
35-39	3,158	6.34
40+	901	1.65

Table 19-3
Marital Status

Status	No.	%
Single	8,153	14.95
Married	41,208	75.56
Common law	875	1.60
Widowed	216	0.40
Divorced	743	1.36
Separated	3,598	6.60

Table 19-4
Maternal Race Distribution

Race	No.	%
White	25,148	46.11
Black	25,612	46.96
Oriental	234	0.43
Puerto Rican	3,511	6.44
Other	290	0.53

Table 19-5
Maternal Parity Distribution

Parity*	No.	%
0	16,267	29.83
1	12,517	22.95
2	8,991	16.49
3	6,186	11.34
4	4,133	7.58
5	2,655	4.87
6	1,581	2.90
7	956	1.75
8	589	1.08
9	362	0.66
10+	408	0.75

* Parity prior to completion of index pregnancy.

Table 19-6
Gestational Duration at Time of Registration

Gestational Duration, wk.	No.	%
0-6	350	0.64
7-10	4,571	8.38
11-14	7,589	13.92
15-18	8,531	15.64
19-22	9,170	16.81
23-26	8,400	15.40
27-30	6,731	12.34
31-34	4,934	9.05
35-36	1,978	3.63
37-38	1,416	2.60
39-40	782	1.43
41-42	216	0.40
43+	85	0.16
"Walk-in"	227	0.42

deliveries (8211 prior to 36 weeks or 14.98%) reinforced our concerns about ensuring that these factors were to be carefully weighed. Additionally, there were quite a number of gravidas whose pregnancy appeared to have been prolonged well beyond term (5095 or 9.30% continued more than 42 weeks); the frequency was well in excess of that expected in the general population, implying that dating errors (specifically as pertaining to the last menstrual period) were common.

The number of prenatal visits (Table 19-8) ranged widely from none for 281 walk-in patients to a maximum of 35. Of interest were the relatively large numbers with few visits (10,062 had less than five or 18.36%), reflecting either late registration or superficial care, or with a large number of visits (4171 had 15 or more, 7.61%), suggesting intercurrent illness requiring special attention. Obstetrical history was available as a set of variables pertaining to antecedent obstetrical experience (Table 19-9), especially prior stillbirths, prior neonatal deaths, prior premature deliveries, and prior abortions. The relatively common occurrence of such events was not anticipated. For example, 1068 (1.95%) had two or more previous perinatal deaths and 2823 (5.15%) had two or more prior abortions.

Difficulty in achieving conception was frequent, 1669 requiring more than 1 year (3.70%) and 838, more than 2 years (1.86%). Actual sterility investigation and care had been undertaken in 1307 of them (2.39%). Smoking was very common

Table 19-7
Gestational Age at Delivery

Gestational Age, wk.	No.	%
<26	454	0.83
26-30	1,083	1.99
31-34	2,830	5.19
35-36	3,844	7.05
37-38	8,532	15.64
39-40	19,721	36.16
41-42	12,993	23.83
43-44	3,295	6.04
45+	1,800	3.30

Table 19-8
Frequency of Prenatal Office Visits

Prenatal Visits, No.	No.	%
0 ("Walk-in")	227	0.42
1-2	3,330	6.11
3-4	6,505	11.93
5-6	8,139	14.92
7-8	9,371	17.18
9-10	9,860	18.08
11-12	7,984	14.64
13-14	5,311	9.74
15-16	2,583	4.74
17-18	917	1.68
19-20	310	0.57
21+	361	0.66

Table 19-9
Prior Obstetrical Experience

	Events No.	No.	%
Prior Abortion			
	0	29,219	53.58
	1	7,280	13.35
	2	1,910	3.50
	3	572	1.05
	4+	341	0.63
Prior Premature Delivery			
	0	30,166	55.37
	1	6,297	11.56
	2	1,880	3.45
	3+	1,015	1.86
Prior Stillbirth			
	0	36,176	66.34
	1	2,692	4.94
	2	340	0.62
	3+	81	0.15
Prior Neonatal Death			
	0	33,812	62.00
	1	1,673	3.07
	2	480	0.88
	3+	167	0.31
Prior Perinatal Loss			
	0	33,812	62.07
	1	4,365	8.01
	2	820	1.51
	3+	306	0.56

among NCPP gravidas, being reported and recorded in 46.75% of them. Of special interest, 8976 (16.38%) smoked at least 20 cigarettes (one pack) per day and 2984 (5.45%), 30 or more per day. In all, more than half (52.13%) had been exposed to some form of irradiation, mostly chest x-ray examination. Abdominal or pelvic x-ray examinations, however, were done in 2658 (4.85%), an unexpectedly high frequency worthy of special note.

Medical Complications

A large variety of maternal, medical, and obstetrical disease factors (pre-existing and intercurrent) were documented in the core patient data files and were available for study. A sampling of this extensive array is shown in Table 19-10. These frequency data were derived from the all-encompassing NCPP systematic codification of the full panoply of conditions that may afflict pregnant women, as detailed in Table 19-11. Those found with sufficient frequency among study gravidas were to be investigated in depth.

Anemia, for example, was present in 12,868 women (28.51%); among them, the anemia was considered severe in 5146 (11.40%), based on very low hematocrit levels. Other commonly encountered disorders included urinary tract infection (5588 or 12.38% in the current pregnancy plus an additional 24.64% with foregoing infections of this nature), vaginitis (10,901 or 24.15% in this pregnancy), and unex-

Table 19-10
Selected Medical and Obstetrical Disorders

| | Relation to Index Pregnancy | | | | | |
| | Prior | | During | | Total | |
	No.	%	No.	%	No.	%
Organic heart disease	874	1.94	109	0.24	983	2.18
Rheumatic fever	1,868	4.14	8	0.02	1,876	4.16
Thrombophlebitis	300	0.66	120	0.27	420	0.93
Active tuberculosis	663	1.47	16	0.04	679	1.50
Pneumonia	-	-	290	0.64	290	0.64
Bronchial asthma	2,255	5.00	89	0.20	2,344	5.19
Anemia	-	-	12,868	28.51	12,868	28.51
Sicklemia	327	0.72	494	1.09	821	1.82
Coagulopathy	31	0.07	17	0.04	48	0.11
Blood dyscrasia	-	-	68	0.15	68	0.15
Diabetes mellitus	631	1.40	151	0.33	782	1.73
Hypothyroidism	-	-	176	0.39	176	0.39
Hyperthyroidism	315	0.70	47	0.10	362	0.80
Syphilis	1,273	2.82	399	0.88	1,672	3.70
Gonorrhea	1,033	2.29	173	0.38	1,206	2.67
Glomerulonephritis	318	0.70	33	0.07	351	0.78
Urinary tract infection	11,123	24.64	5,588	12.38	16,711	37.02
Incompetent cervix	132	0.29	94	0.21	226	0.50
Vaginitis	-	-	10,901	24.15	10,901	24.15
Leiomyomata uteri	379	0.84	399	0.88	778	1.72
Gynecological surgery	9,194	20.37	557	1.23	9,751	21.60
Convulsive disorder	1,252	2.77	33	0.07	1,285	2.85
Psychoneurotic disorder	1,999	4.43	1,060	2.35	3,059	6.78
Gallbladder disease	-	-	90	0.20	90	0.20
Hepatitis	896	1.98	34	0.08	930	2.06
Appendicitis	-	-	63	0.14	63	0.14
Ileitis	146	0.32	44	0.10	190	0.42
Peptic ulcer	412	0.91	35	0.08	447	0.99
Gastrointestinal surgery	-	-	528	1.17	528	1.17
Breast disease	-	-	886	1.96	886	1.96
Hyperemesis gravidarum	-	-	643	1.42	643	1.42
Hydramnios	-	-	1,082	2.40	1,082	2.40
Uterine bleeding, first trimester	-	-	6,123	13.56	6,123	13.56
Uterine bleeding, second trimester	-	-	3,965	8.78	3,965	8.78
Uterine bleeding, third trimester	-	-	7,355	16.29	7,355	16.29

Table 19-11
Systematic Codification of Maternal Disorders*

Code	Condition
	Cardiovascular
001	Organic heart disease
002	No symptoms on exertion
003	Symptoms on ordinary activity
004	Symptoms on limited activity
005	Symptoms on bed rest
006	Rheumatic fever
007	Thrombosis and/or phlebitis
008	Regional increase in body heat

208

009	Fever 100.4° F or above
010	Regional swelling
011	Palpable thrombus
012	Vein tenderness
013	Embolization
014	Other

Pulmonary

015	Tuberculosis, active
016	Positive sputum culture
017	Positive culture, other
018	Positive guinea pig inoculation
019	X-ray evidence of disease
020	X-ray evidence of progression
021	Tuberculosis, inactive
022	Pneumonia
023	Positive culture
024	Viral and/or serological evidence
025	Chest x-ray evidence
026	Bronchial asthma
027	Acute asthma
028	Status asthmaticus
029	Thoracic surgery
030	Other

Blood

031	Anemia
032	Abnormally low serum iron
033	Abnormally high IBC
034	Abnormally high protoporphyrin
035	Abnormal peripheral red cell smear
036	Abnormal bone marrow smear
037	Clinical response to iron therapy
038	Abnormal hemoglobin-S electrophoresis
039	Sickling in peripheral blood
040	Other findings of anemia
041	Coagulation defect
042	Abnormally low prothrombin
043	Abnormally low proconvertin
044	Abnormally low fibrinogen
045	Abnormally low prolonged clotting tiime
046	Clinical response to fibrinogen
047	Other coagulation defects
048	Other

Metabolic and Endocrine

049	Diabetes mellitus
050	Any blood sugar 200 mg.% or more
051	Insulin therapy or oral hypoglycemic analogue
052	Insulin reaction
053	Diabetic coma
054	Ketoacidosis
055	Duration 5 years of more
056	Abnormal glucose tolerance test
057	Hypothyroidism
058	Abnormally low BMR
059	Abnormally low PBI
060	Abnormally low BEI
061	Abnormally low I_{131} uptake
062	Clinical response to thyroid medication
063	Hyperthyroidism
064	Abnormally high BMR
065	Abnormally high PBI
066	Abnormally high BEI
067	Abnormally high I_{131} uptake
068	Clinical response to therapy
069	Thyroid surgery
070	Other

Venereal

071	Syphilis
072	Positive serology
073	Positive cerebrospinal fluid
074	Positive Treponema immobilization test
075	Positive dark field
076	Gonorrhea
077	Positive culture
078	Positive smear
079	Other

Urinary Tract

080	Acute and chronic glomerulonephritis
081	Urinary tract infection
082	Fever 100.4° F or above
083	Costovertebral angle tenderness
084	Positive urine culture
085	Pyuria
086	Hematuria
087	Genitourinary tumor
088	Genitourinary surgery
089	Other

Gynecological

090	Infertility
091	Incompetent cervix
092	Surgery for incompetent cervix
093	Vaginitis
094	Leiomyomata uteri
095	Other gynecologic tumor
096	Gynecologic surgery
097	Other

Neurologic and Psychiatric

098	Convulsive disorder
099	Convulsions during pregnancy
100	Mental retardation
101	Organic brain disease
102	Psychosis or neurosis
103	Other neurologic or neuromuscular disease
104	Alcoholism
105	Drug habituation or addiction
106	Other

Gastrointestinal

107	Cholecystitis
108	Cholelithiasis
109	Hepatitis
110	Appendicitis
111	Colitis, ileitis
112	Hiatus hernia
113	Peptic ulcer
114	Gastrointestinal surgery
115	Gastrointestinal tumor
116	Other

Integument and Appendages

117	Burns, hospitalized
118	Breast disorder
119	Other

Pregnancy Complications

120	Hyperemesis gravidarum
121	Intravenous therapy
122	Acetonuria
123	Hydramnios
151	Placenta previa
152	Abruptio placentae
153	Marginal sinus rupture
124	Uterine bleeding, first trimester
125	Uterine bleeding, second trimester
126	Uterine bleeding, third trimester

```
                    Shock State
        127    Anesthetic
        128    Hemorrhagic
        129    Septic
        130    Positional (vena cava syndrome)
        131    Other
        132    Anesthetic accident, other
        133    Maternal death
                    Pregnancy Infection
        138    Known or presumed viral
        139    Known or presumed bacterial
        140    Known or presumed parasitic
        141    Known or presumed fungal
        142    Type unknown
        143    Attenuated live vaccine, type
        144    Disease and conditions not elsewhere specified
```

*   Based on NCPP form OB-60.

plained vaginal bleeding (concentrated especially in the first and third trimesters). Gynecological surgery was fairly common in this group as well, but most had had such surgery prior to the current pregnancy (9751 or 21.60% overall, but only 557 or 1.23% in this pregnancy).

Less frequent conditions involved many different organ systems. The most prevalent among them were psychiatric or neurotic disorders (3059 or 6.78% in all) and bronchial asthma (2344 or 5.19%, with 89 newly diagnosed cases in the study pregnancy). Among asthmatics, 282 had acute attacks in this pregnancy (0.62%) and 34 were diagnosed as actually having been in status asthmaticus (0.08%).

In addition, such potentially serious problems as organic heart disease in the mother pre-existed the study pregnancy in 874 (1.94%) and was uncovered during this pregnancy in an additional 109 (for a total of 2.18%). Prepregnancy rheumatic fever history was obtained in 1868 (4.14%), but only eight additional cases could be documented in the course of pregnancy, making it very unlikely that we would be able to assess the impact of this gratifyingly rare condition on the fetus. Sickle cell disease was diagnosed in 821 (1.82%), more than half (494 or 1.09%) recognized for the first time in the pregnancy under surveillance.

Obstetrical Disorders

Among obstetrical conditions of relevance were hyperemesis gravidarum (794 or 1.46%), hydramnios (1082 cases or 2.40%), abruptio placentae (945 or 1.73%), placenta previa (541 or 0.99%), and prolapsed cord (488 cases in all or 0.90%, 251 of which were occult). The common obstetrical problem of uterine bleeding has already been mentioned. Pregnancy-induced hypertension occurred in 4604 (9.60%) based on the strict objective classification which had been established earlier for this population.* Rarer obstetrical complications, such as uterine rupture (encountered in only 24 cases or 0.05%), were obviously seen too infrequently to permit us to determine their possible direct effects on offspring or their potential roles as confounding factors.

There were a large number of variables pertaining to the delivery events which should also have been considered intrinsic to the patient and to the fetus (including fetal position and presentation, for example). These were arbitrarily assigned to the list of factors to be investigated later (see chapter 22) as they might apply directly to the effect of the delivery pro-

*Friedman, EA and Neff, RK: *Pregnancy Hypertension: A Systematic Evaluation of Clinical Diagnostic Criteria.* Littleton, Mass, PSG Publishing Co, 1977.

cess on the fetus and infant.

Fetal Variables

Fetal factors were included here if they were uncontrollable in that they pre-existed the onset of labor. Any adverse outcome related to them, therefore, was perhaps the result of an effect already at play. Fetal sex, for example, was examined because of the recognized differences in results, boys tending to do somewhat worse in general than girls for a given birth weight. There were 27,762 (50.75%) males and 26,940 (49.25%) females in the NCPP population. We have already presented the data pertaining to premature and postmature delivery frequencies (see above). There were 1148 multiple pregnancies, including six sets of triplets, and one of quadruplets; these had been excluded from the core index population because the infants were assumed to be at special risk. Their outcome data were available for our investigation, nonetheless. Birth weight, as expected, paralleled gestational age distribution. Discordant cases in which birth weight fell outside the normal range for the gestational age at which they were delivered were classified as either small for gestational age (below the tenth percentile) or large for gestational age (above the 90th percentile).

Major congenital anomalies, especially those incompatible with survival or with normal development, were also taken into account since obviously we wished to ensure that these bad results would not be attributed in any way to the labor and delivery factors being studied. For example, 32 cases of Down's syndrome were diagnosed, nearly all (24) recognized at or soon after birth. In addition, there were 16 with meningomyelocele plus two others with encephalocele. Seventeen had craniosynostosis and 43 were hydrocephalic.

Microcephaly was confirmed in 62, only four of which were apparent at birth, however. This latter situation raised the question as to whether or not the condition arose in most cases as a secondary event, perhaps related more to brain damage during the birth process or subsequently. Other anatomical anomalies not apparently associated with conditions likely to affect growth and development, such as cleft palate (32 cases), were merely noted for completeness. Others, such as congenital heart disease, were divided into those placing the infant at great risk insofar as normal subsequent development was concerned (25 with cyanotic heart disease) and those that did not (121 with acyanotic heart disease).

This process of defining cases according to the presence or absence of each of the aforementioned variables had thus put us into position to group them for purposes of determining the relative frequencies of the outcomes. After such data had been developed, they were then to be compared with the referent rates derived from groups of cases that were similar except for the absence of the intrinsic factor being examined. The comparison was to be done utilizing the same nonparametric paradigm we described earlier (see chapter 7).

CHAPTER 20

Intrinsic Factors and Outcome

Summary

Preliminary bivariate assessments of previously identified intrinsic variables were done to help provide foundational information about those likely to be associated with bad outcomes. Special attention was paid to the impact of such factors as institution at which the delivery occurred, gestational age at time of registration for antepartum care, maternal age and marital status, race, socioeconomic level, parity, height, weight, smoking habit, and obstetrical experience. In addition, fetal sex, gestational age at delivery, birth weight and frequency of prenatal examinations were weighed as were a range of prenatal events and complications. The effects of a large number of maternal conditions and disease states were also examined in great detail.

The spectrum of intrinsic factors displayed in chapter 19 were evaluated for their possible effects on fetal and infant outcomes. They were studied by the same techniques heretofore used for this purpose in this series of investigations. As before, cases were stratified by the variable in question (as to whether it was present or absent) and further substratified by the several categories within each variable whenever such descriptors had been precoded and entered into the data bank. The subsets of case material thus created were examined in detail for outcome statistics.

The derived frequencies of the various outcome results were then subjected to nonparametric testing (Freeman-Tukey deviates, FTD) to ascertain whether the statistical significance of any differences encountered were meaningfully distinct from the overall frequency of occurrence of that outcome variable for the subpopulation being studied. In addition, as in the past, we developed rate ratios to provide quantitation of risk or protective effects, if any, subjecting them in turn to statistical testing as well.

Institutional Effect

Some of these results will be detailed here to demonstrate our approach more clearly. To determine possible institutional effect, for example, we first stratified cases according to the place at which the labor and delivery had occurred. All outcomes were then determined for each institution's population of offspring, frequencies were calculated, and these were then compared with expected rates.

Neonatal deaths, for instance, were tallied in this way (Table 20-1). By contrast with the overall neonatal death rate of 1.95% for all 54,795 infants for whom institutional designations were known, frequencies varied from 1.36% (for institution 50) to 2.71% (for institution 37). FTD values showed two rates to be apparently

protective as a consequence of unexpectedly low rates of infant losses (institutions 05 and 50, with frequencies of 1.62% and 1.36%, respectively) and two to be rather high (institutions 37 and 66, frequencies 2.71% and 2.44%).

We chose institution 05 as the referent index group because it represented the largest single intramural experience in the NCPP data collection activity (and a 22.25% plurality of these cases). Utilizing the neonatal death rate for this hospital unit, we found it a simple matter to assess every other institution's results for heterogeneity.

As fully expected, the three institutions with the greatest relative risks proved to be significantly dissimilar (institutions 37, 66, and 71 with rate ratios of 1.67, 1.51, and 1.36, respectively). It will be shown later that the data for each of these hospitals were also significantly different in regard to other outcomes, whereas no others yielded any form of similar adverse results (see below). While it was understood, of course, that factors other than the institution per se were undoubtedly at play here—including a variety of preselection factors relating to population composition, such as race, socioeconomic status, and so forth, which could explain why such differences occurred—it

Table 20-1
Neonatal Deaths by Institution

Institution Code	Cases No.	Neonatal Death No.	%	Freeman–Tukey Deviate	p	Rate Ratio RR	p
05	12,193	198	1.62	-2.713	0.0033	1.00*	
10	2,348	39	1.66	-1.016		1.02	
15	2,560	49	1.91	-0.112		1.18	
31	2,111	33	1.56	-1.310		0.96	
37	4,057	110	2.71	3.186	0.0007	1.67	1.0×10^{-5}
45	3,322	54	1.63	-1.382		1.01	
50	3,226	44	1.36	-2.571	0.0051	0.84	
55	4,389	89	2.03	0.370		1.25	
60	3,331	69	2.07	0.505		1.28	
66	9,694	237	2.44	3.274	0.00053	1.51	1.6×10^{-5}
71	3,995	88	2.20	1.113		1.36	0.016
82	3,569	61	1.71	-1.050		1.06	

* Referent

214

was clear, nonetheless, from these observations that the institution as a variable could not be ignored for now.

Effect of Registration Date

Similarly, gestational age at registration was examined for purposes of attempting to learn whether or not this variable might also be relevent to outcome. The case material was stratified in four-week intervals from seven through 34 weeks and two-week increments thereafter to 42 weeks; the tail groups (under seven and over 42 weeks) were collapsed. Outcomes were studied within each subset thus formed. Both FTD and rate ratio were derived as before, the latter utilizing the modal gestational age group (those registering at 19 to 20 weeks, the largest subpopulation of NCPP gravidas, consisting of 9170 in all) as the referent.

Our data for neonatal deaths (Table 20-2) revealed that those registering for antepartum care much later in pregnancy, especially from 27 weeks onward, had paradoxically better results than those registering earlier. Fairly constant death rates were encountered in offspring of women presenting for care up to 26 weeks; with each succeeding interval of time beyond that, death rates fell progressively to a low at 35 to 36 weeks. Collapsing all cases in which registration occurred after 30 weeks formed a group of 9411 with a neonatal death rate of 0.86%, a very significantly low frequency (RR 0.37, FTD -9.088, $p < 1.0 \times 10^{-10}$). By contrast, patients who had had no antepartum care at all (constituting the so-called walk-in patients) had the worst death rates of all (3.96%, RR 1.72), but they were not statistically significant.

This quite unexpected effect of late registration was directly contrary to the logical tenets of obstetrics which assert that prenatal care is beneficial and, by inference, delayed pregnancy care is harmful. A similar inverse relationship had previously been disclosed in a parallel study pertaining to the effect of blood pressure levels on outcome; for any given diastolic blood pressure, for example, perinatal mortality rates were found to fall progressively with advancing gestational age.* It was explained by the fact that those enrolling late for care are diminishingly at risk of delivering pre-

---

*Friedman, EA: *Blood Pressure, Edema and Proteinuria in Pregnancy*. New York, Alan R Liss, Inc, 1976, p 136.

Table 20-2
Neonatal Death by Gestational Age at Registration

Gestational age, weeks	Cases No.	Neonatal Death No.	Neonatal Death %	Freeman-Tukey Deviate	Freeman-Tukey p	Rate Ratio RR	Rate Ratio p
0-6	350	6	1.71	-0.231		0.74	
7-10	4,571	101	2.21	1.219		0.96	
11-14	7,589	185	2.44	2.861	0.0021	1.06	
15-18	8,531	198	2.32	2.333	0.0098	1.01	
19-22	9,170	211	2.30	2.292	0.011	1.00*	
23-26	8,400	183	2.18	1.446		0.95	
27-30	6,731	104	1.55	-2.517	0.0059	0.67	
31-34	4,934	49	0.99	-5.595	1.1×10^{-8}	0.43	0.0015
35-36	1,978	11	0.56	-5.695	6.2×10^{-9}	0.24	5.4×10^{-5}
37-38	1,416	13	0.92	-3.222	0.00064	0.40	0.0087
39-40	782	5	0.64	-3.197	0.00069	0.28	0.0064
41-42	216	2	0.93	-1.083		0.40	
43+	85	1	1.18	-0.351		0.51	
"Walk-in"	277	9	3.96	1.402		1.72	

* Referent

215

maturely. The later in pregnancy they surface, the greater the likelihood of a term or near-term delivery. Therefore, there is a smaller risk among late registrants of the newborn infant dying or suffering the kinds of long-term damage to which premature infants are subject.

As to our neonatal death statistics, we recognized here that, if there was any adverse impact from inadequate prenatal care, based on the patient seeking such care late in prenancy, it could not be appreciated from these data. In the interest of further clarification of this issue, more will be said about the subject when we delve into possible effects of the number of prenatal visits (see below). As a factor that reflects simultaneous consideration of both duration and intensity of antepartum care, it may be of greater relevence to our needs as an index of risk than gestational duration at the time of registration.

Maternal Age Effect

Maternal age was examined (Table 20-3) to confirm that age affects outcome, a relationship that has been widely accepted. Specifically, general consensus holds that both the very young and the relatively older gravidas place their fetus at increased risk. Grouping cases by increments of age (based on chronological age at the time of delivery), we found the expected ∪-shaped pattern of neonatal death rates with advancing maternal age. That is to say, the middle range of ages was associated with good outcome as compared with the much poorer results at either extreme.

The Freeman-Tukey deviate for the 20-24 years age group proved to be highly significant (FTD -5.331, p = 4.9×10^{-8}) relative to the overall neonatal death rate, showing a strongly protective effect. Contrastingly, the 30-34 year group demonstrated significantly increased death rates (FTD 2.048, p = .020). By virtue of decreasing number of cases in the tail groups, statistical significance could not be verified here. However, coalescing them showed that the associated increase in the neonatal death rate was probably not just a chance occurrence. For example, the 12,822 teenagers in this series had a neonatal death rate of 1.99% overall (RR 1.36, p = .00025) and those 10,327 gravidas aged 30 years or greater had a 2.23% rate (RR 1.53, p = .027).

Maternal age, therefore, was a factor that would have to be weighed as a possible confounder. Even though the adverse age-related trend was verified here for neonatal death, we were cautioned to bear in mind that other, perhaps more pertinent factors may enter into and explain away the relationship. Specifically, it need not reflect age per se, but rather the recognized increased potential for teenagers to suffer pregnancy-induced hypertension and for elderly gravi-

Table 20-3
Neonatal Death by Maternal Age

Maternal Age, weeks	Cases No.	Neonatal Death No.	%	Freeman–Tukey Deviate	p	Rate Ratio RR	p
11–13	149	4	2.68	0.680		1.84	
14–16	2,860	56	1.96	0.046		1.34	
17–19	9,813	195	1.99	0.248		1.36	0.00070
20–24	19,980	292	1.46	-5.331	4.9×10^{-8}	1.00*	
25–29	11,666	216	1.85	-0.789		1.27	0.0078
30–34	6,268	146	2.33	2.048	0.020	1.60	2.7×10^{-6}
35–39	3,158	64	2.03	0.317		1.39	0.016
40+	901	20	2.22	0.602		1.52	

* Referent

216

das to develop such illnesses of advancing age as chronic hypertensive disease and diabetes mellitus.

Marital Status Effect

Other maternal characteristics were also studied by this approach. Marital status (Table 20-4) was interesting in that married women yielded significantly fewer neonatal deaths (1.83%, FTD -1.869, p = .031) than expected on the basis of the rate for the total population. Offspring of 8153 single and never-married gravidas did not do well by comparison (2.27%), whether related to the overall neonatal death rate (FTD 1.973, p = .024) or to the rate for the referent married group (RR 1.24, p = .0079).

All other marital status groups, except those who had been divorced, showed similar death rates, but only the rate for the group consisting of separated women reached statistical significance (2.64%, FTD 2.743, p = .0030). Thus, never-married and separated gravidas stood apart. This finding was perhaps related to maternal age (that is, unmarried gravidas during the era of this study tended to be quite young, relative to the general population of pregnant women), but it could also have been a reflection of concurrent poor nutrition or anemia, and associated socioeconomic or emotional factors.

Racial Effect

Racial differences in outcome (Table 20-4) were also apparent. Neonatal losses were found to be significantly increased among black gravidas (2.26%, FTD 3.428, p = .00030). This relationship was obviously of major importance to our investigations. It was essential for us to determine in what critical ways black gravidas differed in

Table 20-4
Neonatal Death by Maternal Characteristics

	No.	Neonatal Death No.	%	Freeman–Tukey Deviate	p	Rate Ratio RR	p
Marital Status							
Single	8,152	185	2.27	1.973	0.024	1.24	0.0079
Married	41,208	753	1.83	-1.869	0.031	1.00*	
Common Law	875	19	2.17	0.500		1.19	
Widow	216	5	2.31	0.456		1.26	
Divorced	743	14	1.88	-0.072		1.03	
Separated	3,598	95	2.64	2.743	0.0030	1.44	0.00063
Race							
White	25,148	420	1.67	-3.340	0.00042	1.00*	
Black	25,612	580	2.26	3.428	0.00030	1.35	1.7×10^{-6}
Oriental	234	5	2.14	0.293		1.28	
Puerto Rican	3,511	61	1.74	-0.914		1.04	
Other	290	5	1.72	-0.180		1.03	
Patient Status							
Clinic service	48,370	949	1.96	0.124		1.00*	
Private	2,984	51	1.71	-0.954		0.87	
Socioeconomic Index							
0-19	4,193	90	2.15	0.893		1.08	
20-39	16,699	334	2.00	0.432		1.00*	
40-59	16,505	341	2.07	1.023		1.04	
60-79	10,361	167	1.61	-2.595	0.0047	0.81	0.021
80-95	5,240	72	1.37	-3.236	0.00061	0.69	0.0032

* Referent

217

terms of actuarial, medical, and health care characteristics in order to begin to learn the reasons for such poor outcome data. Only in this way could one hope to improve them substantively. Orientals also had a somewhat increased rate (2.14%, RR 1.28), but this did not prove statistically significant. No other racial group was found to have comparably high rates of neonatal death.

Patient Status and Socioeconomic Effect

Clinic status, although associated with somewhat poorer results than private patient status, failed to yield statistically significant differences in outcome rates (Table 20-4). Socioeconomic attributes had been scored in an index based on education, occupation, and income (see chapter 5), higher scores parallelling greater affluence. Freeman-Tukey deviates were significant for the highest socioeconomic levels only (grouped scores of 60-79 and 80-95). The clear distinction in neonatal death rates in the offspring of these gravidas reflected good outcomes compared with overall population rates. Relative to the rate in the modal group (socioeconomic index 20-39), they demonstrated consistent protection even when coalesced into a single tail group

with socioeconomic index 60+ (1.53% neonatal deaths, RR 0.77, p = .00029).

Parity Effect

Parity effects could be examined, too, seeking verification of the generally accepted risks associated with births in nulliparas and grand multiparas. The 16,267 nulliparas yielded surprisingly few neonatal deaths (1.62%) compared to the overall rate (FTD -3.149, p = .00082). When nulliparas were stratified according to whether or not they had had prior early pregnancy losses (into primigravid versus multigravid nulliparas), however, a rather impressive distinction was disclosed (Table 20-5). True primigravidas did indeed appear to be protected (FTD -4.397, p = 5.5×10^{-6}). Their outcomes contrasted sharply with multigravid nulliparas whose neonatal death rate was very high indeed (FTD 3.087, p = .0010, RR 1.74).

As will be developed in more detail later (see below), prior obstetrical history of pregnancy loss—whether abortion, premature delivery, stillbirth, or neonatal death—impacted unfavorably on future pregnancy outcomes. The good findings for primigravid nulliparas were unexpected because there is a generally held impression that

Table 20-5
Neonatal Death by Parity

Parity	Cases No.	Neonatal Death No.	%	Freeman-Tukey Deviate	p	Rate Ratio RR	p
0 (Gravida 1)	15,091	224	1.48	-4.397	5.5×10^{-6}	0.76	0.0026
0 (Gravida 2+)	1,176	40	3.40	3.087	0.0010	1.74	0.00085
1	12,517	244	1.95	-0.026		1.00*	
2	28,991	182	2.02	0.487		1.04	
3	6,186	115	1.86	-0.520		0.95	
4	4,133	86	2.08	0.397		1.07	
5	2,655	54	2.03	0.323		1.04	
6	1,581	47	2.97	2.621	0.0044	1.52	0.0072
7	956	22	1.75	0.783		0.90	
8	589	18	3.06	1.742		1.57	
9	362	13	3.59	1.934		1.84	
10+	408	16	3.92	2.387	0.023	2.01	0.0053

* Referent

offspring of nulliparas do not fare as well as those of multiparas, at least in terms of perinatal outcome. Surviving offspring of nulliparas, by contrast, can be expected to do better on long-term testing (for example, IQ scores), but it is believed that this may have more to do with rearing differences than with the risk of pregnancy, labor, and delivery. Nonetheless, insofar as these data are concerned, we have been able to distinguish a small subset of nulliparas whose babies do badly (namely, those who have had prior abortion) from the larger population of nulliparas whose offspring do very well. This observation has broad clinical application.

As to women of high parity, we did not encounter the upsurge in poor outcomes we had expected. There was indeed a slight trend toward higher frequencies of neonatal deaths with advancing parity, especially para 6 (that is, women now having their seventh viable delivery) or more, but the trend was unimpressive. Only those para 10 or greater achieved statistical significance; the regression line ($y = 1.45 + 0.199x$) reflected an average increase of 0.20% with each additional pregnancy, but the relatively large standard error of the regression coefficient for the slope (± 0.454) meant that the trend could not be shown to be statistically significant.

Multiple Pregnancy Effect

Multiple pregnancy, as expected on the basis of the high associated risk, impacted very adversely on the infant (Table 20-6). Among 563 twin pairs (1126 babies), the neonatal death rate was found to be nearly six times the overall rate for singletons, an extremely significant difference. The number of triplet and quadruplet sets (six and one, respectively) were insufficient for statistical testing purposes, although it is to be noted that none of these 22 infants died. Factors of prematurity and malpresentation aside, although both conditions are common in multiple pregnancies, it was clear that we were obliged to ensure that considerations of fetal and infant outcome took into account twinning as an important risk factor.

Maternal Height Effect

Maternal height failed to materialize as a variable that could be shown to have any clear adverse relationship to this outcome for the infant (Table 20-7). When gravidas were stratified by height, the only marginally significant findings were the good outcomes for offspring of short women. Those less than 55 inches tall had fewer neonatal deaths than expected (marginally significant rate of 0.71%, FTD -1.655, p = .049). No such comparable benefit was seen for tall women; in fact, there was a suggestion of an adverse effect in their infant outcome results. Examining this group more closely, we encountered a subset of 142 gravidas measuring 71 inches, whose neonatal death rate was very high (4.23%, although just of borderline significance,

Table 20-6
Neonatal Death by Multiple Pregnancy

Plurality	Cases No.	Neonatal Death No.	%	Freeman–Tukey Deviate	p	Rate Ratio RR	p
Singleton	53,647	956	1.78	-2.916	0.0018	1.00*	
Twins	1,126	115	10.21	12.058	$<1.0 \times 10^{-10}$	5.74	$<1.0 \times 10^{-10}$
Triplets	18	0	0.00	-0.552		0.00	
Quadruplets	4	0	0.00	-0.146		0.00	

*   Referent

219

FTD 1.690, p = .046). These observations, while of possible clinical interest, did not raise maternal height to the level of a factor that should have critical concern for our investigational purposes.

Maternal Weight Effect

Maternal weight and weight gain, however, are accepted as important based on much foregoing clinical experience and research activities, including in-depth analysis of these same NCPP data files in the past.* These data demonstrated a clear relationship between large body habitus or obesity (as expressed, for example, in the

---

*Friedman, EA and Neff, RK: *Pregnancy Hypertension: A Systematic Evaluation of Clinical Diagnostic Criteria*. Littleton, Mass, PSG Publishing Co, 1977, pp 73, 128-130.

maximum weight attained in pregnancy) and bad outcome to the fetus. Women over 225 lb had twice the frequency of stillbirths (RR 2.0) as women in the modal weight group (125-149 lb). Moreover, the greater the weight above this level, the worse the results (over 250 lb, RR 2.1; and over 275 lb, RR 3.8, all highly significant).

Although the neonatal death rates in obese women were also increased (Table 20-8), the frequencies did not achieve statistical significance. At the opposite end of the weight range, however, neonatal death rates were very bad for asthenic women. Below 125 lb maximum weight, neonatal death rates rose (1.66% overall for these 2471 women, FTD 3.618, p = .00014, RR 2.1) to a frequency of 3.46% among those 328 gravidas under 110 lb (3.46%, FTD 3.279, p = .00052, RR 4.38).

Data on third trimester rates of weight

Table 20-7
Neonatal Death by Maternal Height

Height, inches	Cases No.	Neonatal Death No.	%	Freeman-Tukey Deviate	p	Rate Ratio RR	p
40-54	282	2	0.71	-1.655	0.049	0.35	
55-59	2,826	60	2.12	0.658		1.03	
60-64	23,269	478	2.05	1.085		1.00*	
65-69	16,212	317	1.96	0.021		0.96	
70-74	441	10	2.27	0.523		1.11	
75+	32	0	0.00	-0.871		0.00	

   * Referent

Table 20-8
Neonatal Death by Maternal Weight

Maximum Weight, lb.	Cases No.	Neonatal Death No.	%	Freeman-Tukey Deviate	p	Rate Ratio RR	p
< 95	9	1	11.11	1.270		14.06	0.00051
95-109	319	10	3.13	3.201	0.0013	3.96	7.7 x 10-6
110-124	2,143	30	1.40	2.409	0.0080	1.77	0.0059
125-149	11,106	88	0.79	-0.740		1.00*	
150-174	8,011	56	0.70	-1.583	0.0057	0.89	
175-199	3,196	16	0.50	-2.401	0.0082	0.63	
200-224	1,029	11	1.07	0.753		1.35	
225+	726	7	0.96	0.382		1.22	

   * Referent

gain (Table 20-9) showed that infants fared poorly in a milieu of weight loss or inadequate weight gain. Weight loss of any magnitude resulted in significant neonatal losses in 2780 cases in which it was observed (0.97%, FTD 1.868, p = .031, RR 1.70).

Smoking Effect

Smoking by pregnant women showed only a negligible overall impact (Table 20-10). Although associated with an 11% relative increase in deaths (RR 1.11), this increase was not quite statistically significant (p = .077). It was found, however, that the group who acknowledged cigarette smoking included a sizable number whose smoking habits could be characterized as light, that is, involving use of relatively few cigarettes daily. Only 13.07%, for example, smoked more than one pack (20 cigarettes) per day, and nearly half (45.92%) smoked ten cigarettes or less.

When stratified by the intensity of smoking (Table 20-11), the data showed that women who smoked more than 1½ packs per day (31 cigarettes or more) placed their infants at increased risk. Their pregnancies resulted in significantly higher neonatal death rates (2.98%, FTD 2.895, p = .0019, RR 1.62). The regression curve, y = 1.535 + 0.056x, describes this relationship; the standard error of its regression coefficient (0.056 ± 0.032) supported a contention that the trend was real (p = .041), reflecting an average increase of 1.12% in neonatal deaths for each pack smoked per day.

Obstetrical History Effect

We alluded in our discussion of parity effects to the apparently adverse impact that prior abortion has in nulliparas (see above). Taking such unfortunate prior obstetrical events into consideration showed this kind of background experience to be especially hazardous to subsequent

Table 20-9
Neonatal Death by Rate of Maternal Weight Gain (or Loss)

Weight Change, lb./wk.	Cases No.	Neonatal Death		Freeman-Tukey		Rate Ratio	
		No.	%	Deviate	p	RR	p
> 1.0 loss	446	6	1.35	1.056		2.37	0.037
0.1–1.0 loss	2,334	21	0.91	0.264		1.60	0.060
0.0–0.9 gain	10,757	61	0.57	-3.561	0.00018	1.00*	
1.0–1.9 gain	4,667	32	0.69	-1.298		1.21	
2.0–2.9 gain	725	4	0.55	-0.853		0.96	
3.0+ gain	109	2	1.83	1.178		3.21	

* Referent

Table 20-10
Neonatal Death by Maternal Smoking

	Cases No.	Neonatal Death		Freeman-Tukey		Rate Ratio	
		No.	%	Deviate	p	RR	p
Nonsmoker	28,878	532	1.84	-1.374		1.00*	
Smoker	25,353	519	2.05	1.052		1.11	
Unknown	304	7	2.30	0.497		1.25	

* Referent

pregnancies (Table 20-12). Any prior early pregnancy loss was associated, for example, with greatly increased neonatal death rates (2.82%, FTD 5.671, p = 7.1×10^{-9}, RR 1.52). Patients with only one prior abortion had about a 50% increase in the death rate over those who had had none (2.75% versus 1.85%, RR 1.49, highly significant statistically). With increasing numbers of abortions (not necessarily successive), there was somewhat of a further increase. The regression equation of this relationship was y = 2.220 + 0.256x, with standard error of the slope (±0.115) clearly demonstrating that this trend was not likely to have been a chance occurrence (p = .013).

Prior stillbirths yielded the same type of bad outcome results, only magnified as to effect (Table 20-12). All women who had had stillbirths collectively yielded more than

Table 20-11
Neonatal Death by Degree of Maternal Smoking

Cigarettes Smoked per day	Cases No.	Neonatal Death		Freeman-Tukey		Rate Ratio	
		No.	%	Deviate	p	RR	p
None	28,878	532	1.84	-1.374		1.00*	
1-5	7,071	126	1.78	-1.039		0.97	
6-10	6,661	134	2.01	0.352		1.09	
11-15	2,116	52	2.46	1.590	0.056	1.34	
16-20	6,191	119	1.92	-0.160		1.04	
21-25	304	6	1.97	0.119		1.07	
26-30	1,097	25	2.28	0.784		1.24	
31-40	781	27	3.46	2.610	0.0045	1.88	0.0010
41-50	86	7	8.14	2.695	0.0035	4.42	1.6×10^{-5}
51+	1,046	23	2.20	0.635		1.20	

* Referent

Table 20-12
Neonatal Death by Prior Obstetrical Event

Obstetrical History	Cases No.	Neonatal Death		Freeman-Tukey		Rate Ratio	
		No.	%	Deviate	p	RR	p
Prior abortion							
None	29,219	542	1.85	-1.223		1.00*	
1	7,280	200	2.75	4.441	4.5×10^{-6}	1.49	1.1×10^{-6}
2	1,910	57	2.98	2.905	0.0018	1.61	0.00049
3	572	18	3.15	1.840	0.033	1.70	0.023
4+	341	10	2.93	1.220		1.58	
Prior stillbirth							
None	36,176	696	1.92	-0.409		1.00*	
1	2,692	93	3.45	4.797	8.1×10^{-7}	1.80	5.5×10^{-8}
2	340	30	8.82	5.793	3.5×10^{-9}	4.59	$<1.0 \times 10^{-10}$
3+	81	5	6.17	1.978	0.024	3.21	0.0054
Prior neonatal death							
None	33,812	587	1.74	-2.948	0.0016	1.00*	
1	1,673	63	3.77	4.457	4.2×10^{-6}	2.17	3.20×10^{-9}
2	480	23	4.79	3.488	0.00024	2.75	5.3×10^{-7}
3+	167	9	5.39	2.413	0.0079	3.10	0.00034

* Referent

twice the expected frequency of neonatal deaths in the index study pregnancy (4.11%, FTD 7.039, p < 1.0×10^{-10}, RR 2.14). One stillbirth almost doubled the subsequent neonatal death rate from 1.92% to 3.45% (RR 1.80, p = 5.5×10^{-8}, a very significant difference); two or more of them more than doubled the adverse impact again to 8.31% (RR 4.33, p < 1.0×10^{-10}).

Gravidas who lost infants in the neonatal period in prior pregnancies were at comparable risk in the future (Table 20-12). Any prior neonatal death nearly tripled the minimal risk as compared to women without this history (4.09% versus 1.74%, FTD 6.040, p = 7.7×10^{-10}, RR 2.35). As with abortions and stillbirths, the greater the number of such prior events, the greater the risk. With each succeeding increment in number, the frequency of neonatal deaths rose. One prior neonatal death yielded 3.77% of neonatal deaths in the index pregnancy (more than twice the expected rate, RR 2.17); two, 4.79% (RR 2.75); and three or more, 5.39% (RR 3.10). The regression equation, y = 2.290 + 1.005x, described this impressive trend and the standard error of the regression coefficient (±0.265) demonstrated its clear-cut statistical significance (p = 7.7×10^{-5}).

Fetal Sex Effect

The baby's gender appeared to be relevant as well (Table 20-13). As anticipated, boys did substantially worse than girls insofar as neonatal death rates were concerned. The difference in death rates, although not large in absolute terms, was nevertheless quite significant (1.75% versus 2.13%, RR 1.22, p = .00070).

Gestational Age and Birthweight Effect

Gestational age at the time of delivery was strongly related to survival rates (Table 20-14), entirely as expected. The inverse relationship between gestational age and neonatal death rates is well recognized and accepted, of course. The shorter the gestational duration, the greater the risk of infant death. In this series, it could be quantitated by the regression equation, y = 85.78 - 2.144x; the standard error of the regression coefficient (±0.489) substantiated the significance of this obvious trend line (p = 5.8×10^{-6}). Birthweight paralleled this pattern almost identically (Table 20-15). Our findings in this regard verified the anticipated correlation of high losses with small babies. Quantitatively, this was described by the equation, y = 51.54 - 0.0128x (standard error of slope ±0.0035, p = .00011).

In both instances, the linearity of these relationships could be challenged. Careful examination showed a parabolic configuration with high frequencies of adverse outcomes at both extremes. The death rate fell rapidly in the 250-g increment groups from the almost uniform fatalities among very small infants to a plateau beyond 2500 g. The very low loss rates were clearly shown by the uniform zone of negative FTD values between 2500 and 4750 g, each subgroup FTD achieving statistical significance independently of the others. The adverse rates in the extreme subsets were much

Table 20-13
Neonatal Death by Fetal Sex

Infant Sex	Cases No.	Neonatal Death No.	Neonatal Death %	Freeman-Tukey Deviate	Freeman-Tukey p	Rate Ratio RR	Rate Ratio p
Male	27,762	591	2.13	2.042	0.021	1.22	0.00070
Female	26,940	471	1.75	-2.476	0.0066	1.00*	

* Referent

223

Table 20-14
Neonatal Death by Gestational Age at Delivery

Gestational Age, weeks	Cases No.	Neonatal Death No.	%	Freeman-Tukey Deviate	p	Rate Ratio RR	p
< 26	454	212	46.70	23.114	1.0×10^{-10}	93.40	1.0×10^{-10}
26–30	1,083	264	24.38	23.271	1.0×10^{-10}	48.76	1.0×10^{-10}
31–34	2,830	159	5.62	10.350	1.0×10^{-10}	11.24	1.0×10^{-10}
35–36	3,844	78	2.03	0.355		4.06	1.0×10^{-10}
37–38	8,532	80	0.92	-7.902	1.0×10^{-10}	1.88	2.0×10^{-5}
39–40	19,721	98	0.50	-19.430	1.0×10^{-10}	1.00*	
41–42	12,993	68	0.52	-15.335	1.0×10^{-10}	1.04	
43–44	3,295	29	0.88	-5.219	9.0×10^{-8}	1.76	0.0066
45+	1,800	18	1.00	-3.303	0.00048	2.00	0.0057

*   Referent

Table 20-15
Neonatal Death by Birth Weight

Weight, grams	Cases No.	Neonatal Death No.	%	Freeman-Tukey Deviate	p	Rate Ratio RR	p
< 1,000	376	348	92.55	31.823	1.0×10^{-10}	154.25	1.0×10^{-10}
1,000–1,249	212	115	54.24	17.302	1.0×10^{-10}	90.40	1.0×10^{-10}
1,250–1,499	284	98	34.51	15.032	1.0×10^{-10}	57.52	1.0×10^{-10}
1,500–1,749	435	67	15.40	10.515	1.0×10^{-10}	26.67	1.0×10^{-10}
1,750–1,999	713	41	5.75	5.351	4.4×10^{-8}	9.58	1.0×10^{-10}
2,000–2,449	1,448	50	3.45	3.526	0.00021	5.75	1.0×10^{-10}
2,500–2,749	7,679	101	1.32	-4.373	6.1×10^{-6}	2.20	1.0×10^{-9}
2,750–2,999	8,680	54	0.62	-11.305	1.0×10^{-10}	1.03	
3,000–3,249	10,890	65	0.60	-13.010	1.0×10^{-10}	1.00*	
3,250–3,499	10,249	49	0.48	-14.254	1.0×10^{-10}	0.80	
3,500–3,749	7,022	22	0.31	-13.966	1.0×10^{-10}	0.52	0.0064
3,750–3,999	3,806	13	0.34	-9.932	1.0×10^{-10}	0.57	
4,000–4,249	1,595	7	0.44	-5.737	4.8×10^{-9}	0.73	
4,250–4,449	759	2	0.26	-4.622	1.9×10^{-6}	0.43	
4,500–4,749	268	1	0.37	-2.271	0.012	0.62	
4,750–4,999	103	2	1.94	0.137		3.23	
5,000+	40	1	2.50	0.383		4.17	

*   Referent

more impressive at the lower end of the scale of birth weights, of course, than at the upper end. Nonetheless, the deleterious impact of very large birth weight cannot be ignored.

As to prolonged or postterm pregnancy, there seems to have been less of a hazard than we have come to expect (albeit statistically significant); moreover, the incidence was somewhat greater than seen in other gravid populations (9.34% occurrence rate over 42 weeks and 3.3% over 44 weeks). These latter observations suggest that the data may not have been truly reflective of the actual prevalence of postdate cases, but were instead perhaps clouded by sizable numbers of cases in which the dating of the pregnancy was suspect.

Prenatal Care Effect

The number of prenatal visits was also

examined (Table 20-16). We studied the outcomes as associated with increasing numbers of office visits for antepartum care, keeping in mind the paradoxically beneficial effect that late registration appeared to have had on the results, as discussed earlier (see above). A contrary relationship was found here, namely, the fewer the visits, the higher the mortality. Compared to the neonatal death rate in the modal group of women who had had nine to ten prenatal visits (0.98%), all those with less than seven visits had a particularly high loss rate over four times expected (3.94%, FTD 15.874, $p < 1.0 \times 10^{-10}$, RR 4.03).

Of course, it was possible that this observation may have been distorted in the other direction by the confounding effects of premature delivery—that is, the reason some gravidas have had so few antepartum visits was that they delivered early (and, therefore, were not pregnant long enough to be able to make many visits). This is confirmed to some extent by the fact that women with no antepartum care at all (walk-in for delivery only) did very badly overall, but not nearly so badly as those who had had up to four prenatal visits (although the difference was not statistically significant).

At the other end of the range of visits, it seemed reasonable to assume that those with many visits undoubtedly represented gravidas who had had recognizable medical illnesses or pregnancy complications that warranted close surveillance. That they did poorly with regard to neonatal outcome, as shown here (those with more than 20 visits had just as bad results as those with few or none), therefore, was not unexpected. Between these extremes, a plateau comparable to that encountered with birth weight trends was found. As before, the stable and uniformly low neonatal death rates were reflected in a homogeneously significant zone of negative FTD values extending between seven and 20 visits.

Effect of Selected Events

Potentially relevant historical events were studied (Table 20-17) to determine whether or not they might have a bearing on infant outcome as well. Whereas women who had had infertility investigations had a somewhat higher neonatal death rate than those who had not, the results could not be shown to be statistically significant.

By contrast, radiation exposure in the index pregnancy did yield significantly more of such deaths, but only if the radiation was directed at the abdomen or pelvis. Radiation of other regions of the body had no apparent comparable effect. It is conceivable, of course, that the results might

Table 20-16
Neonatal Death by Prenatal Visit

Visits No.	Cases No.	Neonatal Death No.	Neonatal Death %	Freeman–Tukey Deviate	Freeman–Tukey p	Rate Ratio RR	Rate Ratio p
"Walk-in"	227	9	3.96	1.832	0.034	4.04	1.3×10^{-5}
1-2	3,330	204	6.13	12.434	$<1.0 \times 10^{-10}$	6.26	$<1.0 \times 10^{-10}$
3-4	6,505	316	4.84	13.007	$<1.0 \times 10^{-10}$	4.96	$<1.0 \times 10^{-10}$
5-6	8,139	189	2.32	2.286	0.011	2.37	$<1.0 \times 10^{-10}$
7-8	9,371	123	1.31	-4.860	3.0×10^{-6}	1.34	
9-10	9,860	97	0.98	-7.609	$<1.0 \times 10^{-10}$	1.00*	
11-12	7,984	55	0.69	-10.104	$<1.0 \times 10^{-10}$	0.70	
13-14	5,311	38	0.72	-7.992	$<1.0 \times 10^{-10}$	0.73	
15-16	2,583	12	0.46	-7.176	$<1.0 \times 10^{-10}$	0.47	0.011
17-18	917	15	1.64	-0.653		1.67	
19-20	310	4	1.29	-0.788		1.32	
21+	361	16	4.43	2.717	0.0033	4.52	$<1.0 \times 10^{-10}$

* Referent

Table 20-17
Neonatal Death by Preexisting or Concurrent Events

Event	Cases No.	Neonatal Death No.	%	Freeman-Tukey Deviate	p	Rate Ratio RR	p
Infertility investigation							
No	52,672	1,000	1.90	-0.918		1.00*	
Yes	1,307	33	2.52	1.418		1.33	
Unknown	237	7	2.96	1.055		1.56	
Radiation in pregnancy							
None	25,109	454	1.81	-1.680	0.047	1.00*	
Abdominal-pelvic	2,658	72	2.71	2.579	0.0050	1.50	0.0012
Other areas only	25,906	492	1.90	-0.631		1.05	
Vaginal bleeding in pregnancy							
No	31,764	458	1.44	-7.018	$<1.0 \times 10^{-10}$	1.00*	
Yes	22,646	598	2.64	6.839	$<1.0 \times 10^{-10}$	1.83	$<1.0 \times 10^{-10}$
Pelvic inlet adequate							
Yes	50,402	887	1.76	-3.200	0.00069	1.00*	
No	1,960	42	2.14	0.619		1.22	
Hydramnios							
No	31,921	516	1.62	-4.513	3.2×10^{-6}	1.00*	
Yes	794	62	7.81	7.869	$<1.0 \times 10^{-10}$	4.82	$<1.0 \times 10^{-10}$

* Referent

reflect the conditions for which the radiation was used—almost exclusively for diagnostic purposes and mostly for gastrointestinal (GI) or genitourinary problems—rather than the radiation effect. This was subsequently examined in detail (see below) and this conjectural hypothesis was verified to some extent.

Vaginal bleeding in pregnancy, although very common (41.62% occurrence rate), did have a very significant negative impact on outcome. Bleeding was also examined by trimester (see below) with very significant results, especially as regards the deleterious association of midtrimester bleeding with neonatal death as well as a host of other short- and long-term results.

The prelabor determination of the adequacy of the pelvic architecture to accommodate the anticipated fetus did appear to matter in terms of infant outcome, although the magnitude of the effect was small (but nonetheless statistically significant). It is possible, of course, that the effect

of this factor was "corrected" to some extent by the confounding influence of the delivery process that was selected. That is to say, a women with a bad pelvis (small, misshapen, or with poor prognostic architectural features) was more likely to have been delivered by cesarean section than others, of course. Therefore, her fetus was at somewhat less risk than it would have been had it been allowed (or forced) to deliver vaginally.

Hydramnios was associated with very high neonatal death rates, as expected on the basis of its common association with fetal anomalies and with maternal diabetes mellitus. There were nearly five times as many neonatal deaths proportionally in cases exhibiting hydramnios than in those without this serious complication. It was clear that it had to be taken into serious account as an intrinsic factor pre-existing the labor-delivery process and one that served as a marker or index of poor prognostic outlook.

Effect of Obstetrical Complications

In the spectrum of identifiable obstetrical complications preceding labor, abruptio placentae, placenta previa, and cord prolapse were demonstrated to have the most devastating effect on the newborn infant (Table 20-18), as expected. Cases with placental abruption yielded about eight times the frequency of neonatal deaths, complete abruptions more than 20 times, both highly significant. Together (partial and complete abruption combined), infant outcome was very poor indeed (14.18% neonatal deaths, FTD 14.541, $p < 1.0 \times 10^{-10}$, RR 8.54).

Placenta previa, whether total or partial, was associated with a 15-fold increase in such infant losses. Rather surprisingly, marginally implanted placentas resulted in just as bad outcomes, if not actually worse. All diagnosed cases considered collectively (total, partial, and marginal) resulted in very significantly, nearly tenfold elevated neonatal death rates (17.24%, FTD 7.809, $p < 1.0 \times 10^{-10}$, RR 9.85). Even more unexpectedly, low placental implantation was also associated with poor infant results. It is possible,

of course, that these latter data reflected reporting biases rather than true effects; that is to say, not all cases of marginal or low implantation were necessarily diagnosed, but those in which bleeding was a prominent manifestation and/or in which the fetus succumbed were much more likely to be recognized and reported as such. The observation of bad effect, nonetheless, carries some clinical significance because marginal or low placental implantation has not heretofore been considered a complication of any great importance.

Prolapse of the umbilical cord was likewise associated with poor infant outcome in all its variants, whether occult or overt, although the latter was clearly a much more serious event insofar as adverse infant impact was concerned. Whereas occult prolapse more than doubled the expected neonatal death rate (RR 2.46, p = .0020), the presence of an intravaginal loop of forelying umbilical cord enhanced the death rate more than 11-fold. In contrast, complete prolapse with an exteriorized loop of cord, while prognostically also extremely serious, did not appear to be associated with nearly

Table 20-18
Neonatal Death by Obstetrical Complication

Condition	Cases No.	Neonatal Death No.	%	Freeman–Tukey Deviate	p	Rate Ratio RR	p
Abruptio placentae							
None	53,085	881	1.66	-5.051	2.2×10^{-7}	1.00*	
Partial	900	118	13.11	13.324	$<1.0 \times 10^{-10}$	7.90	$<1.0 \times 10^{-10}$
Complete	45	16	35.56	5.997	1.0×10^{-9}	21.42	$<1.0 \times 10^{-10}$
Placenta previa							
None	53,370	935	1.75	-3.431	0.00030	1.00*	
Total	70	11	15.71	4.327	1.1×10^{-5}	8.98	$<1.0 \times 10^{-10}$
Partial	72	11	15.28	4.206	1.3×10^{-5}	8.73	$<1.0 \times 10^{-10}$
Marginal	61	13	21.31	4.945	3.8×10^{-7}	12.18	$<1.0 \times 10^{-10}$
Low implantation	130	11	8.46	3.440	0.00029	4.83	6.9×10^{-9}
Cord prolapse							
None	53,196	945	1.78	-3.000	0.0014	1.00*	
Occult	251	11	4.38	2.239	0.033	2.46	0.0020
Intravaginal	151	30	19.87	7.467	$<1.0 \times 10^{-10}$	11.16	$<1.0 \times 10^{-10}$
External	86	10	11.63	3.700	0.00011	6.53	$<1.0 \times 10^{-10}$

* Referent

227

so great a rate of infant losses (RR 6.53 versus 11.16 for intravaginal cord prolapse), although the difference between the two neonatal death rates was not statistically significant. If the latter should actually prove to be less hazardous, it may merely mirror earlier diagnosis and more expeditious intervention.

Neonatal Death Data Summarized

The foregoing results pertaining to the adverse impact of sundry intrinsic variables of neonatal deaths were summarized (Table 20-19) to show the relative risk of each relevant factor and its associated probability (p value) of chance occurrence. The effect of any single item of interest can be read directly from this tabulation. For example, never-married women run a 24% greater risk of having a neonatal death than married women (RR 1.24 based on the data provided in Table 20-4, 2.27% versus the referent rate of 1.83% for married women), a relationship that could be expected to occur by chance 0.8% of the time (p = .008) or about once in 125 times (if this exercise were to be repeated that often). Of course, these data do not yet take into account any confounding factors. To do so will require more sophisticated kinds of analyses to deal with multiple variables simultaneously (see chapter 21).

Table 20-19
Intrinsic Factors Possibly Affecting Neonatal Death

Factor		Rate Ratio	p
Institution	37	1.67	<0.0001
	66	1.51	<0.0001
	71	1.36	0.02
Registration:	> 30 weeks	0.43*	0.002
Maternal age:	< 20 years	1.36	0.0003
	30+ years	1.53	<0.0001
Marital:	Single	1.24	0.008
	Separated	1.44	0.0006
Race:	Black	1.35	<0.0001
Socioeconomic:	High index	0.69*	0.003
Parity:	Primigravid	0.76*	0.003
	Multigravid nullipara	1.74	0.0009
	Para 6+	1.52	0.007
Multiple pregnancy		5.62	<0.0001
Smoking:	> 1½ packs/day	1.62	0.0004
Prior abortion(s)		1.52	<0.0001
Prior stillbirth(s)		2.14	<0.0001
Prior neonatal death(s)		2.35	<0.0001
Male fetus		1.22	0.0007
Gestational age:	< 39	9.47	<0.0001
	> 42	1.84	0.0004
Abruptio placentae		8.54	<0.0001
Placenta previa		9.85	<0.0001
Cord prolapse		2.46	0.002
Birth weight:	< 2,750 g.	7.36	F0.0001
	3,500+ g.	0.52*	0.007
Prenatal visit:	< 7	4.03	<0.0001
	15-16	0.47*	0.01
	> 20	4.52	<0.0001
Pelvic radiation		1.50	0.001
Vaginal bleeding		1.83	<0.0001
Hydramnios		4.82	<0.0001

*   "Protective" effect.

Expansion to Other Outcomes

Before embarking on those analyses, however, we wished to expand the approaches we have used heretofore to detail the effects, if any, of these same factors on the spectrum of other fetal and infant outcomes under surveillance. A sampling of these is displayed for three additional outcomes in Table 20-20 which repeats the convenient shorthand vehicle used for neonatal death for exhibiting large quantities of analytical results. These three factors were representative of immediate, short-term, and long-term outcome variables, similar to others that had been investigated in like manner with comparable results. This tabulation confirmed in large measure both the specific kind of intrinsic variables associated with bad fetal and infant outcomes and the relative impact that each brings to bear (but without accounting for the impact any of the others may bring to bear at the same time).

The data dealing with neonatal deaths, which we detailed so extensively earlier, were thereby verified with only rare modifications here. One new relevant risk variable uncovered at this time was patient status, nonprivate patients demonstrating very impressively adverse eight-month and three-year results. Whereas this factor did not seem to have made any difference in regard to neonatal death or stillbirth rates, late results to offspring of those patients

Table 20-20
Intrinsic Factors Possibly Affecting Other Selected Outcomes

Factor		Stillbirth RR	p	8 Mo. Global Score RR	p	3 Yr. SLH RR	p
Institution:	37	1.41	0.006			3.00	<0.0001
	66					2.76	<0.0001
	71			2.46	<0.0001		
Registration:	> 30 wks.	0.39*	<0.0001				
Maternal age:	< 20					1.46	0.002
	30+	2.05	<0.0001				
Marital:	Single					1.34	<0.0001
	Common law					2.40	<0.0001
Race:	Black	1.19	0.004			1.18	0.005
Socioeconomic:	High index			0.70*	<0.0001	0.49*	<0.0001
Status:	Clinic			1.87	0.0002	4.32	<0.0001
Parity:	Primigravid			0.46*	<0.0001	1.29	0.002
	Multigravid nullipara	1.84	0.0002				
	Para 6+	2.23	<0.0001	1.83	<0.0001	1.64	0.009
Multiple pregnancy		3.46	<0.0001	4.66	<0.0001	3.06	<0.0001
Smoking				1.19	0.004		
Prior premature		1.27	<0.0001	1.63	<0.0001	1.47	<0.0001
Prior abortion		1.32	<0.0001				
Prior stillbirth		3.41	<0.0001	1.46	0.0002	1.52	<0.0001
Male fetus						2.18	<0.0001
Gestational age:	< 39 wks.	8.04	<0.0001	3.15	<0.0001	1.42	<0.0001
	> 42 wks.					1.39	0.0005
Abruptio placentae		13.64	<0.0001	2.80	<0.0001		
Placenta previa		4.64	<0.0001	3.86	<0.0001		
Cord prolapse		9.97	<0.0001				
Prenatal visit:	< 7	4.08	<0.0001	2.34	<0.0001	1.28	0.015
	> 20	2.22	0.013	2.30	0.0001		
Pelvic radiation		1.97	<0.0001	1.66	<0.0001		
Vaginal bleeding		2.07	<0.0001				
Hydramnios		4.08	<0.0001	2.10	0.0003		

* "Protective" effect.

229

with designated clinic status were very significantly worse than among private patients.

Of equal importance, few factors that had been found to have an association with neonatal death rates did not have a comparable effect on stillbirth rates; exceptions included two of the institutions (hospitals 66 and 71), teen age, marital status, socioeconomic index, and smoking. Late results at 3 years showed even greater consistency of deleterious impact among surviving infants; exceptions here encompassed abruptio placentae, placenta previa, cord prolapse, vaginal bleeding, and hydramnios. These latter findings pertaining to placenta and cord complications support those of previously published NCPP studies dealing with the apparent transiency of the impact of some of these conditions.* Vaginal bleeding, when examined more critically by trimester (see below), actually did show long-term adverse outcomes in the four- and seven-year IQ results (but not the three-year speech, language, and hearing results). This applied regardless of the trimester in which it occurred.

Effect of Medical Disorders

A very large series of maternal conditions and disease states was evaluated in the course of this phase of our investigations. This was done to ensure that we were not overlooking any critical intrinsic factors with major pervasive adverse impact on the infant. As before, we intended to determine the fetal and infant outcome results for the offspring of groups of gravidas presenting with a given condition as compared with results for those without that factor. Data from the NCPP code form dealing with the summary of intercurrent maternal disorders (form OB-60) were used for this

---

*Niswander, KR, Friedman, EA and Berendes, H: Do placenta previa, abruptio placentae and cord prolapse cause neurological damage to the infant who survives?, in MacKeith, R and Box, M (eds): *Studies in Infancy*. London, William Heinemann, 1968, pp 78-83.

purpose (see chapter 19).

Significantly adverse neonatal death results (Table 20-21) were disclosed for a variety of such conditions. Some of these relationships were entirely expected, such as the very high infant losses associated with pulmonary embolism, coagulopathy, diabetes mellitus (especially if complicated or poorly controlled), and shock states. The same applied to incompetent cervix and (as noted earlier) to hydramnios. Some, however, were unexpected, including maternal anemia, urinary tract infection, and gastrointestinal tumor.

On the obverse side of the issue, many conditions heretofore felt likely to be deleterious to the infant were not verified as harmful (Table 20-22). These encompassed organic heart disease, thrombophlebitis, pneumonia, sickle cell disease, hypothyroidism, glomerulonephritis, leiomyomata uteri, alcoholism, drug addiction, hepatitis, appendicitis, and a variety of systemic infections. Whereas the neonatal death rates associated with these conditions were well within the normal range, it did not necessarily follow, of course, that other outcomes would be equally favorable. In point of fact, it will be seen that in many the outcome results were indeed unfavorable.

Medical Conditions Surveyed in Depth

Exhaustive examination of most disease states was thus carried out to uncover adverse effects on other outcome measures, studying the range of outcome variables previously detailed. Among the large number of OB-60 codified conditions investigated (Table 20-23), a total of 85 disorders or subcategories of disorders were found to have statistically significant associations with some form of bad outcome; 14 had uncommonly good results—that is, statistically significant protective effects were encountered. In five instances, there were both good and bad effects seen.

Table 20-21
Intercurrent Maternal Diseases in Pregnancy
Significantly Related to Neonatal Death

	RR	p
Cardiovascular		
Embolic disease	6.48	0.030
Pulmonary		
X-ray evidence of tuberculosis	4.01	0.032
Other pulmonary disease	1.58	0.0006
Blood		
Anemia	1.18	0.017
Other anemic manifestation	2.30	0.010
Coagulation defect	12.26	<0.0001
Hypofibrinogenemia	18.94	<0.0001
Prolonged clotting time	10.42	0.003
Response to fibrinogen therapy	20.83	<0.0001
Other blood dyscrasias	3.83	0.001
Metabolic and Endocrine		
Diabetes mellitus	3.67	<0.0001
Insulin-hypoglycemic therapy	3.69	<0.0001
Insulin reaction	4.80	<0.0001
Diabetic coma	20.83	<0.0001
Ketoacidosis	5.82	<0.0001
Diabetes for 5+ years	4.69	<0.0001
Hyperthyroidism	2.15	0.005
Response to thyroid therapy	5.21	0.0007
Venereal disease		
None		
Urinary tract		
Urinary tract infection	1.20	0.013
UTI with fever	1.53	0.045
UTI with CVA tenderness	1.44	0.014
Gynecologic		
Incompetent cervix	19.77	<0.0001
Gynecologic tumor (not fibroid)	1.94	<0.0001
Gynecologic surgery	1.99	0.002
Other gynecologic disorder	1.60	0.003
Hydramnios	4.57	<0.0001
Uterine bleeding, first trimester	1.90	<0.0001
Uterine bleeding, second trimester	4.27	<

Heart Disease

Organic heart disease, for example, which had yielded acceptable neonatal death rates, resulted in a threefold increase in stillbirths and more than twice the expected frequency of perinatal deaths. When stratified by the presence or absence of overt clinical manifestations (vis-à-vis symptoms relating to cardiac decompensation or limitation of activities), the fetal wastage effect was found only in offspring of symptomatic gravidas.

Pulmonary Disorders

Pulmonary embolus led to serious fetal and infant losses, but survivors appeared to have done well as evidenced by the absence of any apparent special relationship with late neurologic or developmental abnormalities. Pneumonia in pregnancy, unexpectedly free of adverse effect on fetal or infant death rates, did seem to impact unfavorably on the more long-term measurements of outcome, particularly as regards eight-month, one-year, and three-year testing results. Bronchial asthma was found to be associated with unexpectedly poor late neurologic and developmental results at three, four, and seven years; only patients with status asthmaticus placed their fetuses at

Table 20-22
Intercurrent Maternal Diseases Not Significantly Related to
Neonatal Death

Cardiovascular
Organic heart disease
Rheumatic fever
Thrombosis-phlebitis
Other cardiovascular disorders

Pulmonary
Clinical tuberculosis
Pneumonia
Bronchial asthma

Blood
Abnormal hemoglobin S
Sicklemia

Metabolic and Endocrine
Abnormal glucose tolerance
Hypothyroidism
Thyroid surgery
Other metabolic condition

Venereal Disease
Syphilis
Gonorrhea
Other venereal disease

Urinary Tract
Acute, chronic glomerulonephritis
Hematuria
GU tumor
GU surgery
Other GU disorder

Gynecologic
Infertility
Vaginitis
Leiomyomata uteri .

Neurologic and Psychiatric
Convulsive disorder
Mental Retardation
Organic brain disease
Psychosis, neurosis
Other neuromuscular disorder
Alcoholism
Drug addiction
Other psychiatric disorder

Gastrointestinal
Cholecystitis
Cholelithiasis
Hepatitis
Appendicitis
Colitis, ileitis
Hiatus hernia
Peptic ulcer
GI surgery
Other GI condition
Hyperemesis gravidarum

Skin and Appendages
Burn
Breast disorder
Other

Shock
Anesthetic
Supine hypotension
Other shock
Anesthesia accident

Infection
    Viral
    Bacterial
    Parasitic
    Fungal
    Other

---

special risk for stillbirths, however.

Blood Conditions

Anemia was related to a range of poor outcomes out to seven years. When manifestations of anemia were examined more closely as an index of severity or type, the very common iron deficiency variety showed mostly poor early results (stillbirth and neonatal depression with some effects still present in the one-year neurologic examination). Interestingly, those anemic patients who were found to have low serum iron levels had particularly bad infant outcomes. Paradoxically, those diagnosed principally by responding well to iron therapy showed an opposite protective effect on the stillbirth rate and no apparent residual effect in the later testing vehicles. Sickle cell disease, whether diagnosed by smear preparation or electrophoresis, was contrastingly related to late adverse effects only. Coagulopathy yielded extreme fetal and infant losses, but the survivors showed no persistent late effect at four and seven years.

Diabetes Mellitus

Maternal diabetes mellitus placed the fetus and infant at especially high risk, as expected, for neonatal death. The more severe classes of diabetics had the worst results, of course. Similarly, the poorer the control, the poorer the outcome. Thus, insulin-dependent diabetics yielded more adverse results than gestational diabetics and those with documented severe hyperglycemia did still worse. Indeed, offspring of gravidas with just an abnormal glucose tolerance test (GTT) did not do badly at all relative to the general population; none of the outcome results were statistically different from those expected in the general obstetrical population. Those who deve-

loped insulin reactions did somewhat worse. Long-standing diabetes impacted even more unfavorably on the fetus or surviving infant. Diabetic coma or ketoacidosis yielded particularly devastating outcomes.

Thyroid Diseases

Hypothyroidism had little consistent effect, except as regards neonatal depression and eight-month results, perhaps because the condition in the mother will prevent pregnancy if it is severe, or it will be readily correctable if diagnosed in pregnancy. Hyperthyroidism showed mixed results: favorable late outcomes overall contrasted with very poor eight-month and three-year results when associated with high basal metabolic rate or elevated serum protein-bound iodine levels. Cases in which clear-cut response to medical therapy (mostly propylthiouracil) was documented—indicating that the diagnosis had probably been correct—did badly with reference to neonatal death, neonatal depression, low eight-month mental scoring, and one-year neurologic abnormality rates.

Genitourinary Conditions

Fetuses and infants of women with urinary tract infections did not do well across the range of outcomes when this condition was associated with high fever. A background of infertility was confirmed as a high-risk condition insofar as the subsequent impact on stillbirths was concerned. Incompetent cervix yielded especially bad results, undoubtedly reflecting the very high rate of premature delivery. Cases in which surgery had been done for cervical incompetence also did poorly, although considerably better than the overall data for these patients.

Table 20-23
Selected Outcomes Significantly Related to Maternal Disorders

Factor	SB	NND	PMR	APG5	GLOB8	MENT8	MOT8	NEUR1	SLH3	IQ4	IQ7
Heart disease	3.09c+		2.46b					1.80a			
No symptoms											
Symptomatic	3.06c		2.10b					8.68b			
Rheumatic fever											
Embolization	10.84d	6.48a	7.73d								
Other cardiovascular	2.22c		1.72b			3.33d	2.01a				
Active tuberculosis				4.22a							
Positive sputum	5.21a			7.01c	9.03b						
X-ray evidence	4.01a			4.51b							
Pneumonia					2.52c	3.44c	5.94b	2.03a	3.87c		
Positive culture					5.37d	5.43b					
Serology					6.04b	6.69a			2.14a	2.65a	1.25a
Bronchial asthma											
Acute asthma	5.16c										
Status		1.62c	2.71a				1.49a	2.28b	1.24c		1.51c
Other pulmonary		1.18a	1.41c				1.47d	2.29a		1.80d	3.50b
Anemia				1.20b							
Low iron	2.23b		1.60a	1.80a							
High IBC	4.90b										
Smear					1.98a						
Bone marrow	2.94a				3.09a						
Iron response	0.58e*		0.58e*								
Electrophoresis									1.73a		
Sickling									1.86c		1.96a
Other		2.30b	2.06b	2.21b	2.18a		2.58a		2.02b		
Coagulopathy	31.23e	12.26d	19.02e	12.58e							
Prothrombin	7.00a										
Fibrinogen	41.67e	18.94d	21.62e	18.87e							
Clotting time	35.36e	10.36b	18.85e	12.58e							
Response	38.90e	20.83e	20.89e / 7.34c	18.87e							
Other	14.14e		4.94e								
Blood disease	6.78e	3.83c		3.39c	3.28b	3.73c	3.83a	2.71d	2.94a		
Diabetes		4.01e				4.03e	5.17e	2.58d		2.13b	1.63a
Blood sugar	4.68e	3.67e	3.83e	2.22e	3.70e	3.31c	4.98e	2.61b		4.46d	3.27c
Insulin		4.20e		2.02d	3.63e		5.34e			3.50c	2.88b
Reaction		4.75e	4.11e		4.11e					6.13d	
Coma	28.01e	20.83e	17.45e	2.87b	5.65e	4.21a	9.79e	3.66e			
Keto-acidosis	10.76e	5.82e	7.56e	2.04c	5.05e	5.18e	6.93e				
5-year duration	5.19e	4.69e	4.63e	1.89a / 2.70b							
Hypothyroid					2.99b	3.05a					
Low PBI											
Low BEI											
Hyperthyroid									4.64a		
High BMR						5.43b	10.78b		2.98a		
High PBI				4.73b			5.56b				
High BEI				3.15a							
Response	4.71b	4.71b	3.08a			6.68b		5.01b			

234

Condition									
Other endocrine	1.22a								
Gonorrhea	2.01d								
Glomerulonephritis						3.86a		1.61b	4.02b
Urinary infection									
Fever	1.53a	1.82d	2.08e	1.61a	0.66a*	1.64a	1.78c	1.60a	1.27a
CVA tenderness	1.44a	1.37b	1.33a		2.08b		1.42a	1.62a	2.77b
Culture	1.80e	1.46c					1.57c	1.25a	1.92c
Pyuria	1.22a	1.19a						1.75b	1.49a
Hematuria	1.64b	1.39b						2.09b	
Other GU disease	2.36d	1.89c						1.07b	1.69a
Infertility	1.94c	1.54b							
Incompetent cervix	7.11e	11.22e	8.87e	5.05d	8.35e	9.96e			
Cerclage	9.62e	5.42e	4.72e	3.23b	5.48c	6.89e			
(Cerclage, cont.)					0.74a*	2.07a			
Vaginitis									
Leiomyomata	2.29c	1.86c	1.64a			1.61a	1.61a	2.58b	1.88a
Gynecological tumor	1.94d	1.49b							
Gynecological surgery	2.67e	2.21e	1.54a			1.49a			
Other gynecologic	1.42a	1.57b	1.49c	1.62a					
Convulsions	2.64b		1.86a	4.80e	3.34b	3.19a	4.66e	2.69c	2.45b
Retardation				4.68e	5.21e	5.29e	4.46e	4.10e	9.19e
Brain disease				3.44a		7.12c	9.52e	8.91e	
Other neurologic	1.61a	1.50a	1.46a			3.74a			
Cholelithiasis	4.12b			3.70b	6.16c	10.26e			
Hepatitis	2.97a	2.76a		4.33b	7.50c				
Appendicitis	6.13b								
GI tumor	6.51b	5.68d							
Other dermatologic				1.32b		1.27a		1.20a	1.32a
Hyperemesis	3.48e	3.80e	3.04e	2.41e	1.94a	2.10b		0.80a*	2.88e
Hydramnios		1.85e	1.49e	2.60e	2.84e	2.94e	1.51a	1.63e	1.11a
Bleeding, first trimester	4.57e	4.08e	3.97e	1.46e	1.44c	1.62c	1.26a	1.58b	2.57d
Bleeding, second trimester	1.90e	1.46e	1.48e		1.43b	1.33b		1.24a	1.22a
Bleeding, third trimester	1.54e								
Shock, anesthetic		0.36b*							
Shock, hemorrhagic	19.64e	11.99e	12.67e	11.18e	6.02c	3.55a			
Shock, septic	25.64e	12.95d	12.34e	7.89c		3.72a			
Shock, other	4.81e		3.44d	4.58e					
Anesthetic accident	0.73a*					0.32a*	0.69c*	0.59b*	
Viral infection									
Bacterial infection	2.48a								
Fungal infection									
Unknown infection			0.18c*	0.16a*	0.58a*	0.59a*			
Live virus vaccine							0.64c*	0.89e*	1.12a
Other conditions	1.34b	1.32c	1.23a						

* Protective effect.

† Data presented as relative risk, compared with referent rate for cases without the factor under consideration.

Code for p-values: a0.05, b0.01, c0.001, d0.0001, e0.00001 or less.

Leiomyomata uteri resulted in increased stillbirth, neonatal depression, low eight-month motor scores, and persistent long-term effects up to seven years. These unexpected findings might also reflect an increased rate of premature births, but the relationship remained to be clarified. Any gynecologic surgery in pregnancy was associated with poor survival rates and frequent neonatal depression, but no apparent residual late adverse impact.

Neurological Disorders

Maternal convulsive disorders, mostly epilepsy (eclampsia was not included here), yielded high stillbirth rates and rather poor long-term results across tests from eight months to seven years. Retardation in the mother, while unassociated with fetal wastage, showed similar (actually rather worse) outcomes extending from the neonatal period (with depression, but not death) all the way to the seven-year IQ scores, a quite unanticipated finding. Organic brain disease, while infrequent in occurrence, yielded similar adverse effects, but these achieved statistical significance only at eight months and one year.

Gastrointestinal Conditions

Hepatitis was particularly harmful to the fetus as shown by the increased stillbirth rate; surviving infants did not fare well either in regard to their very poor showing at eight months and, to a lesser extent, at one year. Appendicitis had not been found to be associated with neonatal deaths, but the frequency of stillbirths was significantly increased. Surviving infants did well, however, with no apparent long-term effect. Gastrointestinal tumors, rare events in pregnancy, yielded especially high fetal losses, probably related to the prematurity associated with the requisite surgical intervention.

Obstetrical Complications

Among intercurrent obstetrically related conditions, hyperemesis gravidarum was associated with acceptable peripartum death and depression rates among infants, but adverse middle-range outcome results (at eight months and one year) were somewhat increased. Long-term residual effect was paradoxically protective at four years and deleterious at seven years. Hydramnios, as aforementioned, yielded high perinatal mortality rates; in addition, surviving infants continued to do badly across the range of outcomes that were studied (except for the seven-year IQs).

Vaginal bleeding in pregnancy, when examined collectively as a single composite variable (see above), did show an adverse short-term fetal and infant effect, but no comparable long-term impact at three years. Stratifying these cases by the trimester in which the bleeding occurred, as shown in Table 20-23, clearly demonstrated the deleterious overall effects of this clinical manifestation as well as the differential effects according to when in pregnancy it took place.

First trimester bleeding, for example, obviously had its impact principally on the fetus and neonate with significant residual effects still seen at four and seven years. Second trimester bleeding resulted in much greater perinatal wastage and neonatal depression, and also showed continuing adverse influence in all subsequent testing. Third trimester bleeding also yielded high perinatal losses, but they were not nearly so great as with bleeding in the first or second trimester. Nonetheless, the deleterious effects continued throughout the seven-year study period.

Hemorrhagic and septic shock states were especially devastating in terms of the greatly elevated perinatal mortality and neonatal depression rates. There were also impressively adverse intervening results at eight months and one year in the hemorrhagic shock subseries. Anesthetic shock was contrastingly unrelated to any discernible effects; in fact, perinatal mortality was unexpectedly low, suggesting a protective effect here. No residual long-term effects were found at four and seven years.

Systemic infections of various kinds

failed to show any consistent adverse impact on offspring, although the data raised questions concerning possible protective effects in some of the test results. The exception was the finding of high stillbirth rates among gravidas with fungal infections, a matter deserving further exploration.

Results by Organ System

By way of summarization of this complex array of data, we coalesced all of the results by organ system, reassessing outcomes simplistically according to the number of maternal manifestations or disorders related to that organ system (Table 20-24). A special added value of this approach was felt to be its potential for uncovering relationships in which multiple manifestations may be additive or synergistic. Significant results may be obtained in this way which might otherwise have been missed by examining a single manifestation alone.

Among the 14 codified items under the cardiovascular rubric (see chapter 19, Table 19-11), for example, all those cases with only one variable present, when studied as a single heterogeneous grouping, failed to show any adverse or beneficial impact on offspring. One should note here that we had already found that some single variables did show such impact (see Table 20-23, above); however, all single variables, including such relatively common ones as asymptomatic heart disease, were now being included, thus diluting out these effects. Despite this, when cases with two factors were examined, neonatal deaths were found to be significantly increased. With three cardiovascular variables present, stillbirths and neonatal depressions surfaced as significant.

Data for other organ systems were of comparable interest, revealing similar kinds of relevant information, mostly reflective of the foregoing single-factor analyses (see above). Of rather special interest, however, were the findings for hematologic, gyneco-logic, and metabolic-endocrine disorders when investigated and displayed in this manner. These systems showed impressive cumulative impact on outcome from multiple concurrent problems.

The data for the metabolic-endocrine conditions are especially noteworthy in this regard. We had already determined that nearly all of the 22 single variables in this group (with the notable exception of abnormal glucose tolerance test alone) had some documentably adverse effect. Here, we found that cases with two factors showed like effects; with three, the adverse impact was further enhanced; and with four or more, it was still worse. The rate ratio of perinatal mortality, for example, with three concurrent manifestations of a metabolic or endocrine condition was 62.7% greater than the risk if only two existed (based on a rate ratio of 2.57 versus one of 1.58, both significantly different from the general population risk and also significantly different from each other, p = .016). Moreover, with four attributes, the risk increased an additional 94.3% (to RR 4.06, again significantly different from the other relative risk values, p = .029) for a total increment in relative risk of 157.0% over that of offspring of uneffected mothers. This effect was apparent not only for perinatal deaths, but extended to eight months and four years as well.

For gynecologic conditions, the incremental increase in perinatal mortality by number of simultaneously acting variables was small, but nonetheless statistically verifiable. One gynecologic factor, all cases considered collectively, increased perinatal mortality by a relative risk of 22.0% (RR 1.22 compared to the referent); two concurrent factors enhanced the adverse effect of a single variable again by 22.1% (RR 1.49 versus 1.22); three factors augmented this by a further 116.4% (RR 2.91) to a total of 138.5% over the one-factor impact. This effect, however, could not be verified beyond the neonatal period for these conditions.

The data for multiple hematologic vari-

Table 20-24
Adverse Outcomes by Summary Classification of Maternal Conditions

Organ System	Number of Conditions	SB	NND	PMR	APG5	GLOB8	MENT8	MOT8	NEUR1	SLH3	IQ4	IQ7
Cardiovascular	2		1.66a									
	3	2.06b†										
Pulmonary	1		1.38c	1.50a	1.61b					1.32b	1.12a	
	2			1.23b								
	3					2.03a		1.76a				
	4+											
Blood	1	1.35d	1.56e	1.43e	4.98d		1.39b	1.60d		1.37d	1.21b	1.16a
	2		0.76a*		1.40e			1.34a		1.27b		1.24a
	3	2.08c		1.50a	1.79b							1.36b
	4	4.90e		3.01e								1.78b
Metabolic-endocrine	2	1.57a	1.63a	1.58b	1.79c	2.31b	2.83a			2.11a	1.27a	
	3	3.55e		2.57e	2.08b	3.58e				1.56a	2.12b	
Venereal	1				1.50c							
	2		4.10e	4.06e			3.75e	4.93e	2.35a		3.02e	
	3	4.52e							2.37c	1.54b	3.11e	
Urinary tract	1				2.30a	1.21b						
	2	1.94e		1.47c								
	3	1.84c		1.74d								
	4+		1.68b									
Gynecologic	1	1.29c	1.16a	1.22d	1.74c	1.67b						
	2	1.53d	1.47c	1.49e	1.12a				1.72b	1.56a	1.40b	1.21a
	3	2.64e	3.40e	2.91e	1.39d						1.44b	1.36b
	4+		4.73e	3.13e	1.84d							
Neurologic-psychiatric	1					1.29b						
	2	1.50a	1.75b	1.60c		1.62a		2.03b	2.49e	2.16b	2.09c	1.90c
	3					2.90b		2.98a	2.83a	2.83b		
	4+	5.39c		3.73b				5.39b				
Gastrointestinal	1						0.65b*					
	2									0.58a*		
Integument-appendages	1	1.52a	1.58a	1.54b		1.24a			2.69a			

* Protective effect.

† Data presented as relative risk, compared with referent rate for cases without the factor under consideration.

Code for p-values: a 0.05, b 0.01, c 0.001, d 0.0001, e 0.00001 or less.

ables were less straightforward. No increment in perinatal mortality rates above that found with one variable was encountered with two or three, but there was a substantive increase with four of 110.5% (RR 3.01 versus 1.43). For stillbirth rates and low seven-year intelligence test scores, the findings paralleled those stepwise increments seen in the other organ systems. One hematologic factor increased the relative risk of fetal deaths 35.0% (RR 1.35 over the referent rate); with three, the relative risk increased 54.1% (RR 2.08); and with four, it rose sharply by an additional 208.9% (RR 4.90) to 263.0% in all above the stillbirth rate for one variable. The enhancement seen in the seven-year results was comparable but of a much lower order of magnitude.

The data thus derived have provided detailed background foundational material on the fetal and infant effects of intrinsic maternal, fetal, and pelvic conditions preceding labor. The relationships thereby uncovered are expected to prove especially useful in permitting future investigations in this project (and others yet to be designed) to assess obstetrical practices in a more meaningful manner than heretofore possible.

CHAPTER 21

Intrinsic Factors: Designation of Risk Variables

Summary

The 271 inherent prenatal variables were studied in depth in 15,169 cases limited by birth weight (2500-4000 g) and exclusive of infants with major congenital disorders. Screening by bivariate and cluster analyses was followed by logistic regression techniques to determine which intrinsic variables retained significant adverse or protective associations with outcome while the influence of all others were being considered at the same time. A total of 59 were found to have such significant residual effects.

The approach utilized for determining those intrinsic variables likely to be most relevant to outcome paralleled the sequence described in chapter 7 and implemented in chapters 14 and 18. The long lists of intrinsic maternal, fetal, and pelvic variables previously alluded to (Table 19-1 and 19-11) were subjected first to Freeman-Tukey bivariate screening, then cluster analysis to reduce redundancy, and finally logistic regression analysis to identify those factors acting to affect the fetus and infant while all others were considered simultaneously. Given the large number of variables now under consideration, the process proved both time-consuming and costly. To recapitulate, we were now addressing a total of 271 discrete variables, consisting of 144 identifiable maternal disorders or variants of disorders plus 13 groupings of diseases by organ system or related groups of conditions, and an additional 114 maternal and fetal factors of possible relevance to outcome. It was felt that the operations were essential, nonetheless, in order to ensure that the basic objectives of the program would be realized.

For uniformity and consistency, it was once again necessary to constrict the index population by deleting those delivering anomalous infants and stratifying by parity and birth weight. The outcome factors were limited to an adverse perinatal vari-

able (death plus severe neonatal depression) and a composite variable (consisting of all definite neurologic or developmental abnormalities recorded through age seven years). The variables to be evaluated were defined (Table 21-1).

Of interest was the need to establish specific definitions for small-for-gestational-age (SGA) and large for gestational age (LGA) that would be directly applicable to the NCPP population itself. To this end, we determined the distribution of birth weights for all deliveries occurring at each successive gestational week. The tenth and 90th percentiles of birth weight for a given

Table 21-1
Intrinsic Variables Defined

Variable	Definition
INST05, INST10, etc.	Institutional codes for 12 collaborating institutions
AGE1	Maternal age less than 20 yr. at delivery
AGE2	Maternal age 19-24 yr.
AGE3	Maternal age 25-29 yr.
AGE4	Maternal age 30-34 yr.
AGE5	Maternal age 35 yr. or more
AGE6	Maternal age less than 18 yr.
AGE7	Maternal age less than 16 yr.
STATUS1	Patient status, clinic service
STATUS2	Patient status, private service
MARIT1	Marital status, single
MARIT2	Marital status, married
MARIT3	Marital status, common law
MARIT4	Marital status, widowed
MARIT5	Marital status, divorced
MARIT6	Marital status, separated
RACE1	Race, white
RACE2	Race, black
RACE3	Race, other
GRAV1	First pregnancy, nullipara for index pregnancy
GRAV2	Gravida 2
GRAV3	Gravida 3
GRAV4	Gravida 4
GRAV5	Gravida 5
GRAV6	Gravida 6+
PARA0	Nullipara for index pregnancy
PARA1	Parity 1-4
PARA2	Grand multipara, parity 5+
PABORT0	No prior abortion
PABORT1	Past history of 1 or more abortions
PPREM0	No prior premature delivery
PPREM1	Past history of 1 or more premature delivery
PSTILLB0	No prior stillbirth
PSTILLB1	Past history of 1 or more stillbirths
PPMR0	No prior perinatal death
PPMR1	Past history of 1 or more perinatal death

241

HGT1	Maternal height 68 in. or over
HGT2	Maternal height under 60 in.
HGT3	Maternal height 60-67 in.
PWGT1	Prepregnancy weight 175 lb. or more
PWGT2	Prepregnancy weight less than 100 lb.
POND1	Ponderal index (HGT/PWGT$^{1/3}$) greater than 13.734 (lean)
POND2	Ponderal index less than 11.891 (obese)
QI1	Quetelet's ponderosity index (PWGT/HGT^2) less than 0.0260 (lean)
QI2	Quetelet's ponderosity index greater than 0.0365 (obese)
WTGAIN1	Weight gain total less than 11 lb.
WTGAIN2	Weight gain 11-13 lb.
WTGAIN3	Weight gain less than 14 lb.
WTGAIN4	Weight gain 39 lb. or more
WTGAIN5	Weight gain 48 lb. or more
SES1	Socioeconomic index under 15
SES2	Socioeconomic index 15-24
SES3	Socioeconomic index 25-34
SES4	Socioeconomic index 35-44
SES5	Socioeconomic index 45-54
SES6	Socioeconomic index 55-64
SES7	Socioeconomic index 65-74
SES8	Socioeconomic index 75-84
SES9	Socioeconomic index 85+
VISIT1	Prenatal care office visits fewer than 7
VISIT2	Prenatal visits 8-14
VISIT3	Prenatal visits 15-16
VISIT4	Prenatal visits 17-20
VISIT5	Prenatal visits 21+
GREG	Gestational age at registration over 28 wk.
GDEL1	Gestational age at delivery under 34 wk.
GDEL2	Gestational age at delivery under 36 wk.
GDEL3	Gestational age at delivery under 38 wk.
GDEL4	Gestational age at delivery over 41 wk.
GDEL5	Gestational age at delivery over 42 wk.
GDEL6	Gestational age at delivery over 43 wk.
GDEL7	Gestational age at delivery over 44 wk.
BW1	Birth weight 2500-2749 g.
BW2	Birth weight 2750-2999 g.
BW3	Birth weight 3000-3249 g.
BW4	Birth weight 3250-3499 g.
BW5	Birth weight 3500-3749 g.
BW6	Birth weight 3740-3999 g.
MALE	Male infant
FEMALE	Female infant
STERIL	Prior sterility evaluation
RADN1	Abdominal or pelvic radiation in this pregnancy
RADN2	Radiation to other areas
RADN3	Radiation to abdomen-pelvis and other areas
RADN4	No radiation in pregnancy
VAGBLD	Vaginal bleeding in first trimester
RHSENS	Rh isoimmunization
SMOKE0	Nonsmoker
SMOKE2	Smoker, duration 10 yr. or more
SMOKE3	Smoker, more than 30 cigarettes per day
SMOKE4	Smoker, 10-30 cigarettes per day
SMOKE5	Smoker, less than 10 cigarettes per day
ABRUPT	Abruptio placentae
PREVIA	Placenta previa
PIH1	Pregnancy-induced hypertension, diastolic 95+ torr only
PIH2	PIH, diastolic 85+ torr and proteinuria 1+ or more
PIH3	PIH, proteinuria 2+ or more only
PIH4	Pregnancy hypotension, diastolic less than 65 torr maximum

HYDRAM	Hydramnios, polyhydramnios
UTRUP	Uterine rupture
PROLAP	Cord prolapse
PELV1	Summary of pelvic capacity, adequate
PELV2	Pelvic contracted
PELV3	Pelvic borderline

week were then assigned as the cut points for defining SGA and LGA (Table 21-2). All infants falling outside these limits were designated accordingly.

Screening Analysis

Study populations remained at the same level for this analysis as before, namely 6688 nulliparas and 8481 multiparas. Freeman-Tukey deviates and rate ratios were determined for each variable in isolation. Exclusive of disease states, those showing measurably significant association with outcome are shown in Table 21-3. Institutional differences were rather apparent, some appearing to be protective (INST05 and INST10) and others deleterious (INST60 and INST71). Whether or not these findings reflected the confounding effects of differences in population make-up in regard to concentration of high-risk factors remained to be determined.

Maternal age seemed relevant, median groups (especially AGE2, 19-24 years) showing protection, while older (AGE5, 35 or more) and younger (AGE6, under 18, and AGE5, under 16) showed adverse effects. Patient status demonstrated the expected benefit of private care (STATUS2), although it was not unlikely that this reflected factors relating to general health and well-being rather than to the care being rendered. Marital status focused on the apparent adverse effect of being single (MARIT1) or divorced (MARIT5) in contrast to the protection afforded by marriage (MARIT2). Again, these may merely have served as markers for some other factor, such as socioeconomic status (see SES below).

Racial associations were as previously observed with protection among white gravidas (RACE1) and adverse outcomes for others (both RACE2, black, and RACE3, other). Gravidity showed little relation to results, except for some degree of benefit for first pregnancies (GRAV1) and an inexplicable adverse effect in third pregnancies (GRAV3). Nulliparity (PARA0) yielded an inconsistent effect, perhaps because the group contained subsets of both primigravidas and multigravidas.

Past history of fetal wastage showed the expected adverse effects on the current pregnancy, including prior premature birth (PPREM1), stillbirth (PSTILLB1) and perinatal death (PPMR1). There was some consistent increase in bad outcomes among those with prior abortion (PABORT1), but none attained statistical significance. Maternal height was relevant in cases in which short stature prevailed (HGT2, under 60 inches); offspring of tall women (HGT1, over 67 inches) did unexpectedly well. Both ponderal measurements of maternal body mass revealed that obese women seemed to place their infants at risk (POND2, low ponderal index, and QI2, high ponderosity index). Those gaining excessively in pregnancy showed a similar effect (WTGAIN4, 39 lb or more, and WTGAIN5, 48 lb or more). Offspring of nulliparas who failed to gain adequately (WTGAIN1, less than 11 lb) also did poorly in the perinatal period.

The impact of socioeconomic status was confirmed. Indigent gravidas (SES1-4, scores below 45) were associated with bad results; this stood in sharp contrast to outcomes for affluent women (SES8 and SES9, indices over 74) who showed a marked protective effect. Data for the number of prenatal visits demonstrated a comparable adverse effect from too few (VISIT1, less than 7) and too many (VISIT4 and VISIT5, more than 16). The former possibly

Table 21-2
Fetal Growth Parameters for Retardation and Macrosomia Defined

Variable	Gestational Age, weeks	Birthweight Limit* grams
SGA, Small for gestational age		
	42+	2835
	41	2807
	40	2722
	39	2608
	38	2438
	37	2381
	36	2211
	35	2128
	34	1953
	33	1755
	32	1525
	31	1411
	30	1380
LGA, Large for gestational age		
	42+	3997
	41	3884
	40	3742
	39	3629
	38	3544
	37	3572
	36	3597
	35	3487
	34	3517
	33	3432
	32	3572
	31	3674
	30	3385

* Based on tenth and ninetieth percentiles of the distribution of weights for infants delivered at each gestational age for the full 42,972 case data base.

Table 21-3
Effect of Intrinsic Variables on Outcome by Parity

Variable	Perinatal Outcome		Composite Outcome	
	Nulliparas	Multiparas	Nulliparas	Multiparas
INST05	0.55C	0.79	0.55F	0.77B
INST10	0.79	0.49A	0.63A	0.50E
INST15	1.64	0.96	1.43	1.50C
INST37	1.52	1.39	1.65F	1.25A
INST45	1.96B	0.87	1.58C	1.14
INST60	1.75A	1.37	2.06F	1.71F
INST71	1.01	1.67A	1.38A	1.50C
INST82	1.01	0.63	1.13	0.70B
AGE1	1.17	0.81	1.16B	1.11
AGE2	0.78A	0.92	0.84B	1.00
AGE5	1.00	1.66C	0.46	1.06
AGE6	1.18	1.44	1.30E	1.06
AGE7	1.79B	2.11	1.35A	1.69
STATUS2	0.70	0.47A	0.67A	0.48E
MARIT1	1.28A	1.13	1.25D	0.95

MARIT2	0.88	0.90	0.90A	0.97
MARIT5	1.00	2.66C	1.00	1.54A
RACE1	0.72B	0.76A	0.86B	1.02
RACE2	1.33B	1.09	1.28F	1.05
RACE3	1.14	1.63	0.57D	0.71B
GRAV1	0.96	0.87	0.99	0.87A
GRAV3	1.16	1.30	2.02A	1.19A
PARA0	1.34	0.90	1.13	0.85B
PARA1	0.96	0.84	0.99	1.23B
PPREM1	1.35	1.40B	1.14	1.29E
PSTILLB1	1.34	1.49A	1.13	1.25A
PPMR1	1.00	1.56	1.00	1.27B
HGT1	0.39A	0.89	0.90	1.02
HGT2	1.64A	1.98C	1.30A	1.23
POND2	2.07E	1.22	1.43C	1.27A
QI2	1.71B	1.20	1.25A	1.26A
WGT1	2.04C	0.70	1.18	1.01
WGT4	1.98D	1.22	1.54E	1.13
WGT5	2.76C	1.64A	1.63A	1.17
SES1	1.58A	1.01	1.53D	1.57C
SES2	0.97	1.15	1.39C	1.20A
SES3	1.42	1.25	1.50F	1.13
SES4	1.67D	1.12	1.15	1.15A
SES8	0.95	0.41A	0.61C	0.50C
SES9	0.27C	0.44A	0.27F	0.46D
VISIT1	1.03	0.98	1.09	1.21D
VISIT4	0.89	2.42C	0.86	1.47A
VISIT5	2.32	1.58	1.34	2.37A
GREG	0.69	0.95	0.96	1.21C
GDEL1	1.27	2.19B	1.10	1.38
GDEL2	1.67A	1.79B	1.41B	1.38B
GDEL3	1.30	1.56C	1.24A	1.35E
GDEL5	1.45B	1.19	0.99	1.05
GDEL6	1.45A	1.35	1.05	1.16
GDEL7	1.43A	1.31	1.02	1.14
BW1	1.14	1.47A	1.05	1.18
MALE	1.31C	1.21A	1.18D	1.13C
VGBLD	1.32	2.43F	0.97	1.42B
RHSENS	0.00	5.68E	0.00	2.43C
SMOKE2	2.31C	1.11	1.05	0.94
SMOKE3	1.54	0.94	2.46D	1.06
ABRUPT	2.45B	4.00F	1.14	1.44A
PIH1	1.18	2.13C	1.07	1.32
PIH2	1.45A	1.80A	1.54B	1.17
HYDRAM	1.60	3.99F	1.93	2.07E
PROLAP	1.90	5.53F	2.35C	2.31D
PELV2	1.48	3.01C	1.19	1.52A
SGA	1.32A	1.42A	1.23	1.02
LGA	1.68A	0.80	1.25	1.12

---

* Only variables found to be significant by Freeman-Tukey analysis are included. Data expressed in rate ratios. Probability code: A 0.05, B 0.01, C 0.005, D 0.001, E 0.0005, F 0.0001 or less.

reflected inadequate care and the latter, concurrent illness.

Late registration for antepartum care (GREG) showed some late adverse effect, as did early delivery (GDEL1-3, prior to 38 weeks). These observations were especially pertinent in light of the fact that this analysis was limited to study of a population of cases delivering babies weighing 2500-4000 g. Prolonged or postdate pregnancies (GDEL5-7, deliveries beyond 42 weeks) showed adverse perinatal impact only, especially in nulliparas. Those at the lowest end of the birth weight scale (BW1, 2500-2749 g) had significantly poorer outcomes than any other birth weight group. Male babies (MALE) did significantly worse than females in both perinatal and composite outcomes for both parity groups.

Neither prior infertility problems (STERIL) nor prenatal exposure to radiation (RAD1-4) was found to have any demonstrable adverse effect. Early pregnancy bleeding (VAGBLD) gave rise to poor results. Rh-isoimmunization (RHSENS) was, as expected, a serious adverse factor in multiparas only. Cigarette smoking for 10 years or more (SMOKE2) or at a rate of at least one and a half packs per day (SMOKE3) was associated with significantly poor results. Placental abruption (ABRUPT) was an expectedly adverse factor. Pregnancy-induced hypertension was significant in the presence of elevated diastolic blood pressure (PIH1 and PIH2). Persistent hypotensive levels of blood pressure in pregnancy (PIH4, less than 65 torr maximum diastolic) also showed increases in bad outcomes, but not to significant levels when assessed statistically.

Hydramnios (HYDRAM) showed impressively bad outcome results. It should be recalled in this regard that fetal anomalies—and therefore many cases of hydramnios with which such anomalies were associated—were excluded from consideration here. Uterine rupture (UTRUP) was too rare an event to be studied meaningfully. Cord prolapse (PROLAP) was especially deleterious, as expected. Pelvic

inadequacy proved to be a disadvantage, particularly with documented contracted pelvis (PELV2); it was associated with significantly poorer outcomes than the general population. Both intrauterine growth retardation (SGA) and fetal macrosomia (LGA) were verified to have adverse effects despite the narrow birth weight constraints imposed by patient selection criteria.

Screening was done for all 144 variables pertaining to maternal disorders, designated in sequence as DIS1 through DIS144 (Table 19-11), plus 13 summary variables encompassing all diagnosed disorders for a given organ system or a related group of conditions (SDIS1 through SDIS13). Those found to be significantly related to outcome are listed in Table 21-4 with their rate ratios and coded p values for both perinatal and composite outcomes, separately for nulliparas and multiparas.

Maternal cardiac disease (DIS1) was associated with adverse outcome, more prominently in multiparas than nulliparas. Of interest was the observation that women with organic heart disease who had symptoms on ordinary physical activity (DIS3) yielded even worse results, suggesting that a patient's functional status was an important prognostic index for her fetus.

Pulmonary tuberculosis, if active in pregnancy (DIS15), had a very serious impact; inactive tuberculosis (DIS21) did not, and it may have even been somewhat protective, albeit inconsistently so (RR = 0.45 in multiparas for composite outcome, just short of statistical significance). Pneumonia documented by chest x-ray findings (DIS25) appeared to have a bad perinatal impact which did not continue beyond the neonatal period. Diagnoses of pneumonia made by other means (DIS22) showed similar findings, but they were not statistically significant (RR = 2.22 for perinatal outcome in multiparas, an elevated but not significant ratio). Acute bronchial asthma in pregnancy (DIS27) showed almost identical results as documented pneumonia. If they share a common mechanism in regard to fetal damage, it is more likely to be maternal

Table 21-4
Effects of Maternal Disorders on Outcome by Parity*

Variable		Perinatal Outcome		Composite Outcome	
		Nulliparas	Multiparas	Nulliparas	Multiparas
DIS1	Organic heart disease	1.19	1.76A	0.84	1.52A
DIS3	Cardiac, symptoms with activity	1.70	3.41A	1.42	2.86C
DIS15	Tuberculosis, active	---	8.87C	---	2.37A
DIS25	Pneumonia	---	3.41A	---	0.82
DIS27	Acute bronchial asthma	---	2.61A	---	1.04
DIS32	Anemia, iron deficiency	2.08A	2.02A	1.82A	2.02A
DIS38	Sicklemia	1.39	2.50A	1.82A	0.96
DIS49	Diabetes mellitus	1.60A	4.43F	1.60A	2.71F
DIS50	Blood sugar over 200 mg.%	2.00A	5.53F	2.39A	2.97F
DIS51	Insulin therapy	2.60A	6.52F	2.84A	3.85F
DIS52	Insulin reaction	1.66	3.69	1.42	4.24E
DIS55	Diabetes 5 yr. or more	3.00	7.39D	3.83B	7.63F
DIS60	Hypothyroidism	2.77A	5.54A	1.71	3.95C
DIS71	Syphilis	1.29	1.99A	0.34A	1.09
DIS79	Other venereal diseases	---	4.03B	---	1.98A
DIS80	Glomerulonephritis	---	9.85F	---	3.95C
DIS82	Pyelonephritis	2.28A	1.55A	1.94C	1.36A
DIS99	Seizures in pregnancy	2.96A	2.00A	2.69A	1.85A
DIS100	Mental retardation	12.31F	1.39	7.21F	3.23F
DIS103	Neurological disorder	2.69A	2.42A	1.42	2.37C
DIS111	Colitis, ileitis	0.00	5.54B	4.25A	3.95B
DIS126	Late bleeding	0.72	1.42A	0.86	1.25B
DIS127	Anesthetic shock	0.52	2.61A	0.96	1.29A
DIS128	Hemorrhagic shock	---	19.00F	---	4.45C
DIS130	Supine hypotension	3.69A	5.11D	2.04A	1.32A
DIS131	Other shock	6.33A	6.33A	3.19A	1.32A
SDIS2	Pulmonary disorders	0.63	1.41A	0.78	1.05
SDIS3	Blood disorders	1.21	1.30A	1.15A	1.05
SDIS5	Venereal diseases	1.36	1.76B	1.42A	1.38B

* See Table 21-3 for criteria and coding. Data omitted for subsets represented by insufficient numbers of cases.

hypoxemia than infection or hyperthermia.

Iron deficiency anemia (DIS32) was associated with poor outcomes. This was paralleled in anemic cases diagnosed just on the basis of their response to iron therapy (DIS37), but not to the same magnitude or level of significance. Sickle cell disease (DIS38), as diagnosed by electrophoresis, showed the expected adverse effect on the fetus and infant, but the effect was inconsistent.

The most impressive and repetitively uniform results were found with maternal diabetes mellitus (DIS49). Both short-term and long-term effects were quite apparent in the two parity groups. The effect was magnified by features reflecting severity of the condition (such as the need for insulin, DIS51, and disease of long duration, DIS55) as well as poor control (for example, high blood sugar levels, DIS50, and insulin reaction, DIS52). When the fact that these data were derived from a series of cases that had excluded anomalous infants and both small and large birth weights is taken into account, these results must be considered especially noteworthy.

Other metabolic disorders also showed adverse effects, but only hypothyroidism (DIS60) reached statistical significance in regard to the magnitude of effect on the offspring. Syphilis (DIS71) had an unexpected deleterious association, but other sexually transmitted diseases were not consistent. Babies born to women with gonorrhea (DIS76) generally did well, except for suggestively poor results in the composite variable (RR = 1.56, not statistically significant), whereas those with other venereal diseases (DIS79) showed adverse outcomes. It is conjectured that these conditions might merely serve as markers for socioeconomic status or other more pervading influences.

Acute and chronic glomerulonephritis (DIS80), although not found in large numbers and limited almost exclusively to multiparas, yielded particularly poor outcomes. Cases with pyelonephritis (DIS82) had bad results as well, although they were not as impressively adverse as glomerulonephritis. The broader diagnosis of urinary tract infection (DIS81), encompassing the more common condition of cystitis, failed to show a comparable effect.

Offspring of women with diagnosed neurologic and neuromuscular conditions (DIS103) did poorly across the range of outcomes. The most common condition among them was epilepsy, suggesting the possibility that this finding might have reflected the anticonvulsive agent rather than the disorder itself. Countering this were the results for cases with past history of seizures (DIS98) but without seizures in the current index pregnancy; outcomes among this group of cases was about as expected for the general population. Infants delivered of mothers who had seizures in pregnancy (DIS99) did badly. While such effects may have resulted from either the underlying hypertensive diathesis or the causative neurologic disorder, hypoxia or acute drug effects may have been contributory instead during the seizure or in the immediate postictal state.

Of rather special interest here was the observation that mentally retarded gravidas (DIS100) placed their infants at very high risk of death or damage. This unanticipated finding clearly deserves more intensive study than it could be given in this investigation. Those babies delivered of psychotic or psychoneurotic women (DIS102), by contrast, did as well as the general population group.

Regional ileitis and ulcerative colitis (DIS111) were associated with particularly bad results. This was not duplicated with other gastrointestinal disorders, however. The only exception was severe hyperemesis gravidarum (requiring intravenous therapy, DIS121), which showed a marginally significant adverse effect in the composite outcome for multiparas (RR = 2.16).

Several types of shock states took their toll, as anticipated. The supine hypotension syndrome (DIS130) was quite unexpectedly associated with very bad outcomes. This suggested the condition to be either a much more serious clinical entity than heretofore appreciated or, more likely, an indicator of some underlying deleterious maternal state which in turn places fetuses at serious risk.

The data for summary groupings by organ system mirrored the results of the individual conditions contributing to their composition. Thus, the pulmonary disease group (SDIS2) showed the expected impact previously seen for tuberculosis, pneumonia, and acute bronchial asthma; and the blood disease group (SDIS3) reflected the effects of anemia and sickle cell disease. Similarly, the results for the sexually transmitted disease group (SDIS5) echoed those of syphilis and other venereal diseases.

Other groupings failed to show comparable outcome data because of the admixture of conditions that did not cause damage with those that did. The adverse effect of organic heart disease associated with functional impairment, for example, was diluted by the much larger number of cases without symptoms (DIS2), giving the grouped data (SDIS1) good overall results. Even the major effects of severe, long-standing, or poorly controlled diabetes mellitus were lost when they were combined with cases showing only abnormal glucose tolerance tests (DIS56) to form the metabolic-endocrine grouping (SDIS4).

Our screening operations to this point had studied the 271 intrinsic variables and found 145 of them to be significantly associated in bivariate isolation with bad fetal and infant outcomes. Among these, 39 were common to both parity groups; 46 occurred only in nulliparas and 60 only in multiparas. Thus, there were a total of 85 intrinsic variables found to be significant among nulliparas and 99 among multiparas. We were now ready to proceed with cluster analyses to ascertain similarities of informational content so as to determine if any of the variables could be legitimately deleted from further consideration.

Cluster Analysis

As described in detail for the labor progression variables (chapter 14) and the adjunctive drug variables (chapter 18), we next undertook aggregative hierarchical clustering analysis of the entire set of 145 intrinsic factors remaining to be considered on the basis of the foregoing bivariate screening procedure. We were searching for clusters of items containing essentially the same information about outcome. Redundancy could thereby be eliminated by utilizing only a single member of such a cluster as a representative variable for all members.

The analysis was carried out separately for nulliparas and multiparas. Figure 21-1 shows a portion of the resulting cluster tree for nulliparas. In general, most of the vari-

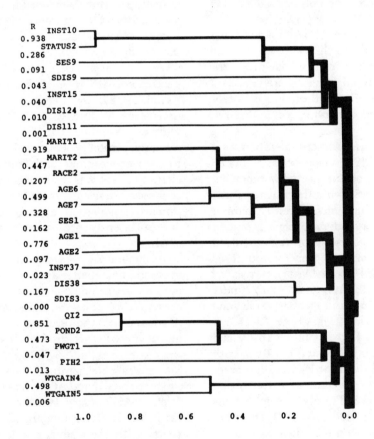

Figure 21-1. Cluster analysis of intrinsic maternal, fetal, and pelvic variables in nulliparas showing a portion of the cluster tree to illustrate some of the relevant relationships. Note the strong association between INST10 and STATUS2, MARIT1 and MARIT2, AGE1 and AGE2, and QI2 and POND2. Horizontal axis represents the correlation coefficient (*R*) between variables and subclusters.

ables were either unclustered or grouped in such weakly correlated clusters as to signify only the most tenuous relationships. These latter fell to the right of the cluster tree because of their very low correlation coefficients. An example of a cluster with such a low index of similarity in regard to informational content is seen in Figure 21-1, namely INST15, DIS124 (early pregnancy bleeding), and DIS111 (ileitis and colitis), seemingly representing just a chance association.

By contrast, some were strongly interrelated. INST10 and STATUS2 (private), for example, were very highly correlated (r = .938). In fact, only private patients were selected for the NCPP data collection at INST10. Moreover, no other collaborating institution included any private patients in their sampling frame. Thus, it followed that INST10 and STATUS2 should perforce have been highly correlated as study variables. Either could serve, therefore, as a marker for the other without loss of potentially important data on outcome. We felt justified as a consequence in deleting INST10 from further consideration as a risk variable. SES9 (socioeconomic score 85 or more) was not unexpectedly somewhat correlated (r = .286) with the private patient status cluster, but not sufficiently to merit elimination as a study variable.

Similar types of close correlations, albeit not quite so strong, were encountered between MARIT1 and MARIT2 (single and married, r = .919); AGE6 and AGE7 (under 18 and under 16 years, r = .499); AGE1 and AGE2 (age under 20 and age 19-24, r = .776); QI2 and POND2 (ponderosity and ponderal indices of obesity, r = .851), both related as a subcluster to PWGT1 (prepregnancy weight 175 lb or more, r = .473); and WTGAIN4 and WTGAIN5 (weight gains exceeding 39 and 48 lb, r = .498). These are all illustrated in Figure 21-1.

In addition, two large clusters showed the anticipated similarity among related features of diabetes mellitus (DIS49-52 and DIS55, namely diabetes mellitus, blood sugar 200 mg/dL or more, insulin therapy, insulin reaction, and duration 5 years or more, r = .825) and upper urinary traction infections (DIS82-85, fever 100° F or more, costovertebral angle tenderness, positive urine culture, and pyuria, r = .501). Another paired cluster consisted of the variables GDEL2 and GDEL3 (delivery prior to 36 and 38 weeks, r = .645).

Since none of these was inconsistent with clinical information or recognized clinical relationships, it was felt acceptable to proceed to delete a number of variables that were clearly redundant. Accordingly, MARIT2 (married) was eliminated and MARIT1 (single) retained. The impact of one undoubtedly reflected the mirror image effect of the other, that is, the good results seen in offspring of married gravidas stood as an index of the absence of the adverse results characteristic of the unmarried population.

A secondary cluster association of this subcluster with RACE2 (black) and with AGE6, AGE7, and SES1 (young gravidas under age 18 and very indigent women with socioeconomic index less than 15) indicated the capability of this analytic approach to uncover meaningful relationships. However, no effort was made to constrict these clustered variables because their degrees of similarity, while rather suggestive, were not sufficiently strong to warrant any deletions.

AGE6 and AGE7 were exceptions; they appeared to be correlated well enough to permit the pruning operation to take place. Since AGE7 cases were included within AGE6 (but not the reverse), they were not mutually exclusive variables. It was logical, therefore, to exclude AGE7 and keep AGE6 for future consideration. The correlated cluster of AGE1 and AGE2 was resolved by deleting AGE2 (aged 19-24 years) so as to retain an index of young gravidas (under 20 years) with their adverse effects on offspring as a preferable choice over that of the somewhat older (and much more common) group with their contrastingly good results.

QI2 was similarly omitted because it contained the same outcome data as POND2, both reflecting large body mass relative to height. The association of both these variables with PWGT1, as noted, was not quite close enough to warrant eliminating this latter factor. Nonetheless, WTGAIN5 was deleted in favor of WTGAIN4 because they had such similar informational content and because cases falling into the first set were incorporated into the second.

A similar procedure permitted us to retain just one representative variable (DIS49) for the five that had addressed various aspects of diabetes mellitus, and one composite variable (DIS82) to serve for the four upper urinary tract infection factors. In addition, GDEL3 was tabled in favor of GDEL2.

When the same technique was applied to the multiparous data, the results were almost identical. INST10 and STATUS2, for example, were very closely correlated (r = .975) and both were subclustered with SES9 (r = .440). QI2 was clustered with POND2 (r = .852), as before. The cluster representing diabetes mellitus was also much the same (DIS49-55). For these and others, it was possible to reduce the numbers of variables as described for nulliparas.

New relationships were disclosed that had not been encountered earlier. Variables dealing with thrombophlebitis, for example, were tightly clustered (DIS7-10, r = .816). A single factor (DIS7) was, therefore, chosen to represent them all. VISIT1 and VISIT2 (office visits less than seven and seven to 14) were also correlated (r = .847), reflecting complementary effects; the latter, being much more common, was deleted.

Overall, cluster analyses had thus enabled us to delete a number of redundant intrinsic variables so that we were left with a total of 70 in nulliparas (from the original group of 85) and 78 in multiparas (from 99). This paring operation was felt to provide a satisfactory means for reducing the large number of intrinsic variables to a more workable size. In this way, we were able to diminish the anticipated onerous task of logistic regression analysis somewhat.

Logistic Regression Analysis

Composite Outcome Data

Logistic regression analysis was used to study the effects of each intrinsic factor on outcome while the effects of all the others were being simultaneously considered. The results of the full analysis for the composite outcome (any definite adverse effect from before birth to 7 years) are shown in Tables 21-5 and 21-6 for nulliparas and multiparas, respectively. Strong associations were found for 18 of the 70 variables tested in nulliparas and 31 of the 78 in multiparas.

Many variables, previously designated as relevant by bivariate screening, failed to retain a significant relationship to adverse outcome when examined in the presence of associated factors. Examples include maternal age, patient and marital status, and race (except other than black and white). The analysis demonstrated that the variables were thus probably mere confounders— that is, their impact probably reflected or masked that of other, more fundamental, underlying adverse or protective factors. Of even greater importance were those variables continuing to show effects under this form of intensive scrutiny. Among them were obesity, heavy smoking, and excessive weight gain in nulliparas and prior fetal wastage, short stature, and low socioeconomic index in multiparas. Male infants fared especially poorly in both parity groups.

Perinatal Outcome Data

When the logistic regression analysis was applied to data for perinatal outcome (death plus severe neonatal depression), the results were somewhat different among the 18 significant items for nulliparas (Table 21-7) and the 24 for multiparas (Table 21-8). In nulliparas, offspring of black women (RACE2) and those with low socioeconomic indices (SES3 and SES4) did rather badly. Excessive and insufficient weight gain were both adverse factors, as were macrosomia (LGA) and postterm delivery (GDEL4). Factors with effects

Table 21-5
Logistic Regression Analysis of Intrinsic Variables in Nulliparas
for Composite Outcome*

Variable		Regression Coefficient	Standard Error	t-Statistic	Relative Risk	p-Value
Constant		-3.010	0.203	-14.81		
INST31	Hospital 31	0.614	0.230	2.67	1.85	0.010
INST37	Hospital 37	0.441	0.172	2.57	1.55	0.013
INST45	Hospital 45	0.457	0.199	2.29	1.58	0.026
INST60	Hospital 60	0.810	0.189	4.28	2.25	0.000084
INST71	Hospital 71	0.429	0.210	2.04	1.54	0.047
MARIT1	Single	-0.224	0.124	-1.81	0.80	0.073
RACE3	Other race	-0.813	0.232	-3.51	0.44	0.00096
GRAV3	Gravida 3	0.828	0.465	1.78	2.29	0.078
POND2	Obese	0.386	0.178	2.17	1.47	0.034
PWGT1	175+ lb.	-0.580	0.342	-1.70	0.56	0.092
SES3	Index 25-34	0.384	0.163	2.36	1.47	0.022
SES9	Index 85+	-1.338	0.314	-4.26	0.26	0.000090
BW2	2750-2999 g.	0.254	0.118	2.14	1.29	0.037
MALE	Male infant	0.427	0.097	4.38	1.53	0.000061
SMOKE3	> 30 per day	1.133	0.364	3.11	3.11	0.0031
WTGAIN4	39+ lb.	0.402	0.154	2.61	1.49	0.010
WTGAIN5	48+ lb.	0.723	0.234	3.09	2.06	0.0025
LGA	Macrosomia	0.318	0.189	1.68	1.37	0.096
DIS48	Blood disorder	2.869	1.020	2.81	17.61	0.0071
DIS63	Hyperthyroidism	1.492	0.882	1.69	4.45	0.097
DIS87	GU umor	3.838	1.429	2.69	46.42	0.0097
DIS100	Mental retardation	2.288	0.470	4.87	9.85	0.000012
DIS111	Colitis, ileitis	2.372	0.923	2.57	10.72	0.013

*   Only those variables with p-values of 0.10 or less from among the 70 tested.

comparable to those encountered in the composite outcome data included cigarette smoking (heavy habit in one, long duration in the other), excessive weight gain, and male fetus, as well as maternal mental retardation, colitis-ileitis, and hyperthyroidism. Obesity (POND2) was no longer significantly adverse and high socioeconomic index (SES9) no longer protective.

In multiparas, there was greater similarity with the results for composite outcomes for such conditions as prior fetal wastage, short stature, Rh isoimmunization, diastolic blood pressure elevation, male infant, diabetes mellitus, glomerulonephritis, late bleeding, and venereal disease. Low socioeconomic index, by contrast, was no longer relevant and the data for some medical conditions, previously flagged, were not significant; these included maternal anemia and mental retardation. A newly significant factor that surfaced at this time was vaginal bleeding in early pregnancy.

Step-up Logistic Modelling

Step-up modelling of logistic regression was pursued next, as previously described (see chapter 14). For composite outcomes, separate analyses were done for nulliparas (Table 21-9) and multiparas (Table 21-10). The base model for nulliparas was constructed from the 23 items previously found to have been significant at the 10% probability level in the full logistic regression analysis that had examined all 70 intrinsic variables simultaneously (Table 21-5).

Comparison with rate ratios in the full model showed some shifts, most notably reductions in the effects of variables such as SMOKE3 (more than 30 cigarettes daily) and several of the disease states (DIS48,

252

Table 21-6
Logistic Regression Analysis of Intrinsic Variables in Multiparas
for Composite Outcome*

Variable		Regression Coefficient	Standard Error	t–Statistic	Relative Risk	p–Value
Constant		-3.093	0.143	-21.62		
INST15	Hospital 15	0.384	0.194	1.97	1.47	0.050
INST55	Hospital 55	0.303	0.172	1.76	1.35	0.080
INST60	Hospital 60	0.619	0.141	4.37	1.86	0.000063
INST71	Hospital 71	0.584	0.190	3.08	1.79	0.0034
INST82	Hospital 82	-0.368	0.182	-2.01	0.69	0.047
AGE3	25-29 yr.	-0.221	0.099	-2.23	0.80	0.030
RACE3	Other race	-0.559	0.193	-2.90	0.57	0.0046
PARA2	Grand multipara	0.314	0.116	2.72	1.37	0.0077
PABORT1	Prior abortion	-0.180	0.103	-1.75	0.84	0.083
PPREM1	Prior premature	0.249	0.099	2.52	1.28	0.013
PPMR1	Prior death	1.204	0.687	1.75	3.33	0.0083
HGT2	Short stature	0.298	0.168	1.78	1.35	0.078
RHSENS	Rh disease	1.224	0.430	2.84	3.40	0.0054
SES1	Index < 15	0.438	0.180	2.43	1.55	0.017
SES4	Index 35-44	0.208	0.103	2.02	1.23	0.046
VISIT4	17-20 visits	0.621	0.250	2.48	1.86	0.014
PIH1	Diastolic increase	0.359	0.205	1.75	1.43	0.080
BW5	3500-3799 g.	-0.191	0.114	-1.68	0.83	0.096
MALE	Male infant	0.317	0.082	3.85	1.37	0.00021
DIS21	Tuberculosis, active	-0.919	0.522	-1.76	0.40	0.080
DIS32	Low serum iron	0.741	0.445	1.66	2.10	0.099
DIS49	Diabetes mellitus	0.843	0.334	2.52	2.32	0.013
DIS75	Syphilis	2.554	1.445	1.77	12.86	0.079
DIS80	Glomerulonephritis	1.816	0.755	2.40	6.15	0.018
DIS100	Mental retardation	1.056	0.442	2.39	2.87	0.019
DIS103	Neurological disease	0.847	0.371	2.28	2.33	0.025
DIS111	Colitis, ileitis	1.480	0.800	1.85	4.39	0.067
DIS126	Late bleeding	0.258	0.110	2.34	1.29	0.021
DIS128	Hemorrhagic shock	1.570	0.830	1.89	4.81	0.065
SDIS5	Venereal diseases	0.266	0.151	1.77	1.31	0.079

* Only those variables with p-values of 0.10 or less from among the 78 tested are tabulated.

DIS87, and DIS111, namely blood, genitourinary, and gastrointestinal disorders). There were increases in others, including POND2 (obesity) and DIS100 (mental retardation). One variable, MARIT1 (single), which previously had been marginally significant but was nonetheless included because it fell below the 10% probability level (p = .073), was now clearly insignificant (t = 1.06, p = .54); it will become apparent that in the subsequent step-up models, it did not improve its standing in this regard.

Testing was done of all 47 remaining intrinsic variables to determine if any could serve as candidates for inclusion in a step-up model composed of 24 variables. Ten were flagged as contenders, using a cutoff of p < .10. The most promising of these were: INST05 (p = .0006), RACE2 (p = .0039), MARIT5 (p = .0174), SMOKE4 (p = .0248), and SES8 (p = .0372). The rest had p values greater than 0.045. INST05, when added to the base model to form the first step-up model (Table 21-9), was found to be significantly protective. At the same time, it served to reduce the impact of all five of the institutional variables uniformly in both magnitude and significance level. In fact, the effect of one of them (INST71) became insignificant by this operation (t = 1.69, p = .094). The protective effect of RACE3 was

Table 21-7
Logistic Regression Analysis of Intrinsic Variables in Nulliparas
for Perinatal Outcome

Variable		Regression Coefficient	Standard Error	t-Statistic	Relative Risk	p-Value
Constant		-5.765	0.430	-13.42		
INST45	Hospital 45	0.795	0.337	2.36	2.21	0.022
RACE2	Black	0.453	0.271	1.67	1.57	0.098
SES3	Index 25-34	0.658	0.339	1.94	1.93	0.055
SES4	Index 35-44	0.909	0.314	2.89	2.48	0.0047
SES8	Index 75-84	0.896	0.409	2.19	2.45	0.031
MALE	Male infant	0.685	0.189	3.62	1.98	0.00046
SMOKE3	Smoking 10+ yr.	1.242	0.401	3.10	3.46	0.0025
WTGAIN1	< 11 lb. gain	0.911	0.306	2.97	2.49	0.0037
WTGAIN4	39+ lb. gain	0.630	0.261	2.41	1.88	0.018
LGA	Macrosomia	0.824	0.314	2.62	2.28	0.0097
GDEL4	Delivery after 41 wk.	0.651	0.206	3.15	1.92	0.0022
DIS63	Hyperthyroidism	3.045	0.996	3.06	21.01	0.0028
DIS74	Syphilis	3.725	1.732	2.15	41.49	0.034
DIS86	Pyelonephritis	0.748	0.442	1.69	2.11	0.094
DIS97	Other gyn disorder	0.914	0.404	2.26	2.49	0.026
DIS100	Mental retardation	2.625	0.629	4.18	13.80	0.000063
DIS107	Cholecystitis	3.047	1.229	2.48	21.06	0.014
DIS140	Parasitic infection	1.801	0.794	2.27	6.06	0.025

Table 21-8
Logistic Regression Analysis of Intrinsic Variables in Multiparas
for Perinatal Outcome

Variable		Regression Coefficient	Standard Error	t-Statistic	Relative Risk	p-Value
Constant		-5.153	0.306	-16.85		
INST31	Hospital 31	-1.121	0.594	-1.89	0.33	0.064
INST71	Hospital 71	0.674	0.388	1.74	1.96	0.088
MARIT5	Divorced	0.979	0.416	2.35	2.66	0.023
RACE3	Other race	0.638	0.347	1.84	1.89	0.072
PARA2	Grand multipara	0.506	0.233	2.17	1.66	0.034
PPREM1	Prior premature	0.344	0.196	1.76	1.41	0.084
HGT2	Short stature	0.609	0.283	2.15	1.84	0.036
RHSENS	Rh disease	2.509	0.561	4.48	12.30	0.000044
VAGBLD	Early pregnancy bleeding	0.782	0.275	2.84	2.19	0.0065
VISIT4	17-20 visits	0.841	0.420	2.00	2.32	0.049
PIH1	Diastolic increase	0.940	0.348	2.70	2.56	0.0094
MALE	Male infant	0.492	0.170	2.89	1.63	0.0057
DIS15	Tuberculosis, active	3.174	1.228	2.59	23.90	0.013
DIS37	Other pulmonary	0.471	0.241	1.95	1.60	0.051
DIS49	Diabetes mellitus	1.471	0.534	2.75	4.36	0.0083
DIS80	Glomerulonephritis	3.445	0.856	4.03	31.35	0.00019
DIS126	Late pregnancy bleeding	0.424	0.215	1.98	1.53	0.049
DIS128	Hemorrhagic shock	2.647	0.913	2.90	14.12	0.0055
DIS130	Supine hypotension	1.860	0.731	2.54	6.42	0.014
SDIS5	Venereal diseases	0.561	0.274	2.05	1.75	0.045

Table 21-9
Step-Up Logistic Regression Analysis of Intrinsic Variables
for Composite Outcome in Nulliparas*

Variable		Initial Model		Step-Up Model 1		Step-Up Model 2		Step-Up Model 3	
		RR	t	RR	t	RR	t	RR	t
INST31	Hospital 31	1.90	3.02C	1.65	2.33A	1.65	2.31A	1.64	2.30A
INST37	Hospital 37	1.80	3.71E	1.59	2.89C	1.60	2.93C	1.58	2.84B
INST45	Hospital 45	1.84	3.20C	1.63	2.52A	1.64	2.54A	1.60	2.44A
INST60	Hospital 60	2.36	5.12F	2.07	4.24F	2.13	4.42F	2.08	4.27F
INST71	Hospital 71	1.60	2.47A	1.39	1.69	1.39	1.71	1.37	1.62
MARIT1	Single	1.06	0.61	0.98	-0.18	0.97	-0.26	0.95	-0.47
RACE3	Other race	0.52	-3.18C	0.47	-3.66E	0.47	-3.67E	0.46	-3.77D
GRAV3	Gravida 3	2.30	1.81	2.20	1.72	2.26	1.80	2.28	1.78
PWGT1	175+ lb.	0.56	-1.73	0.56	-1.72	0.55	-1.80	0.54	-1.82
POND2	Obese	1.63	2.92C	1.60	2.83B	1.65	2.98C	1.62	2.90C
SES3	Index 25-34	1.48	3.15C	1.43	2.90C	1.42	2.84B	1.39	2.64B
SES9	Index 85+	0.29	-4.36F	0.30	-4.28F	0.30	-4.30F	0.28	-4.46F
BW2	2750-2999 g.	1.36	2.68B	1.33	2.46A	1.33	2.48A	1.32	2.42A
MALE	Male infant	1.53	4.41F	1.52	4.38F	1.52	4.37F	1.52	4.37F
SMOKE3	> 30 cigarettes per day	2.69	2.84B	2.95	3.08C	2.98	3.10C	3.00	3.12C
WTGAIN4	39+ lb.	1.55	2.89C	1.50	2.68B	1.48	2.62B	1.48	2.62B
WTGAIN5	48+ lb.	2.06	3.14C	2.04	3.09C	2.03	3.08C	2.02	3.05C
LGA	Macrosomia	1.32	1.51	1.34	1.56	1.36	1.67	1.36	1.66
DIS48	Blood disorder	16.10	2.85C	18.30	2.91C	18.42	2.91C	18.00	2.89C
DIS63	Hyperthyroidism	4.40	1.77	4.69	1.82	4.71	1.82	4.70	1.81
DIS87	GU tumor	35.32	2.46A	37.16	2.54A	37.29	2.54A	36.10	2.51A
DIS100	Mental retardation	13.84	6.01F	13.45	5.94F	13.45	5.94F	13.14	5.89F
DIS111	Colitis, ileitis	9.80	2.54A	9.29	2.49A	9.26	2.49A	9.63	2.53A
INST05	Hospital 05			0.62	-3.33D	0.62	-3.33D	0.63	-3.17C
MARIT5	Divorced					0.00	-1.33	0.00	-1.33
SES8	Index 75-84							0.70	-1.76

*   Probability code: A 0.05, B 0.01, C 0.005, D 0.001, E 0.0005, F 0.0001 or less.

enhanced (RR 0.52 to 0.47), as were the adverse effects SMOKE3 (RR 2.69 to 2.95) and some diseases (especially DIS48, DIS63, and DIS87).

Another set of tests for variables to be considered for a 25-factor step-up model disclosed that only four remained in contention, namely MARIT5 (p = .0179), SES8 (p = .0697), SMOKE4 (p = .0833), and RACE2 (p = .0865). Accordingly, MARIT5 (divorced) was added to create the second step-up model (Table 21-9), where it failed to achieve statistical significance (t = -1.33, p = .19). Moreover, the new model showed very little difference in the relative impact of each of the other variables vis-a-vis the effects they had shown in the prior models.

Repeat testing of all remaining variables was done seeking candidates for the next step-up model to be made up of 26 factors. Three candidates emerged: SES8 (p = .0675), SMOKE4 (p = .0883), and RACE2 (p = .0920). SES8 (index 75-84) was, therefore, incorporated into the third step-up model (Table 21-9). It fell short of statistical significance itself (t = 1.76, p = .082) and had only negligible effects on the other variables in the model with regard to their relationship to composite outcome. When retesting was done to determine whether any other variables could be entertained for inclusion in another step-up model, none surfaced at the 10% probability level. This concluded the process.

Among multiparas, the base model was composed of the 30 variables previously determined to be significant (at or below p = .10) from among the 78 intrinsic variables

255

Table 21-10
Step-up Logistic Regression Analysis of Intrinsic Variables for
Composite Outcome in Multiparas*

Variable		Initial Model		Step-Up Model 1		Step-Up Model 2		Step-Up Model 3		Step-Up Model 4		Step-Up Model 5		Step-Up Model 6	
		RR	t	RR	t	RR	t	RR	t	RR	t	RR	t	RR	t
INST15	Hospital 15	1.68	2.89C	1.67	2.86C	1.61	2.65C	1.71	2.94C	1.65	2.75C	1.67	2.80C	1.63	2.65B
INST55	Hospital 55	1.37	2.01A	1.35	1.92	1.32	1.76	1.38	2.02A	1.36	1.94	1.38	2.01A	1.39	2.05A
INST60	Hospital 60	2.12	5.96F	2.02	5.55F	1.96	5.28F	2.06	5.58F	2.02	5.41F	2.03	5.46F	2.02	5.42F
INST71	Hospital 71	1.92	3.71E	1.89	3.63E	1.86	3.54D	1.97	3.81E	1.96	3.79E	1.98	3.84E	1.96	3.78E
INST82	Hospital 82	0.77	-1.52	0.73	-1.84	0.71	-2.00A	0.75	-1.63	0.73	-1.82	0.74	-1.77	0.73	-1.80
AGE3	Age 25-29 yr.	0.80	-2.39A	0.80	-2.35A	0.81	-2.24A	0.81	-2.21A	0.82	-2.14A	0.82	-2.12A	0.81	-2.18A
RACE3	Other race	0.58	-2.90C	0.58	-2.91C	0.57	-2.98C	0.58	-2.89C	0.57	-2.98C	0.57	-2.96C	0.57	-2.96C
PARA3	Grand multipara	1.40	3.21C	1.39	3.18C	1.39	3.13C	1.38	3.08C	1.38	3.08C	1.38	3.09C	1.43	3.34D
PABORT1	Prior abortion	0.89	-1.28	0.90	-1.10	0.90	-1.12	0.89	-1.18	0.89	-1.18	0.89	-1.23	0.84	-1.69
PPREM1	Prior premature	1.40	3.61E	1.38	3.44D	1.36	3.33D	1.35	3.24C	1.35	3.18C	1.34	3.16C	1.31	2.85C
HGT2	Short stature	1.37	1.94	1.38	1.99A	1.37	1.91	1.37	1.91	1.36	1.87	1.35	1.82	1.35	1.82
RHSENS	Rh disease	3.11	2.70B	3.14	2.73B	3.02	2.63B	3.15	2.73B	3.18	2.74B	3.20	2.77B	3.14	2.72B
PPMR1	Prior death	4.34	2.14A	4.20	2.09A	4.10	2.06A	3.93	2.01A	4.01	2.04A	4.12	2.09A	3.67	1.90
SES1	Index < 15	3.46	1.70	3.52	1.71	3.59	1.73	3.64	1.74	3.54	1.71	3.56	1.72	3.46	1.68
SES4	Index 35-44	1.27	2.48A	1.26	2.37A	1.23	2.10A	1.22	1.99A	1.27	2.39A	1.27	2.39A	1.27	2.38A
VISIT4	17-20 visits	1.56	1.84	1.69	2.16A	1.76	2.32A	1.72	2.22A	1.75	2.29A	1.73	2.26A	1.74	2.27A
PIH1	Diastolic increase	1.42	1.77	1.43	1.82	1.42	1.77	1.45	1.86	1.44	1.86	1.46	1.91	1.43	1.78
BW5	3500-3799 g.	0.80	-2.05A	0.81	-1.86	0.81	-1.89	0.82	-1.82	0.81	-1.84	0.81	-1.83	0.81	-1.86
MALE	Male infant	1.38	4.00F	1.38	3.96E	1.38	3.94E	1.38	3.94E	1.38	3.98E	1.38	4.00F	1.39	4.03F
DIS21	Tuberculosis, active	0.42	-1.71	0.43	-1.67	0.43	-1.71	0.42	-1.74	0.41	-1.77	0.41	-1.78	0.40	-1.81

Code		1	2	3	4	5	6	7	8	9	10	11	12	13	14
DIS32	Low serum iron	2.38	2.12A	2.31	2.06A	2.26	2.00A	2.35	2.09A	2.35	2.10A	2.37	2.12A	2.36	2.11A
DIS49	Diabetes mellitus	3.00	3.46E	3.09	3.73E	3.01	3.64E	2.97	3.60E	2.95	3.58E	2.63	3.11C	2.60	3.08C
DIS74	Syphilis	12.37	1.76	13.25	1.80	12.76	1.77	11.83	1.71	12.50	1.74	12.85	1.77	13.24	1.79
DIS80	Glomerulonephritis	7.27	2.73B	6.98	2.66B	6.78	2.63B	6.70	2.59B	6.72	2.58B	6.77	2.59B	6.73	2.58B
DIS100	Mental retardation	3.06	2.66B	3.04	2.66B	2.98	2.61B	2.92	2.57B	2.82	2.48A	2.85	2.51A	2.90	2.55A
DIS103	Neurological disease	2.19	2.27A	2.22	2.31A	2.26	2.35A	2.25	2.34A	2.25	2.34A	2.25	2.33A	2.26	2.34A
DIS111	Colitis, ileitis	3.54	1.61	3.74	1.68	3.68	1.66	3.77	1.68	3.88	1.72	3.91	1.73	3.96	1.75
DIS126	Late bleeding	1.35	2.82B	1.36	2.84B	1.37	2.92C	1.35	2.75B	1.34	2.73B	1.35	2.75B	1.35	2.75B
DIS128	Hemorrhagic shock	5.56	2.20A	5.71	2.24A	5.93	2.29A	6.18	2.34A	5.96	2.30A	5.30	2.08A	5.02	2.02A
SDIS4	Venereal diseases	1.40	2.28A	1.40	2.25A	1.37	2.14A	1.34	1.96A	1.32	1.87	1.32	1.86	1.30	1.77
VISIT1	< 7 visits			1.30	3.08C	1.26	2.70B	1.28	2.72B	1.27	2.76B	1.27	2.78B	1.27	2.71B
STATUS2	Private					0.59	-2.49A	1.39	-2.24A	1.37	-2.13A	0.64	-2.09A	0.64	-2.07A
INST37	Hospital 37								2.25A	1.30	2.17A	1.35	2.04A	1.33	1.95
SES2	Index 15-24										2.05A	1.30	2.08A	1.28	1.96A
DIS123	Hydramnios												1.80	1.62	1.77
GRAV1	First pregnancy													1.24	1.71

* Probability coding: A 0.05, B 0.01, C 0.005, D 0.001, E 0.0005, F 0.0001 or less.

in the full logistic model (Table 21-6). Examining these variables in isolation increased the effects of variables such as PPMR1 (RR 3.33 to 4.34), SES1 (RR 1.55 to 3.46), DIS49 (RR 2.32 to 3.00), and DIS128 (RR 4.81 to 5.56), and decreased those of others, particulary RHSENS (RR 3.40 to 3.11), VISIT4 (RR 1.86 to 1.56), and DIS111 (RR 4.39 to 3.54). The protective effect of INST82 diminished in magnitude (RR 0.69 to 0.77) and became statistically insignificant (p .047 to .13).

A series of tests was undertaken to determine which of the residual 48 variables might be used for subsequent step-up logistic models. Ten candidates emerged, including VISIT1 (p = .0024), STATUS2 (p = .0032), GREG (p = .0107), SES2 (p = .0164), INST37 (p = .0210), SES9 (p = .0217), GRAV1 (p = .0320), and DIS123 (p = .0599). The first step-up model (Table 21-10) incorporated VISIT1 (< seven antepartum visits). The effects of the variable proved quite significant in the 31-factor model. Most variables retained their prior relation to outcome, but a few diminished it (such as PPMR1 and DIS80) and some enhanced it (for example, VISIT4, DIS75, DIS111, and DIS128).

The next set of tests for additional candidates for another step-up model revealed seven, all previously identified by prior testing (see above) but now excluding GREG and PARA2. The variable with the lowest p value, STATUS2 (p = .0103), was added to form the second step-up 32-member model (Table 21-10). It also had a significant protective effect relative to composite outcome, while minimally altering the effects of the other variables in the model.

Another set of tests disclosed five factors still contesting for a place in the next step-up model, all as before, except for SES9 which no longer pertained at the 10% probability level. INST37 (p = .0371) was added to the third set-up model made up of 33 variables (Table 21-10). This process modified some of the relationships among the variables in regard to their effects on outcome. The impact of PPMR1, for example,

which had been slowly falling in each successive step-up model (and will be seen to continue to fall in the subsequent ones), dropped more acutely here (RR 4.34, 4.20, and 4.10 to 3.93 in this third model); an upward trend for DIS111 was now evident as well (and will continue later). Rising trends for SES1 and DIS128 were also noted (but these will not progress beyond this model).

Further testing for additional step-up models was done. Four variables proved suitable for the fourth 34-factor model, and SES2 (p = .0451) was incorporated. Except for the aforementioned continuing trend, it had little effect either overall or on individual variables. Ensuing tests allowed us to develop two other step-up models containing 35 and 36 variables, respectively, by adding DIS123 (p = .0849) and GRAV1 (p = .0931) in sequence. The unimpressive effects of these step-up processes are illustrated in Table 21-10. No other variables proved significant at the 10% probability level, terminating the operation.

The same procedure was repeated for perinatal outcome (death plus severe depression). In nulliparas, the initital model was composed of the same 18 significant variables derived for the full logistic regression analysis model (Table 21-7). When these items were examined as a base model without consideration for all other intrinsic variables, the data shown in Table 21-11 were produced.

The effects of some were diminished, such as SMOKE2 (duration 10 years or more), WTGAIN1 (less than 11 lb gain), LGA (macrosomia), and GDEL4 (postterm delivery), plus syphilis, cholecystitis, and hyperthyroidism. Others showed stronger impact, including low or high socioeconomic indices, male infant, and maternal mental retardation. Most of these had stronger confirmation in terms of statistical significance.

RACE2 (black), which had previously been included because it fell just within the 10% probability cutoff, was now well within the statistically significant group (t =

Table 21-11
Step-Up Logistic Regression Analysis of Intrinsic Variables for Perinatal Outcome in Nulliparas*

Variable		Initial Model RR	t	Step-Up Model 1 RR	t	Step-Up Model 2 RR	t	Step-Up Model 3 RR	t	Step-Up Model 4 RR	t
INST45	Hospital 45	2.08	2.33A	2.03	2.26A	2.07	2.32A	1.98	2.18A	1.97	2.16A
RACE2	Black	1.59	2.52A	1.49	2.12A	1.51	2.19A	1.33	1.48NS	1.30	1.36NS
SES3	Index 25-34	1.83	2.45A	1.70	2.15A	1.70	2.15A	1.63	1.97A	1.64	1.99A
SES4	Index 35-44	2.33	3.87E	2.15	3.49D	2.19	3.55D	2.13	3.41D	2.15	3.47D
SES8	Index 75-84	1.80	1.84	1.61	1.47N	1.74	1.72	1.85	1.89	1.89	1.96A
MALE	Male infant	1.97	3.62E	1.97	3.64E	1.99	3.69E	1.99	3.69E	1.98	3.66E
SMOKE2	Smoking 10+ yr.	2.50	2.54A	2.63	2.68B	2.76	2.79B	2.87	2.88C	2.72	2.72B
WTGAIN1	< 11 lb. gain	2.69	3.34D	2.63	3.26C	2.66	3.29D	2.64	3.26C	2.50	3.04C
WTGAIN4	39+ lb. gain	2.01	2.72B	1.99	2.70B	2.02	2.76B	1.94	2.58B	1.92	2.54A
LGA	Macrosomia	2.19	2.58B	2.25	2.66B	2.23	2.63B	2.26	2.67B	2.21	2.59B
GDEL4	Delivery after 41 wk.	1.82	3.03C	1.81	3.00C	1.80	2.98C	1.81	2.98C	1.77	2.87B
DIS63	Hyperthyroidism	11.64	2.59B	12.23	2.63B	15.82	2.78B	16.86	2.78B	18.03	2.87C
DIS74	Syphilis	31.52	2.21A	30.25	2.19A	29.64	2.17A	28.38	2.14A	30.74	2.20A
DIS86	Pyelonephritis	2.10	1.78	2.14	1.82	2.10	1.77	2.04	1.70	2.01	1.66
DIS97	Other gyn disorders	2.36	2.16A	2.31	2.10A	2.35	2.14A	2.42	2.23A	2.47	2.28A
DIS100	Mental retardation	19.56	5.30F	18.66	5.23F	18.66	5.23F	17.84	5.16F	17.50	5.09F
DIS107	Cholecystitis	15.19	2.36A	18.07	2.45A	18.19	2.45A	19.96	2.53A	20.29	2.54A
DIS140	Parasitic infection	7.54	2.63B	7.70	2.65B	7.81	2.66B	7.27	2.55A	7.15	2.53A
SES9	Index 85+			0.38	-1.86	0.38	-1.86	0.39	-1.76	0.40	-1.69
DIS94	Leiomyoma					0.01	-1.17N	0.00	-0.87NS	0.00	-0.85NS
INST05	Hospital 05							0.61	-1.84	0.61	-1.83
POND2	Obesity									1.61	1.86

* Probability code: A 0.05, B 0.01, C 0.005, D 0.001, E 0.0005, F 0.0001 or less; NS not significant, p > 0.10.

2.52, p = .014), even though the rate ratio remained essentially unchanged. This last variable should be kept in mind as the rest of this step-up operation is evolved for perinatal outcome because it will be seen to undergo an interesting transformation as confounding effects are taken into account.

Testing for 19-factor possible models showed four variables to be contenders for inclusion, namely INST05 (p = .052), POND2 (obesity, p = .052), SES9 (high index, p = .042), and DIS94 (leiomyomata, p = .051). SES9 was, therefore, added to the first step-up model as the variable with the best (that is, lowest) p value. This had the effect, shown in Table 21-11, of decreasing the magnitude of effect and statistical significance of all other SES variables as well as RACE2 and DIS100 (maternal mental retardation). At the same time, it increased the influence of SMOKE2, LGA, cholecystitis, and hyperthyroidism. The effect of cholecystitis was especially enhanced (RR 15.19 to 18.07), but it was not much more significant than it had been before (t = 2.45, p = .018).

Exploration for the 20-factor modelling yielded the same variables for consideration: INST05 (p = .058), POND2 (p = .065), and DIS94 (p = .051). When DIS94 (leiomyomata) was incorporated, the logistic regression analysis produced a second step-up model (Table 21-11) with essentially the same configuration as the first. The newly introduced factor failed to achieve or even approach statistical significance when considered concurrently with all the other variables in the model (t = -1.17, p = .25). Negligible changes occurred in regard to the other factors, except for DIS63 (hyperthyroidism), which increased its rate ratio from 12.23 to 15.82 but retained about the same level of statistical significance (t = 2.78, p = .0076).

Further testing for 21-factor models reintroduced the aforementioned variables of INST05 (p = .056) and POND2 (p = .073). Incorporation of INST05 yielded a third step-up model (Table 21-11) with findings in large measure comparable toq those seen

in earlier models. The impact of DIS63 (hyperthyroidism) and DIS107 (cholecystitis) had increased again, whereas that of RACE2 (black), DIS74 (syphilis), and DIS100 (mental retardation) had diminished. Indeed, it was now quite apparent that the trends in all five of these variables had been consistent across all step-up models thus far for this subset of data.

Of special interest, as noted above, was the diminishing impact of RACE2 (black) on perinatal outcome. The rate ratio had fallen from 1.59 (t = 2.52, p = .012) to reach 1.33; the relationship had become increasingly less significant when subjected to scrutiny by statistical testing until it had actually become quite insignificant in this third step-up model (t = 1.48, p = .14).

There was a clear demonstration that it was not race per se that invoked the adverse effect observed earlier, but rather the confounding by other factors commonly associated with this population group. Incorporating SES9 (high socioeconomic index) and INST05 into the model in sequence had largely reduced the impact of RACE2 by accounting for much of its deleterious effect. In actuality, all these added step-up factors thus far exhibited protective effects, indicating that it was probably their negative association with RACE2 that caused the changes encountered here. Thus, in the case of SES9, for example, it accounted for the absence of a strong beneficial effect, as previously shown.

Parallel trends seen for DIS74 (syphilis) and DIS100 (mental retardation) could be supported logically on the same basis. Similarly, the reverse trends (reflected by increasingly strong relationships) for DIS63 (hyperthyroidism) and DIS107 (cholecystitis) were defensible.

Exploration of the remaining variables to determine if any others could be utilized helped create still another (fourth) step-up model revealed only POND2 (obesity) to be a candidate (p = .074). Inclusion of this variable into the 22-factor model (Table 21-11) enhanced all of the aforementioned relationships. The effect of RACE2 became even weaker (RR = 1.30) and less significant (t = 1.36, p = .20).

This reaffirmed the implication, stated above, that RACE2 was not necessarily an adverse factor in its own right, but served instead as a marker in this study population of the presence of various deleterious variables or the absence of some beneficial ones. Had it been feasible to continue this form of analysis further (on the basis of larger numbers of cases), other relevant factors would undoubtedly have been disclosed.

Further testing for additional variables to be incorporated into a fifth step-up model containing 23 factors, however, failed to identify any even at the 10% probability level. Accordingly, we were unable to pursue this most interesting avenue of investigation any further.

The logistic regression modelling was also applied to the study of the effects of intrinsic factors on perinatal outcome in multiparas. To begin with, a 21-factor initial or base model was developed utilizing those variables determined to be most significant in regard to their impact on the offspring (Table 21-12). The list was entirely comparable to that previously displayed for the full model logistic regression analysis (Table 21-8), but the relative effects were modified by examining only those selected factors unencumbered by all the remaining intrinsic variables.

The effects of MARIT5 (divorced), RACE3 (other), VAGBLD (early bleeding), DIS49 (diabetes mellitus), and DIS128 (hemorrhagic shock) were augmented, as was their statistical significance (markedly so for the last three of these variables). Reduced effects were found for PARA2 (grand multipara), RHSENS (Rh-isoimmunization), PIH1 (diastolic pressure increase), DIS126 (late bleeding), and SDIS5 (venereal

Table 21-12
Step-Up Logistic Regression Analysis of Intrinsic Variables for Perinatal Outcome in Multiparas*

Variable		Initial Model		Step-Up Model	
		RR	t	RR	t
INST31	Hospital 31	0.34	-1.96A	0.35	-1.94A
INST71	Hospital 71	1.99	2.00A	2.04	2.07A
MARIT5	Divorced	2.95	2.75B	3.02	2.81C
RACE3	Other race	2.25	3.41D	2.25	3.41D
PARA2	Grand multipara	1.53	2.06A	1.52	2.02A
PPREM1	Prior premature	1.41	1.87	1.41	1.87
HGT2	Short stature	1.88	2.34A	1.92	2.42A
RHSENS	Rh disease	9.57	4.27F	9.77	4.31F
VAGBLD	Early bleeding	2.27	3.10C	2.27	3.10C
VISIT4	17-20 visits	2.23	2.03A	2.23	2.03A
PIH1	Diastolic increase	2.38	2.65B	2.42	2.69B
MALE	Male infant	1.62	2.90C	1.62	2.89C
DIS15	Tuberculosis, active	16.31	2.36A	16.60	2.37A
DIS37	Response to iron	1.71	2.40A	1.69	2.34A
DIS49	Diabetes mellitus	4.48	3.18C	4.56	3.21C
DIS80	Glomerulonephritis	27.97	4.02F	28.54	4.04F
DIS126	Late bleeding	1.47	1.87	1.47	1.84
DIS128	Hemorrhagic shock	17.51	3.36D	18.00	3.40D
DIS130	Supine hypotension	6.29	2.55A	6.44	2.58B
SDIS5	Venereal diseases	1.71	1.99A	1.69	1.94
DIS38	Sicklemia			3.33	2.24A

*   Probability code: A 0.05, B 0.01, C 0.005, D 0.001, E 0.0005, F 0.0001 or less.

diseases) with comparable diminution in statistical significance. Smaller impact was also seen for VISIT4 (17-20 visits) and DIS130 (supine hypotension), but without change in the associated p value.

Only one viable candidate was disclosed for a possible 22-factor step-up model. It was DIS38 (sickle cell disease, p = .053). Inclusion of this variable in a step-up model for this subset produced the logistic regression analysis results shown in Table 21-12. The new factor easily achieved statistical significance (t = 2.24, p = .027), but its incorporation caused relatively little alteration in the relationships established in the base model. The only variable showing any reduction of impact was DIS37 (anemia showing response to iron), an effect that could have been anticipated.

Enhancement of effect, while not very impressive, was encountered for such diverse variables are MARIT5, HGT2 (short stature), PIH1, DIS15 (active tuberculosis), DIS49, DIS80 (glomerulonephritis), DIS128, and DIS130. All except DIS15 and DIS80 also increased their statistical significance somewhat (that is, reduced their p values). No other variables were found as possible contenders for another step-up analysis (at the 10% probability level) when testing was carried out for 23-factor models. The process was, therefore, concluded at this point.

Summary of Risk Variables
Among Intrinsic Factors

The data derived thus far have shown a number of the intrinsic factors we have been studying here to be significantly associated with adverse or beneficial outcome results for the fetus and infant. They are summarized in Table 21-13. From the original collection of 271, we can now recognize 59 intrinsic variables as important contributors to such outcome. Alternatively, of course, some might present mere markers of closely interrelated or confounding factors. Clarification in this regard awaits analysis of these residual factors in conjunction with those flagged as probable risk factors from the other groups of variables under investigation.

We had thus accomplished the objectives of the third major phase of the investigation, having derived those intrinsic maternal, fetal, and pelvic variables carrying the greatest probability of impacting on the fetus and infant. Our studies examined the large array of these variables and identified those clearly relevant to outcome when all were being considered simultaneously. The next step was to repeat these complex procedures for the fourth and last group of variables, namely those pertaining to the delivery process itself. Selected factors for labor progression, adjunctive drugs, and intrinsic factors will then be combined with those determined to be equivalently important in regard to the delivery for the final collective evaluation of this program (chapter 25). In this way, we anticipated achieving our goal of ascertaining which among them was most critical to outcome, quantitating their effects while simultaneously taking the effects of all other factors into account.

Table 21-13
Summary of Significant Intrinsic Variables by Logistic Regression*

Variable	Full Model				Initial Model				Step-Up Model			
	Composite		Perinatal		Composite		Perinatal		Composite		Perinatal	
	N	M	N	M	N	M	N	M	N	M	N	M
INST15						C			B			
INST31	B				C			a	A			a
INST37	A				E				B			
INST45	A		A		C		A		A		A	
INST55						A				A		
INST60	F	F			F	F			F	F		
INST71	A	B			A	E		A		E		A
INST82		a										
AGE3		a				a				a		
STATUS2										a		
MARIT5				A				B				C
RACE2							A					
RACE3	d	c			c	c		D	d	c		D
PARA2		B		A		C		A		D		A
PPREM1		A				E				C		
PPMR1		B				A						
HGT2				A				A				A
POND2	A				C				C			
WTGAIN1		C					D				C	
WTGAIN4	B	A			C	B			B	A		
WTGAIN5	C				C				C			
SES1		A										
SES3									A			
SES3	A				C		A		B		A	
SES4		A	C			A		E		A	D	
SES8		A									A	
SES9	f				f				f			
VISIT1									B			
VISIT4		A		A				A		A		A
GDEL4		C					C				B	
BW2	A				B				A			
BW5						a						
MALE	F	E	E	B	F	F	E	C	F	F	E	C
LGA		B				B				B		
VAGBLD				B				C				C
RHSENS		B		F				F				F
SMOKE2		C				A				B		
SMOKE3	C				B				C			
PIH1				B				B				B
DIS15				A				A				A
DIS32						A				A		
DIS37								A				A
DIS38												A

	C1	C2	C3	C4	C5	C6	C7	C8	C9	C10	C11	C12
DIS48	B				C				C			
DIS49		A		B		E		C		C		C
DIS63			C				B				C	
DIS74		A					A				A	
DIS80		A		E		B		F		B		F
DIS87	B				A				A			
DIS97		A					A				A	
DIS100	F	A	F		F	B	F		F	A	F	
DIS103		A					A				A	
DIS107		A					A				A	
DIS111	A				A				A			
DIS126		A		A		B				B		
DIS128				B		A		D		A		D
DIS130				A				A				B
DIS140			A				B				A	
SDIS4				A		A		A				

* Significance code: A 0.05, B 0.01, C 0.005, D 0.001, E 0.0005, F 0.0001 or less. Protective relationships designated by lower case coding; adverse, by capital letter coding. N nulliparas, M multiparas.

264

CHAPTER 22

Delivery Factors

Summary

An extensive, all-encompassing survey was undertaken to delineate as many delivery-related variables as feasible among 59,584 cases constituting the full NCPP population. A total of 287 groups of variables was disclosed, encompassing 1980 separate items pertaining to the delivery process for consideration. Those determined to occur in sufficient numbers to warrant further study were identified. A detailed data file was established for assessing their potential impact on offspring.

A major component of these investigations involved examination of delivery events. Stepwise, this required identification of a broad range of relevant delivery variables and then isolating them within the context of the NCPP data files for purposes of determining and describing their frequencies of occurrence and distribution among study gravidas. Subsequently, it would be necessary to stratify index cases according to the presence or absence of each of these variables. Once this was accomplished, the next phase was to ascertain the impact of such factors on the fetus and infant as measured by the series of outcomes we had earlier chosen as representative, ranging all the way from stillbirths to low seven-year IQ scores. The data thus derived were to be analyzed to flag those relationships with adverse outcomes that remained intact under statistical scrutiny. In this way, we felt we could identify those delivery variables that were worthy of further intensive and closely focused consideration in more sophisticated multivariate analyses.

The delivery factors we sought were widely scattered in the NCPP data bank, having been collected from a variety of sources. The latter included codified data from several of the obstetrical forms in the project, most pertinently OB-33, OB-34, OB-55, and ADM-50 (see chapter 3). Special difficulties were encountered due to the incompatible nature of some of the different coding systems used at different times in the project. Changes in the coding, done for purposes of ensuring greater detail and accuracy in the collected information, left us with incomplete segments of data for earlier case registrants, for example. It will be seen that some of the variables we explored encompassed very extensive proportions of the NCPP population, while others involved only a fraction. Those available areas of interest considered potentially important insofar as the objectives of this program were concerned are broadly characterized in Table 22-1. Collectively, they constituted 287 discrete groups of variables all relating to the delivery process. Individually, there were 1980 separately coded factors that could be identified for study.

Each of these was tallied to provide information on incidence rates. Every gravida presenting with a given specified variable was assigned to the special group represented by that variable. Within the subsets of individuals thus identified for each of the variables, we examined the outcome frequencies. The entire NCPP population of 59,584 women and their offspring was utilized for this series of analyses. Parity stratification was done preliminarily. Although it was later realized that differences in outcome effects between parity groups were for the most part negligible, the parity separations were nonetheless maintained.

Among core cohort cases, 94.42% were delivered vaginally and the remainder, 5.58%, by cesarean section (Table 22-2). There were 3.28% breech presentations

Table 22-1
Delivery Variables Under Surveillance

NCPP Source (Form: Card)	Variable
OB55:1355	Type of delivery
	Status of attendant
	Labor: spontaneous/induced
	Fetal position: admission/delivery
	Fetal station: admission/delivery
	Change in fetal position
	Change in fetal station
	Compound presentation
	Amniotomy: duration to delivery
	Amniotomy: indication
OB55:2355	Oxytocic use
	Mechanical induction
	Induction attempts
	Reactions to stimulants
	Induction: indications
	Augmentation: indications
	Arrest of labor
OB55:3355	Vertex: delivery control
	Fundal pressure
	Manual rotation
	Manual rotation: difficulty
	Conversion: manual
	Conversion: forceps
	Forceps: station
	Forceps: rotation
	Forceps: type

266

	Forceps: axis traction
	Forceps: difficulty
	Forceps: indication
	Vacuum extractor: dilation
	Vacuum extractor: position
	Vacuum extractor: station
	Vacuum extractor: pressure
	Vacuum extractor: failure
	Vacuum extractor: indication
OB55:4355	Breech: version
	Breech: indication
	Breech: attitude
	Breech: complications
	Breech: fundal pressure
	Breech: forceps to head
	Breech: delivery type
	Breech: difficulty
OB55:5355	Cesarean: incision
	Cesarean: placental site
	Cesarean: head delivery
	Cesarean: body delivery
	Cesarean: difficulty
	Cesarean: indication
OB55:6355	Cord stripped
	Cord prolapse: degree
	Cord prolapse: treatment
	Nuchal cord
OB55:7355	External version
	Amniocentesis
	Labor inhibitor
	Shoulder dystocia
OB33:0333	Forceps traction: duration
	Body delivered: delay
OB34:1334	Type of delivery
	Attempt before section
	Labor before section
	Fetal presentation
	Fetal position
	Conversion
	Rotation: difficulty
	Rotation: type
	Delivery: control
	Forceps: station
	Forceps: difficulty
	Breech: type
	Breech: delivery
	Breech: head control
	Breech: forceps to head
	Version: indication
OB34:2334	Nuchal cord
	Induction of labor
	Induction: method
	Amniotomy
	Oxytocic use
	Oxytocic reaction
	Version
	Manual dilatation
	Dührssen's incisions
	Cord prolapse: degree
	Cord prolapse: treatment
	Uterine rupture
OB34:3334	Cesarean: after labor
	Cesarean: indication
	Cesarean: type
	Cesarean: head delivery

delivered as such per vaginam; these constituted 3.49% of all vaginal deliveries. Vaginal vertex deliveries were further divisible into those 54.78% delivered spontaneously (Table 22-3) and those delivered either by forceps (44.90%) or by vacuum extractor (0.32%).

Strict definitions were used to define forceps applications according to fetal station and position. True low forceps procedures (designated class I or outlet forceps) were those in which the fetal scalp was visible at the introitus without separating the labia, the fetal cranium having actually reached the perineal floor with the sagittal suture in the anteroposterior diameter of the pelvic outlet. Midforceps operations were subdivided into those in which the fetal head had descended to the pelvic floor at station +3 or +4 but did not completely fulfill all the other criteria of low forceps (class II), and those in which the fetus was just engaged in the maternal midpelvis at station 0 to +2 (class III). Rarely executed and clinically unacceptable high forceps were designated class IV.

Low and low midforceps (classes I and II) constituted 34.57% of cases (or 76.46% of all forceps operations); true low or outlet forceps of the class I variety totalled 18.11% (40.06% of the forceps procedures done). The more difficult class III midforceps included 10.61% in all (23.46% of forceps). There were 5.94% forceps rotations of 90° or more in vertex presentations; they represented 13.43% of all forceps deliveries, about equally divided between rotations from occiput transverse positions and those from occiput posterior positions (7.09% and 6.34%, respectively). Additionally, there were rare forceps conversions of face and brow presentations (0.11%).

The types of forceps used (Table 22-4) varied considerably, of course; of those utilized most commonly (more often than 500 cases of each in this series), in descending order of frequency, were Irving (13.78%), Simpson (9.45%), Luikart (7.34%), Elliott (4.32%), DeLee (2.28%), Kielland (1.82%), and Tucker-McLane (1.59%). Multiple forceps applications (Table 22-5) were attempted in 8.71% of these cases, almost exclusively limited to the midforceps cases.

The difficulty of various aspects of the operative vaginal procedures was evaluated

Table 22-2
Type of delivery

Delivery Type	No.	%	% of Vaginal Deliveries
Vaginal vertex	53,288	90.96	96.34
Vaginal breech	2,026	3.46	3.66
Cesarean section	3,271	5.58	

Table 22-3
Forceps Delivery

Forceps Procedure	No.	%	% of Forceps Deliveries
Forceps not used	26,793	54.78	
Class I (low forceps)	8,859	18.11	40.06
Class II	8,051	16.46	36.40
Class III	5,188	10.61	23.46
Class IV (high forceps)	19	0.04	0.09

Table 22-4
Type of Forceps Used

Forceps Type	No.	%	% of Forceps Deliveries
Barton	48	0.14	0.32
DeLee	733	2.28	5.16
DeWees	382	1.13	2.56
Elliott	1,468	4.32	9.77
Gillespie	41	0.12	0.27
Haig-Ferguson	44	0.13	0.29
Hawks-Dennen	84	0.24	0.54
Irving	4,679	13.78	31.16
Kielland	618	1.82	4.12
Luikart	2,492	7.34	16.60
Luikart-Tucker	162	0.48	1.09
Piper	22	0.07	0.15
Simpson	3,209	9.45	21.37
Tucker-McLane	541	1.59	3.60
Other	176	0.52	1.17

Table 22-5
Frequency of Attempts to Apply Forceps Blades

No. Attempts*	No.	%	% of Forceps Deliveries
0	18,859	55.54	
1	60	0.18	0.40
2	11,875	34.97	78.66
3	749	2.21	4.97
4	1,387	4.09	9.20
5	197	0.58	1.30
6	245	0.72	1.62
7	232	0.68	1.53
8+	147	0.43	0.97

* Refers to the number of tries to apply a single forceps blade; thus, 2 signifies the usual successful first application of 2 forceps blades to the fetal head.

as objectively as possible by disinterested trained observers during the delivery and before the condition of the infant was known, thereby to reduce any possible bias on this basis. Gradations into (1) average difficulty, (2) difficult, (3) very difficult, and (4) failed at all attempts were used for assessing the application and traction as well as rotation and conversion, if applicable to the situation (Table 22-6). Forceps applications were deemed to be of average difficulty in 40.04% (or 92.23% of the 14,741 forceps applications); they were very difficult or so difficult that they failed in 1.00% overall (or 2.30% of those attempted). Similar frequencies were derived for traction difficulty (0.73% overall were very difficult or failed, or 1.71% of the forceps attempts). Rotations of 90° or more were fewer in number and were felt to be particularly difficult in 0.59% (or 10.02% of the 2026 attempted rotations). Conversions were rarely done (only 17 cases), but the relative frequencies of difficulty or failure was about the same.

Manual rotations of 90° or more occurred in 1012 cases (2.98%). The majority (1.84%) were accomplished by rotation from an occiput posterior position (including left and right occiput posterior positions). All but a few of the remaining were rotated from an occiput transverse position (1.11%). The rest were those rare cases involving rotation of face or brow presentations (0.03%).

As noted, there were only a small number of vacuum extractor procedures. Among the 86 cases included in the core population, 29 or 33.72% failed to achieve the objectives of application (8.14%), rotation (4.65%), descent (12.79%), or delivery (8.14%). In passing, it was of interest to note that the cervix was not yet fully dilated when the vacuum extractor was applied in

26 (30.23%); indeed, in 15 (17.44%) it was less than 9.0 cm dilated.

Among the 2166 cesarean sections, 68.78% were done via lower uterine segment transverse incisions, 22.33% low vertical incisions, and 7.04% by classical (vertical miduterine) incisions. In a small number (1.43%), a vertical T-extension was added to a low cervical transverse incision. Combined cesarean section and hysterectomy were rarely done (0.28%). In all but 1.33%, the cesarean section was undertaken without a preceding failed operative attempt to effect vaginal delivery.

The attendant at the delivery (specifically designated as the "hands-on" person actually performing the procedure rather than the responsible party, although they were often the same individual) was of interest (Table 22-7). Residents and interns

Table 22-6
Relative Difficulty of Forceps Procedures

| Manuever | Average | | Degree of Difficulty | | | | | |
| | | | Difficult | | Very Difficult | | Failed | |
	No.	%*	No.	%*	No.	%*	No.	%*
Application	13,596	40.04 (92.23)	805	2.37 (5.46)	248	0.73 (1.68)	92	0.27 (0.62)
Traction	13,034	38.38 (90.41)	1,136	3.34 (7.88)	235	0.69 (1.63)	12	0.04 (0.08)
Rotation	1,542	4.54 (76.11)	281	0.83 (13.87)	120	0.35 (5.92)	83	0.24 (4.10)
Conversion	12	0.04 (76.47)	2	0.01 (11.76)	1	0.00 (5.88)	1	0.00 (5.88)

* Percentages in parentheses represent frequencies with reference to denominator for row totals.

Table 22-7
Attendant at Delivery

Status	No.	%
Obstetrician	2,897	7.87
Resident	13,451	36.56
Intern	13,558	36.85
Medical student	5,698	15.49
Nurse, nurse-midwife	643	1.75
Other*	545	1.48

* Includes physician generalist, emergency personnel, and unattended.

in training delivered the majority of NCPP babies, together totalling 73.41%, with medical students (15.49%), and staff obstetricians (7.87%) trailing well behind. A relatively small number was managed by nurses or nurse-midwives (1.75%). In consideration of the large proportion of nonprivate patients in the index population, this breakdown was not unexpected.

We had previously examined utilization of uterotonic agents for induction and augmentation of labor (see chapters 15-17). Here, our interest went beyond the pharmacologic agent to encompass all inductions regardless of method (Table 22-8) and to examine indications as well (see below). We learned, for example, that 3.02% had no labor at all. Of those who experienced labor, it was spontaneous in onset in 92.64%. Thus, there were 7.36% inductions (or 7.14% overall). Of special interest, the first attempt at induction failed in 16.35% (and 4.37% needed three or more tries). Identifiable complications—other than the commonly seen failed induction—included sustained uterine contraction in 0.39%, uterine hypertonus in 0.26%, fetal heart rate abnormality in 0.74%, and tumultuous labor in 0.50%.

Nonpharmacologic inductions included principally amniotomy (1.69%) and membrane stripping (1.81%). Other aspects of membrane status were also examined to yield information to the effect that only 56.45% ruptured spontaneously (Table 22-9). Aside from those left intact until ruptured artificially at delivery (20.56%), most of the remaining cases had surgical amniotomy done ostensibly for purposes of augmenting a labor already in progress (21.30%). In this latter regard, it does strain credulity to consider that this large proportion of cases (48.91% of all amniotomies) might actually have had some form of labor aberration requiring such intervention. The duration of rupture of membranes prior to delivery was stratified by increments of time (Table 22-10). As seen, nearly two thirds of cases had membranes intact to within six hours of the delivery and nearly four fifths (78.59%) within 12 hours. It is of interest that 10.81% had rupture exceeding 24 hours and only 4.12% for more than 48 hours.

Fetal presentations and positions showed the expected distributions (Table 22-11) as well as the anticipated kind of dynamic change with time. The changing mix of fetal

Table 22-8
Onset of Labor

Labor	No.	%	% of Patients With Labor
No labor	1,117	3.02	
Spontaneous onset	33,261	89.84	92.64
Induced labor	2,644	7.14	7.36

Table 22-9
Amniotomy and Membrane Status Before and During Labor

Status	No.	%	% of Amniotomies
Spontaneous rupture	20,428	56.45	
Amniotomy at delivery	7,440	20.56	47.21
Amniotomy for induction	612	1.69	3.88
Amniotomy for augmentation	7,709	21.30	48.91

271

position, of course, may have resulted from inherent alterations in fetal-maternal relationships in labor. An example is the rotational change that normally accompanies the physiologic cardinal movements of internal rotation in vertex presentation. However, positional changes with time may also have reflected clarification or correction of unknown, uncertain, or erroneous diagnoses of presentation and position as the cervix opened and the fetal presenting part became more accessible to palpation. Undetermined vertex positions, for example, fell in frequency from 47.33% at the time of the first examination in labor to 1.61% at the time of delivery. Simultaneously, recognized occiput anterior positions increased from 19.44% to 85.83%, reflecting both the increased rate of diagnosis and the associated rotation with time of occiput transverse and occiput posterior positions to occiput anterior (from 15.66% and 8.89% to 0.27% and 2.47%, respectively).

A similar trend, albeit less obvious, was seen with the positional variants of breech presentation. Face presentations remained stable in number over the course of labor, increasing at delivery in inverse proportion

Table 22-10
Duration of Membrane Rupture Prior to Delivery

Duration, hr.	No.	%	Cum %
< 6.0	22,504	62.19	100.00
6.0-11.9	5,937	16.41	37.81
12.0-17.9	2,578	7.12	21.40
18.0-23.9	1,256	3.47	14.28
24.0-29.9	1,015	2.80	10.81
30.0-35.9	504	1.39	8.01
36.0-41.9	658	1.82	6.62
42.0-47.9	246	0.68	4.80
48.0-71.9	647	1.79	4.12
72.0-95.9	302	0.83	2.33
96.0+	543	1.50	1.50
Total	36,189	100.00	

Table 22-11
Fetal Presentation and Position

Presentation Position	At First Examination		Before Operative Maneuver		At Delivery	
	No.	%	No.	%	No.	%
Occiput anterior (LOA to ROA)	7,228	19.44	12,169	32.73	31,914	85.83
Occiput transverse (LOT, ROT)	5,822	15.66	1,675	4.51	100	0.27
Occiput posterior (LOP to ROP)	3,304	8.89	1,944	5.23	918	2.47
Vertex, position undetermined	17,601	47.33	1,031	2.77	599	1.61
Sacrum anterior (LSA to RSA)	197	0.53	373	1.00	625	1.68
Sacrum transverse (LST, RST)	128	0.34	248	0.67	111	0.30
Sacrum posterior (LSP to RSP)	64	0.17	114	0.31	57	0.15
Breech, position undetermined	738	1.98	402	1.08	437	1.18
Transverse lie	105	0.28	123	0.33	2	0.01
Face	48	0.13	48	0.13	68	0.18
Brow	18	0.05	22	0.06	4	0.01
Compound	24	0.06	30	0.08	49	0.13
Unknown	835	2.25	629	1.69	162	0.44

to the simultaneous fall in brow presentations, undoubtedly reflecting conversions of brow to face. Interestingly, although few in number, compound presentations increased somewhat over the course of labor. This latter perhaps mirrored the better diagnostic capabilities of obstetrical attendants for this condition in late labor as well as the greater potential for a compound presentation to occur and to be recognized as a labor complication at that time.

Breech attitudes (Table 22-12) were distributed about as expected, with frank breech leading in number (35.99% of breech presentations or 51.59% of those with known attitudes) and full or complete breech presentations occurring least often (5.27%). Among them, delivery was spontaneous in 45.22%, by partial extraction (assisted breech delivery) in 31.00%, and by total extraction in the other 23.79%. The aftercoming head was delivered spontaneously or manually aided in 82.18% (usually by a Mauriceau-type maneuver) and by forceps in 17.82% (almost always with Piper forceps). Nuchal arms were encountered in 3.25% and a hyperextended fetal head in 0.42% (one case had both).

Pressure was applied to the uterine fundus (Kristeller expression) to aid in effecting delivery in 8574 cases (25.54%). In most instances (Table 22-14), the degree of force used was slight to moderate as judged by the trained objective observer (22.93% overall or 89.21% of those in which expression was used). In 2.61%, the pressure employed was considered to be strong on the basis of the intensity of effort and the strength of the individual or individuals involved.

Precipitate vertex delivery—that is, uncontrolled delivery of the fetal head—was recorded in 1117 gravidas (3.29%). The standard modified Ritgen maneuver was used for control in 54.58% (Table 22-14). In the rest (42.13%), some form of instrumental control was employed either alone or in combination with the aforementioned manual technique. Nearly all of these cases were forceps deliveries; only a fraction

Table 22-12
Breech Attitudes

Attitude*	No.	%	% of Known Attitudes
Frank	957	35.99	51.59
Full or complete	140	5.27	7.55
Single footling	224	8.42	12.08
Double footling	534	20.08	28.79

* Excludes 804 breech presentations (30.24%) in which the fetal attitude was unknown or unrecorded.

Table 22-13
Delivery of the Fetal Head

Delivery Control	No.	%
Uncontrolled	1,117	3.30
Manual control	18,532	54.83
Instrumental control*	14,151	41.87

* Includes forceps and vacuum extractor.

Table 22-14
Use of Kristeller Expression

Degree*	No.	%	% of Expression Cases
None	24,771	74.29	
Slight	3,516	10.54	41.01
Moderate	4,133	12.39	48.20
Strong	870	2.61	10.15

* Excludes 55 cases (0.16%) in which fundal pressure was administered, but in which degree was unrecorded.

(0.32%, as previously noted) involved use of the vacuum extractor.

Indications for the various therapeutic or interventive measures were studied (Table 22-15), especially concentrating on those invoked for induction or augmentation of labor, forceps use, and cesarean delivery. The physician's stated indication was accepted, provided it could be substantiated by documentable facts in the record, of course. Elective inductions (that is, those done for patient or physician convenience without clear-cut logical justification on the basis of any medical or obstetrical reason) were done in 974 cases, constituting 2.62% of the NCPP gravid population and 35.19% of all inductions that were done. Among those with documentable indications, premature rupture of the membranes was the most common reason given (2.83% overall, 39.97% of inductions, and 58.58% of the ostensibly indicated inductions). Cases with pregnancy-induced hypertension (12.83% of inductions), diabetes mellitus (6.65%), and Rh isoimmunization (4.30%) were also induced, but only in moderate numbers, and there were rather infrequent inductions for a variety of other conditions as well, such as intrauterine infection (1.26%) and abruptio placentae (1.01%).

Labor augmentation was done electively in 3327 cases, a reflection of the kind of aggressive obstetrical practices then prevailing (8.94% overall and 44.80% of the augmentations that were done in the Project patients). Among indicated augmenta-tions, again premature rupture of the membranes led the list (4.33% overall, 21.69% of augmentations, and 39.30% of those that were indicated). Distinctively, arrested labor was the next most frequently invoked indication (3.28%, 16.42% of augmentations, and 29.74% of those indicated). A diverse potpourri of other indications trailed with relatively few cases of each; the most frequent of these less common reasons for augmenting labor included pregnancy-induced hypertension (4.55% of augmentations), diabetes (2.18%), uterine dysfunction (1.83%), and postmaturity (1.82%). When all labor-related disorders for which augmentation was used were considered together, they totalled 34.28% of the indicated augmentations (18.92% of all augmentation cases).

Forceps operations were undertaken electively in 12,699 cases, constituting 37.40% of the NCPP population or 85.12% of all forceps usage. Fetal distress (diagnosed on the basis of auscultatory evidence only) was by far the most common reason given for undertaking a forceps procedure in this series, totaling 1.83% of the entire population, 4.16% of forceps operations, and 27.93% of indicated cases of forceps use. Persistent occiput posterior followed in order of frequency (2.78% of forceps). Next came anesthesia (1.86%)—that is, forceps done to effect delivery because the terminal expulsive effects had been interfered with by the anesthesia given in anticipation of the delivery—and transverse arrest

Table 22-15
Primary Indications for Procedures

Indication	Induction No.	Induction %*	Augmentation No.	Augmentation %*	Forceps No.	Forceps %*	Cesarean Section No.	Cesarean Section %*
Elective	974	35.19	3,327	44.80	12,699	85.12		
Ruptured membranes	1,051	37.97	1,611	21.69			33	1.07
Preeclampsia	355	12.83	338	4.55	122	0.82	89	2.90
Diabetes mellitus	184	6.65	162	2.18			295	9.60
Erythroblastosis fetalis	119	4.30	84	1.13			31	1.01
Intrauterine infection	35	1.26	80	1.08			8	0.26
Pyelonephritis	17	0.61	14	0.19			3	0.10
Abruptio placentae	28	1.01	95	1.28	21	0.14	86	2.80
Placenta previa	5	0.18	21	0.28			114	3.71
Arrested labor			1,219	16.42	81	0.54	7	0.23
Vaginal bleeding			41	0.55	17	0.11	9	0.29
Uterine dysfunction			136	1.83	21	0.14	108	3.51
Fetal distress			38	0.51	620	4.16	224	7.29
Prolapsed cord			5	0.07	14	0.09	64	2.08
Transverse arrest			14	0.19	267	1.79		
Anesthesia			36	0.48	278	1.86		
Postmaturity			135	1.82				
Fetal death			70	0.94				
Cephalopelvic disproportion					87	0.58	512	16.66
Malpresentation					14	0.09	89	2.90
Cardiac disease					27	0.18		
Prolonged second stage					136	0.91		
Persistent occiput posterior					415	2.78		
Prematurity					100	0.67		
Transverse lie							72	2.34
Maternal age							27	0.88
Obstetrical history							78	2.54
Obstructing tumor							22	0.72
Cervical cancer							32	1.04
Previous vaginal surgery							22	0.72
Previous myomectomy							18	0.59
Previous cesarean section							1,131	36.79

* Percentages based on incidence among those undergoing the procedure (by column).

(1.79%). In addition, a range of other indications existed, although none was seen often, including prolonged second stage (0.91%), pregnancy-induced hypertension (0.82%), and prematurity (0.67%). Labor progression problems, collectively considered, were involved as indications in 58.51% of all indicated forceps cases (14.88% of all forceps operations).

Cesarean section was done most often because of a prior cesarean section (1131 cases, 3.33% overall, 36.79% of the cesarean sections done). Among primary cesarean sections, common indications included cephalopelvic disproportion (26.35% of primary sections), diabetes (15.18%), and fetal distress (11.53%). Placenta previa (5.87%) and uterine dysfunction (5.56%) were next in order of frequency, and a large variety of other indications followed. In all, there were only 37.98% of primary cesarean sections done for indications related to disordered labor progression.

In addition to this extensive sampling of the large number of variables related to the delivery process which we have tabulated thus far, there were a great many more which were available for study. Those occurring in sufficient number were indeed examined along with those detailed above. Where relevant outcome information was uncovered, especially insofar as adverse effects were concerned, they were incorporated into our more sophisticated multivariate analyses (see chapter 24). At this point, having created a utilitarian file of delivery factors seemingly worthy of examination, we proceeded directly to determine frequencies of bad outcome and to flag those variables among them that could be shown on a statistical basis to be significantly associated with and, therefore, perhaps causative of such untoward results.

CHAPTER **23**

Delivery Factors and Outcome

Summary

A series of exploratory analyses was undertaken to study the effects, if any, of a number of delivery-related variables on fetal and infant outcome utilizing nonparametric analytic methods. The index population consisted of 36,479 gravidas for whom adequate delivery information was available; the investigation focused on eight principal types of outcome from stillbirth to 7-year IQ results. Rates of adverse outcomes associated with each variable were compared with overall outcome rates. A number of delivery variables were flagged as probably contributing to untoward results when examined in isolation.

Continuing our analyses of outcome effects, the array of delivery factors available for study in depth were examined to ascertain their potential impact on offspring. The same paradigm was followed as had earlier proved so effective for our needs in comparable investigations dealing with other relevant variables. Applying nonparametric statistical tests seriatim to the frequencies of adverse outcomes associated with each of the delivery factors allowed us to flag those that appeared to place the fetus and infant at significantly increased risk. On that basis, the kinds of delivery characteristics, complications, and practices likely to have a deleterious effect could be identified for later assessment by somewhat more sophisticated techniques of multivariate analysis. These approaches were expected to help weigh the relative influences of such factors while taking all the others into simultaneous account. For now, however, our interest focused on the large number of individual delivery variables reviewed in the preceding chapter.

Type of Delivery

The general type of delivery, for example, divided gravidas into three groups, namely those delivered per vaginam in either vertex or breech presentation and those delivered by cesarean section. The outcomes for these broad categories were very different. Neonatal deaths (Table 23-1) occurred considerably more frequently among those delivered by cesarean section as compared with vaginal vertex deliveries by a factor of more than threefold in nulliparas (RR 3.05) and fourfold in multiparas (RR 4.51), both highly significant findings. Even more impressive was the neonatal death rate among infants delivered vaginally as breech births; the frequency multiplied over 12 times in both nulliparas and multiparas. It must be pointed out, of course, that these data did not account for such obvious hidden influences as the reason the operation was undertaken (for cesarean section) or the major factor of prematurity (recognized to be highly correlated with breech delivery). Nonetheless,

the results showed remarkable differences insofar as this outcome variable was concerned.

Other fetal and infant outcomes were examined in the same way by delivery category (Table 23-2). Cesarean section was found associated with such adverse results as stillbirth (but achieving significance only in multiparas) and neonatal depression, showing a consistency in regard to poor immediate impact on the fetus and newborn infant. In multiparas, there was some continuing adverse effect as late as the eight-month Bayley examinations. However, neither nulliparas nor multiparas showed any subsequent persistence of permanent, long-term residua. To the contrary, there appeared to be some protective effect encountered at the three-year speech, language, and hearing studies, but this did not persist into the four- and seven-year testing vehicles.

Breech babies did particularly badly in the perinatal period with very high frequencies of death and depression. In multiparas, deleterious results were seen over the entire range of outcomes up to seven years of age, all statistically significant. This was not the case among offspring of nulliparas, however, only a transient residual effect being found in the eight-month mental

Table 23-1
Neonatal Death by General Category of Delivery

Delivery	Cases	Neonatal Deaths		Freeman–Tukey		Rate Ratio	
	No.	No.	%	Deviate	p	RR	p
Vaginal vertex							
Nulliparas	10,634	100	0.94	-3.361	0.00039	1.00*	
Multiparas	22,684	280	1.23	-8.603	1.0×10^{-10}	1.00*	
Vaginal breech							
Nulliparas	274	32	11.68	7.516	1.0×10^{-10}	12.43	1.0×10^{-10}
Multiparas	780	121	15.51	14.177	1.0×10^{-10}	12.61	1.0×10^{-10}
Cesarean section							
Nulliparas	522	15	2.87	2.595	0.0047	3.05	2.0×10^{-5}
Multiparas	1,585	88	5.55	7.644	1.0×10^{-10}	4.51	1.0×10^{-10}

* Referent

Table 23-2
Outcome by General Category of Delivery

	No.	SB	NND	APG5	MENT8	MOT8	SLH3	IQ4	IQ7
Vaginal vertex									
Nulliparas	10,634	1.00(1.09)*	1.00(0.94)	1.00(2.68)	1.00(0.43)	1.00(0.56)	1.00(6.68)	1.00(2.04)	1.00(2.16)
Multiparas	22,684	1.00(1.03)*	1.00(1.23)	1.00(1.89)	1.00(0.99)	1.00(0.98)	1.00(5.67)	1.00(2.20)	1.00(2.11)
Vaginal breech									
Nulliparas	274	16.75e	12.43e	5.08e	3.80a	0.54	0.36	1.24a	0.98
Multiparas	780	13.14e	12.61e	9.91e	5.36e	6.34e	1.93a	1.36a	1.22a
Cesarean section									
Nulliparas	522	1.78	3.05d	2.77d	0.57	0.42	0.00a	0.99	1.06
Multiparas	1,585	2.90d	4.51e	3.66e	1.98a	2.27b	0.00a	1.02	0.98

* Data presented as rate ratios, relative to referent rate in parentheses.

Code for p-value: a 0.05, b 0.01, c 0.001, d 0.0001, e 0.00001or less.
Outcomes: SB, stillbirth; NND, neonatal death; APG5, low Apgar score at 5 minutes; MENT8 and MOT8, abnormal scores at 8 months on Bayley mental and motor tests, respectively; SLH3, abnormal 3-year communications; IQ4 and IQ7, low scores at ages 4 and 7 years.

279

scores and, to a statistically significant degree, in the four-year IQ scores; the latter was no longer present at seven years.

These parity differences perhaps reflected the great concern for and care of nulliparas with breech presentation, resulting in stricter selection of cases for vaginal delivery and more liberal use of cesarean section for breech presentation. This contrasted with the more permissive attitude among obstetricians in the past to allow vaginal breech births in multiparas on the assumption (sometimes mistaken as suggested by these data) that the fetal risk was negligible. There can be no doubt that these two general types of delivery (cesarean section and vaginal breech birth) must be weighed as high risk factors that could possibly impact unfavorably on the child.

Fetal Head Control

Among vaginally delivered fetuses in vertex presentation, the control of the fetal head was studied as an index of potential trauma to intracranial structures. Cases were divided into those delivered spontaneously by the standard form of modified Ritgen maneuver, those in which forceps were used to maintain control, and those in which delivery of the head was uncontrolled. The last usually occurred in association with precipitate delivery over an unsterile field. The spectrum of outcomes was examined for all infants according to the applicable head control group (Table 23-3).

Unexpectedly, forceps control appeared to yield much better results than manual control. The benefit associated with forceps use was found in both nulliparas and multiparas and was statistically significant in nearly all the early outcomes (up to eight months) that were examined. The good results persisted in multiparas through seven years. Nulliparas, by contrast, showed no continuing good effect beyond eight months and a counterbalancing adverse effect at three years.

While it is possible that delivery of the fetal head was actually benefitted by forceps control, before grasping at this concept to support promulgation for clinical application, we felt it essential to ensure first that forceps use did not merely serve as an indicator for preselection of cases that are likely to turn out well. It seemed reasonable, for example, to consider the possibility that such cases were more likely to involve normal term-size fetuses and healthy mothers who were perhaps in the private practice sector than those delivered by manual control or precipitately without control. Whether correct or not, it was important to examine forceps deliveries in greater depth (see below) before drawing conclusions that might prove inappropriate.

Class of Forceps Delivery

To illustrate, stratification by class of forceps delivery was accomplished and outcomes were determined for each group. Definitions of the four classes have been detailed earlier (see chapter 22). The numbers of class IV forceps deliveries were gratifyingly negligible and proved insufficient for meaningful statistical analysis; however, it was rather clear, even without such formal testing, that the infant outcomes were so poor as to warrant continuing the categorical interdiction against this procedure. The separation of midforceps operations into two varieties (class II for those in which the fetal head had descended to the pelvic floor as distinguished from class III in which it had not) was retained in an effort to learn about the relative impact, if any, of these procedures on the infant. This was felt to be particularly relevant to clinical practice because of the contention expressed in some obstetrical circles that the class II variant of midforceps delivery was innocuous and should, therefore, not be included with those class III type midforceps operations that were acknowledged to be more difficult and, as a consequence, more likely to be hazardous.

At first glance, the data for neonatal deaths (Table 23-4) served to confirm that

Table 23-3
Outcome by Fetal Head Delivery Control*

	No.	SB	NND	APG5	MENT8	MOT8	SLH3	IQ4	IQ7
Manual control									
Nulliparas	3,094	1.00(2.04)	1.00(1.40)	1.00(3.95)	1.00(0.91)	1.00(0.79)	1.00(3.91)	1.00(2.00)	1.00(2.12)
Multiparas	15,183	1.00(1.08)	1.00(1.34)	1.00(1.84)	1.00(1.64)	1.00(1.53)	1.00(7.08)	1.00(2.18)	1.00(2.08)
Uncontrolled									
Nulliparas	176	6.14e	6.34e	2.61c	0.00	2.36	0.00	1.38	1.46
Multiparas	888	3.34e	2.95e	2.77e	2.15a	2.62a	1.46	1.22	1.34a
Forceps control									
Nulliparas	7,370	0.21e	0.41c	0.50d	0.31a	0.41	2.91a	0.97	0.94
Multiparas	6,659	0.54d	0.54e	0.95	0.58c	0.75b	1.10	0.80b	0.78b

* See footnote, Table 23-2.

class II midforceps did not yield significantly increased mortality rates, even though the frequencies of losses were somewhat elevated in both nulliparas and multiparas when compared with class I low forceps results (RR 1.22 and 1.48, neither statistically significant). The poor neonatal outcomes associated with class III midforceps, however, stood as strong confirmation of their adverse impact, acknowledging that the reasons for undertaking the procedure had not yet been taken into consideration here. The frequency of neonatal deaths was nearly three times the rate accompanying class I forceps delivery for both nulliparas and multiparas (RR 2.74 and 2.92, respectively, both statistically significant, but especially so in nulliparas).

Examined over the range of outcomes under surveillance (Table 23-5), uniformly consistent bad results were disclosed for class III midforceps, showing significant long-term, apparently permanent, residual damage through age seven years. These findings paralleled those reported in a prior comparable study.* Moreover, class II forceps procedures likewise showed long-term deleterious impact; this proved statistically significant, albeit not of the same magnitude of effect as for class III forceps. As will be seen later, cases stratified by the fetal station reached just prior to any manipulation (Kristeller expression, vacuum extraction, manual rotation, or forceps) showed very similar outcome results, specifically demonstrating adverse effects occurring in relationship to high station. Indeed, the higher the station at delivery, the worse the outcome (see below).

Type of Forceps Instrument

As to the various types of forceps instruments utilized to effect delivery, we recognized that specific varieties were often used under widely different circumstances. Some were generally invoked only in cases presenting the conditions for which they were designed, such as Kielland forceps for occiput transverse or posterior arrest in an anthropoid pelvis. Others, including most of the classical Simpson and Elliot type variants, were used principally for elective class I forceps delivery but were also employed for forceps rotations and other more difficult operative manipulations. Thus, it was understood that evaluation of their individual impact on offspring was likely to be difficult to interpret at best.

Nonetheless, the outcome data (Table 23-6) were examined for each instrument used in sufficient numbers of cases to allow analysis to be carried out plausibly. The referent for the Freeman-Tukey analysis in this instance was chosen as the overall frequency of the specific adverse outcome for all forceps cases, as distinct from the frequencies derived from the total index population (which, of course, included a large proportion delivered without such instrumentation).

For the rate ratios, however, no optimal group was readily identifiable to serve as referent. Accordingly, we arbitrarily selected that group which represented the largest single subset, namely those delivered by Irving forceps, as the referent. It should be noted in passing that these cases were principally managed at a single NCPP collaborating institution (hospital 05). Close examination of the data for adverse outcome rates showed that the results derived were not necessarily representative in that they fell well below expected rates for the gravid population at large in nearly all aspects (some significantly so). Because the referent data were not truly representative, therefore, the rate ratio data derived for other forceps groups should be interpreted with caution—that is, while the p values based on Freeman-Tukey deviates were probably valid in this set of analyses, the rate ratios may have exaggerated the magnitude of effect unduly.

---

*Friedman EA, Sachtleben MR, Bresky PA: Dysfunctional labor: XII. Long-term effects on infant. *Amer J Obstet Gynecol* 1977; 127:779; Friedman EA, Sachtleben-Murray M, Dahrouge D, Neff RK: Long-term effects of labor and delivery on offspring: A matched-pair analysis. *Amer J Obstet Gynecol* 1984; 150:941.

Table 23-4
Neonatal Death by Class of Forceps Delivery

Forceps Class	Cases No.	Neonatal Deaths		Freeman-Tukey		Rate Ratio	
		No.	%	Deviate	p	RR	p
I (Low)							
Nulliparas	2,774	11	0.397	-1.098		1.00*	
Multiparas	2,127	11	0.517	-1.261		1.00*	
II (Mid)							
Nulliparas	3,294	16	0.486	-0.451		1.22	
Multiparas	2,616	20	0.765	0.150		1.48	
III (Mid)							
Nulliparas	1,745	19	1.089	2.343	0.010	2.74	0.0053
Multiparas	2,328	27	1.160	1.692	0.045	2.92	0.020

* Referent

These caveats in mind, we were nevertheless impressed by an especially strong relationship between delivery by Kielland forceps and bad results across the full range of outcome variables studied (Table 23-6). This mirrored and enlarged upon short-term data previously reported from other sources.* It undoubtedly reflected the procedure most often undertaken with these forceps (midforceps rotation) rather than the forceps instrument itself.

At the other extreme on the scale of results, DeWees forceps were associated with no demonstrable adverse effects. Furthermore, some outcome measures suggested a protective effect with frequencies of adverse outcomes significantly lower than expected relative to the overall rate for forceps cases. Some were even significantly lower than the already low referent rates for Irving forceps.

The Simpson forceps group (admittedly consisting of an admixture of procedures, as noted earlier) showed a bad effect in nulliparas and a paradoxically good effect in multiparas. The disparate conditions pre-

ceding forceps use in nulliparas and multiparas, respectively, might explain these apparently conflicting findings—that is, use of these forceps in a nullipara was much more likely to have been undertaken for a compelling reason, such as dystocia, than in a multipara. At the same time, for cases in which equivalent indications may have existed, the forceps operation in a nullipara was likely to have been more difficult to accomplish. The issue of difficulty of the procedure will be addressed in more detail (see below).

Cases in which Luikart forceps were employed did well with regard to short-term outcome, although there was a suggestion (not statistically significant) of an increased perinatal mortality among offspring of multiparas. Late measures of outcome at four and seven years showed unexpectedly poor results in both parity groups, supported in nulliparas by even worse data in the three-year testing vehicle.

For Elliot forceps, data for offspring of nulliparas were almost identical with those seen after Simpson forceps delivery. The outcome in multiparas delivered by Elliot forceps, however, did not show the same kind of apparent benefit found among multiparas in the Simpson forceps subseries. DeLee forceps use yielded the similarly

*Hughey MJ, McElin TW, Lussky R: Forceps operations in perspective: I. Forceps rotation operations. *J Reprod Med* 1978; 20:253; Chiswick ML, James DK: Kielland's forceps: Association with neonatal morbidity and mortality. *Brit Med J* 1979; 1:7.

Table 23-5
Outcome by Class of Forceps Delivery*

Class	No.	SB	NND	APG5	MENT8	MOT8	SLH3	IQ4	IQ7
I (Low)									
Nulliparas	2,774	1.00(0.36)	1.00(0.40)	1.00(1.94)	1.00(0.30)	1.00(0.39)	1.00(7.29)	1.00(2.12)	1.00(2.02)
Multiparas	2,127	1.00(0.75)	1.00(0.52)	1.00(1.11)	1.00(0.80)	1.00(1.38)	1.00(4.33)	1.00(1.98)	1.00(2.00)
II (Mid)									
Nulliparas	3,294	1.51	1.22	1.05	1.62a	1.54a	1.32a	1.44a	1.26a
Multiparas	2,616	0.97	1.48	1.29	1.26	1.12	1.24a	1.60b	1.48a
III (Mid)									
Nulliparas	1,745	0.78	2.74b	1.46a	1.77b	2.00b	2.47b	2.35b	1.87b
Multiparas	2,328	0.52	2.92a	2.48c	1.58a	1.88b	2.67b	2.01b	1.99b

* See footnote, Table 23-2.

Table 23-6
Outcome by Type of Forceps Instrument*

Type	No.	SB	NND	APG5	MENT8	MOT8	SLH3	IQ4	IQ7
Irving									
Nulliparas	2,047	1.00(0.29)	1.00(0.34)	1.00(1.73)	1.00(0.19)	1.00(0.25)	1.00(1.44)	1.00(2.03)	1.00(1.92)
Multiparas	2,604	1.00(0.50)	1.00(0.42)	1.00(1.24)	1.00(0.87)	1.00(1.03)	1.00(2.68)	1.00(2.40)	1.00(1.97)
Simpson									
Nulliparas	1,683	2.63b	0.87	1.21	3.44a	2.82	5.59b	2.70b	2.55a
Multiparas	1,506	2.04	1.10	1.26	0.86	0.59a	0.89a	0.90a	0.92
Luikart									
Nulliparas	1,516	0.68	1.16	1.12	1.68	1.90	6.16b	2.31a	3.11d
Multiparas	961	1.48	1.72	1.27	1.64	1.23	1.13	1.66e	4.02e
Elliot									
Nulliparas	612	2.24	2.39	2.75d	2.30	3.59a	6.98b	1.90	2.02
Multiparas	846	0.84a	1.68	1.51	1.20	1.33	2.01	1.11	2.17a
DeLee									
Nulliparas	615	0.56a	1.90	1.13	1.03	2.24	3.56a	1.86	3.22a
Multiparas	157	0.80	1.71	0.62b	2.01a	1.56	0.48a	1.59c	4.01e
Kielland									
Nulliparas	267	1.30	6.57b	2.26a	2.40	1.80	7.55b	2.28a	4.10b
Multiparas	345	2.76a	4.11b	4.53d	1.27	1.35	4.06b	2.38b	3.51d

Tucker-McLane									
Nulliparas	293	3.49a	1.01	0.84	2.08	1.58	2.37	1.83	2.04
Multiparas	244	1.96	4.84a	2.37	0.86a	0.88	2.57	1.17	2.64a
DeWees									
Nulliparas	305	1.12	0.96	0.68a	0.80	0.60a	2.04	1.04	0.98
Multiparas	76	0.93	0.99	1.04	0.88	1.52	0.90	0.87	1.47
Luikart-Tucker									
Nulliparas	89	0.00	0.00	0.00a	0.00	0.00	2.63	2.29	4.09a
Multiparas	73	0.00	0.00	0.00	0.00	0.00	2.79	1.20	3.64
Hawks-Dennen									
Nulliparas	75	0.00	0.00	0.00	0.00	1.48	3.90	2.68	3.26
Haig-Ferguson									
Nulliparas	37	0.00	0.00	4.04b	3.71	3.60	0.00	2.23	4.04

* See footnote, Table 23-2.

poor long-term outcome in nulliparas as with the other classical instruments. Moreover, it was found to have an impressively adverse impact in the seven-year results for both nulliparas and multiparas.

Similarly, delivery by Tucker-McLane forceps was associated with statistically significant bad effects only in multiparas (and only insofar as neonatal death and low seven-year IQ scores were concerned), with an inexplicably counterbalancing, apparently protective effect in the eight-month Bayley scales. Infants of nulliparas delivered with Tucker-McLane forceps did not seem to do badly; this applied even though the rate ratios were uniformly increased when outcomes were compared with those of the referent Irving forceps group (see above). The exception here was the rather high stillbirth rate (3.5 times the referent rate but only marginally elevated over that of the total population, $p = .049$).

Other forceps types were used in relatively few cases, most insufficient to permit reliable statistical testing. Some of the data pertaining to use of Luikart-Tucker, Hawks-Dennen, and Haig-Ferguson forceps are displayed in Table 23-6. They show persistent late effects even among infants in apparently acceptable condition earlier (as evidenced by their uniformly good five-minute Apgar and eight-month Bayley scores). Not shown are the data for forceps used even more infrequently, some of which were found to be associated with particularly bad outcomes. Indeed, the outcome rates achieved statistical significance despite the small numbers, most notably with Piper forceps, but this of course is more relevant to breech delivery and management of the aftercoming head (see below).

Forceps Manipulation

Various kinds of forceps manipulation were examined separately as related to application, traction, and rotation (90° or more). Conversion—principally involving flexion to make the presenting fetal head

diameters more favorable for delivery in deflexed attitudes associated with sincipital or brow presentations—was done too infrequently to allow reliable statistical analysis. Forceps application to and subsequent traction on the fetal head were, of course, almost always concurrent, but not universal. In 1.75% of forceps applications in nulliparas and in 3.72% of applications in multiparas, traction was never actually undertaken. These cases usually represented those in which application failed or misapplication was recognized and subsequent attempts to effect vaginal delivery by this means were abandoned. We felt it worthwhile, therefore, to study outcomes for forceps application separately from traction.

Utilizing the data for the application group as the referent (Table 23-7), we determined that there was no real difference from the results for traction cases but rather impressively adverse effects among those subjected to rotation. The greatest impact appeared in the neonatal death and depression rates. Follow-up studies did uncover residual effects on the offspring. There was uniform persistence of significantly deleterious findings through seven years in both nulliparas and multiparas (with the exception of paradoxical eight-month scores).

Difficulty of Forceps Procedure

Assessment of the degree of difficulty encountered in the several types of forceps operations was done next. It will be recalled (chapter 22) that the degree of difficulty of a given procedure was based on as objective an interpretation of the technical skill, expediency, and especially force as it was possible to obtain prior to the birth by a trained observer. Three degrees of difficulty—average, moderate, and very difficult—were assigned, plus a category for failed attempts. The last often also reflected very difficult procedures, of course, but were not included in the mutually exclusive subsets.

The outcome data for difficulty of for-

Table 23-7
Outcome by Forceps Manipulation*

Procedure	No.	SB	NND	APG5	MENT8	MOT8	SLH3	IQ4	IQ7
Application									
Nulliparas	7,672	1.00(0.43)	1.00(0.51)	1.00(2.16)	1.00(0.40)	1.00(0.56)	1.00(7.06)	1.00(1.77)	1.00(2.04)
Multiparas	7,037	1.00(0.62)	1.00(0.74)	1.00(1.80)	1.00(0.95)	1.00(1.14)	1.00(3.78)	1.00(1.67)	1.00(1.96)
Traction									
Nulliparas	7,538	0.96	0.99	0.97	1.02	0.96	1.01	0.99	1.00
Multiparas	6,775	0.91	0.98	0.96	0.95	0.99	1.06	0.99	1.00
Rotation									
Nulliparas	890	0.79	2.43c	1.69b	0.68	0.94	1.10	1.46a	1.82b
Multiparas	1,127	0.58	1.92b	1.52b	0.46	0.49	1.40b	1.59a	1.66a

* See footnote, Table 23-2.

ceps application (Table 23-8) showed that the more difficult the application, the greater the adverse infant impact. Relative to those applied with average difficulty, moderate difficulty yielded significantly increased perinatal mortality and neonatal depression as well as long-term residual deficits, the latter having been noted especially in multiparas. Very difficult application resulted in still worse results in the same pattern of distribution. Although the numbers of failed applications were small, their great adverse effect was nonetheless demonstrable in this series. The very high stillbirth rate in multiparas (more than tenfold increase) was unexpected; results to liveborn infants, however, were almost identical in magnitude and distribution to those seen after very difficult applications.

This approach had thus permitted us to further stratify cases of forceps application into those in which traction was applied and those in which the forceps were abandoned. Relative to the usual combination of application followed by traction, cases in which no traction was done because the application failed fared poorly. This did not necessarily mean that desisting from traction was inappropriate; rather, it suggested that failed forceps applications served as markers for complications related to bony and positional dystocia. Similarly, many of those applications that proved to be difficult may have had the same connotation.

As to traction difficulty (Table 23-9), too few cases (12 in all) of traction failure were recorded to allow meaningful interpretation of results to the infant. Therefore, they were incorporated into those designated as having been very difficult. As anticipated from the foregoing study of application difficulty, the more difficult the traction, the worse the outcome. Short-term and medium-term adverse results through eight months were clearly demonstrated in both nulliparas and multiparas after both moderate and very difficult traction. Subsequently, there were hints of continuing deficits in the offspring. Statistical significance of the adverse result was achieved inconsis-

tently however.

The difficulty of accomplishing forceps rotation enhanced the inherent apparent risk of the procedure. The outcome data (Table 23-10) revealed that moderate difficulty increased perinatal mortality and neonatal depression in both parity subgroups, while greater degrees of difficulty not only unfavorably affected the perinatal results but had a lasting impact as well (significantly so in multiparas).

It is important to recognize that the rate ratios shown in Table 23-10 flag the augmenting influence of moderate difficulty or worse in accomplishing forceps rotation as related to forceps rotations of average difficulty. The underlying adverse effect of forceps rotations as compared to forceps delivery without prior rotation, as shown in Table 23-7, was not taken into account here. Instead, these data dealt only with the additional effect that any associated difficulty had on the bad effect that already existed.

For example, the neonatal death rate for offspring of nulliparas delivered after forceps rotation of average difficulty was actually more than twice that for babies delivered by forceps without preceding rotation (RR 2.14, p = .00092); this increased to more than fourfold if the rotation had been moderately difficult (RR 4.17, p = 4.2×10^{-5}) and remarkably to sixfold after difficult or failed rotation (RR 6.10, p < 1.0×10^{-10}). Thus, the adverse impact of forceps rotation was augmented considerably if the rotation proved to be difficult to accomplish.

Indication for Forceps Use

Stratification of forceps delivery by the indication for which it was done allowed us to examine the differential effects of the underlying problem which ostensibly justified the procedure (Table 23-11). Relative to forceps operations undertaken electively, outcome results show significantly increased perinatal mortality and neonatal depression rates for infants subjected to forceps

Table 23-8
Outcome by Difficulty of Forceps Application*

Difficulty of Application	No.	SB	NND	APG5	MENT8	MOT8	SLH3	IQ4	IQ7
Average									
Nulliparas	6,983	1.00(0.40)	1.00(0.43)	1.00(1.85)	1.00(0.39)	1.00(0.53)	1.00(6.44)	1.00(1.90)	1.00(2.01)
Multiparas	6,514	1.00(0.57)	1.00(0.74)	1.00(1.50)	1.00(0.96)	1.00(1.18)	1.00(4.03)	1.00(2.09)	1.00(1.98)
Moderate									
Nulliparas	492	2.53d	1.42b	2.34c	1.92a	1.78a	1.81b	1.12	1.20
Multiparas	306	1.15a	2.28b	2.24b	1.23	0.68	0.45	1.28a	1.41b
Very difficult									
Nulliparas	157	0.00	5.93e	3.55d	0.00	1.48a	2.22a	1.56c	1.58c
Multiparas	91	1.93b	0.00	7.59e	0.00	0.00	1.77a	1.70b	2.23d
Failed									
Nulliparas	42	0.00	11.05e	6.59e	0.00	0.00	0.00	2.01	2.31a
Multiparas	49	10.76e	4.95c	9.95e	0.00	0.00	0.00	2.20a	3.03b

* See footnote, Table 23-2.

Table 23-9
Outcome by Difficulty of Forceps Traction*

Difficulty of Traction	No.	SB	NND	APG5	MENT8	MOT8	SLH3	IQ4	IQ7
Average									
Nulliparas	6,628	1.00(0.32)	1.00(0.42)	1.00(1.87)	1.00(0.37)	1.00(0.49)	1.00(7.10)	1.00(1.94)	1.00(2.10)
Multiparas	6,316	1.00(0.57)	1.00(0.74)	1.00(1.64)	1.00(0.91)	1.00(1.20)	1.00(3.86)	1.00(2.04)	1.00(2.14)
Moderate									
Nulliparas	741	3.41e	1.61b	1.62b	0.91	1.37a	1.23	1.19	1.30
Multiparas	387	0.90	1.12	1.29a	0.72	0.90	1.67a	1.10	1.06
Very difficult or failed									
Nulliparas	172	3.82d	6.89e	3.75d	5.97e	4.32e	0.92	1.49	1.40
Multiparas	72	2.43a	1.87a	4.24c	2.34b	0.86	0.00	1.67a	1.43

* See footnote, Table 23-2.

Table 23-10
Outcome by Difficulty of Forceps Rotation*

Difficulty of Rotation	No.	SB	NND	APG5	MENT8	MOT8	SLH3	IQ4	IQ7
Average									
Nulliparas	615	1.00(0.33)	1.00(1.30)	1.00(2.99)	1.00(0.30)	1.00(0.39)	1.00(8.89)	1.00(2.12)	1.00(2.09)
Multiparas	921	1.00(0.22)	1.00(1.19)	1.00(2.32)	1.00(0.53)	1.00(0.53)	1.00(4.11)	1.00(2.08)	1.00(2.01)
Moderate									
Nulliparas	162	1.89a	1.95a	1.45a	3.77a	3.76a	0.92	1.09	1.37
Multiparas	118	0.00	2.13a	1.22a	0.71	0.68	0.99	1.21	1.30
Very difficult or failed									
Nulliparas	112	0.00	2.85b	2.11b	0.00	0.00	0.98	1.22	1.26
Multiparas	88	10.38c	1.90a	5.39b	0.00	0.00	0.00	1.54a	1.65a

*   See footnote, Table 23-2.

Table 23-11
Outcome by Indication for Forceps*

Indication	No.	SB	NND	APG5	MENT8	MOT8	SLH3	IQ4	IQ7
Elective									
Nulliparas	6,472	1.00(0.37)	1.00(0.42)	1.00(1.79)	1.00(0.36)	1.00(0.47)	1.00(6.74)	1.00(1.67)	1.00(1.92)
Multiparas	6,129	1.00(0.54)	1.00(0.51)	1.00(1.40)	1.00(0.84)	1.00(1.02)	1.00(3.99)	1.00(1.50)	1.00(1.71)
Fetal distress									
Nulliparas	338	3.196	1.43	2.46d	2.07	3.17d	0.25a	1.60a	1.55
Multiparas	278	1.36	4.26d	3.74e	1.09	1.40	0.00	1.79b	1.88b
Prolonged second stage									
Nulliparas	115	2.35	0.00	1.99	0.00	0.00	0.00	1.19	1.23
Multiparas	21	0.00	18.82e	3.41b	0.00	0.00	0.00	1.40	2.11a
Transverse arrest									
Nulliparas	148	0.00	6.48e	3.06d	0.00	0.00	2.47a	1.24	1.18
Multiparas	118	1.59	3.35a	1.93	0.00	0.00	0.00	1.42	1.31
Cephalopelvic disproportion									
Nulliparas	54	4.99a	2.00	2.21	7.91b	0.00	3.71a	1.82	2.12
Multiparas	33	0.00	0.00	0.00	0.00	0.00	0.00	2.02	1.18
Arrested labor									
Nulliparas	60	0.00	4.00	3.85c	5.23a	7.80d	0.00	4.07a	2.70
Multiparas	21	0.00	18.82e	11.30e	6.61a	5.47a	0.00	3.18	3.05
Preeclampsia									
Nulliparas	99	0.00	0.00	1.16	0.00	0.00	0.74	1.67	1.88
Multiparas	23	0.00	0.00	6.82c	0.00	0.00	0.00	1.70	2.46b

* See footnote, Table 23-2.

delivery for fetal distress, as expected. In nulliparas, surviving children showed statistically significant residual adverse impact to four years of age, and in multiparas to seven years.

Forceps procedures indicated for labor disorders had been variously designated to distinguish prolonged second stage (roughly equivalent to inertial dystocia) from transverse arrest (referring to persistent occiput transverse fetal position, or positional dystocia) and both of these from cephalopelvic disproportion (representing a trial of forceps in association with bony dystocia); in addition, another group included those with arrested labor in which the pathogenic mechanism was unclear or unstated. Data for each of these subsets yielded information on the possible influence on the condition for which the forceps were used or for the procedure itself when done under these particular circumstances.

When a forceps delivery was undertaken for prolonged second stage in multiparas, for example, the rates of neonatal death and depression were very severely affected, with continuing bad results among survivors at seven years of age as well. The impact in nulliparas appeared to be related only to stillbirth and neonatal depression, but neither was found to be statistically significant. Moreover, there were only suggestive residual effects seen in the four- and seven-year follow-up data pertaining to these infants.

Forceps for transverse arrest resulted in similar exceptionally high neonatal death rates plus frequent low five-minute Apgar scores. Long-range permanent damage was suggested by the late results, particularly the three-year communications skills data in offspring of nulliparas. Adverse results were found to be associated with forceps done in conjunction with cephalopelvic disproportion among nulliparas. Very high stillbirth rates were encountered along with elevated (but not statistically significant) neonatal death and depression frequencies plus some poor residual effects at eight months and three years. There was also some later impact discerned from these data at four and seven years in both nulliparas and multiparas, but it was not statistically significant.

Forceps for arrested labor showed surprisingly good stillbirth rates, but they were counterbalanced by particularly bad neonatal death and depression data. This latter effect was still very apparent at eight months in both Bayley mental and motor scores. Later effects were also seen at four and seven years, but they were not statistically significant except in nulliparas for the four-year IQ results.

Instrumental delivery for pregnancy-induced hypertension did not result in any perinatal deaths; however, neonatal depression was augmented (significantly so in multiparas) and there was some residual late effect at four and seven years (also significant in offspring of multiparas).

Status of Delivery Attendant

Moving on to other matters, we tried to learn if the status of the attendant at delivery might affect outcome. The results (Table 23-12) suggested at first glance that it did. Relative to infants delivered by staff obstetricians, those attended by residents and nurses fared rather poorly, while those delivered by interns and medical students did paradoxically well. These findings were especially noteworthy for offspring of multiparas among whom the adverse results were consistent through the seventh year of life.

The good short-term results for interns and medical students stood in inexplicable contrast to the bad long-term results in these same cases. The latter observation raised the question of comparability among the several data subsets. Indeed, the basic issue of population preselection could readily explain the differences seen here. If the gravidas at greatest risk for developing complications were more likely to be cared for and delivered in a nonprivate setting and be delivered by a resident physician, then it would perforce follow that the out-

Table 23-12
Outcome by Delivery Attendant*

Attendant	No.	SB	NND	APG5	MENT8	MOT8	SLH3	IQ4	IQ7
Obstetrician									
Nulliparas	929	1.00(2.48)	1.00(1.74)	1.00(3.26)	1.00(0.41)	1.00(0.40)	1.00(3.53)	1.00(1.90)	1.00(1.78)
Multiparas	1,900	1.00(1.74)	1.00(2.05)	1.00(2.33)	1.00(1.01)	1.00(1.33)	1.00(1.82)	1.00(2.01)	1.00(1.98)
Resident									
Nulliparas	4,803	0.76	0.82	1.10a	1.03	1.49a	2.12b	1.99b	1.84a
Multiparas	8,355	1.36b	1.37b	1.67e	1.46b	1.24b	3.36c	2.28c	1.98b
Intern									
Nulliparas	4,507	0.41b	0.46b	0.77a	1.15	1.36a	3.09c	2.01b	2.14b
Multiparas	8,901	0.57c	0.76a	0.97	1.13	0.77a	5.31d	2.23b	2.25b
Medical student									
Nulliparas	962	0.46a	1.02	1.00	1.27	1.28	0.58a	1.93a	2.31b
Multiparas	4,672	0.50b	0.45c	0.60b	0.61b	0.44c	2.79c	2.28b	2.53b
Nurse, nurse-midwife									
Nulliparas	35	4.62a	1.80	0.96	0.00	0.00	7.08b	2.51a	4.59c
Multiparas	601	0.49a	1.30	1.73a	0.88	0.84	3.73c	2.22a	2.47a

* See footnote, Table 23-2.

come would be expected to be worse. Contrastingly, if the normal, healthy, uncomplicated case was preferentially referred for delivery by the intern or medical student, the results must be better (barring problems introduced by the attendant, of course). It was not unexpected, therefore, that residents' data were bad, while interns' and students' were good. One could also explain the contrastingly poor late results in the student and intern groups by the ethnic biases inherent in intelligence testing vehicles, again reflecting differences in population make-up rather than the impact of the delivery attendant.

Regrettably, we are unable to account for the apparently poor data for deliveries by nurses and nurse-midwives because comparable preselection of low-risk cases should have yielded just as good perinatal results for them as for interns and medical students. One would have to consider that if preselection biases were acting here, they would require nurses to be delivering a group that was somehow especially at risk; such might be the case in regard to deliveries characterized as rapid, unanticipated, or precipitate. We have already seen (Table 23-3) that the outcome for uncontrolled delivery was suboptimal, although not quite to the same degree as found here. We were, therefore, left with an essentially unanswered concern that deserves closer study.

Fetal Position

Having already demonstrated that breech delivery of a fetus carries a substantially worse prognosis than vaginal vertex delivery (Table 23-2), we felt it reasonable to dissect fetal vertex positions still further so as to determine if differences in outcome could be uncovered on this basis. As will be recalled (chapter 22), data were available for fetal position early in labor, fetal position prior to any form of manual or instrumental manipulation or intervention, and for fetal position at the actual moment of delivery. Examination of early labor fetal position failed to reveal any meaningful trends, apparently because positional change was so common as labor evolved (see above). Therefore, we concentrated exclusively on the remaining two data sets. Because information on position prior to intervention had not been collected until the study was well under way, this subset did not encompass all NCPP gravidas, thus making the two groups dissimilar in size. Nonetheless, the impressive results to offspring were deemed to be representative as a major population sampling and, therefore, reflective of relationships that were probably true.

Before intervention (Table 23-13), those fetuses in occiput transverse or occiput posterior positions did significantly worse than those in occiput anterior with regard to neonatal death and depression. Occiput transverse positions fared less well than occiput posterior. Stillbirths rates were poorer as well, but achieved statistical significance only in those born to nulliparas. Long-term follow-up showed persistently bad outcomes, especially in offspring of multiparas.

Fetal position at delivery (Table 23-14) had the same pattern of adverse effect, except that the relative magnitude was enhanced considerably. Occiput posterior positions were associated with greatly increased perinatal mortality. Stillbirth rates, for example, were 2-2.5 times those for fetuses in occiput anterior position, regardless of parity. Occiput transverse deliveries multiplied the fetal deaths by an additional factor of three to yield a more than sixfold relative increase over occiput anterior deliveries. Similarly, significantly increased neonatal death and depression rates were found with both occiput posterior and occiput transverse positions. Adverse effects persisted to four and seven years.

While very significant statistically, those actually delivered as occiput transverse (especially among nulliparas) were too few in number to permit useful comparisons. Nonetheless, the findings were very impressive and strongly reflected the likeli-

Table 23-13
Outcome by Fetal Position and Presentation Before Intervention for Delivery*

Position Presentation	No.	SB	NND	APG5	MENT8	MOT8	SLH3	IQ4	IQ7
Occiput anterior (LOA to ROA)									
Nulliparas	6,520	1.00(0.43)	1.00(0.41)	1.00(1.76)	1.00(0.38)	1.00(0.50)	1.00(6.19)	1.00(2.20)	1.00(2.28)
Multiparas	5,555	1.00(0.63)	1.00(0.56)	1.00(1.49)	1.00(1.00)	1.00(1.12)	1.00(3.59)	1.00(2.31)	1.00(2.37)
Occiput transverse (LOT, ROT)									
Nulliparas	675	1.40a	4.29e	3.90e	1.46a	1.42a	2.14b	1.11	1.03
Multiparas	981	1.14	2.74d	2.10d	0.79	1.05	1.10	1.16b	1.32b
Occiput posterior (LOP to ROP)									
Nulliparas	762	1.83b	1.59a	2.47e	0.82	1.25a	1.22	1.13	1.27a
Multiparas	1,162	1.10	1.70b	1.98e	1.06	0.94	2.06	1.26b	1.77e

* See footnote, Table 23-2.

Table 23-14
Outcome by Fetal Position and Presentation at Delivery*

Position	No.	SB	NND	APG5	MENT8	MOT8	SLH3	IQ4	IQ7
Occiput anterior (LOA to ROA)									
Nulliparas	10,147	1.00(0.81)	1.00(0.77)	1.00(2.49)	1.00(0.39)	1.00(0.55)	1.00(6.73)	1.00(2.11)	1.00(2.20)
Multiparas	21,424	1.00(0.82)	1.00(1.05)	1.00(1.74)	1.00(1.96)	1.00(0.95)	1.00(5.52)	1.00(2.24)	1.00(2.37)
Occiput transverse (LOT, ROT)									
Nulliparas	22	6.81d	18.18e	7.66d	0.00	0.00	4.94	1.38	1.86
Multiparas	73	6.43a	3.92a	1.77a	2.11	0.00	0.00	1.55a	1.80a
Occiput posterior (LOP to ROP)									
Nulliparas	293	2.06a	3.55d	2.40a	2.16	1.48	0.82	1.43a	1.68b
Multiparas	605	2.52a	2.04a	2.19a	1.17	1.09	1.51	1.19	1.33

* See footnote, Table 23-2.

hood that occiput transverse delivery was a major risk factor. At a lesser order of magnitude, occiput posterior position also appeared to impact unfavorably on the fetus. The results in both delivery malpositions were somewhat worse than for children stratified according to the position prior to intervention. This was particularly the case for perinatal death data.

Those still in an occiput posterior position at delivery consisted of a composite of those in whom attempts to rotate had failed plus those in whom no attempts had been made, less those who had spontaneously rotated or had been successfully rotated manually or instrumentally. The composition is further complicated by the recognition that the group contained both cases delivered spontaneously and those delivered by forceps as occiput posterior. This set of data does not help distinguish among these kinds of cases, but it does raise questions concerning the relative merits and risks of forceps rotation (Table 23-10) versus those of spontaneous or forceps delivery of the occiput posterior fetal head as such.

Fetal Station

Fetal station at the onset of labor or early in its course had been found to be a utilitarian index of possible cephalopelvic disproportion in nulliparas and of subsequent disordered labor in both nulliparas and multiparas.* Our interest in early labor fetal station extended here to determining potential impact on the fetus. Data on fetal station, as previously noted (chapter 22), were available based on admission and delivery observations and recordings. Those obtained at the time of admission represented a range of time frames insofar as the labor pattern was concerned, of course, but were concentrated principally in the latent phase. The groups stratified

*Friedman EA, Sachtleben MR: Station of the fetal presenting part: II. Effect on the course of labor. *Amer J Obstet Gynecol* 1965; 93:530.

according to fetal station at the first observation in labor, therefore, were not perfectly homogeneous. Nonetheless, the outcome data derived from them (Table 23-15) were most interesting. Comparisons were made to those at zero station, the modal group which served for reference purposes.

Among stations cephalad to the referent group, there was a very strong relationship between admission station and outcome: the higher the station, the worse the outlook. Perinatal death and depression rates for those first seen with a floating presenting part (stations -4 and -5) were startlingly elevated, and the deleterious long-term outcomes reflected the same for surviving infants. This confirmed the earlier findings pertaining to bony dystocia and dysfunctional labor which could be expected to yield poor fetal and infant results. Quite unanticipated was the observation that this applied to both nulliparas and multiparas alike. Moreover, the more caudad station groups disclosed results that had not previously been encountered, namely a significant increase in adverse outcomes for cases presenting with very low stations. It was unclear what this may have represented, although it was conjectured that prematurity may have played a contributory role here; this finding needed elucidation.

Outcomes related to fetal station just prior to delivery, specifically prior to any manipulation or operative intervention, were of equal interest. While the group at high stations just before delivery was effected did contain individuals delivered spontaneously (perhaps after manual rotation and/or Kristeller expression), most constituted forceps deliveries. The results, therefore, principally reflected the latter influence and verified the effects previously encountered for midforceps procedures. Here, the data were fractionated more finely by the actual station at which the forceps were applied rather than broadly grouping cases by standardized definitions of forceps classes that encompassed a range of stations.

Table 23-15
Outcome by Fetal Station at First Observation in Labor*

Station	No.	SB	NND	APG5	MENT8	MOT8	SLH3	IQ4	IQ7
-4, -5									
Nulliparas	333	4.37e	7.18e	4.33c	6.94e	2.36	1.41	1.20d	1.63e
Multiparas	1,536	6.67e	4.89e	3.75e	1.83b	1.35	1.84a	1.20e	1.41e
-3									
Nulliparas	572	1.88a	2.19b	1.74	0.62	0.45	1.26	1.10b	1.43e
Multiparas	2,000	2.65e	2.92e	2.53e	0.75	0.85	0.75	1.11e	1.16d
-2									
Nulliparas	1,358	1.45	1.06	1.29	1.80	1.86	1.16	1.06a	1.26e
Multiparas	3,732	1.61b	1.25	1.67d	0.78	0.95	0.87	1.08d	1.15e
-1									
Nulliparas	2,731	0.93	0.84	1.23	1.13	1.28	1.56	1.02	1.19e
Multiparas	5,722	1.08	1.14	1.32a	0.86	0.93	0.92	1.02	1.07a
0									
Nulliparas	3,768	1.00(1.12)	1.00(0.88)	1.00(2.51)	1.00(0.36)	1.00(0.48)	1.00(5.24)	1.00(2.00)	1.00(2.12)
Multiparas	6,034	1.00(0.78)	1.00(1.03)	1.00(1.61)	1.00(1.07)	1.00(1.09)	1.00(5.97)	1.00(1.94)	1.00(2.20)
+1									
Nulliparas	1,610	0.72	0.92	1.02	1.05	0.77	1.09	0.96	0.93
Multiparas	2,423	1.11	1.08	1.20	1.01	0.94	0.77	1.05a	0.96
+2									
Nulliparas	503	1.07	1.36	0.41	0.00	0.00	1.74	1.09a	0.82a
Multiparas	964	1.87a	2.02c	1.26	1.45	1.89a	1.01	1.14d	1.20d
+3									
Nulliparas	104	2.59	3.29a	1.59	3.70	2.65	0.00	1.11	1.48c
Multiparas	272	0.96	2.50b	1.20	1.44	0.90	0.00	1.29e	1.29e
+4									
Nulliparas	90	3.09a	7.59e	1.94	0.00	3.09	0.00	1.11	1.08
Multiparas	436	1.80	3.12e	1.71a	1.45	1.73	3.05	1.19d	1.52e

* See footnote, Table 23-2.

As expected, the outcomes for deliveries undertaken at high stations yielded poor fetal and infant results (Table 23-16). The lower the station, the better the outcome. This relationship held across the entire range of outcome variables through seven years of age. In the short-term results, the trend was nearly linear; for example, neonatal deaths were related to predelivery station by the regression equations

$$y = 4.46 - 1.66x \text{ and } y = 3.41 - 0.81x$$

in nulliparas and multiparas, respectively (both slopes statistically significant, standard errors 0.390 and 0.218, t values 4.25 and 3.73). Contrary to the adverse effects seen with low station at first examination (see above), low station at delivery was uniformly beneficial to the fetus.

Breech Position and Station

Earlier, we saw that vaginal breech delivery was associated with pervasively poor outcomes (see Table 23-2). Data were available to help determine whether high-risk aspects of breech presentation could be identified. Among relevant factors for study were fetal position, attitude, delivery procedure, and accompanying complications. Stratifying by fetal station just prior to any intervention or manipulation to effect delivery (Table 23-17) failed to show any consistent impact of this factor on the fetus and infant.

Contrary to expectations, fetuses in sacrum posterior positions did not fare worse than those with sacrum anterior position; although the numbers were small and the results not statistically significant, those in sacrum posterior positions actually seemed to do somewhat better when compared to the more commonly encountered anterior fetal position. For nulliparas with offspring in sacrum transverse position, results were still better, achieving statistical significance in several of the outcome variables; data for multiparas, however, did not show a parallel trend.

Breech Attitude

Breech attitude, similarly examined, showed much more impressive effects (Table 23-18). Babies delivered in frank breech presentation served as the referent group for comparison purposes, accepting that outcomes among them were considerably worse overall than in vertex presentations. Both single and double footling delivery significantly enhanced the already adverse effects of breech presentation. The deleterious impact was especially noteworthy in the frequencies of neonatal death and depression, and there were apparent long-term effects as well (although they did not consistently show statistical significance).

To illustrate, we found the neonatal death rate in nulliparous frank breech fetuses to have been 4.3 times greater than in similar vertex presentations delivered vaginally (4.03% versus 0.94%, RR 4.29, p = 7.1 x 10^{-5}), while single footling breech increased the rate by more than an additional fourfold increment (to 17.64%, RR 4.38 relative to frank breech and 18.77 relative to vertex) and double footling by fivefold (to 20.31%, RR 5.04 and 21.61, respectively).

Full or complete breech attitude was also associated with poor outcomes relative to frank breech results. Here the neonatal death rate was three times that for frank breech (12.12%, RR 3.01 and 12.89). Although principally demonstrated in short-term effects, the adverse impact persisted over the range of the study, achieving statistical significance in the four-year IQ scores only in offspring of multiparas.

Breech Delivery Type

The type of breech delivery also provided interesting data pertaining to outcome (Table 23-19). Relative to spontaneous breech delivery, babies born by assisted breech maneuvers (partial extraction after spontaneous birth to the umbilicus) fared poorly. There were significant increases in

Table 23-16
Outcome by Fetal Station Preceding Manipulation or Operative Intervention*

Station	No.	SB	NND	APG5	MENT8	MOT8	SLH3	IQ4	IQ7
-1 and cephalad									
Nulliparas	291	2.90b	4.34d	2.88d	1.47	1.46	1.34	1.23e	1.69e
Multiparas	965	1.47b	7.23e	2.91e	2.29b	2.42b	1.21	1.31e	2.22e
0									
Nulliparas	138	1.22	3.14b	2.49a	4.74c	3.57b	3.46a	1.42c	1.38b
Multiparas	298	1.08	4.59d	3.36d	1.74a	2.56a	2.02a	1.30b	2.29e
+1									
Nulliparas	176	1.12	4.11b	2.48a	1.81a	1.48	1.22	1.24a	1.31a
Multiparas	485	1.09	1.54a	1.35a	1.62a	1.49	2.00a	1.26a	1.94d
+2									
Nulliparas	1,021	0.98	1.84a	1.57a	1.39	1.95a	1.51	1.15	1.44b
Multiparas	1,390	1.06	1.94a	1.44a	1.43	1.44	1.89a	1.25b	1.63b
+3									
Nulliparas	2,173	0.91	1.11	1.08	1.17	1.08	1.38	1.12	1.48e
Multiparas	1,651	0.97	1.08	1.10	1.06	1.11	1.39	1.18a	1.40d
+4 and caudad									
Nulliparas	4,628	1.00(1.03)	1.00(0.69)	1.00(2.40)	1.00(0.40)	1.00(0.49)	1.00(5.78)	1.00(1.90)	1.00(2.06)
Multiparas	4,104	1.00(1.09)	1.00(0.81)	1.00(2.71)	1.00(0.99)	1.00(1.05)	1.00(3.57)	1.00(1.86)	1.00(2.02)

* See footnote, Table 23-2.

302

Table 23-17
Outcome by Fetal Position in Breech Presentation Before Delivery Intervention*

Position	No.	SB	NND	APG5	MENT8	MOT8	SLH3	IQ4	IQ7
Sacrum anterior (RSA to LSA)									
Nulliparas	119	1.00(13.45)	1.00(7.21)	1.00(12.15)	1.00(1.30)	1.00(1.32)	1.00 (0.00)	1.00(3.03)	1.00(2.61)
Multiparas	230	1.00 (7.11)	1.00(9.13)	1.00(12.68)	1.00(2.78)	1.00(2.04)	1.00(12.00)	1.00(4.17)	1.00(2.79)
Sacrum transverse (RST, LST)									
Nulliparas	79	0.00d	0.18	0.21b	0.00c	0.00	0.00	1.19	1.06
Multiparas	154	1.30	1.14	0.97	1.07	3.81a	0.52	1.50	1.09
Sacrum posterior (RSP to LSP)									
Nulliparas	35	0.21	0.77	0.50	0.00a	0.00	0.00	1.04	1.12
Multiparas	73	0.82	1.20	1.01	0.00	0.00	2.78	1.13	1.24

* See footnote, Table 23-2.

Table 23-18
Outcome by Attitude of Breech Presentation*

Attitude	No.	SB	NND	APG5	MENT8	MOT8	SLH3	IQ4	IQ7
Frank									
Nulliparas	164	1.00(12.81)	1.00 (4.03)	1.00 (4.97)	1.00(0.86)	1.00(0.85)	1.00(0.00)	1.00(3.02)	1.00(2.40)
Multiparas	367	1.00(11.72)	1.00(10.24)	1.00(13.65)	1.00(3.77)	1.00(4.29)	1.00(4.35)	1.00(3.09)	1.00(2.64)
Full									
Nulliparas	35	1.34	3.01a	4.41c	0.00	0.00	0.00	1.12	1.16
Multiparas	65	1.30	2.25c	2.09c	0.00	1.46	0.00	1.43c	1.20
Single footling									
Nulliparas	17	0.98	4.38b	7.11e	0.00	0.00	0.00	1.35	1.92
Multiparas	85	1.00	1.15	1.54	0.47	0.93	15.33e	1.14	1.21
Double footling									
Nulliparas	68	1.95b	5.04d	3.47c	3.63	0.00	0.00	1.45a	1.35
Multiparas	208	1.26	2.16d	1.58b	1.88	2.16a	3.06	1.15	1.37a

* See footnote, Table 23-2.

Table 23-19
Outcome by Type of Breech Delivery*

Delivery	No.	SB	NND	APG5	MENT8	MOT8	SLH3	IQ4	IQ7
Spontaneous									
Nulliparas	303	1.00(8.58)	1.00(3.82)	1.00(5.84)	1.00(0.45)	1.00(0.90)	1.00(11.36)	1.00(2.96)	1.00(3.03)
Multiparas	504	1.00(9.13)	1.00(7.29)	1.00(6.49)	1.00(1.47)	1.00(2.05)	1.00 (3.70)	1.00(3.23)	1.00(3.45)
Assisted (partial extraction)									
Nulliparas	149	1.03	2.70c	2.47c	2.66	1.23	0.34	0.98	1.26
Multiparas	388	0.99	1.99d	2.95e	3.28b	2.78b	3.31a	0.97	1.25a
Extraction (total extraction)									
Nulliparas	106	0.98	2.62a	1.38	8.93a	0.00	0.00	1.09	1.17
Multiparas	305	1.00	1.54a	2.28d	4.72d	4.09d	3.60a	1.01	1.32a

* See footnote, Table 23-2.

neonatal death and depression among both nulliparas and multiparas. The adverse effect persisted to seven years, remaining statistically significant among offspring of multiparas. Total extraction yielded comparably bad results; except for the eight-month data, the deleterious impact of total extraction was unexpectedly found to be about equivalent to that of assisted breech births.

Once again, it should be noted in passing that the referent levels (for outcomes of spontaneously delivered breech babies) were considerably higher than for vaginal vertex deliveries. Thus, the neonatal death rate in multiparous offspring was four times greater with a spontaneous breech delivery (3.82% versus 0.94%, RR 4.06, p = 8.7 x 10^{-7}); for assisted breech, the increment in death rate was further enhanced to nearly 11-fold (10.29%, RR 2.70 relative to spontaneous breech and RR 10.96 relative to vertex) and for breech extraction, about the same (RR 2.62 and 10.64, respectively).

Breech Complication

Identifiable breech complications were studied in an attempt to determine their effect on the infant, but the numbers generally proved too small to permit meaningful analyses. The most frequently reported complication associated with breech birth was nuchal arms, appearing in only 48 cases. When the outcome in them was contrasted with that of infants delivered by uncomplicated breech delivery, low Apgar scores surfaced as significantly increased in both nulliparas and multiparas, as did three-year speech, language, and hearing results in multiparas (Table 23-20). The poor four- and seven-year IQ results failed to reach statistical significance.

Only seven cases had documentably extended fetal heads (an incidence in this series of 0.40% or one per 251 vaginal breech births). Among them, however, four were stillborn (57.1%), a remarkable frequency indeed, and two of the remaining three had persistent major neurologic defi-cits at age seven years. The total of dead and damaged infants in this small series was thus 85.7%. Since specific intrapartum efforts had not routinely been made to ascertain head extension in breech presentations during the era of this study, we cannot determine the true frequency of this complication. Nonetheless, the results for those few in which the diagnosis was actually made proved to be so devastating that there can be little doubt as to its seriously adverse effect, verifying current opinions in this regard.*

Labor Induction

There were 7.9% inductions of labor in this series (7.15% in nulliparas and 8.27% in multiparas). Without considering method, indication, or number of attempts, we determined that induction was associated with a substantially increased stillbirth rate, but had little, if any, negative effect on the surviving infant (Table 23-21). By comparison to fetuses involved with spontaneous onset labor, those subjected to inductions had nearly three times the chance of dying before birth (for nulliparas 3.90% versus 1.36%, RR 2.87, p = 7.5 x 10^{-8}; for multiparas, 3.42% versus 1.32%, RR 2.59, p $<$1.0 x 10^{-10}). Other than the increase in low Bayley mental scores among offspring of nulliparas at eight months of age, no other evidence of poor outcome was observed. If anything, there appeared to have been a protective effect for babies delivered after induced labor in the long-term results, especially in seven-year IQ scores.

These paradoxical findings suggested that induction might have been invoked selectively for cases in which intrauterine fetal death had occurred at or near term; alternatively (and perhaps additionally),

---

*Abroms IF, Bresnan MJ, Zuckerman JE, et al: Cervical cord injuries secondary to hyperextension of the head in breech presentations. *Obstet Gynecol* 1973; 41:369; Ballas S, Toaff R, Jaffa AJ: Deflexion of fetal head in breech presentation: Incidence, management and outcome. *Obstet Gynecol* 1978; 52:653.

Table 23-20
Outcome by Breech Complication*

Complication	No.	SB	NND	APG5	MENT8	MOT8	SLH3	IQ4	IQ7
None									
Nulliparas	550	1.00(10.36)	1.00 (6.45)	1.00 (7.82)	1.00(1.04)	1.00(0.77)	1.00(7.06)	1.00(3.00)	1.00(2.40)
Multiparas	1,137	1.00 (8.90)	1.00(10.91)	1.00(12.36)	1.00(3.48)	1.00(4.24)	1.00(8.33)	1.00(3.27)	1.00(2.54)
Nuchal arm(s)									
Nulliparas	12	0.00	1.29	3.49b	0.00	0.00	0.00	1.46	1.37
Multiparas	48	0.26	0.96	2.07c	0.96	0.85	6.00a	1.60	1.84

* See footnote, Table 23-2.

Table 23-21
Outcome by Spontaneous Versus Induced Onset of Labor*

Onset	No.	SB	NND	APG5	MENT8	MOT8	SLH3	IQ4	IQ7
Spontaneous									
Nulliparas	10,578	1.00(1.36)	1.00(1.23)	1.00(3.11)	1.00(0.45)	1.00(0.57)	1.00(6.42)	1.00(2.07)	1.00(2.19)
Multiparas	22,890	1.00(1.32)	1.00(1.81)	1.00(2.53)	1.00(1.16)	1.00(1.17)	1.00(5.84)	1.00(2.25)	1.00(2.13)
Induced									
Nulliparas	851	2.87e	0.81	1.00	1.23e	0.64	1.10	1.12	0.88
Multiparas	2,124	2.59e	0.99	1.20	0.66	0.89	0.88	0.96	0.54e

* See footnote, Table 23-2.

307

those who had labor preferentially induced may have been gravidas with attributes associated with high infant IQ scores such as affluent, white nulliparas at term. Needless to say, these potentially confounding factors had to be investigated simultaneously.

Induction Attempts

To examine the impact of labor induction more closely, we stratified the cases by the number of times induction was attempted prior to delivery. The largest proportion had only one such attempt, of course (90.54% of all induced nulliparas and 85.47% of induced multiparas), but moderate numbers had two (10.69% and 12.97%, respectively) and even three tries (2.33% and 3.66%). The outcome data (Table 23-22) confirmed the high stillbirth rate after even one attempt at inducing labor compared to cases in which no such attempts had been made; there were more than twice the expected frequency of fetal deaths in this group, a statistically very significant observation.

Still more impressively, two induction attempts yielded an even greater proportion of stillbirths, reaching about seven times that of uninduced nulliparous labors and more than three times in multiparas. Three or more attempts (up to a maximum of six in this series) yielded more than eightfold fetal mortality in nulliparas and more than fourfold in multiparas.

We could thus demonstrate a progressive increase in stillbirth rates with each succeeding attempt at induction. To illustrate this, we calculated the rate ratios based on comparison with results for the group in which only one induction attempt had been tried (Table 23-22). Utilizing the data from this group as referent, we found nulliparas had a 2.6-fold increase in stillbirths after two attempts and 3.1-fold more after three or more, whereas multiparas had 1.4 and 1.8 times more, respectively (only the nulliparous increments proved statistically significant, however).

Contrary to expectations, there was no accompanying increase in neonatal death rates or low Apgar scores with multiple induction attempts, either when examined in comparison with noninduced cases or when viewed in contrast to single attempts to induce labor. The paradoxical good effect of induction on long-term results, alluded to above, was replicated here in the significantly diminished frequencies of low seven-year IQ scores associated with one induction attempt in both nulliparas and multiparas and with two attempts in nulliparas only.

Relative to the data for a single attempt, however, we uncovered an apparent adverse impact for three or more induction attempts. While the increases in low IQ scores was equivalent in both nulliparas and multiparas (RR 1.29 and 1.32), they achieved statistical significance only in multiparas because of the larger number of cases involved.

Earlier, we had noted that infants delivered by induction did better overall than those who had not, suggesting a possible preferential preselection of cases for induction from among gravidas whose offspring could be expected to score well on intelligence testing vehicles. We now find that this ostensible benefit is counterbalanced by an adverse effect from multiple inductions which would likely have remained hidden had we not examined the two factors separately.

Indication for Induction

Outcomes examined by the reason the induction was undertaken (Table 23-23) were compared with outcomes for cases of elective induction. Children delivered by nulliparas induced for premature rupture of the membranes did uniformly well, but those of multiparas did rather badly. There were nearly three times the expected perinatal mortality rate and frequency of neonatal depression, all highly significant findings. Scores at eight months were about the same and there was still some

Table 23-22
Outcome by Number of Attempts to Induce Labor*

Attempts	No.	SB	NND	APG5	MENT8	MOT8	SLH3	IQ4	IQ7
Data relative to noninduced labors									
None									
Nulliparas	10,578	1.00(1.36)	1.00(1.23)	1.00(3.11)	1.00(0.45)	1.00(0.57)	1.00(6.42)	1.00(2.07)	1.00(2.19)
Multiparas	22,890	1.00(1.32)	1.00(1.81)	1.00(2.53)	1.00(1.16)	1.00(1.17)	1.00(5.84)	1.00(2.25)	1.00(2.13)
One									
Nulliparas	737	2.63e	0.85	1.14	1.60	0.93	1.23	0.91b	0.65e
Multiparas	1,753	2.32e	1.20	1.35b	0.63	0.81	0.93	0.92d	0.74e
Two									
Nulliparas	87	6.84e	0.00	1.26	0.00	0.00	2.14	0.92	0.64a
Multiparas	266	3.33e	1.20	1.37	1.28	1.68	0.00	0.94	0.90
Three or more									
Nulliparas	27	8.27e	0.00	0.00	0.00	0.00	3.21	0.97	0.83
Multiparas	105	4.22d	0.52	1.23	0.00	1.09	1.22	0.91	0.97
Data relative to one induction attempt only									
One									
Nulliparas	737	1.00	1.00	1.00	1.00	1.00	1.00	1.00	1.00
Multiparas	1,753	1.00	1.00	1.00	1.00	1.00	1.00	1.00	1.00
Two									
Nulliparas	87	2.61b	0.00	1.10	0.00	0.00	1.73	1.01	0.99
Multiparas	266	1.44	1.00	1.01	2.04	2.06	0.00	1.02	0.64a
Three or more									
Nulliparas	27	3.14a	0.00	0.00	0.00	0.00	2.60	1.06	1.29
Multiparas	105	1.82	0.43	0.91	0.00	1.35	1.31	1.00	1.32a

* See footnote, Table 23-2.

Table 23-23
Outcome by Indication for Induction of Labor*

Indication	No.	SB	NND	APG5	MENT8	MOT8	SLH3	IQ4	IQ7
Elective									
Nulliparas	239	1.00(2.09)	1.00(0.43)	1.00(3.69)	1.00(1.10)	1.00(0.54)	1.00(9.80)	1.00(2.23)	1.00(1.89)
Multiparas	731	1.00(0.69)	1.00(0.82)	1.00(1.85)	1.00(0.35)	1.00(0.34)	1.00(5.92)	1.00(2.10)	1.00(1.26)
Ruptured membranes									
Nulliparas	315	0.61	0.75	0.55	0.00	0.00	0.76	1.06	0.89
Multiparas	757	3.50c	3.86d	2.49c	2.98	5.32b	1.08	1.14a	1.15a
Preeclampsia									
Nulliparas	145	2.31	4.92a	1.56	1.55	3.11	1.13	1.26a	1.60c
Multiparas	203	5.75d	0.62	2.80b	0.00	0.00	0.77	1.33d	1.59e
Pyelonephritis									
Nulliparas	92	10.90e	10.21c	2.71	0.00	0.00	0.00	1.18	1.11
Multiparas	224	4.56c	3.88b	5.22e	7.18b	5.09a	0.73	2.01e	1.04
Erythroblastosis fetalis									
Nulliparas	58	0.89	8.09a	0.52	0.00	0.00	2.92	1.25	0.74
Multiparas	216	7.44e	4.02c	3.11c	1.71	1.78	0.00	0.94	0.85a
Diabetes mellitus									
Nulliparas	41	5.83d	6.35a	1.55	2.94	6.17	2.55	1.08	0.58
Multiparas	140	6.26d	2.67	1.66	2.64	5.62a	0.00	0.99	0.94
Amnionitis									
Nulliparas	16	5.98c	15.65c	5.61d	0.00	0.00	0.00	1.33	0.33
Multiparas	35	8.34c	6.96c	7.10e	1.97a	0.00	0.00	1.25	1.09
Abruptio placentae									
Nulliparas	9	21.24e	39.12e	0.00	0.00	0.00	0.00	1.81a	0.00
Multiparas	24	30.41e	21.18e	10.27e	0.00	24.80e	0.00	1.69c	0.85

* See footnote, Table 23-2.

residual effect disclosed in the IQ scores at both four and seven years.

Inductions done for the various disorders heretofore recognized to be associated with fetal hazard were, of course, confirmed to yield poor results. Inductions for pregnancy-induced hypertension, for example, showed adverse effects over the range of outcome variables that were studied. These effects were undoubtedly related directly to the impact of the pre-eclamptic condition with added impact from prematurity as well. Whether or not labor induction had a further additive (or beneficial) effect could not be ascertained from these data, however.

The same invidious influence was seen for children delivered after inductions for pyelonephritis, except for somewhat less of a residual late effect (significant only in the four-year IQ data for multiparas). Interestingly, inductions for Rh isoimmunization, while yielding poor early outcomes, failed to demonstrate any adverse long-range persistent effect; in fact, there appeared to have been somewhat of a protective action among surviving infants by age seven years (statistically significant in offspring of multiparas).

Although the numbers of inductions for amnionitis were small, the high perinatal death and neonatal depression rates were impressive and contrasted sharply with the relatively good results for survivors. Labor inductions done for abruptio placentae, also few in number, took a particularly great toll in stillbirths and neonatal deaths, as expected, along with significantly poor outcomes at age four years (but inexplicably, not at seven years).

Reaction to Induction Agent

Reactions following upon the administration of uterotonic agents were studied to assess their possible impact on the fetus and infant. Cases in which such agents had been given were stratified according to whether or not there was evidence of persistently increased basal uterine tonus, tetanic uterine contraction, or tumultuous contractile pattern, on the one hand, or no documentable uterine response to the drugs, on the other. Fetal heart rate changes, especially as regards marked irregularity and/or bradycardia, were also surveyed separately, recognizing that the data were collected before current electronic fetal heart rate monitoring capabilities were available. Those given oxytocin, but who had no such reaction, served as controls. Their outcome results represented referent rates for comparison purposes.

Persistent hypertonus (Table 23-24) was associated with markedly increased rates of perinatal mortality and neonatal depression. In multiparas, this effect continued among surviving infants throughout the seven-year follow-up period. Tetanic contractions in nulliparas yielded an increased stillbirth rate and some residual late effects. In multiparas, however, they were associated with consistently poor outcomes across the range of the study without exception. A similar deleterious effect was seen with tumultuous labor. Infants of nulliparas (who were rather few in number) fared considerably worse than those of multiparas in the perinatal period and at three years, but the adverse four- and seven-year results were about the same in both parity groups.

Although there was a suggestion that the perinatal results for cases with no uterine response were adverse, none of the rate ratios achieved statistical significance; nonetheless, late results were especially bad in both nulliparas and multiparas (with the unanticipated exception of the four-year IQ score data). Abnormal fetal heart rate variations following oxytocin resulted in rather few stillbirths; indeed, there was apparent protection in this regard among multiparas. However, the frequencies of neonatal death and depression were clearly enhanced and this bad effect re-emerged at eight months and three and seven years of age.

Table 23-24
Outcome by Reaction to Uterotonic Stimulation*

Reaction	No.	SB	NND	APG5	MENT8	MOT8	SLH3	IQ4	IQ7
None									
Nulliparas	2,144	1.00(2.30)	1.00(1.12)	1.00(2.83)	1.00(0.23)	1.00(0.28)	1.00(0.79)	1.00(2.19)	1.00(1.84)
Multiparas	3,032	1.00(3.13)	1.00(2.51)	1.00(3.76)	1.00(0.91)	1.00(0.97)	1.00(0.74)	1.00(2.08)	1.00(1.22)
Persistent hypertonus									
Nulliparas	44	4.94d	0.00	3.82c	0.00	0.00	0.00	1.13	1.07
Multiparas	49	3.26c	2.54a	1.77	6.49c	6.08c	15.10d	1.15	1.66
Sustained uterine contraction(s)									
Nulliparas	59	2.21a	0.00	0.63	0.00	0.00	0.00	1.47	1.60a
Multiparas	83	1.54	1.46	2.33b	1.75a	3.23b	24.70e	1.70a	1.88a
Tumultuous labor									
Nulliparas	17	5.12c	10.51e	6.63d	0.00	0.00	14.05e	1.64	2.81a
Multiparas	166	0.96	0.49	1.23	0.85	1.63a	0.00	1.80a	2.17b
No uterine response									
Nulliparas	136	1.60	0.00	1.44	3.71a	3.00a	17.56e	0.57e	2.16e
Multiparas	301	0.75	1.19	1.04	1.41	1.34	6.57d	0.91	1.96e
Significant variation in fetal heart rate									
Nulliparas	107	0.81	1.67	3.43e	4.82a	0.00	5.75a	0.94	1.89c
Multiparas	162	0.21a	1.97a	2.86e	1.76	1.69	12.35e	0.96	1.35

* See footnote, Table 23-2.

Membrane Status

Data on the status of the membranes with particular reference to spontaneous rupture versus surgical amniotomy were available for investigation as well. The latter group was further divisible according to intent—that is, whether done for labor induction or stimulation (or inadvertently as recorded in response to formal inquiry at the time). Outcome data for those in whom rupture occurred spontaneously were utilized for purposes of developing referent values (Table 23-25).

Cases in which the membranes remained intact throughout the course of labor (with spontaneous or artificial rupture at the time of delivery) were found to be associated with significantly higher neonatal death rates than expected in nulliparas, an adverse effect that continued through age seven years. The impact was not so clearly defined in multiparas, although the isolated three-year communication and four-year intelligence testing results were poor among their offspring.

Surgical amniotomy for induction purposes yielded impressively increased stillbirth rates in both nulliparas and multiparas plus elevated neonatal death rates in nulliparas. However, there was no lasting effect in either parity group. There were actually suggestions of a protective effect seen in these data. This paralleled the apparently beneficial impact of induction with oxytocin which we had encountered earlier (see Table 23-21) and which we had conjectured might be attributable to case selection.

Amniotomy for labor enhancement was unassociated with any adverse effects at all. Quite the contrary, protective effects were pervasive throughout, once again raising the question of preferential utilization of this practice in otherwise uncomplicated cases. The absence of a comparable beneficial effect from unintentional amniotomy supported this view. That significantly adverse results were actually found for several of the outcome variables, ranging from stillbirth to seven-year results, adds still more weight to the argument.

Duration of Membrane Rupture

Examination of outcome results by duration of membrane rupture (Table 23-26) showed increasingly bad neonatal results with increasingly prolonged durations. Duration prior to delivery was incrementally stratified, shown here for three-hourly intervals. Within each subgroup of cases thus formed, outcome data were derived for comparison with the overall rate and the rate in the appropriate referent group (designated here as those with membranes ruptured less than six hours at the time of delivery). Consistently low death rates were encountered among offspring of gravidas with membranes ruptured less than 24 hours (with the single exception of those in the nine- to 11-hour group). The neonatal death rate averaged 1.44% under 24 hours (FTD -3.357, p = .00017). The rate doubled in the next 18-hour increment to a mean of 2.87% (FTD 1.763, p = .039) and almost doubled again beyond 42 hours to 4.78% (FTD 4.122, p = 1.9×10^{-5}). Rather impressively good outcomes were seen in cases with short durations under six hours in length. Long-term results were far more inconsistent.

While these trends suggest that rupture of the membranes for more than 24 hours is harmful, one must be cautioned to recognize that this analysis has not as yet taken into account the factor of prematurity. Correcting for the confounding effect of premature labor and delivery, so commonly associated with prolonged premature rupture of the membranes, may markedly affect these results. Nonetheless, it was clear that prolonged duration of membrane rupture was a factor to be dealt with in these analyses either as a risk factor itself or perhaps as a marker of infant risk.

These and other comparable data have thus been developed to help us assess the possible fetal and infant effects of the extensive array of delivery-related factors available for investigation. We recognized

313

Table 23-25
Outcome by Amniotomy*

Status of Membranes	No.	SB	NND	APG5	MENT8	MOT8	SLH3	IQ4	IQ7
Spontaneous rupture									
Nulliparas	6,358	1.00(1.59)	1.00(1.31)	1.00(3.24)	1.00(0.44)	1.00(1.21)	1.00(5.11)	1.00(2.11)	1.00(2.15)
Multiparas	13,703	1.00(1.53)	1.00(1.99)	1.00(2.96)	1.00(0.54)	1.00(1.24)	1.00(5.29)	1.00(2.24)	1.00(2.12)
Intact until delivery									
Nulliparas	1,228	0.88	2.05d	1.23	2.21a	1.73a	2.53c	1.85a	2.08a
Multiparas	6,083	0.95	1.20	0.90	0.96	1.16	1.58b	1.34a	1.12
Amniotomy for induction									
Nulliparas	183	3.44e	1.73a	0.90	0.00	0.00	0.00	1.06	0.90a
Multiparas	416	2.52d	0.74	0.43a	0.00a	0.50	0.00	0.89c	1.08
Amniotomy for augmentation									
Nulliparas	3,366	0.80	0.48c	0.79	0.75	0.85	1.35	1.09	0.98
Multiparas	4,261	0.74a	0.52e	0.65d	0.63a	0.71	0.93	0.62a	0.89b
Unintentional amniotomy									
Nulliparas	259	1.70	1.49	1.65	1.10	0.87	2.30a	1.08	1.30c
Multiparas	457	2.44d	1.22	1.58a	0.78	0.26a	1.50	1.67a	2.35c

* See footnote, Table 23-2.

Table 23-26
Neonatal Death and Duration of Ruptured Membranes Prior to Delivery

Duration, hr.	Cases No.	Neonatal Death No.	Neonatal Death %	Freeman-Tukey Deviate	Freeman-Tukey p	Rate Ratio RR	Rate Ratio p
< 6	8,135	111	1.36	-3.518	0.00022	1.00*	
6–8	1,348	19	1.41	-1.239		1.04	
9–11	798	18	2.27	0.851		1.67	0.040
12–14	541	8	1.48	0.598		1.09	
15–17	391	2	0.51	-2.342	0.0096	0.38	
18–20	265	6	2.26	0.540		1.66	
21–23	189	4	2.12	0.353		1.56	
24–26	228	8	3.51	1.588		2.58	0.0068
27–29	139	4	2.88	0.867		2.12	
30–32	97	2	2.06	0.278		1.52	
33–35	85	3	3.53	1.024		2.60	
36–41	149	3	2.01	0.254		1.48	
42–47	89	4	4.49	1.474		3.30	0.012
48–71	234	4	1.71	-0.057		1.26	
72–95	109	6	5.50	2.075		4.20	0.00027
96–119	58	3	5.17	1.426		3.80	0.014
120+	138	13	9.42	3.989	3.3×10^{-5}	6.93	2.3×10^{-9}

* Referent

that we were viewing each of them essentially in isolation with little, if any, consideration for other important and perhaps closely related variables. Some of those relevant relationships have been addressed directly or hinted at indirectly in the foregoing material. It was clear that simultaneous consideration of many of these concurrently acting factors (and all of them, if feasible) would have to be pursued before we could obtain meaningful information about their true relative impact on offspring. The tabular analyses completed to this point have nonetheless been valuable in placing us in a favorable position to embark on such multivariate studies.

CHAPTER **24**

Delivery Factors: Designation of Risk Variables

Summary

All 1980 delivery-related variables were studied in sequence by bivariate cluster and logistic regression methods to determine which among them had significant adverse impact on the fetus and infant and to help quantitate the risk to which they exposed the offspring. The designated study population was limited to those 15,169 women who delivered infants without serious congenital anomalies and weighing 2500–4000 g. Outcomes were collapsed into a small number of manageable groups. In all, only 47 of the original spectrum of variables were found to maintain a statistically verifiable effect when all were weighed concurrently.

Numerous factors pertaining to the delivery process have been listed and explored in chapters 22 and 23. Having examined them in some detail, we were now in a position to quantitate their impact more precisely using the paradigm that proved so effective for variables identified for labor progression (chapter 14), adjunctive agents (chapter 18), and intrinsic maternal, fetal, and pelvic factors (chapter 21).

The variables to be assessed were designated in detail. The population of offspring to be investigated was carefully restricted so as to avoid confounding by the major effects of birth weight and congenital anomalies, limiting further study at this point to those weighing 2500-4000 g at birth and free of definable malformations obviously unrelated to the labor and delivery process.

Outcome results were analyzed by the nonparametric bivariate Freeman-Tukey screening techniques to flag those variables most likely to have some impact on the fetus and infant. Cluster techniques were then applied to find redundant variables, thereby reducing the number to be evaluated collectively by the multivariate approach. Linear regression analyses followed to identify those factors that placed the infant at greatest risk and to quantitate the degree of risk when that risk was considered in conjunction with that of all other flagged risk factors at the same time.

The 287 groups of delivery-related variables, broadly categorized in Table 24-1, included 1980 coded items of possible relevance. The size of the task exceeded that for all other study variables combined. All were screened preliminarily by bivariate testing. Table 24-1 lists the codes and definitions of the 224 principal items of interest. They represent those occurring in suitable numbers or determined to be strongly deleterious or beneficial to offspring. The index population in which they were studied included 6688 nulliparas and 8481 multiparas, constituted as previously described (see chapter 14).

Screening Analysis

The Freeman-Tukey analysis of the entire range of delivery variables yielded the information summarized in Tables 24-2 and 24-3 for nulliparas and multiparas separately. Items not listed included those appearing in negligible numbers or deviating minimally from the mean outcome for the index population under study—that is, those with RR at or about 1.00.

It was apparent, for example, that infants who were delivered by an obstetrician (OBTYPE1) did considerably better than those delivered by residents or interns

in training (OBTYPE2-3). It was equally clear, however, that the patients' hospital and perhaps her socioeconomic status were reflected in the attendant at delivery. Moreover, the complexity of the case in regard to complications may also have influenced the choice of attendant. This may have accounted for the much better results for medical student deliveries (OBTYPE4) than for those involving residents. The paradoxical data for intern deliveries is noted for interest. It is difficult to rationalize why the good perinatal results were reversed in later childhood.

Induction of labor (ONSET2), as noted previously (see chapter 18), was associated with poorer outcomes than labors beginning spontaneously (ONSET1), but this may be related more to the indication for the induction than to the induction technique or procedure itself. The latter contention was confirmed by the data, presented below, showing elective induction to be essentially free of adverse consequences overall in this study population. This is not meant to imply that induction is necessarily always innocuous, of course, but rather that its bad effects can probably be minimized if it is conducted optimally.

Further, the data suggested that the harmful effects of some of the conditions militating for the induction were worse by far than those of the induction process itself. Unfortunately, this study was not designed to assess the merits or pitfalls of the specific circumstances prevailing at the time such inductions were undertaken. It is not possible, therefore, to determine the effects of attempting induction under suboptimal conditions, for example, although the data presented earlier (chapter 23) showing the impact of multiple induction attempts did indirectly address the issue somewhat.

Fetal presentation and position at delivery were studied in detail. Despite the tight birth weight constraints invoked here, infants in both breech and face presentations (PRES5-8 and PRES10) had particularly bad perinatal outcomes. Long-term

Table 24-1
Delivery Variables Defined

Variable Code	Definition
OBTYPE1-6	Status of attendant: 1 Obstetrician; 2 resident; 3 intern; 4 medical student; 5 generalist; 6 nurse or nurse-midwife
ONSET1-2	Onset of labor: 1 Spontaneous; 2 induced
PRES1-12	Fetal presentation: 1-4 Vertex; 5-8 breech; 9 transverse; 10 face; 11 brow; 12 compound (see Table 22-11)
ROM1-11	Duration ruptured membranes: 1 <1 hr.; 2 1-2 hr.; 3 3-4 hr.; 4 4-5 hr.; 5 6-8 hr.; 6 9-12 hr.; 7 13-18 hr.; 8 19-24 hr.; 9 25-30 hr.; 10 31-36 hr.; 11 >36 hr.
CONTROL1-3	Delivery of fetal head: 1 Manual control; 2 uncontrolled; 3 instrumental
FUNDAL0-3	Kristeller fundal pressure: 0 None; 1 slight; 2 moderate; 3 strong; 4 failed
MANROT1-2	Manual rotation: 1 Successful; 2 failed
AMNIO1-3	Indication for amniotomy: 1 induction; 2 augmentation; 3 other
INDUCT1-9	Indication for induction: 1-9 See Table 22-15
AUGMENT1-18	Indication for augmentation: 1-18 See Table 22-15
FORCEPS0-4	Forceps: 0 Not used; 1 Class I (+4); 2 Class II (+3); 3 Class III (+2); 4 Class IV (+1, 0)
FORAPP1-4	Forceps application: 1 Average difficulty; 2 difficult; 3 very difficult; 4 failed
FORTRAC1-4	Forceps traction: 1-4 Same as FORAPP1-4
FORROT1-4	Forceps rotation: 1-4 Same as FORAPP1-4
FORCONV1-4	Forceps conversion: 1-4 Same as FORAPP1-4
FORIND1-16	Forceps indication: 1-16 See Table 22-15
FORTYPE1-15	Forceps type: 1-15 See Table 22-4
FORAXIS1-4	Axis traction forceps: 1-4 Same as FORAPP1-4
FORFREQ0-8	Frequency of forceps attempts: 0-8 See Table 22-5
VACEXT0-4	Vacuum extractor: 0-4 Same as FORCEPS0-4
VACTRAC1-4	Vacuum traction: 1-4 Same as FORAPP1-4
BREECH1-4	Breech attitude: 1 Frank; 2 full or complete; 3 single footling; 4 double footling
BRVERS0-4	Version of breech: 0 Not done; 1-4 Same as FORAPP1-4
BRCOMP0-2	Breech complication: 0 None; 1 nuchal arm; 2 hyperextended head

318

BRDELIV0-3	Breech delivery procedure: 0 Spontaneous; 1 decomposition; 2 assisted; 3 extraction
BRFACH0-4	Forceps to aftercoming head: 0 not used; 1-4 Same as FORAPP1-4
CSINDIC1-12	Cesarean section indication: 1-23 See Table 22-15
CSINCIS1-4	Cesarean incision: 1 low transverse; 2 low vertical; 3 classical; 4 extraperitoneal
CSVAG	Cesarean after attempted vaginal delivery
CSHEAD1-2	Delivery of head at cesarean: 1 Manual; 2 forceps
REACT0-5	Reaction to oxytocin: 0 None; 1 no response; 2 sustained contraction; 3 increased tone; 4 fetal heart alteration; 5 tumultuous labor
PROLAP	Cord prolapse
PREVIA	Placenta previa
ABRUPT	Abruptio placentae
SHOULD	Shoulder dystocia
NUCHAL	Nuchal cord
DIL0-10	Prelabor cervical dilatation: 0-10 cm.
STA1-7	Prelabor fetal station: 1-4, -1 to -4; 5, zero; 6, +1; 7, +2 to +4

adverse outcome was especially apparent for breech presentations in nulliparas, but not in multiparas. The results for brow presentation and transverse lie were equally poor, but the numbers of cases were too small to permit meaningful statistical analysis.

Of special interest among vertex presentations were the consistently adverse perinatal effects of occiput transverse and occiput posterior positions (PRES2 and PRES3). In relative terms, occiput transverse had a worse impact than occiput posterior, but neither effect appeared to persist into later life. Of relevance in regard to these malpositions was the influence of the delivery procedure. As will be seen, manual rotation (MANROT1) enhances the negative aspects of the fetal position somewhat (in nulliparas, but not in multiparas), and difficult forceps rotations (FORROT2-3) augment it even more (in both nulliparas and multiparas).

The effect of duration of ruptured membranes was studied in various ways. Considerable effort was expended to calculate the precise duration from rupture of the membranes to onset of labor and to delivery, and then to group patients according to incremental divisions of time. The outcome data for the various subgroups proved quite comparable within the limited index study populations. No definite differences were detectable except as noted for multiparas with membranes ruptured just prior to or at delivery (ROM1). It is doubtful that this reflected the effect of the short duration of membrane rupture or of maintaining the membranes intact; more likely, the confounding influence of the precipitate labor which was so frequently associated was mirrored in these results. The adverse effect of excessively rapid labors has been shown earlier (see chapter 14).

Kristeller pressure was associated with significantly adverse effects if applied more

Table 24-2
Outcome by Delivery Variables in Nulliparas

Variable		Perinatal				Infancy				Childhood			
		Definite		Suspect		Definite		Suspect		Definite		Suspect	
		RR	p	RR	p	RR	p	RR	p	RR	p	RR	p
OBTYPE1	Obstetrician	0.88		0.43	0.0047	0.49		0.92		0.25	$<10^{-6}$	0.41	$<10^{-6}$
OBTYPE2	Resident	1.23	0.10	1.08		1.03		0.93		1.09		0.97	
OBTYPE3	Intern	0.69	0.070	0.92		1.00		0.84		1.54	0.000054	1.28	$<10^{-6}$
OBTYPE4	Student	0.88		0.94		1.61		1.13	0.040	0.88		1.22	0.0028
ONSET1	Spontaneous labor	0.98		0.99		0.95	0.10	1.00		0.99		1.00	
ONSET2	Induced	1.29		1.17		1.72	0.037	0.87		1.23		0.98	
PRES1	Occiput anterior	0.78	0.017	0.80	0.00024	0.96		0.99		0.99		1.00	
PRES2	Occiput transverse	1.90	0.0018	1.43	0.014	1.20		0.98		0.93		1.12	0.10
PRES3	Occiput posterior	1.76	0.0065	1.62	0.00020	1.05		0.84		0.88		0.90	
PRES1-4	All vertex	0.98		0.95		1.00		1.00		0.99		1.01	
PRES5-8	All breech	2.42	0.065	2.89	0.000018	1.42		1.47		1.77	0.096	1.01	
PRES10	Face	3.79	0.10	3.77	0.011	3.20		1.00	0.10	1.00		1.30	
ROM1	Membranes ruptured <1 hr.	0.97		1.15	0.087	0.95		1.15	0.014	1.02		1.04	
FUNDAL0	No fundal pressure	0.64	0.0026	0.71		0.83		0.90	0.042	0.84		0.98	
FUNDAL1	Light	1.25		1.08	0.000042	1.22		1.08		1.27	0.036	0.97	
FUNDAL2	Moderate	2.05	0.0016	1.45	0.024	2.06	0.0027	0.79		1.62	0.0029	1.15	0.080
FUNDAL3	Strong	3.19	0.00066	2.55	0.00011	1.01		0.55		1.88	0.044	1.18	
MANROT1	Rotation	1.78	0.093	1.71	0.010	1.97	0.063	1.31		1.13		0.67	0.0044
AMNIO1	Induction	1.13		1.27		1.92		1.15		1.00		1.13	
AMNIO2	Augmentation	0.98		0.91		0.63	0.0064	0.93		0.94		1.02	
INDUCT1	Elective induction	0.96		0.95		1.00		0.93		1.00		1.01	
INDUCT2	Ruptured membranes	0.36		1.31		1.49		0.79		0.51		0.92	
INDUCT3	Preeclampsia	4.17	0.00044	1.63	0.000011	1.92		0.54		1.77		0.84	
INDUCT4	Diabetes	2.00		5.44		6.39	0.023	1.70		2.26		0.54	
INDUCT6-9	Other	4.17	0.0065	1.13		3.41	0.067	0.64		1.62		1.08	
AUGMENT1	Elective	1.17		0.79		0.85		0.90		1.27		1.23	0.015
AUGMENT2	Ruptured membranes	1.01		1.60	0.014	1.49		0.82		0.93		0.97	
AUGMENT3	Preeclampsia	1.87		1.40		2.25		0.70		1.66		0.99	
AUGMENT10	Arrested labor	2.10	0.0021	2.04	1.2×10^{-6}	0.86		0.87		1.06		0.81	0.052
AUGMENT11-18	Other	2.19	0.10	1.25		1.42	0.073	0.98		1.07		0.94	
FORCEPS0	Forceps not used	0.63	0.10	0.78	0.018	0.70		1.02		0.99		1.07	
FORCEPS1	Class I	0.72	0.075	0.78	0.017	0.91		1.03		1.04		1.05	
FORCEPS2	Class II	1.16	0.049	1.31	0.012	1.13		0.87		1.16		0.96	
FORAPP1	Application average	0.57	0.00046	0.70	0.000057	0.82		0.93		0.93		1.04	

320

Code	Description												
FORAPP2	Difficult	2.00	0.017	1.56	0.027	1.05		0.88		1.45	0.061	0.78	0.041
FORAPP3	Very difficult	3.91	0.00027	1.98	0.043	2.09		0.64		2.12	0.038	1.30	
FORTRAC1	Traction average	0.65	0.00071	0.78	0.00051	0.81		1.03		1.01		1.04	
FORTRAC2	Difficult	1.32	0.037	1.49	0.0084	1.28	0.096	0.72	0.044	1.15		1.01	
FORTRAC3	Very difficult	2.63	0.0071	1.94	0.0094	2.37	0.040	0.66		1.53		0.87	
FORROT1	Rotation average	1.19	0.048	1.16		1.06	0.027	1.09		1.12		1.00	
FORROT2	Difficult	1.42	0.031	1.73	0.0028	1.61	0.017	1.07		0.81		1.07	
FORROT3	Very difficult	2.60	0.015	4.08	1.2x10-6	1.07		2.04	0.059	4.71	0.040	0.97	
BREECH1	Frank breech	0.70		1.30		1.01		1.57		3.77	0.026	0.72	
BREECH2	Full	8.33	0.010	5.43	0.0054	1.00		1.23		1.41		1.01	
BREECH3	Single footling	3.63	0.048	2.61	0.039	1.12		2.49	0.0047	1.54		1.06	
BREECH4	Double footling	2.10		2.04		1.60		1.05		2.83		1.08	
BRDELIV0	Spontaneous breech	0.93		1.96	0.014	1.10		0.78		0.68		0.63	0.029
BRDELIV2	Assisted	0.90		2.20	0.028	1.00		2.05	0.0061	1.07		0.59	0.027
BRDELIV3	Extracted	2.91	0.049	1.81	0.064	1.32		1.63		1.25		0.90	
BRFACH0	Manual	3.09	0.089	1.74		1.01		2.94	0.00056	1.62		1.08	
BRFACH1	Forceps average	1.46	0.085	2.07	0.030	0.87		1.50		0.98		0.59	
BRFACH2	Difficult	2.00		2.72	0.082	1.80		1.47		1.62		0.72	
BRFACH1-3	All aftercoming forceps	1.63	0.060	2.14	0.011	0.91		1.49		0.99		0.64	0.024
CSVAG	Failed vaginal delivery	8.33	0.00028	3.26	0.068	4.26	0.031	1.47		2.00		1.08	
REACT2	Tetany	8.77	<10-6	2.02		1.16		0.98		1.88		1.72	
REACT3	Hypertonus	4.44	0.00022	2.61	0.0036	1.01		0.64		0.97		0.87	
SHOULD	Shoulder dystocia	1.35		2.33	0.044	1.47		0.83		2.82	0.023	1.80	0.068
PROLAP	Cord prolapse	1.90	0.048	1.45		2.32	0.042	1.02		1.49		0.97	
ABRUPT	Abruptio placentae	2.45	0.014	1.54		0.91		0.80		0.60		0.85	
DIL0	Prelabor dilatation <1 cm.	1.67	0.013	1.68	0.011	0.72		1.01		1.23		1.15	
DIL1-3	1-3 cm.	0.70	0.014	0.93		0.77	0.033	0.97		1.03		0.92	
DIL4-10	4+ cm.	0.80		0.47	0.10	1.05		0.58	0.072	0.27	0.028	0.83	
STA7	Station +2 to +4	0.67		0.56		0.48		0.90		0.87		0.84	
STA6	+1	0.79		0.67	0.067	0.75		1.07		0.84		0.89	
STA5	0	0.82		0.70	0.0056	1.01		0.88		0.96		0.97	
STA1	-1	1.52	0.092	1.44	0.071	0.57		0.93		0.98		1.03	
STA2	-2	1.96	0.037	1.39		1.25		1.03		1.36		1.08	

Table 24-3
Outcome by Delivery Variables in Multiparas

	Perinatal				Infancy				Childhood			
Variable	Definite RR	p	Suspect RR	p	Definite RR	p	Suspect RR	p	Definite RR	p	Suspect RR	p
OBTYPE1 Obstetrician	0.45	0.061	0.69		0.36	0.0043	0.74	0.0052	0.25	$<10^{-6}$	0.38	$<10^{-6}$
OBTYPE2 Resident	1.24		1.00		0.73	0.051	0.85	0.0092	1.06		1.05	
OBTYPE3 Intern	0.70	0.080	0.94		0.70	0.035	0.94		1.39	0.0060	1.26	$<10^{-6}$
OBTYPE4 Student	0.37	0.0034	0.75		0.97		1.03		0.89		1.15	0.0011
ONSET1 Spontaneous labor	0.93		0.97		0.98		0.98		1.00		1.00	
ONSET2 Induced	1.68	0.0095	1.26		1.25	0.081	1.16		1.04		0.97	
PRES1 Occiput anterior	0.70	0.00039	0.82	0.0048	0.98		0.98		0.98		1.00	
PRES2 Occiput transverse	2.34	4.1×10^{-6}	1.42	0.062	0.91		1.05		1.11		1.03	
PRES3 Occiput posterior	1.34		1.49	0.013	1.02		1.01		0.84		0.97	
PRES1-4 All vertex	0.90		0.94		0.98		0.99		0.98		1.01	
PRES5-8 All breech	7.39	$<10^{-6}$	4.13	1.4×10^{-6}	1.86	0.10	1.43		0.94		0.63	0.048
PRES10 Face	3.55	0.053	1.12		2.58		1.32		1.13		1.11	
ROM1 Membranes ruptured <1 hr.	1.29	0.043	1.39	0.0034	1.41	0.00077	1.14	0.0056	1.13		0.99	
FUNDAL0 No fundal pressure	0.55	0.000084	0.66	0.00013	0.64	0.00014	0.90	0.0081	0.75	0.0043	0.96	0.00012
FUNDAL1 Light	0.61		0.78		0.90		0.82		1.36	0.016	1.30	
FUNDAL2 Moderate	0.84		1.09		0.60	0.069	0.87		1.16		1.06	
FUNDAL3 Strong	2.96	0.0023	2.03	0.038	0.99		0.99		0.85		0.99	
MANROT1 Manual rotation	0.90		0.87	0.029	1.68	0.10	1.32		1.00		1.00	
AMNIO1 Induction	2.10	0.0043	0.83	0.071	1.02		1.01		1.63	0.027	0.98	
AMNIO2 Augmentation	0.97		0.82		0.60		0.95		0.81		0.97	
INDUCT1 Elective induction	0.98		1.11		0.80		1.04		0.60		0.87	
INDUCT2 Ruptured membranes	1.15		1.36		0.71		1.12		1.30		1.06	
INDUCT3 Preeclampsia	2.96	0.046	0.63		1.37		1.84	0.052	1.70		1.11	
INDUCT4 Diabetes	4.75	0.0026	1.99		1.02		1.47		1.00		1.11	
INDUCT5 Rh disease	6.33	0.00021	2.68						1.13		0.83	
INDUCT6-9 Other indication	0.73	0.0064	0.88		0.73	0.00054	0.90		0.90		1.01	
AUGMENT1 Elective augmentation	0.55	0.067	0.91		0.73	0.021	0.70		1.02		1.00	
AUGMENT2 Ruptured membranes	1.95	0.040	1.05		1.33		0.80		1.47		1.02	
AUGMENT3 Preeclampsia	4.67	0.00060	1.04		1.00		1.01		1.13		0.63	
AUGMENT10 Arrested labor	3.75	2.6×10^{-6}	1.89	0.049	0.64	0.076	0.66		1.24		0.97	
AUGMENT11-18 Other indication	4.70	5.1×10^{-6}	2.09	0.084	0.87		1.02		0.97		0.78	
FORCEPS0 Forceps not used	0.59	0.068	0.91		0.58		0.96		1.02		0.93	
FORCEPS1 Class I	0.99		1.01		0.63	0.025	0.91	0.037	0.70	0.054	0.91	
FORCEPS2 Class II	1.15		1.23		0.77	0.052	0.83	0.053	1.11		0.77	0.00023
FORAPP1 Application average	0.48	0.0028	0.73	0.048	0.46	0.00017	0.88		0.70	0.0070	0.80	0.0044

FORAPP2	Difficult	1.88		1.84		0.67		0.32	0.0068	0.70		0.70	0.092
FORAPP3	Very difficult	3.55	0.053	4.79	0.000079	1.04		0.69		1.15		0.85	
FORTRAC1	Traction average	0.71	0.043	0.97		0.64	0.0017	0.91	0.054	0.81	0.044	0.88	0.00079
FORTRAC2	Difficult	1.69		1.60		0.70		0.83		1.15		0.67	0.026
FORTRAC3	Very difficult	7.39	0.000038	5.65	0.000067	1.04		0.91		1.26		0.82	0.063
FORROT1	Rotation average	1.26		1.26		0.85		0.79		1.03		1.03	
FORROT2	Difficult	3.27		3.45		1.62		1.34		1.57		0.64	0.071
BREECH1	Frank breech	4.25	0.00079	3.53	1.4x10-6	1.00		1.32		0.88		0.51	0.0079
BREECH2	Full	3.69	0.000025	2.23	0.000014	1.37		1.12		1.94		0.67	
BREECH3	Single footling	5.54	0.042	8.94	0.061					1.00		0.95	
BREECH4	Double footling	2.00	0.0058	6.71	0.0014	7.30	0.00074	1.02		6.79	0.00067	2.21	
BRDELIV0	Spontaneous breech	0.94		1.26		0.98		0.69	0.091	1.47		1.08	
BREDELIV2	Assisted	1.93	0.024	4.13	<10-6	1.11	0.025	0.99	0.041	1.03		0.82	
BREDELIV3	Extracted	10.70	<10-6	5.75	1.1x10-6	3.29		1.83		1.36		0.70	
BRFACH0	Manual	1.08		1.34		1.01		0.73		1.43		1.14	
BRFACH1	Forceps average	3.59	0.017	5.11	<10-6	1.37		0.38		0.90		0.70	
BRFACH1-3	All aftercoming forceps	5.16	0.000035	5.59	<10-6	1.19		0.98		0.85		0.66	
CSVAG	Failed vaginal delivery	29.55	<10-6	2.00	<10-6	1.60		2.96	0.034	1.34		1.10	
REACT2	Tetany	2.00		2.98		1.16		0.93		2.04		0.92	
REACT3	Hypertonus	1.20		1.02		1.26		0.96		0.97		0.74	
SHOULD	Shoulder dystocia	10.70	<10-6	4.13	0.0017	1.82		4.40		1.01		0.86	
PROLAP	Cord prolapse	5.54	<10-6	3.35	0.00021	0.89		0.92		1.17		0.84	0.056
ABRUPT	Abruptio placentae	4.00	<10-6	3.19	1.2x10-6	0.95		0.94		0.64	0.084	0.67	0.0081
DIL0	Prelabor dilatation <1 cm.	1.22		1.02		1.46	0.10	1.34	0.0046	1.17		1.13	
DIL1-3	1-3 cm.	0.73		0.82		0.59	0.019	0.91		0.81		0.99	
DIL4-10	4+ cm.	0.49	0.053	0.79		0.47	0.012	0.78	0.013	0.77		1.03	
STA6	Station +1	0.60		1.06		0.68		0.84		0.54	0.093	1.13	
STA5	0	0.51	0.020	0.53	0.0036	0.83		0.82	0.016	0.71	0.043	0.95	
STA1	-1	0.46	0.0050	0.79		0.70		0.92		0.83		0.96	
STA2	-2	0.64		0.83		0.48		0.80		0.82		0.96	
STA3	-3	1.45		0.82		0.62		1.06		0.99		1.06	

than lightly, based on evaluative interpretations by a disinterested trained observer. The impact of both moderate and strong fundal pressure (FUNDAL2-3) appeared to persist into later childhood among offspring of nulliparas, but this was not duplicated in children delivered of multiparas. Assessment of this factor in isolation neglected to take into account other concurrent confounding variables that might have had a similar deleterious effect. Such factors include disordered labor, fetal malposition, cephalopelvic disproportion, or even instrumental delivery, all of which are commonly associated with fundal pressure.

Amniotomy undertaken for the ostensible purpose of augmenting a labor already in progress (AMNIO2) had no documentably consistent adverse or beneficial effect. When done for induction (AMNIO1), by contrast, some bad results were encountered; these achieved statistical significance in multiparas only. This observation again raised the issue of distinguishing the effect of the procedure from the effect of the condition for which the procedure was being done.

Clarification came in the form of the data based on stratification of labor inductions and augmentations by indication. As previously stated, elective induction of labor (INDUCT1) proved generally risk-free (reiterating the caveat pertaining to the need to ensure ideal conditions in order to minimize potential risk). Inductions done for pregnancy-induced hypertension, diabetes mellitus, and Rh isoimmunization (INDUCT3-5), however, were especially troublesome in regard to perinatal outcome; some adverse long-term effect was also seen, but it did not attain statistical significance in this series.

Induction for ruptured membranes (INDUCT2) in multiparas showed some adverse effect as well, but the outcome data did not fall into the statistically significant range. Other indications taken collectively (INDUCT6-9) yielded significantly bad results for nulliparas and contrastingly good results for multiparas; these encom-

passed inductions undertaken primarily for amnionitis, pyelonephritis, and abruptio placentae.

The effect of labor augmentation also varied according to the indication. Elective stimulation of labor (AUGMENT1) proved generally innocuous in multiparas. In nulliparas, there was some adverse effect in both the perinatal period and in childhood; only the latter proved significant. The deleterious perinatal effects of labor augmentation in multiparas was magnified when indicated, regardless of the indication.

Very impressive results were found for cases in which uterotonic stimulation was done for pregnancy-induced hypertension (AUGMENT3) and arrested labor (AUGMENT10) as well as for the composite of all other indications (AUGMENT11-18). Similar results were derived for nulliparas (except for AUGMENT2, augmentation for ruptured membranes), but the magnitude of effect and the degree of significance were much smaller than for multiparas.

Forceps use yielded poorer overall results than nonuse (FORCEPS0). True low forceps (FORCEPS1), as defined in this study, were innocuous. Midforceps falling into class II category (FORCEPS2), consisting of applications with the fetal head just off the pelvic floor and the saggital suture not aligned anteroposteriorly, had clear adverse effects in nulliparas. A similar impact was seen in multiparas, but it did not reach statistical significance. The numbers of class III midforceps (FORCEPS3) were too small for effective analysis, but the deleterious influence was nonetheless magnified. In multiparas, for example, the rate ratio of bad definite perinatal outcome was 14.75 (p = .00029).

Dissection of forceps operations into their component parts revealed interesting relationships. Ignoring the issue of difficulty for a moment, we observed that forceps application (FORAPP1) served as a much better prognostic index for good outcome than traction (FORTRAC1), and both in turn, had less impact on the offspring

324

than rotation (FORROT1), as might be expected.

Adding the dimension of the difficulty of the process was of considerable importance. One should recall that the assessment of difficulty was not made by the obstetrical attendant or in retrospect, but rather by a trained observer and before the infant was actually delivered. For each aspect of the forceps process, the greater the degree of difficulty the worse the outcome, without exception.

In nulliparas, forceps applications considered to be difficult (FORAPP2) doubled the adverse perinatal outcome (RR = 2.00), a significant finding reflecting more than 3.5 times the effect seen with applications of average difficulty (relative to FORAPP1, RR = 0.57). Very difficult forceps applications (FORAPP3) almost doubled the bad effects once again (RR = 3.91). The data for forceps applications in multiparas paralleled these findings with rate ratios of 0.48 for FORAPP1, 1.88 for FORAPP2, and 3.55 for FORAPP3. These reflected sequential increases in adverse effects of 3.9 and 1.9 times, respectively.

The multiplier effect of difficulty was seen with forceps traction as well. It doubled with difficult traction (FORTRAC2 versus FORTRAC1) and doubled again with very difficult traction (FORTRAC3 versus FORTRAC2) in nulliparas, and increased 2.4 and 4.4 times in multiparas.

Although the more difficult forceps rotations (FORROT2-3) were associated with significantly poorer results than those with average difficulty (FORROT1), the multiplier effects were smaller, namely 1.2 and 1.8 times in nulliparas, and 2.6 and 1.4 times in multiparas. This reflected the fact that there was already an adverse effect seen with rotations of average difficulty (relative to those by forceps without rotation, FORAPP1). Given that the denominator (FORROT1) outcome results were increased, the incremental impact related to increasing difficulty of rotation was necessarily small in a comparative sense.

The clear-cut perinatal effects of forceps delivery continued beyond the newborn period, although not homogeneously or with consistent statistical significance. In nulliparas, for example, both difficult and very difficult forceps applications (FORAPP2-3) showed bad long-term results. Difficult and very difficult traction (FORTRAC2-3) showed comparable outcomes, but they were not statistically significant. Very difficult forceps rotations (FORROT3) yielded significantly poor childhood results. Those for difficult rotations (FORROT2) were also bad at a level reaching statistical significance. The data for multiparas demonstrated similar trends, but none so strong as to be statistically verifiable.

Thus, the analysis demonstrated essentially the same or somewhat better results for spontaneous delivery (FORCEPS0) as for true low forceps (FORCEPS1). These data contrasted with much worse outcomes after midforceps (FORCEPS2-3) and after forceps procedures deemed difficult or very difficult by a trained objective observer, whether related to application (FORAPP2-3), rotation (FORROT2-3), or traction (FORTRAC2-3).

Results for breech presentation showed good short-term outcomes for those in frank breech attitude (BREECH1) among nulliparas and corresponding bad results among multiparas. Much greater intergroup consistency (between parity groups, that is) was found for all other breech attitudes, with full or complete (BREECH2) and single footling breech (BREECH3) showing the worst effects.

Spontaneous (BRDELIV0) and assisted breech deliveries (BRDELIV2) were associated with comparable outcome results in nulliparas, but those multiparas delivered by assisted breech maneuvers had babies in much worse condition. Total breech extraction (BRDELIV3) proved to be an especially serious hazard, consistent with clinical experience. Long-term effects were similar, although without statistical significance.

Use of forceps to deliver the aftercoming head (BRFACH1-3) was associated with significantly increased adverse outcome. This was especially marked in multiparas, in whom there was a fivefold overall increment in bad perinatal results relative both to the general index population and to those delivered with manual control of the head (BRFACH0, Mauriceau maneuvers). In nulliparas, by contrast, manual delivery of the aftercoming head was associated with much greater risk than forceps. Increased difficulty in the use of forceps for this purpose (BRFACH2-3) not unexpectedly yielded still poorer results. No long-term persistent effect was demonstrated.

A variety of other variables were studied in detail. Some of those showing significant results are presented in Tables 24-2 and 24-3. Rather impressively bad outcomes were disclosed for infants delivered by cesarean section after a failed attempt to effect vaginal delivery (CSVAG). The highly significant adverse perinatal results in these cases persisted into infancy and early childhood, although they became less significant with time.

Patients who had documented reactions to uterotonic stimulation in labor did badly, especially as a consequence of uterine tetany (REACT2) or hypertonus (REACT3). The effects of prolonged uterine contractions persisted into later life, but those of hypertonus apparently did not. Similar effects were seen with tumultuous labor, but they were not as strong and did not reach statistical significance.

Shoulder dystocia was especially devastating in multiparas. It was much less so in nulliparas, although still showing adverse short- and long-term effects. The impact of shoulder dystocia was unexpected in view of the constricted birthweight limits (2500-4000 g) of the index population for this analysis. These results emphasized not only that shoulder dystocia can occur with infants of average size, but that the condition was just as serious when encountered among them as with macrosomic infants.

Cord prolapse (PROLAP) and premature separation of the placenta (ABRUPT) were both associated with bad perinatal results.

Outcomes were much worse in offspring of multiparas than of nulliparas, suggesting that expeditious delivery by cesarean section, more likely to have been undertaken in nulliparas without further trial of labor, may have helped salvage affected fetuses in these cases. The adverse effects did not persist over the course of the study, however, except for some suggestive, but insignificant, long-term results after a prolapsed cord.

The status of the cervix and that of the fetal station at the onset of labor was felt to be a factor determining the labor process to follow. Therefore, they warranted evaluation as variables that might affect fetal and infant well-being. In both parity groups, patients beginning labor with negligible cervical dilatation (DIL0) had infants with increased perinatal difficulties (significant in nulliparas only). The effect persisted into the late follow-up period, but was no longer statistically significant. Uniformly good overall results were encountered for moderate prelabor dilatation of 1-3 cm (DIL1-3). Still greater dilatation was followed by even better end results over the course of the study, especially in multiparas.

Fetal station at labor onset showed almost no definable relationship to outcome in multiparas. In nulliparas, there were generally good results in cases with the fetal head engaged prior to onset of labor (STAT5-7). Indeed, there appeared to be a trend toward progressively better outcome with lower prelabor stations. Contrariwise, unengaged fetuses (STAT1-4) in nulliparas fared badly in the perinatal period. Those at station -2 showed persistence of effect into later time frames, although the data were no longer statistically significant. Similar findings were duplicated at still higher stations, but the numbers were too small for the analysis to be considered reliable.

Outcome data were also derived by bivariate screening for the entire range of delivery variables incorporating all definite bad results into a single composite variable. Our objective in this regard was to ensure that delivery factors carrying subtle, but continuing adverse or beneficial effects might be identified more readily. Those found to be significant (at p < .05) are listed in Table 24-4, which provides quantitation of the effect of each of the variables in terms of its rate ratio and its degree of statistical significance.

The apparent advantage of being delivered by a staff obstetrician (OBTYPE1) was verified and proved statistically significant in multiparas. However, the previous finding of poor results in the hands of residents was not confirmed. Induction of labor, without regard for indication or method (ONSET2), was again shown to be associated with bad composite outcomes.

Table 24-4
Effects of Delivery Variables on Outcome by Parity*

Variable		Perinatal Outcome		Composite Outcome	
		Nulliparas	Multiparas	Nulliparas	Multiparas
OBTYPE1	Obstetrician				0.51D
OBTYPE2	Resident	1.23B			
OBTYPE4	Student		0.37C		
ONSET2	Induced		1.68B	1.35A	1.29A
PRES1	Occiput anterior	0.78A	0.70E		0.92A
PRES2	Occiput transverse	1.90C	2.34F		
PRES3	Occiput posterior	1.76B			1.37B
PRES5-8	Breech		7.39F		2.34E
PRES11	Brow				4.31D
ROM1	Membranes ruptured <1 hr.		1.29A		1.14A
FUNDAL0	No fundal pressure	0.64C	0.55F	0.80C	0.77F
FUNDAL1	Light			1.44B	
FUNDAL2	Moderate	2.05C		1.62E	
FUNDAL3	Strong	3.19D	2.96C	1.73A	
AMNIO1	Induction	2.10A			
INDUCT1	Elective induction			1.67A	
INDUCT3	Preeclampsia	4.17E	2.96A	2.55D	2.06A
INDUCT4	Diabetes		4.75C		
INDUCT5	Rh disease		6.33E		2.79A
INDUCT6-9	Other indication	4.17B	0.73B	2.71C	
AUGMENT1	Elective augmentation				0.67A
AUGMENT2	Ruptured membranes		1.95A		1.65C
AUGMENT3	Preeclampsia		4.67D		2.18A
AUGMENT10	Arrested labor	2.10C	3.75F		1.61A
AUGMENT11-18	Other		4.70F		1.95A
FORCEPS0	Forceps not used				0.77A
FORCEPS2	Class II	1.16A		1.30C	
FORAPP1	Application average	0.57E	0.48C	0.78D	0.67E
FORAPP2	Difficult	2.00A		1.69C	
FORAPP3	Very difficult	3.91E		2.10B	
FORTRAC1	Traction average	0.65D	0.71A	0.84C	0.78C
FORTRAC2	Difficult	1.32A			
FORTRAC3	Very difficult	2.63B	7.39F	2.03D	
FORROT1	Rotation average	1.19A		1.25A	
FORROT2	Difficult	1.42A	3.27D		
FORROT3	Very difficult	2.60A			
BREECH1	Frank breech		4.25F		1.84A
BREECH2	Full	8.33B	3.69A	3.65A	
BREECH3	Single footling	3.63A	5.52B		3.95B
BRDELIV2	Assisted breech		1.93A		
BRDELIV3	Extracted	2.91A	10.70F		3.73F
BRFACH1	Forceps average		3.59A		1.98B
BRFACH1-3	All aftercoming forceps		5.16F	1.46A	
CSVAG	Failed vaginal delivery	8.33E	29.55F	1.50B	7.91F
REACT2	Tetany	8.77F		2.69A	
REACT3	Hypertonus	4.44E			

Code	Description				
SHOULD	Shoulder dystocia		10.70F		3.23F
PROLAP	Cord prolapse	1.90A	5.54F	2.34B	2.31D
ABRUPT	Abruptio placentae	2.45A	4.00F		
DIL0	Prelabor dilatation <1 cm.	1.67A			
DIL1-3	1-3 cm.	0.70A			0.71C
DIL4-10	4+ cm.				0.69A
STA6	Station +1				0.53A
STA5	0		0.51A		0.74A
STA1	-1		0.46C		0.78A
STA2	-2	1.96A		1.31A	0.74A

* Probability code: A 0.06, B 0.01, C 0.005, D 0.001, E 0.0005, F 0.0001 or less.

Occiput transverse fetal positions (PRES2) yielded damaged babies; this was significant in multiparas only. Occiput posterior positions (PRES3) did the same, but the relationship was not strong enough in regard to this outcome variable to reach statistical significance.

The adverse effect of breech presentation (PRES5-8) was reconfirmed, and it proved especially noteworthy in offspring of multiparas. Fetuses in brow presentation (PRES11), not previously shown to be significantly affected in this study, did very badly, especially in multiparas.

The duration of rupture of the membranes prior to delivery had little impact on outcome, as previously found, although very brief duration (ROM1) appeared to be deleterious in multiparas. This perhaps reflected the effect of short, tumultuous labors instead.

The adverse influence of Kristeller pressure (FUNDAL1-3) was clearly verified again in nulliparas, increased degrees leading to worse outcomes. Amniotomy, whether done for induction or augmentation of labor (AMNIO1-2), failed to show the adverse effect that had been seen earlier.

Elective induction (INDUCT1), which previously appeared entirely innocuous, was shown to yield poor composite outcome in infants delivered of nulliparas. Inductions undertaken for a variety of medical or obstetrical indications were associated with bad outcome in general. This was expected on the basis of the impact of the condition for which the induction was done, such as pregnancy-induced hypertension (INDUCT3) and Rh isoimmunization (INDUCT5). Although inductions for diabetes mellitus (INDUCT4) were similarly affected, the rate ratio was not statistically significant for the composite variable.

Labor augmentation did not appear to be harmful if undertaken electively (AUGMENT1). In fact, it appeared to be significantly beneficial. If done for documentable indication, however, labor stimulation showed consistently adverse effects. These proved significant in multiparas.

The series of relationships between forceps use and outcome, detailed earlier, were reconfirmed more or less completely with the composite variable. Midforceps (FORCEPS2) showed a significantly adverse effect. Average degrees of difficulty in forceps application or traction (FORAPP1 and FORTRAC1) conferred an apparent advantage, whereas more difficult application or traction (FORAPP2-3 and FORTRAC2-3) were decidedly hazardous, as shown in nulliparas. Forceps rotation yielded poor results even when done with average difficulty (FORROT1); the data were significant in nulliparas. Similar trends were seen for the more difficult forceps rotations (FORROT2-3), but they did not reach statistical significance because of the relatively small numbers of cases.

Breech outcomes for the composite variable also paralleled those encountered in the preceding set of bivariate analyses. The results for breech delivery were significantly worse than for the general population. Relative to the optimal frank breech attitude (BREECH1), much greater risk was found for full and footling varieties (BREECH2-3). Delivered by breech extractions (BRDELIV3) fared much worse than either spontaneous or assisted breech deliveries (BRDELIV0 and BRDELIV2). Forceps used to deliver the aftercoming fetal head (BRFACH1-3) had an overall adverse impact, as previously shown.

Failed attempts to effect vaginal delivery (CSVAG) again yielded consistently bad results. Uterine tetany in response to an oxytocic agent (REACT2) was once more shown to be a significantly adverse factor. Shoulder dystocia (SHOULD) and cord prolapse (PROLAP) were also reconfirmed to cause fetal harm, but not abruptio placentae (ABRUPT). The advantage of ample prelabor cervical dilatation (DIL1-3 and DIL4-10) was verified in multiparas. Failure of the fetal head to engage before labor (STA1-2) was again shown to be a potential peril in nulliparas.

The bivariate screening process had thus surveyed all 1980 coded items, concentrating on 224 deemed to be of primary relevance. It had succeeded in identifying 71 variables among nulliparas and 114 among multiparas with documentable statistical significance in regard to adverse or beneficial fetal and infant outcome. The next step was to proceed with cluster analysis for purposes of assessing for possible redundancy prior to undertaking multivariate analysis.

Cluster Analysis

The aggregative hierarchical clustering technique was applied to all delivery variables heretofore identified by bivariate screening as having potential impact on the infant. As previously explained, this was done to ascertain if any of them contained informational content of sufficient similarity to others to permit their deletion. Because factors containing very similar content can be considered redundant, one member of a highly correlated cluster may be chosen to serve as a representative

marker of them all. Economy of scale can thereby be achieved in the complex multivariate analyses to follow.

Several interesting clusters were disclosed by this approach (Figure 24-1). They supported the value of the technique for reducing the number of variables necessary to be retained for later investigation. Equally important, they pointed to some relationships between variables that might prove clinically relevant. In nulliparas, for example, cases delivered by forceps in which traction and/or application proved difficult or very difficult (FORTRAC2-3 and FORAPP2-3) were clustered with shoulder dystocia (SHOULD) insofar as adverse outcome results were concerned. Although none of these variables was correlated strongly enough to shoulder dystocia to warrant assigning it as a marker, the clustering did indicate that there was some interrelationship among them. An association between difficult instrumental delivery and shoulder dystocia is thus demonstrated. It is perhaps mediated by the common factor of cephalopelvic disproportion shared by both.

A strong relation was found between the more difficult forceps procedures (class III, FORCEPS3) and failed forceps traction (FORTRAC4). This subcluster was associated in turn with cesarean section after failed attempt at vaginal delivery (CSVAG) and failed forceps rotation (FORROT4), but with lesser degrees of correlation. These findings were not unexpected. Diabetics whose labors were induced (INDUCT4) were very closely clustered with those whose labors were augmented (AUGMENT4). Inductions and augmentations for pregnancy-induced hypertension (INDUCT3 and AUGMENT3) showed the same pattern, at a lower level of correlation. Such observations reinforced a contention that the effect of the maternal disorder on the offspring far exceeded that of the uterotonic stimulation used to induce or enhance the labor.

In multiparas, a large number of variables representing normal states clustered

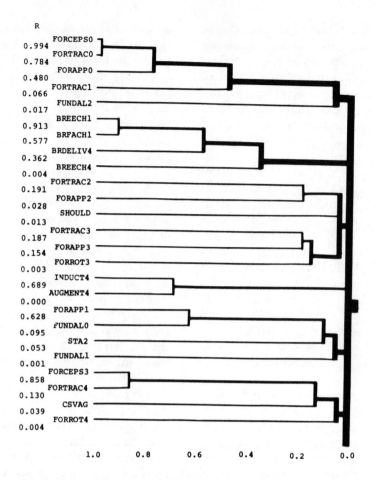

R

0.994	FORCEPS0
0.784	FORTRAC0
0.480	FORAPP0
0.066	FORTRAC1
0.017	FUNDAL2
0.913	BREECH1
0.577	BRFACH1
0.362	BRDELIV4
0.004	BREECH4
0.191	FORTRAC2
0.028	FORAPP2
0.013	SHOULD
0.187	FORTRAC3
0.154	FORAPP3
0.003	FORROT3
0.689	INDUCT4
0.000	AUGMENT4
0.628	FORAPP1
0.095	FUNDAL0
0.053	STA2
0.001	FUNDAL1
0.858	FORCEPS3
0.130	FORTRAC4
0.039	CSVAG
0.004	FORROT4

1.0   0.8   0.6   0.4   0.2   0.0

Figure 24-1. Cluster analysis of delivery variables in nulliparas, showing a portion of the resulting tree. Close correlation is seen between no-forceps-use (FORCEPS0), no-forceps-traction (FORTRAC0), and no-forceps-application (FORAPP0), as would be obvious. This warrants deletion of all but one of these variables because of their similarity of informational content. The same applies for frank breech (BREECH1) and use of forceps to the aftercoming head (BRFACH1, average difficulty), and to mid-forceps (class III, FORCEPS3) and failed forceps traction (FOR-TRAC4) which are also highly correlated. The relation of shoulder dystocia to a number of variables pertaining to difficult forceps operations is suggested (see text).

together. These included all those pertaining to the absence of potential perilous factors, such as the range of medical and obstetrical disorders for which induction was done. In addition, the same type of close clustering seen in nulliparas for induction and augmentation for diabetes and pregnancy-induced hypertension was repeated among multiparas and extended to many of the other stipulated indications as well. Very few of the clusters of delivery variables pertaining to the mode of delivery and the delivery processes, which had been so evident in the cluster analysis for nulliparas, was duplicated here, however.

Cluster analysis thus permitted us to delete eight of the 71 delivery variables in nulliparas and 46 of the 114 in multiparas on the basis of the aforementioned redundancy as reflected in their high degree of similarity of informational content. This reduced the number of variables remaining to be evaluated by the multivariate technique to a workable total of 63 for nulliparas and 68 for multiparas. We were now in a favorable position to proceed with the more sophisticated logistic regression analysis for purposes of determining which was truly significant when the confounding effects of all the others were taken into account at the same time.

Logistic Regression Analysis

The logistic regression modelling technique was applied to those variables identified thus far as warranting further investigation in depth. The technique was the same as has been detailed for the preceding subsets of data variables (see chapters 7 and 14). All delivery variables remaining after bivariate screening and cluster analysis were examined simultaneously. Subsequently, step-up analyses were to be undertaken as well to test the possible

significance of adding those variables not found to be significant back into the core or base model composed of significant variables only.

Composite Outcome Data

The results of the primary logistic regression analysis for the 63 delivery variables in offspring of nulliparas as related to the composite outcome variable (any definitely adverse effect or combination of effects over the entire course of the investigation up to seven years) are shown in Table 24-5. Because of the large number of variables involved here, only those 14 factors yielding p values less than .10 are presented. The relative impact of each of these delivery variables on this index of outcome can be readily seen from the relative risk. The relative risk here refers to the frequency of risk in comparison to the referent frequency for the entire nulliparous population.

Thus, FORCEPS3 (class III forceps delivery from station 0 to +2) had a 12-fold adverse impact on offspring when all the other delivery factors were taken into

Table 24-5
Logistic Regression Analysis of Delivery Variables in
Nulliparas for Composite Outcome*

Variable	Regression Coefficient	Standard Error	t-Statistic	Relative Risk	p-Value
Constant	-2.510	0.514	-4.882		
FORCEPS3	2.491	1.045	2.382	12.07	0.021
FORTRAC2	0.944	0.396	2.384	2.57	0.021
FORTRAC3	1.154	0.631	1.829	3.17	0.073
FORAPP1	-0.397	0.226	-1.757	0.67	0.085
FORROT1	-0.420	0.202	-2.079	0.66	0.043
INDUCT3	0.878	0.456	1.926	2.41	0.059
INDUCT6	1.115	0.464	2.398	3.05	0.020
AUGMENT6	2.132	0.799	2.666	8.43	0.010
BREECH3	1.854	0.999	1.857	6.39	0.069
FUNDAL2	0.403	0.237	1.704	1.50	0.094
FUNDAL3	0.542	0.230	2.360	1.72	0.022
PROLAP	0.909	0.386	2.356	2.48	0.022
ROM11	2.611	1.423	1.835	13.62	0.072
STA1-2	0.277	0.158	1.756	1.32	0.085

* Results listed only for those factors determined to have p-values less than 0.10 among the 63 variables included in the full model based on data from offspring of 6,688 nulliparas.

account simultaneously. The p value indicates this could have occurred by chance only 2.1% of the time. Similarly, FORTRAC2 and FORTRAC3 (difficult and very difficult forceps traction) increased the risk 2.6 and 3.2 times, respectively, although the latter was not statistically significant (p = .073) because of the small number of cases involved.

Contrastingly, FORAPP1 (application of average difficulty) appeared to be somewhat protective (RR = 0.67), but this relationship fell outside the statistically significant range (p = .085). Nonetheless, such protection might have mirrored the effect seen earlier, namely that infants delivered by forceps seemed to do better overall than those delivered spontaneously, perhaps more attributable to patient selection than to the procedure itself. This remained to be investigated more carefully in connection with subsequent studies that will examine the effects of these delivery variables together with those of intrinsic and other factors which may be confounding.

In multiparas, application of the logistic regression analytic method disclosed only four delivery factors with p values less than 0.10, and surprisingly, none less than .05 for the composite outcome variable (Table 24-6). Only PRES5-8 (breech presentations) even approached statistical significance (p = .058), despite the impressively

high relative risk (RR = 18.65), indicating more than an 18-fold adverse effect when all other delivery variables were being simultaneously considered. ROM11 (prolonged rupture of the membranes beyond 36 hours) was also an adverse factor, showing nearly 15 times the bad results expected (although this was not quite statistically significant, p = .066). By contrast, those delivered by an obstetrician (OBTYPE1) did well; this was also only marginally significant, p = .067, paralleling the protective effect seen earlier for this factor (see chapter 23).

FORTRAC3 (forceps traction considered very difficult) yielded a high relative risk (RR = 3.53), but this relationship was not a strong one (p = .10) because the sample size was so small. Results for AUGMENT2 (labor stimulation for ruptured membranes) were similar, but here it is more likely that the high p value reflected a weak correlation with outcome (RR = 1.58) since the case numbers were substantial.

Perinatal Outcome Data

When perinatal outcome (death plus severe neonatal depression) was used as the index for the logistic regression model, the analytical results were somewhat different. Those derived for nulliparas are shown in Table 24-7. Eleven delivery factors surfaced, only six of which had been identified

Table 24-6
Logistic Regression Analysis of Delivery Variables in Multiparas for Composite Outcome*

Variable	Regression Coefficient	Standard Error	t-Statistic	Relative Risk	p-Value
Constant	-2.246	1.224	-1.835		
FORTRAC3	1.260	0.811	1.653	3.53	0.10
AUGMENT2	0.454	0.273	1.662	1.58	0.099
OBTYPE1	-0.528	0.283	-1.870	0.59	0.067
ROM11	2.692	1.449	1.857	14.75	0.066
STA6	-0.515	0.314	-1.640	0.60	0.10
PRES5-8	2.926	1.528	1.914	18.65	0.058

* Results listed only for those factors determined to have p-values less than 0.10 among the 68 variables included in the full model based on data from offspring of 8,481 multiparas.

in offspring of nulliparas by the same method using composite outcome (see Table 24-5). The impact of each of these latter six factors was markedly increased. This was especially apparent with BREECH3 (single footling, RR 6.39 to 19.14, although both were only marginally significant, p .069 and .062), FORTRAC3 (very difficult forceps traction, RR 3.17 to 6.29, p .073 to .039), and INDUCT3 (induction for pregnancy-induced hypertension, RR 2.41 to 4.23, p .059 to .032). INDUCT6, AUGMENT6 (induction and augmentation for amnionitis), and FUNDAL2 (moderate Kristeller pressure) showed lesser degrees of enhancement.

New factors included FORROT2 and FORROT3 (difficult and very difficult forceps rotations) with impressively high relative risks (RR 6.29 and 8.76, p .059 and .023). AUGMENT9 and AUGMENT10 (labor stimulation for placenta previa and for arrested labor) had significantly adverse perinatal effects as well (RR 14.01 and 2.03, p .046 and .036). PRES3 (occiput posterior position) was also identified as having a deleterious effect (RR = 2.14, p = .030).

Perinatal outcomes in multiparas were examined in the same way to determine the effects of delivery factors. Table 24-8 illustrates the much larger number of delivery variables that could be shown to affect the infant during the perinatal period, as compared with the preceding analysis which had studied composite outcome instead (see Table 24-6). Only one of these factors was common to both analyses, namely FOR-TRAC3 (very difficult forceps traction); although its impact proved much stronger in the perinatal data (RR 3.53 to 5.64), neither was statistically significant (p .10 and .086), again related to the small numbers of cases.

Among the 17 delivery factors flagged by this approach, seven dealt with forceps and five with labor induction or stimulation. In addition to the aforementioned FOR-TRAC3 variable, FORAPP3 (very difficult forceps application), FORROT2-4 (difficult, very difficult, and failed forceps rotations), and CSVAG (cesarean section after failed attempt to effect vaginal delivery) were clearly hazardous to the fetus and newborn infant.

FORAPP3 sharply contrasted with FORAPP1 (application of average difficulty), the latter showing a protective effect (RR = 0.47, p = .056), the former a delete-

Table 24-7
Logistic Regression Analysis of Delivery Variables in Nulliparas for Perinatal Outcome*

Variable	Regression Coefficient	Standard Error	t-Statistic	Relative Risk	p-Value
Constant	-4.020	1.010	-3.980		
FORTRAC3	1.838	0.879	2.091	6.29	0.039
FORROT2	2.170	1.136	1.910	8.76	0.059
FORROT3	1.996	0.866	2.303	7.36	0.023
INDUCT3	1.487	0.696	2.136	4.43	0.035
INDUCT6	1.616	0.738	2.190	5.03	0.032
AUGMENT6	2.432	1.144	2.126	11.38	0.038
AUGMENT9	2.643	1.305	2.025	14.05	0.046
AUGMENT10	0.709	0.329	2.152	2.03	0.036
BREECH3	2.952	1.563	1.888	19.14	0..062
FUNDAL2	0.744	0.404	1.841	2.10	0.069
PRES3	0.762	0.346	2.199	2.14	0.030

* Results listed only for those factors determined to have p-values less than 0.10 among the 63 variables included in the full model based on data from offspring of 6,688 nulliparas.

Table 24-8
Logistic Regression Analysis of Delivery Variables in
Multiparas for Perinatal Outcome*

Variable	Regression Coefficient	Standard Error	t-Statistic	Relative Risk	p-Value
Constant	-9.148	12.150	-0.753		
FORTRAC3	1.729	0.998	1.733	5.64	0.086
FORAPP1	-0.749	0.388	-1.930	0.47	0.056
FORAPP3	1.617	0.952	1.699	5.04	0.092
FORROT2	0.986	0.484	2.036	2.68	0.044
FORROT3	1.516	0.624	2.427	4.55	0.017
FORROT4	2.425	0.930	2.607	11.30	0.011
INDUCT4	1.269	0.718	1.766	3.56	0.080
INDUCT5	2.182	0.779	2.800	8.86	0.0061
INDUCT6	1.293	0.598	2.163	3.64	0.033
AUGMENT6	3.563	0.955	3.731	35.25	0.00032
AUGMENT10	1.257	0.424	2.964	3.51	0.0038
BRDELIV3	2.380	0.978	2.434	10.80	0.017
CONTROL2	0.992	0.489	2.026	2.70	0.045
PROLAP	0.873	0.517	1.687	2.39	0.093
SHOULD	2.585	0.512	5.047	13.26	2.0×10^{-6}
ABRUPT	1.356	0.404	3.349	3.88	0.0011
CSVAG	3.785	1.009	3.749	44.02	0.00030

* Results listed for those factors determined to have p-values less than 0.10 among 68 variables included in full model based on data from offspring of 8,481 multiparas.

rious one (RR = 5.04, p = .092). Although neither actually achieved statistical significance at the 5% level, they were markedly different from each other by a factor of nine.

The incremental increases in adverse effects from FORROT2 to FORROT4 constituted an impressive trend (RR 2.68 to 4.55 and 11.30) and each was statistically significant by itself (p .044, .017 and .011). Failed vaginal delivery attempts (CSVAG), consisting nearly always of failed forceps, were especially devastating (RR = 44.02). They were obviously harmful in the extreme and achieved a very strong level of significance even though their numbers were not large (p = .00030).

Interesting relations were seen among the remaining factors in this model. BRDELIV3 (breech extraction), for example, was associated with particularly poor outcomes (RR = 10.80, p = .017). An even more adverse association was found for SHOULD (shoulder dystocia, RR = 13.26, p = 2.0×10^{-6}). The impact of labor induction and augmentation reflected the condition for which these practices were undertaken, especially as regards diabetes mellitus (INDUCT4), erythroblastosis fetalis (INDUCT5), amnionitis (INDUCT6 and AUGMENT6), and arrested labor (AUGMENT10).

Step-Up Logistic Modelling

Step-up logistic regression techniques were also applied to these data, as before. The initial model for the composite outcome in offspring of nulliparas (Table 24-9) displayed the same 14 variables as the full model had (see Table 24-5), but the magnitude of effect was somewhat different. In general, the impact of forceps use was less than it had been, although still in the same range, order, and direction. The adverse effect of FUNDAL2 and FUNDAL3 (moderate and strong Kristeller expression) had increased both in magnitude and in significance.

The remaining 49 delivery variables (of the 63 originally designated as potentially significant in nulliparas) were tested seriatim to determine if any could serve as contenders for inclusion in a 15-factor step-up model. Two were identified at a 10% probability cutoff level: INDUCT1 (elective induction, p = .0862) and FORROT2 (difficult forceps rotation, p = .0826).

The latter was thus added to the first step-up logistic model (Table 24-9). Its effect (RR = 1.48) fell short of statistical significance (p = .073). It enhanced the impact of FORCEPS3 (class III, midforceps at 0 to +2) slightly and simultaneously reduced that of FORTRAC2 and FORTRAC3 (difficult and very difficult forceps traction).

Further testing for a 16-factor model showed only INDUCT1 to be significant (p = .0851). When added to the second step-up model (Table 24-9), this variable had an adverse effect (RR = 1.73), but it did not quite achieve statistical significance (p = .070). The only change it produced in the other relations in the logistic model was a further enhancement of the effect of FORCEPS3 (RR = 10.88). No other variables were found to be possible candidates for inclusion in a 17-factor model at the 0.10 probability level, although CSVAG (cesarean section after failed vaginal delivery attempt) came close (p = .1077).

Parallel step-up modelling was done for composite outcome in multiparas. The six delivery factors previously identified were utilized to create the initial or base model (Table 24-10). All but PRES5-8 (breech presentations) were approximately the same in regard to the magnitude of risk effect and their significance level. Breech presentations, by contrast, yielded a very marked increase in adverse effect (RR 18.65 to 28.12, p .058 to .0077). Both FORTRAC3 and ROM11 had somewhat diminished effects, but the differences were small.

Testing was carried out to ascertain possible additional variables for inclusion in a seven-factor step-up model from among the residual group of 62 delivery variables under surveillance here for multiparas. Twelve surfaced as potentially valuable in this regard below the 10% probability cutoff level. In ascending order of p value, they included: INDUCT6 (induction for amnionitis, p = .014), CONTROL3 (forceps control for delivery of the fetal head, p = .0157), FORTRAC2 (difficult forceps traction, p = .0195), BREECH3 (single footling, p = .0206), DIL3 (3 cm cervical dilatation at onset of labor, p = .0206), STA7 (+2 station, p = .0361), FORCEPS2 (class II forceps at station +3, p = .0479), AUGMENT1 (elective induction, p = .0524), FORAPP2 (difficult forceps application, p = .0571), STA5 (zero station, p = .0636), BRCOMP1 (nuchal arm, p = .0946), and BRDELIV3 (breech extraction, p = .0966).

INDUCT6 was added to form the seven-factor step-up logistic model (Table 24-10), where it proved to have very little overall effect and failed to reach statistical significance on its own (RR = 1.62, p = .090). Further testing reconfirmed the candidacy of all eleven residual delivery variables, as previously identified. CONTROL3 (p = .0172) was, therefore, added to the second step-up model containing eight delivery variables. It proved protective at a statistically significant level (RR = 0.78, p = .022). Its inclusion enhanced the effect of PRES5-8 (RR = 28.75) and ROM11 (RR = 14.96), without altering the effects of other variables in the model.

The next series of tests for candidates in a nine-factor model yielded only six, namely DIL3 (p = .0174), BREECH3 (p = .0246), STA7 (p = .0308), AUGMENT1 (p = .0599), STA5 (p = .0831), and FORTRAC4 (failed forceps traction, p = .0958). DIL3 was included in the third step-up model (Table 24-10) and was demonstrated to be significantly protective (RR = 0.62, p = .024). Its incorporation did not alter the relationships encountered for the other delivery variables in the nine-factor model.

A fourth set of tests again disclosed six variables as potential contenders for a ten-factor model, deleting FORTRAC4 and STA5, but adding BRDELIV3 (p = .0875),

Table 24-9
Step-Up Logistic Regression Modelling of Delivery Variables
for Composite Outcome in Nulliparas*

Variable	Initial Model		Step-Up Model 1		Step-Up Model 2	
	RR	t	RR	t	RR	t
FORCEPS3	10.61	2.35A	10.78	2.37A	10.88	2.38A
FORTRAC2	2.28	3.29D	2.08	2.84C	2.06	2.79B
FORTRAC3	2.92	1.89	2.84	1.84	2.86	1.85
FORAPP1	0.61	-4.97F	0.61	-4.96F	0.61	-5.02F
FORROT1	0.71	-2.07A	0.72	-2.03A	0.72	-1.99A
INDUCT3	2.75	2.85C	2.76	2.85C	2.79	2.89C
INDUCT6	3.33	2.74B	3.30	2.72B	3.35	2.75B
AUGMENT6	9.01	2.93C	8.87	2.88C	8.44	2.78B
BREECH3	4.36	1.75	4.44	1.77	4.47	1.78
FUNDAL2	1.64	2.94C	1.63	2.91C	1.60	2.79B
FUNDAL3	1.89	3.97E	1.87	3.90E	1.86	3.89E
PROLAP	2.84	2.78B	2.85	2.79B	2.88	2.82B
ROM11	13.46	1.83	13.64	1.84	13.69	1.84
STA1-2	1.32	1.85	1.33	1.88	1.31	1.80
FORROT2			1.48	1.81	1.49	1.82
INDUCT1					1.73	1.83

*   Probability of chance occurrence (p-value) coded as follows:

A 0.05, B 0.01, C 0.005, D 0.001, E 0.0005, F 0.0001 or less.

NS not significant at p > 0.10.

DIL4 (p = .0688), and DIL5 (p = .0731) to the previous list. BREECH3 (p = .0247), when added to form the ten-factor model (Table 24-10), demonstrated its strongly adverse impact (RR = 6.26, p = .012). This step had no effect at all on the other factors in the model.

Still more testing for an 11-factor model showed four remaining candidate variables. They were: STA7 (p = .0633), DIL4 (p = .0743), DIL5 (p = .0772), and AUGMENT1 (p = .0874). The fifth step-up model was created by incorporating STA7, which was shown to be protective, but not significantly so (RR = .074, p = .084). This addition served to enhance the adverse impact of PRES5-8 considerably (RR = 30.17, p = .0067) without affecting the other variables to any extent. The process was concluded when it was determined that no other variables would yield any relevant effect.

The complex step-up modelling procedures were repeated for perinatal outcome. In nulliparas, eleven variables made up the initial model (Table 24-11). The results of the logistic regression analysis carried out on this model differed somewhat from those found earlier (see Table 24-7). The impact of some delivery variables were magnified, such as FORTRAC3 (very difficult forceps traction, RR 6.29 to 9.84, p .039 to .0010), FORROT2 (difficult forceps rotation, RR 8.76 to 10.89, p .059 to .032), and AUGMENT9 (stimulation for placenta previa, RR 14.05 to 16.96, p .046 to .032). In others it was diminished, including FORROT3 (very difficult forceps rotation, RR 7.36 to 5.65, p .023 to .040), INDUCT6 (induction for amnionitis, RR 5.03 to 3.86, p 0.32 to .037), and BREECH3 (single footling, RR 19.14 to 13.61, p .062 to .022).

Tests for the next step-up model flagged 15 variables as possible candidates within the 10% probability cutoff. The most promising among these were: FORAPP1 (forceps application of average difficulty, p < 10^{-5}), FORTRAC1 (forceps traction of average difficulty, p < 10^{-5}), CONTROL2 (manual

Table 24-10
Step-Up Logistic Regression Modelling of Delivery Variables for
Composite Outcome in Multiparas*

Variable	Initial Model		Step-Up Model 1		Step-Up Model 2		Step-Up Model 3		Step-Up Model 4		Step-Up Model 5	
	RR	t	RR	t	RR	t	RR	t	RR	t	RR	t
FORTRAC3	3.20	1.66	3.19	1.60NS	3.24	1.69	3.30	1.72	3.33	1.74	3.39	1.77
AUGMENT2	1.64	2.10A	1.63	2.07A	1.65	2.14A	1.64	2.12A	1.62	2.05A	1.66	2.15A
OBTYPE1	0.48	-3.09C	0.48	-2.96C	0.56	-2.27A	0.58	-2.09A	0.58	-2.09A	0.60	-1.95
ROM11	14.06	1.87	13.97	1.86	14.96	1.91	14.47	1.88	14.51	1.89	14.22	1.87
STA6	0.58	-1.91	0.57	-1.86	0.59	-1.75	0.62	-1.58	0.63	-1.57NS	0.61	-1.67
PRES5-8	28.12	2.72B	27.94	2.72B	28.75	2.74B	27.79	2.71B	27.88	2.71B	30.17	2.77B
INDUCT6			1.62	-1.71	1.62	-1.70	1.62	-1.71	1.62	-1.70	1.62	-1.70
CONTROL3					0.78	-2.34A	0.77	-2.39A	0.78	-2.33A	0.77	-2.40A
DIL3							0.62	-2.28A	0.70	-2.28A	0.73	-2.03A
BREECH3									6.26	2.57B	6.27	2.57B
STA7											0.74	-1.79

* See Table 24-9 for probability code.

337

Table 24-11
Step-Up Logistic Regression Modelling of Delivery Variables
for Perinatal Outcome in Nulliparas*

Variable	Initial Model RR	t	Step-Up Model 1 RR	t	Step-Up Model 2 RR	t	Step-Up Model 3 RR	t	Step-Up Model 4 RR	t	Step-Up Model 5 RR	t
FORTRAC3	9.84	3.39D	7.22	2.92C	6.11	2.67B	5.72	2.53A	6.01	2.59C	5.41	2.43A
FORROT2	10.89	2.17A	8.06	1.89	10.14	2.09A	10.29	2.10A	10.56	2.13A	9.36	2.01A
FORROT3	5.65	2.08A	5.57	2.06A	5.05	1.94	5.36	2.01A	5.59	2.06A	5.41	2.02A
INDUCT3	4.00	2.66B	4.05	2.63B	3.71	2.46A	3.56	2.38A	3.69	2.44A	3.72	2.44A
INDUCT6	3.86	2.12A	4.85	2.39A	4.85	2.39A	5.04	2.45A	5.12	2.47A	5.04	2.42A
AUGMENT6	10.38	2.37A	8.34	2.05A	8.11	2.03A	8.57	2.08A	8.69	2.09A	7.27	1.86
AUGMENT9	16.96	2.27A	13.22	2.07A	12.72	2.04A	13.48	2.09A	14.18	2.13A	14.19	2.12A
AUGMENT10	1.92	2.26A	2.23	2.71B	2.03	2.38A	1.99	2.30A	2.05	2.40A	1.91	2.13A
BREECH3	13.61	2.33A	10.07	2.05A	8.32	1.88	8.67	1.92	5.40	1.45NS	5.73	1.50NS
FUNDAL2	2.26	3.10C	2.34	3.19C	2.15	2.84C	2.23	2.98C	2.33	3.12C	2.29	3.05C
PRES3	1.98	2.79B	1.84	2.47A	1.91	2.61B	1.83	2.44A	1.83	2.44A	1.97	2.70B
FORAPP1			0.41	-4.49F	0.54	-2.73B	0.54	-2.75B	0.54	-2.69B	0.55	-2.68B
FORTRAC1					0.59	-2.60B	0.61	-2.42A	0.65	-2.11A	0.65	-2.12A
FUNDAL3							2.74	2.40A	2.88	2.51A	2.63	2.28A
CONTROL2									2.27	2.04A	2.26	2.02A
PRES4											1.63	1.91

* See Table 24-9 for probability code.

338

control of head, p = .0010), FUNDAL3 (strong Kristeller pressure, p = .0031), CSVAG (p = .0055), CONTROL3 (forceps control of head delivery, p = .0073), and FUNDAL2 (moderate Kristeller pressure, p = 010), all at or below the 1% p value.

FORAPP1 was added to the first step-up 12-factor model (Table 24-11) where it was shown to be significantly protective (RR = 0.41, p = .000019). Its inclusion diminished the effects of FORTRAC3 (RR 9.84 to 7.22) and FORROT2 (RR 10.89 to 8.06) as well as AUGMENT6 (RR 10.38 to 8.34) and AUGMENT9 (RR 16.96 to 13.22), while enhancing that of INDUCT6 (RR 3.86 to 4.85) and, to a lesser extent, AUGMENT10 (RR 1.92 to 2.23).

Testing of the remaining variables for the 13-factor model demonstrated seven candidates, including FORTRAC1 (p = .0085), FUNDAL3 (p = .0186), and CONTROL2 (p = .0275). The second step-up model incorporated FORTRAC1 (Table 24-11) and showed its protective effect (RR = 0.59, p = .011). It also further reduced the impact of FORTRAC3 (RR 7.22 to 6.11) and FORROT3 (RR 5.57 to 5.05).

Retesting yielded only three candidates among the residual variables, namely FUNDAL3 (p = .0320), PRES3 (occiput posterior, p = .0420), and CONTROL2 (p = .0777). All three were subsequently included in the next three sequential step-up logistic models (Table 24-11). Each had demonstrably adverse effects.

Adding FUNDAL3 to form the third step-up 14-factor model augmented the effects of many of the delivery variables already in the model, except FORTRAC3, which was diminished somewhat (RR 6.11 to 5.72). The addition of CONTROL2 further enhanced the effects of a number of variables in the fourth step-up 15-factor model. In this model, the downward trend for FORTRAC3 was temporarily reversed, its effect increasing somewhat (RR 5.72 to 6.01). The impact of BREECH3 was markedly reduced in this model (RR 8.67 to 5.40) and became statistically insignificant at this time.

The final step-up model, containing 16 factors, was formed by adding PRES3. The process diminished the effects of several of the other variables in this model, especially FORTRAC3 (RR 6.01 to 5.41), continuing its downward trend which had been interrupted transiently only in the fourth step-up model. Again, the procedure ended when no more potentially significant candidate variables could be identified.

In multiparas the step-up modelling process for perinatal outcome results started with an initial model containing the 17 variables previously identified as significant in the full 68-factor model (see Table 24-9). Several noteworthy changes in effects were revealed in the logistic regression analysis of this core model. Five variables showed markedly increased effects. They were FORAPP3 (RR 5.04 to 11.19), FORROT3 (RR 4.55 to 7.78), FORROT4 (RR 11.30 to 15.32), AUGMENT6 (RR 35.25 to 64.71), and SHOULD (RR 13.26 to 15.17). One factor considerably diminished its effect, namely BRDELIV3 (RR 10.80 to 7.19).

Testing for candidates to include in an 18-factor step-up model flagged five delivery variables at p values of 0.10 or less. They included PRES2 (occiput transverse, p = .0242), FORTRAC2 (p = .0300), PRES4 (vertex presentations, p = .0344), PRES5-8 (breech presentations, p = .0525), and PRES1 (occiput anterior position, p = .0645). All five remained significant on serial testing as each was entered in sequence into the series of five step-up models shown in Table 24-12. No further variables could be identified as contributory at the p = .10 level after the fifth or 27-factor step-up model had been constructed. No especially meaningful trends were apparent as a result of the stepwise enlargement of the logistic models for this outcome in multiparas.

Summary of Risk Variables Among Delivery Factors

The results of this series of logistic regression analyses yielded information pertaining to a number of delivery vari-

Table 24-12
Step-Up Logistic Regression Modelling of Delivery Variables
for Perinatal Outcome in Multiparas*

Variable	Initial Model RR	t	Step-Up Model 1 RR	t	Step-Up Model 2 RR	t	Step-Up Model 3 RR	t	Step-Up Model 4 RR	t	Step-Up Model 5 RR	t
FORTRAC3	6.03	1.99A	6.34	2.06A	5.65	1.82	5.92	1.88	5.91	1.88	5.94	1.89
FORAPP1	0.49	-2.36A	0.47	-2.51A	0.47	-2.54A	0.46	-2.58B	0.45	-2.62B	0.45	-2.63B
FORAPP3	11.19	3.09C	8.17	2.60B	8.08	2.59B	8.48	2.67B	8.33	2.64B	8.53	2.67B
FORROT2	3.71	3.05C	3.10	2.59B	2.96	2.47A	2.90	2.43A	2.89	2.42A	3.03	2.55A
FORROT3	7.78	3.61E	6.27	3.16C	6.34	3.19C	5.77	2.96C	5.79	2.97C	5.86	2.99C
FORROT4	15.32	3.08C	14.55	3.05C	14.86	3.08C	14.94	3.08C	14.93	3.08C	15.05	3.08C
INDUCT4	3.12	1.68	3.32	1.77	3.41	1.81	3.40	1.80	3.25	1.73	3.82	1.98A
INDUCT5	9.82	3.38D	9.72	3.30D	9.80	3.31D	8.78	2.94C	8.67	2.91C	9.33	3.03C
INDUCT6	4.03	2.46A	4.26	2.56B	4.29	2.57B	4.34	2.59B	4.41	2.61B	4.16	2.49A
AUGMENT6	64.71	4.79F	63.71	4.70F	64.23	4.71F	65.19	4.73F	63.64	4.68F	63.31	4.66F
AUGMENT10	4.40	3.88E	4.25	3.77E	4.29	3.79E	4.16	3.69E	4.36	3.81E	4.29	3.77E
BRDELIV3	7.19	3.58E	7.25	3.58E	7.27	3.58E	7.30	3.59E	10.31	3.90E	9.41	3.72E
CONTROL2	3.06	3.07C	3.14	3.12C	3.09	3.06C	3.09	3.05C	2.73	2.64B	3.02	2.91C
PROLAP	2.08	1.55NS	2.23	1.70	2.33	1.79	2.33	1.79	2.28	1.71	2.31	1.73
SHOULD	15.17	5.66F	14.23	5.48F	14.35	5.50F	13.80	5.30F	13.91	5.32F	14.42	5.44F
ABRUPT	3.60	3.36D	3.50	3.30D	3.42	3.23C	3.47	3.26C	3.44	3.23C	3.74	3.44D
CSVAG	61.41	4.30F	45.90	4.00F	40.22	3.73E	41.64	3.77E	41.55	3.76E	42.55	3.78E
PRES3			1.82	2.38A	1.87	2.48A	1.77	2.22A	1.75	2.18A	1.67	1.97A
PRES5-8					6.96	2.22A	6.93	2.21A	6.92	2.21A	5.96	2.00A
FORTRAC2							5.98	2.19A	5.95	2.18A	6.07	2.20
PRES2									0.01	-1.11NS	0.01	-1.09NS
PRES1											0.40	1.61NS

* See Table 24-9 for probability code.

ables, indicating their possible impact on offspring. The findings are summarized in Table 24-13 for all delivery variables determined to have significant impact on the fetus and infant when studied in this way, every other relevant delivery variable having been considered simultaneously. The tabulation allows comparison of effects by significance level for both composite and perinatal outcome by parity groupings.

These analyses conclude the last of the foundational surveys of the four large groups of variables comprising this investigation. We have thus derived four subsets of highly significant variables from each of the master groups involving those dealing with labor progression, adjunctive drugs, intrinsic factors, and delivery variables. At this point, we are ready to embark on a further series of analyses using the same paradigm as heretofore, but collectively encompassing all four subsets of significant variables together. We will proceed seriatim with cluster and logistic regression analyses, just as we have done before for each of the separate groups of variables, seeking to determine if any are redundant and to ascertain finally which have the greatest impact on the offspring when all the others are considered simultaneously.

Table 24-13
Summary of Significant Delivery Variables by Logistic Regression*

Variable	Full Model Composite		Perinatal		Initial Model Composite		Perinatal		Step-Up Model Composite		Perinatal	
	N	M	N	M	N	M	N	M	N	M	N	M
FORCEPS3	A				A				A			
FORTRAC1											a	
FORTRAC2	A				D				B		A	A
FORTRAC3			A				D	A	A			
FORAPP1					f			a	f		b	b
FORAPP3								C				B
FORROT1	a				a				a			
FORROT2				A			A	C			A	A
FORROT3			A	A			A	E			A	C
FORROT4				B				C				C
INDUCT3			A		C		B		C		A	
INDUCT4												A
INDUCT5								D				C
INDUCT6	A		A	A	B		A	A	B		A	A
AUGMENT2						A				A		
AUGMENT6	B		A	E	C		A	F	B			F
AUGMENT9			A				A				A	
AUGMENT10			A	C			A	E			A	E
BREECH3							A			B		
BRDELIV3				B				E				E
FUNDAL2					C		C		B		C	
FUNDAL3	A				E				E		A	
CONTROL2				A				C			A	C
CONTROL3										a		
CSVAG				E				F				E
PROLAP	A				B				B			
SHOULD				F				F				F
ABRUPT				D				D				D
DIL3										a		
PRES3			A				B				B	A
PRES5-8		A				B				B		A
OBTYPE1						c						

* Significance code: A 0.05, B 0.01, C 0.005, D 0.001, E 0.0005, F 0.0001 or less.

Protective in lower case; adverse in capital letter codes.

N nulliparas, M multiparas.

CHAPTER 25

Aggregated Risk Factors

Summary

All of the 129 variables flagged by the four antecedent complex analyses of labor, drug, intrinsic, and delivery factors were studied collectively. When interactional and confounding effects were taken into account by cluster and logistic regression analyses, many were found to lose their adverse impact on outcome. Based on these results, 86 variables were identified as retaining some significant residual effects on the fetus and infant, including four labor, 12 drug, 45 intrinsic, and 25 delivery variables taken from the original 2441 studied.

The results of the four parallel investigational efforts were ready to be combined and assessed at this point. To recapitulate, we had separately studied variables dealing with (1) labor progression and its disorders, (2) adjunctive pharmacologic agents and anesthesias, (3) intrinsic maternal, fetal, and pelvic factors, and (4) the delivery process. Among these four major groups, we had identified a number of variables significantly associated with adverse or beneficial outcomes. These subsets had been extensively tested to eliminate informational redundancy and to determine the degree of verifiable significance of their relation to outcome which remained when modifying or confounding factors were taken into account simultaneously.

We had begun with more than 2000 variables (actually 2441), each of which was examined separately in two population subgroups, namely nulliparas and multiparas. Of these, simple nonparametric bivariate screening by the Freeman-Tukey technique (applied 4882 times) showed 326 factors to be of potential significance in regard to their impact on fetal and infant outcome. Cluster analyses demonstrated high degrees of similarity of informational content in 70. These correlations served to permit us to reduce the number of variables to be examined to 256. When studied by logistic regression modelling methods, only 129 were determined to be significantly associated with fetal and infant outcomes. These latter, summarized in Table 25-1, included eight labor, 15 drug, 59 intrinsic, and 47 delivery variables.

Our task at this juncture was to repeat the complex analytical approach for the entire amalgam of 129 residual variables, again to eliminate redundancy, if any, between correlated variables with similar informational content and to determine the risk to which each variable exposes the fetus and infant when all others are considered at the same time. To this end, we proceeded just as we had before through the sequence of cluster and logistic regression analyses.

Cluster Analyses

The index population for this segment of the investigation included those 6688 nulliparas and 8481 multiparas from the full NCPP data base who had delivered infants weighing 2500-4000 g at birth and did not have major congenital anomalies incompatible with survival or with normal development. Two outcome variables were used as definitive endpoints, namely (1) adverse perinatal outcome and (2) adverse composite outcome. The former included perinatal death or severe neonatal depression based on low five-minute Apgar score; the latter encompassed any definite bad result from the perinatal period through the battery of neurologic, psychological, and developmental testing at 8 months and 1, 3, 4, and 7 years.

Four hierarchical cluster analyses were performed for the collective series of previously flagged risk variables. They dealt separately with the data for offspring of nulliparas and multiparas and, within each parity group, separately for perinatal and composite outcomes. Not unexpectedly, the intercorrelations that were encountered were found to be rather weak. This demonstrated that the original groupings of the four subsets of variables had been well chosen—that is, the variables under study fell into distinctive categories with little relationship to each other in regard to risk across group boundaries. Nonetheless, certain interesting clusters of variables were identified even though none was sufficiently well correlated to justify flagging one member to serve as the marker for the next (with a single exception, see below).

Two full cluster trees are illustrated here for nulliparas, one pertaining to the composite outcome data (Figure 25-1), the other to the perinatal outcome (Figure 25-2). The cluster results for multiparas were similar, especially in regard to the observation that the correlations were generally not strong. The most highly correlated cluster in the composite outcome data for nulliparas, as shown in Figure 25-1, involved PWGT1 (prepregnancy weight of 175 lb or more) and POND2 (ponderal index less than 11.9, clearly showing obesity). This was subclustered in turn with RACE3 (other than white or black) and WTGAIN5 (weight gain of 48 lb or more). Within this cluster of four variables, however, only the first two even approached significant correlation ($r = .473$). Disregarding statistical significance, we found there was an inescapable clinical logic to the association suggested by the clustering.

Further down the cluster tree, we encountered a set of seven variables beginning with INST71. It related the impact of FUNDAL2 and FUNDAL3 (moderate and strong Kristeller pressure) to STATUS2 (private patient) at that institution. It further suggested INDUCT1 and INDUCT2 (elective induction and induction for ruptured membranes) were associated with the effects of REACT3 (uterine hypertonus). Once again, the correlation was weak, but the relationships may be clin-

Table 25-1
Recapitulation of Analytic Processes for Determining Critical Variables

Variable Group	Total Number of Variables	Insignificant by Bivariate Screening	Subset of Significant Variables	Redundant by Cluster Analysis	Subset of Significant Variables	Insignificant by Logistic Regression	Residual Significant Variables
Labor Progression							
Nulliparas	22	12	10	2	8	2	6
Multiparas	22	9	13	1	12	7	5
Total*	22	7	15	2	13	5	8
Adjunctive Drug							
Nulliparas	168	151	17	0	17	4	13
Multiparas	168	145	23	0	23	15	8
Total*	168	137	31	0	31	16	15
Intrinsic							
Nulliparas	271	186	85	15	70	33	37
Multiparas	271	172	99	21	78	42	36
Total*	271	126	145	26	119	60	59
Delivery							
Nulliparas	1980	1909	71	8	63	37	26
Multiparas	1980	1866	114	46	68	34	34
Total*	1980	1845	135	42	93	46	47
Collective							
Nulliparas	2441	2258	183	25	158	76	82
Multiparas	2441	2192	249	68	181	98	83
Grand Total*	2441	2115	326	70	256	127	129

* Totals are not additive because subgroups share common variables.

345

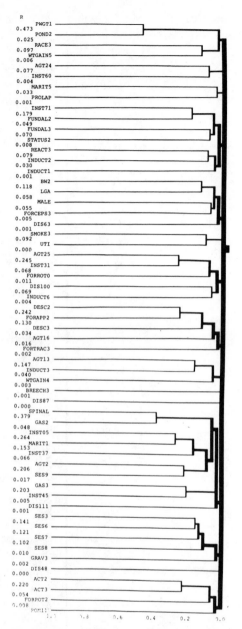

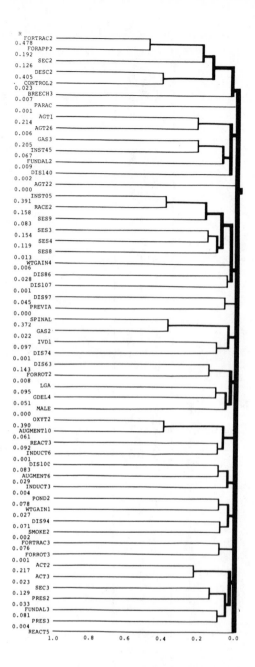

Figure 25-1. Cluster analysis of aggregated variables for composite outcome in nulliparas. Although there is relatively little overall intercorrelation between the clusters of variables derived from the subgroups (labor, drug, intrinsic, and delivery variables, respectively), some variables show evidence of similar informational content. PWGT1 and POND2 relate to each other and to the subcluster of RACE3 and WTGAIN5, for example. Other relationships of possible clinical relevance are also shown.

Figure 25-2. Results of cluster analysis of aggregated variables for perinatal outcome in offspring of nulliparas. FORTRAC2 and FORAPP2 correlate moderately well; they relate somewhat in turn to SEC2 and to the subcluster of DESC2 and CONTROL2. Additional clusters illustrate correlative relationships between risk variables derived from the foregoing series of analyses all considered collectively.

ically meaningful. Still further down, BW2 (2750-2999 g) and LGA (macrosomia) were related to MALE and FORCEPS3 (class III midforceps).

DESC2 (protracted descent) and FORAPP2 (forceps application of moderate difficulty) correlated somewhat with DESC3(precipitate descent), use of AGT16 (Vistaril), and more distantly to FOR-TRAC3 (very difficult forceps traction). A small cluster followed which included AGT13 (phenobarbital), INDUCT3 (induction for pregnancy-induced hypertension), and WTGAIN4 (39 lb or more gain). Then there was a cluster of ten variables beginning with SPINAL and GAS2 (continuous use of inhalation anesthesia). It showed linkage of effect to MARIT1 (unmarried), SES9 (highest socioeconomic index), AGT2 (Nisentil), and GAS3 (continuous and intermittent use) at three of the study hospitals (INST05, INST37, and INST45). At the bottom, ACT2 and ACT3 (short and long active phase durations) related to each other and to FORROT2 (difficult forceps rotation) and, less so, to ROM11 (prolonged rupture of the membranes).

For perinatal outcome in offspring of nulliparas, the cluster analysis showed similar types of potentially important relationships (Figure 21-2), but no correlation strong enough to warrant deleting any of the variables being studied. The closest correlation, signifying the greatest similarity of informational content with regard to adverse perinatal outcome, was between FORTRAC2 (difficult forceps traction) and FORAPP2 (difficult forceps application). This cluster fell short of statistical significance ($r = .478$). It was related in turn to SEC2 (short second stage duration) and the combination of DESC2 (protracted descent) and CONTROL2 (uncontrolled delivery of the fetal head).

The next cluster unexpectedly related AGT1 (Demerol) with AGT26 (magnesium sulfate) and these in turn with GAS3 (both intermittent and continuous inhalation anesthesia) at INST45 (a subcluster identical to that seen earlier in the cluster analysis addressing composite results, with the same level of correlation) as well as with FUNDAL2 (moderately strong Kristeller pressure). A stronger correlation was found between INST05 and RACE2 (black) and these factors were related to four of the relevant socioeconomic variables.

As before, SPINAL and GAS2 retained their association and were found to be somewhat correlated with IVD1 (intravenous anesthesia agent use). DIS63 (hyperthyroidism) and FORROT2 (difficult forceps rotation) were clustered with LGA (macrosomia), GDEL4 (delivery beyond 41 weeks), and MALE, although all had low correlation coefficients. OXYT2 (oxytocin augmentation of labor) related well to AUGMENT10 (enhancement for arrested labor), as expected, and the cluster they formed was associated with REACT3 (uterine hypertonus) and INDUCT6 (induction for amnionitis).

POND2 (obesity) and WTGAIN1 (less than 11 lb) were weakly clustered together and were more distantly associated with DIS94 (leiomyomata uteri) and SMOKE2 (cigarette smoking for 10 years or more). Just as in the composite data cluster, ACT2 and ACT3 (short and long active phase durations) were somewhat correlated with each other and with the subcluster of SEC3 (prolonged second stage) and PRES2 (occiput transverse position) as well as that of FUNDAL3 (strong Kristeller pressure) and PRES3 (occiput posterior).

The cluster analyses for outcome data in multiparas yielded similar results. With only one exception, no strong correlations were encountered, but a number of clusters suggested the existence of clinical relationships of possible importance. For composite outcome in multiparas, the results of the cluster analysis showed good correlation ($r = .896$) between STATUS2 (private) and OBTYPE1 (obstetrician). This was not unexpected and warranted accepting STATUS2 as the representative variable for both members of this cluster, deleting OBTYPE1 from further consideration.

Other, less well correlated clusters were

encountered, suggesting possible relationships. For example, INST55 and RACE3 (other than black or white) formed a cluster with a correlation coefficient which just attained statistical significance ($r = .607$). Clarification of this association came from the observation that 59.2% of the NCPP study population at INST55 was Puerto Rican (plus 0.3% other races). Only one other collaborating hospital had a sizable population of RACE3 patients, namely INST31, where the proportion totalled 27.8% Puerto Rican and 2.8% other races. No other instituion had numbers even approaching these, the largest frequency being 5.2% at INST45.

Another interesting, but not statistically significant cluster ($r = .338$) encompassed DEC2 (foreshortened deceleration phase), DESC3 (precipitate descent), and SEC2 (short second stage), confirming clinical impressions. AGT18 (triflupromazine) was associated somewhat with PARAC (paracervical block) at INST60 and INST82, reflecting prevailing clinical practices there ($r = .273$).

In the cluster dealing with perinatal outcome for offspring of multiparas, DESC2 (protracted descent) was related to CONTROL3 (forceps control for delivery of the fetal head), athough the correlation did not quite achieve statistical significance ($r = .432$). As might be expected, DIS49 (diabetes mellitus) correlated well with INDUCT4 (induction for diabetes) at a level approaching statistical significance ($r = .510$), and both were clustered in turn with OXYT1 (induction by oxytocin). A similar association was seen for RHSENS (Rh isoimmunization) and INDUCT5 (induction for Rh disease), and this cluster was in turn found related to all three of the variables signalling problems with bleeding in pregnancy, namely VAGBLD (bleeding in early pregnancy), ABRUPT (abruptio placentae), and DIS126 (third trimester bleeding).

SPINAL and FORAPP1 (forceps application of average difficulty) were also clustered together ($r = .518$), and both were tied

to INST71. A large cluster was formed of eight correlated variables, including the following pairs: OXYT2 (oxytocin for augmentation) and AUGMENT10 (stimulation for arrested labor); ARRS3 (arrest of descent) and ACT3 (prolonged active phase); and FORROT3 (very difficult forceps rotation) and PRES2 (occiput transverse).

This series of cluster analyses did not help reduce the total number of risk factors to be assessed by logistic regression techniques. The only exception was OBTYPE1 insofar as composite outcome in offspring of multiparas was concerned. However, the analyses did show quite clearly that our antecedent preliminary exploratory efforts had successfully selected variables from the several major categories, such variables apparently acting independently of others—that is, their informational content was sufficiently dissimilar from all others to justify retaining them for more in-depth evaluation as to impact on fetus and infant. A secondary gain of these analyses was the identification of a series of relationships between variables, some of which were admittedly obvious but others more subtle and of potential importance.

Logistic Regression Analyses

The objectives, concepts, and methods pertaining to logistic regression analysis have been reviewed extensively (see chapters 7 and 14). The technique was applied to the entire combined set of variables from the four major preceding studies. Four separate analyses were conducted to assess the impact of all variables acting concurrently on two measures of outcome (adverse composite and perinatal results) and two parity populations (nulliparas and multiparas).

The full model containing all relevant variables previously determined to be significant for each parity-outcome group was evaluated first to determine which of the many variables retained their significant relationships to fetal and infant outcomes when all were considered simultaneously.

Following this, a base model was constructed of those variables identified as statistically significant by the full model (the criterion was a p value of .10 or less). Their collective effects were then assessed.

A sequence of step-up models was subsequently created by adding single variables seriatim. These latter variables were selected on the basis of a series of tests of each of the residual variables to ascertain their suitability for inclusion. Each successive model was analyzed by the logistic regression method in order to determine the changing effects of the variables incorporated therein. When no additional variables could be shown to add significantly more information to the larger step-up models, the process was terminated.

Composite Outcome Data

The results of the full model logistic regression analysis of the entire set of variables as they affected offspring of nulliparas, measured by the composite outcome variable (any definite adverse effect from the perinatal period to seven years), are detailed in Table 25-2. A total of 26 of the 53 variables studied in this single analytic process was found to be statistically significant at the 5% probability level, 36 at the 10% level. It was clear that this approach had shown that some of these variables, previously determined to have significant effects on offspring whn considered alone or in conjunction with like variables of their category, were no longer relevant in this regard. The influence they appeared to have had before did not pertain when examined concurrently with that of other interactive or confounding factors. For others, the effects were enhanced by this process. These observations re-emphasized the critical nature of interrelational studies such as this, while stressing the potential shortcomings of investigations that only address the impact of factors in isolation.

Some of the more clinically relevant transformations became apparent when we compared the results of the foregoing logistic regression analyses with this one.

Among adjunctive drug variables, for example, the data in Table 18-8 contrast with those in Table 25-2 in several important ways. SPINAL (spinal anesthesia) had earlier been shown to have a significantly protective effect (RR = 0.77, p = .019), confirmed by the step-up modelling process (see Table 18-12, RR = 0.79, p = .025). The more generalized logistic regression analysis, incorporating intrinsic, labor, and delivery variables simultaneously, now revealed SPINAL to have no effect whatever (RR = 0.98, p = .85), either adverse or beneficial.

Similarly, the effects of GAS2 and GAS3 (continuous and combined continuous and intermittent inhalation anesthesia) were attenuated somewhat in magnitude and statistical significance; indeed, GAS3 was no longer statistically significant at the 5% probability level (RR 1.94 to 1.61, p .0071 to .058). AGT2 (Nisentil), previously shown to be rather protective (RR = 0.48, p = .014), an effect confirmed by step-up modelling (RR = 0.56, p = .023), no longer had any effect at all (RR = 0.92, p = .77). This was in contradistinction to the adverse effects seen before with AGT13 (phenobarbital), AGT16 (hydroxyzine), and AGT24 (oxytocin), which persisted essentially unchanged in terms of levels of relative risk and statistical significance.

A number of institutions appeared to be correlated with composite outcome in the earlier studies of intrinsic variables. Now that other factors were being considered simultaneously, some of the institutional effects vanished. INST05, for example, had previously been shown on step-up logistic regression analysis to be significantly protective (see Table 21-9, RR = 0.63, p = .0020); in the current analysis, its effect was no longer significant although still somewhat protective (RR = 0.79, p = .14). The adverse impact attributed to three other hospitals, namely INST31, INST45, and INST71, were now considerably diminished and none was statistically significant any longer.

Only two institutions retained their prior relation to composite outcome. One of

Table 25-2
Logistic Regression Analysis of All Residual Variables in
Nulliparas for Composite Outcome

Variable	Regression Coefficient	Standard Error	t-Statistic	Relative Risk	p-Value
ACT2	0.257	0.125	2.06	1.29	0.042
ACT3	0.118	0.128	0.92	1.13	
DESC2	-0.028	0.151	-0.19	0.97	
DESC3	-0.350	0.141	-2.48	0.71	0.015
SPINAL	-0.022	0.118	-0.19	0.98	
GAS2	0.330	0.139	2.38	1.39	0.019
GAS3	0.479	0.251	1.91	1.61	
AGT2	-0.084	0.292	-0.29	0.92	
AGT13	0.554	0.320	1.73	1.74	
AGT16	0.701	0.309	2.27	2.02	0.025
AGT24	0.832	0.377	2.21	2.30	0.029
AGT25	0.448	0.419	1.07	1.56	
INST05	-0.241	0.162	-1.48	0.79	
INST31	0.383	0.235	1.63	1.47	
INST37	0.346	0.172	2.01	1.41	0.047
INST45	0.322	0.205	1.57	1.38	
INST60	0.817	0.179	4.56	2.26	1.5×10^{-5}
INST70	0.234	0.209	1.12	1.26	
MARIT1	-0.091	0.110	-0.83	0.91	
MARIT5	-5.659	3.766	-1.50	0.60	
RACE3	-0.733	0.211	-3.47	0.48	0.00077
GRAV3	0.874	0.474	1.85	2.40	
PWGT1	-0.645	0.346	-1.86	0.52	
POND2	0.376	0.173	2.18	1.46	0.032
SES3	0.249	0.130	1.92	1.28	
SES8	-0.495	0.214	-2.31	0.61	0.023
SES9	-1.318	0.293	-4.50	0.27	1.8×10^{-5}
BW2	0.289	0.118	2.45	1.34	0.016
MALE	0.440	0.098	4.47	1.55	2.1×10^{-5}
SMOKE3	0.976	0.376	2.60	2.65	0.011
WTGAIN4	0.320	0.156	2.05	1.38	0.042
WTGAIN5	0.709	0.233	3.04	2.03	0.0030
LGA	0.290	0.189	1.54	1.34	
DIS48	2.810	1.048	2.68	16.62	0.0086
DIS63	1.463	0.869	1.68	4.32	
DIS87	3.960	1.441	2.75	52.44	0.0071
DIS100	2.275	0.459	4.95	9.73	3.0×10^{-6}
DIS111	2.414	0.914	2.64	11.17	0.0096
FORCEPS3	2.157	1.017	2.12	8.65	0.037
FORTRAC2	0.769	0.278	2.77	2.16	0.0067
FORTRAC3	0.917	0.620	1.48	2.50	
FORAPP1	-0.286	0.111	-2.57	0.75	0.012
FORROT1	-0.129	0.171	-0.75	0.88	
FORROT2	0.238	0.225	1.06	1.27	
INDUCT1	0.381	0.328	1.16	1.46	
INDUCT3	0.765	0.393	1.95	2.15	
INDUCT6	1.044	0.499	2.09	2.84	0.039
AUGMENT6	1.373	0.846	1.62	3.95	
BREECH3	1.607	0.889	1.81	4.99	
FUNDAL2	0.392	0.182	2.16	1.48	0.033
FUNDAL3	0.461	0.173	2.67	1.59	0.0089
PROLAP	0.996	0.400	2.49	2.71	0.014
ROM11	2.604	1.471	1.77	13.52	
STA1-2	0.306	0.159	1.93	1.36	

these, INST37 was now only marginally significant even though it had previously been more strongly correlated with bad results (RR 1.58 to 1.40, p .0055 to .047). Only the effect of INST60 remained highly significant, its relative risk and p value persisting at about the same level it had reached before. It was clear from these findings that nearly all effects attributable to the delivery site (except INST60) could be accounted for by factors other than the institution itself.

Effects of most of the other intrinsic factors were unchanged. Two showed markedly diminished relative risk. The first of these, SES3 (socioeconomic index 25-34), became statistically significant (RR 1.47 to 1.28, p .022 to .056); the other, SMOKE3 (more than 30 cigarettes per day), remained an impressively adverse factor (RR 3.11 to 2.65, p .0031 to .011). Only SES8 (socioeconomic index 75-84), which had not previously been determined to be a meaningful factor in the step-up logistic model of intrinsic variables (see Table 21-9), enhanced its protective effect into the statistically significant range (RR 0.70 to 0.61, p .080 to .023).

Delivery effects were modified to a very limited extent when compared with those seen earlier when the delivery factor effects were weighed without simultaneous consideration of all other relevant variables (see Table 24-5 and 24-9). The effect of FORCEPS3 (class III midforceps at station 0 to +2), for example, was reduced somewhat (RR from 10.88 and 12.07 to 8.65), but it was still impressively adverse and carried about the same level of statistical significance as before (p = .037). FORTRAC2 (difficult forceps traction) slightly increased its adverse impact on offspring relative to data from the prior step-up logistic model (RR 2.06 to 2.16), but with unchanged statistical significance (p = .0067).

The effects of most of the other delivery variables were either unaltered or slightly diminished. In this latter regard, the deleterious effects of INDUCT3 (induction for pregnancy-induced hypertension) on outcome was no longer statistically significant at the 5% probability level (RR 2.79 to 2.15, p .0047 to .053). The same applied to AUGMENT6 (labor augmentation for amnionitis), the effect of which was markedly reduced (RR 8.44 to 3.95, p .0065 to .11). The only delivery variable to have enhanced its impact was BREECH3 (single footling), although the increase was not quite enough to achieve statistical significance (RR 4.47 to 4.99, p .077 to .072).

The same technique was applied to the examination of the results of the full model logistic regression analysis as it reflected the relationship between all the relevant variables and the composite outcome of the offspring of multiparas. The data yielded by this investigation are detailed in Table 25-3. In all, 25 of the 55 variables were determined to have a statistically significant effect at the level of p = .05 or less; 42 were significant at p values between 0.05 and 0.10. Thus, a number of variables which had previously been shown to have a significant impact on outcome when considered only in association with related variables lost their effects by this more critical approach. By examining them in conjunction with the entire set of variables, we found the earlier impact to be dissipated. This again showed how important it was to pursue such sophisticated types of analyses. Much more meaningful results were likely to be derived here as compared with those of studies that fail to account for the confounding effects of other variables.

Among labor progression variables, the results of the logistic regression analysis for the collective set of the four groups of variables for composite outcome in multiparas (Table 25-3) showed little change in the effects that had been demonstrated earlier for some of the variables (see Table 18-11 and 18-13), such as DEC2 (foreshortened deceleration phase). However, there were somewhat reduced effects in SEC2 (short second stage duration) and DESC2 (protracted descent), neither of which was statistically significant any longer.

For adjunctive drugs and anesthesias, the impact of OXYT1 and OXYT3 (oxy-

Table 25-3
Logistic Regression Analysis of All Residual Variables in
Multiparas for Composite Outcome

Variable	Regression Coefficient	Standard Error	t-Statistic	Relative Risk	p-Value
DEC2	0.267	0.133	2.00	1.31	0.048
SEC2	0.042	0.090	0.47	1.04	
DESC2	0.227	0.136	1.67	1.26	
OXYT1	0.219	0.299	0.73	1.25	
OXYT3	0.176	0.207	0.85	1.19	
SPINAL	-0.204	0.134	-1.52	0.82	
PUDEND	0.229	0.101	2.26	1.26	0.026
AGT18	-1.158	1.010	-1.14	0.31	
AGT23	-0.509	0.291	-1.74	0.60	
AGT27	2.488	1.344	1.85	12.04	
INST15	0.464	0.187	2.48	1.59	0.015
INST37	0.286	0.151	1.90	1.33	
INST55	0.291	0.162	1.80	1.34	
INST60	0.566	0.138	4.10	1.76	8.4×10^{-5}
INST71	0.829	0.184	4.51	2.29	1.8×10^{-5}
INST82	-0.200	0.180	-1.11	0.82	
AGE3	-0.216	0.096	-2.26	0.81	0.026
STATUS2	-0.210	0.238	-0.88	0.81	
RACE3	-0.564	0.188	-3.00	0.57	0.0034
PARA2	0.352	0.108	3.27	1.42	0.0015
PABORT1	-0.177	0.103	-1.72	0.84	
PPREM1	0.268	0.096	2.79	1.31	0.0063
HGT2	0.286	0.166	1.73	1.33	
RHSENS	1.105	0.440	2.51	3.02	0.014
PPMR1	1.220	0.676	1.80	3.39	
SES1	0.478	0.180	2.66	1.61	0.0091
SES2	0.227	0.130	1.74	1.25	
SES4	0.251	0.102	2.44	1.28	0.016
VISIT1	0.216	0.088	2.44	1.24	0.016
VISIT4	0.584	0.248	2.36	1.79	0.020
PIH1	0.378	0.201	1.88	1.46	
BW5	-0.214	0.114	-1.88	0.81	
MALE	0.330	0.083	3.99	1.39	0.00013
GRAV6	0.159	0.129	1.24	1.17	
DIS21	-1.051	0.539	-1.95	0.35	0.052
DIS32	0.780	0.409	1.91	2.18	
DIS49	0.859	0.328	2.62	2.36	0.010
DIS74	2.283	1.464	1.56	9.81	
DIS80	1.947	0.744	2.62	7.01	0.010
DIS100	1.048	0.424	2.47	2.85	0.015
DIS103	0.732	0.350	2.09	2.08	0.039
DIS111	1.428	0.805	1.77	4.17	
DIS123	0.400	0.279	1.43	1.49	
DIS126	0.290	0.110	2.64	1.34	0.0096
DIS128	1.510	0.852	1.77	4.53	
SDIS5	0.242	0.151	1.61	1.27	
FORTRAC3	0.047	0.117	0.40	1.05	
INDUCT6	-0.678	0.584	-1.16	0.51	
AUGMENT2	0.637	0.243	2.62	1.89	0.010
BREECH3	1.381	0.750	1.84	3.98	
ROM11	2.809	1.439	1.95	16.59	0.052
DIL3	-0.259	0.143	-1.82	0.77	
STA6	-0.559	0.284	-1.97	0.57	0.050
STA7	-0.272	0.153	-1.78	0.76	
PRES5-8	3.488	1.341	2.60	32.71	0.011

tocin induction and combined induction and augmentation of labor) was markedly diminished (RR 4.15 to 1.25 and 3.13 to 1.19), making variables that were highly significant before quite insignificant now (p .00046 to .47 and .00034 to .40). PUDEND (pudendal block) retained its effect intact both as to magnitude and statistical significance, but the protective effect of SPINAL (spinal anesthesia) was essentially gone (RR 0.75 to 0.82, p .0063 to .13). A similar change was found for AGT27 (antibiotics other than penicillin, Achromycin, streptomycin, and chloramphenicol (Chloromycetin), RR 20.44 to 12.04, p .020 to .085).

Many of the intrinsic variables remained significant influences on outcome at about the same level as before (see Table 21-10). They included INST60, INST71 (the impact of which had actually increased, RR 1.96 to 2.29), RACE3 (other than black or white), AGE3 (25-29 years), PARA2 (grand multipara), PPREM1 (prior premature birth), RHSENS (Rh isoimmunization), SES4 (socioeconomic index 35-44), VISIT1 (< 7 antepartum visits), VISIT4 (17-20 visits), MALE (male infant), DIS21 (active tuberculosis), DIS49 (diabetes mellitus), DIS80 (glomerulonephritis), DIS100 (mental retardation), DIS103 (neurologic disease), and DIS126 (late pregnancy bleeding).

Reduced effects were encountered for SES1 (index < 15, RR 3.46 to 1.61), although this was actually associated with an impressive improvement in the level of statistical significance (p .096 to .0091). The diminished influence of a few intrinsic variables neutralized previous statistical significance; they included INST55, STATUS2 (private patient), SES2 (index 15-24), DIS32 (low serum iron), and DIS128 (hemorrhagic shock).

Only four delivery variables among those previously deemed relevant (see Table 24-10) survived this critical analytical approach, namely AUGMENT2 (labor stimulation for ruptured membranes, RR 1.66 to 1.89), ROM11 (membranes ruptured for more than 36 hours, RR 14.22 to 16.59), STA6 (station +1 at onset of labor, a protective factor), and PRES5-8 (breech, RR 30.17 to 32.71). All of them showed increased effects. The impact of BREECH3 (single footling breech) was reduced somewhat (RR 6.27 to 3.98), and the effects of FORTRAC3 (very difficult forceps traction, RR 3.39 to 1.05) and INDUCT6 (labor induction for amnionitis, RR 1.62 to 0.51) were diminished markedly. Other delivery variables retained about the same relationship they had earlier.

Perinatal Outcome Data

Logistic regression analysis of the full collective set of 52 variables for perinatal outcome in offspring of nulliparas (Table 25-4) yielded 23 factors with significant effects at the 5% probability level and 27 at 10% probability. As with the other logistic models described above, this operation altered the relationship of many of the variables which had previously shown significant adverse or beneficial effects. All labor progression variables, for example, showed reduced neonatal effects, without exception. Diminution in impact had also taken place in the parallel logistic regression analysis involving the composite outcome for offspring of nulliparas (Table 25-2), but the changes seen then were negligible. They were much more impressive here.

The effect of ACT2 (foreshortened active phase duration) was much less than it had been before (see Table 14-10, RR 1.92 to 1.68, p .0034 to .031) and that of ACT3 (prolonged active phase) was even more suppressed (RR 2.12 to 1.57, p .0052 to .057). This trend applied so strongly to SEC2 (foreshortened second stage duration), in fact, that it became quite insignificant (RR 1.40 to 0.97, p .088 to .89). SEC3 (prolonged second stage), which had just managed to achieve statistical significance in the step-up model (see Table 14-3, RR = 1.84, p = .050), was now without any meaningful impact at all (RR = 1.42, p = .34); the same applied to DESC2 (protracted descent), which had fallen short of statistical significance before and was now well outside the range (RR 1.55 to 0.80, p .056 to

353

Table 25-4
Logistic Regression Analysis of All Residual Variables in
Nulliparas for Perinatal Outcome

Variable	Regression Coefficient	Standard Error	t-Statistic	Relative Risk	p-Value
ACT2	0.517	0.236	2.19	1.68	0.031
ACT3	0.452	0.236	1.92	1.57	
SEC2	-0.032	0.223	-0.14	0.97	
SEC3	0.353	0.370	0.95	1.42	
DESC2	-0.225	0.328	-0.69	0.80	
OXYT2	0.476	0.227	2.09	1.61	0.039
SPINAL	-0.276	0.231	-1.19	0.76	
PARAC	0.715	0.358	1.99	2.04	0.047
GAS2	0.606	0.253	2.39	1.83	0.019
GAS3	0.719	0.403	1.78	2.05	
IVD1	1.220	0.524	2.33	3.39	0.022
AGT1	0.407	0.234	1.74	1.50	
AGT22	1.825	1.013	1.80	6.20	
AGT26	-4.987	4.402	-1.13	0.01	
INST05	-0.256	0.297	-0.86	0.77	
INST45	0.673	0.338	1.99	1.96	0.048
RACE2	0.204	0.211	0.97	1.23	
POND2	0.390	0.275	1.42	1.48	
SES3	0.592	0.260	2.28	1.81	0.025
SES4	0.896	0.233	3.85	2.45	0.00021
SES8	0.691	0.343	2.01	1.99	0.046
SES9	-0.693	0.561	-1.24	0.50	
MALE	0.693	0.195	3.55	2.00	0.00059
SMOKE2	0.871	0.400	2.18	2.39	0.032
WTGAIN1	1.075	0.313	3.43	2.93	0.00088
WTGAIN4	0.431	0.278	1.55	1.54	
LGA	0.838	0.322	2.60	2.31	0.011
GDEL4	0.497	0.211	2.35	1.64	0.021
DIS63	3.047	1.169	2.61	21.05	0.010
DIS74	2.163	1.951	1.11	8.70	
DIS86	0.598	0.455	1.31	1.82	
DIS94	-5.821	6.620	-0.88	0.00	
DIS97	1.082	0.414	2.62	2.95	0.010
DIS100	2.573	0.651	3.95	13.10	0.00015
DIS107	3.419	1.194	2.86	30.54	0.0052
DIS140	2.110	0.808	2.61	8.25	0.010
FORTRAC1	-0.290	0.232	-1.25	0.75	
FORTRAC3	1.099	0.839	1.31	3.00	
FORAPP1	-0.315	0.243	-1.30	0.73	
FORROT2	2.113	0.874	2.42	8.27	0.017
FORROT3	0.244	2.725	0.09	1.28	
INDUCT3	1.193	0.604	1.98	3.30	0.049
INDUCT6	1.126	0.803	1.40	3.08	
AUGMENT6	0.743	1.218	0.61	2.10	
AUGMENT9	1.490	1.477	1.01	4.44	
AUGMENT10	-0.072	0.389	-0.19	0.93	
BREECH3	1.926	1.422	1.36	6.86	
CONTROL2	0.601	0.514	1.17	1.82	
FUNDAL2	0.704	0.297	2.37	2.02	0.020
FUNDAL3	0.508	0.487	1.04	1.66	
PRES3	0.582	0.287	2.03	1.79	0.044
PRES4	0.438	0.287	1.53	1.55	

.49).

Some of the previously described drug effects were also markedly reduced; others were augmented. Those undergoing reduction in adverse effects were: OXYT2 (oxytocin stimulation of labor, see Table 18-10, RR 1.94 to 1.61, p .00085 to .039), GAS2 (RR 2.17 to 1.83, p .0012 to .019), GAS3 (RR 2.69 to 2.05, p .0096 to .077), and AGT22 (Apresoline, RR 8.41 to 6.20, p .056 to .074). SPINAL (spinal anesthesia) showed a marked reduction in its ostensibly protective effect (RR 0.58 to 0.76, p .010 to .24). This alteration was similar to that encountered earlier for the composite outcome data in nulliparas (see Table 25-2). A somewhat enhanced effect was seen for PARAC (paracervical block, RR 1.83 to 2.04, p .056 to .047); this applied to a degree to IVD1 (intravenous anesthesia, RR 2.99 to 3.39, p .017 to .022) as well.

The intrinsic variables also showed a range of effect, mostly in the form of reductions. Almost all institutional impact vanished, including INST05 (see Table 21-11, RR 0.61 to 0.77, p .070 to .39) and INST45 (see Table 21-7, RR 2.21 to 1.96, p .022 to .048). The minimal effect of RACE2 (black) disappeared altogether (RR 1.59 to 1.23, p .098 to .33). A similar trend was seen with SES8 (socioeconomic index 75-84, RR 2.45 to 1.99, p .031 to .046) and SES9 (index 85+, RR 0.40 to 0.50, p .094 to .22). The adverse impact of SMOKE2 (smoking for 10 years or more) persisted, but at a lower level of impact (RR 3.46 to 2.39, p .0025 to .032). The same pertained for the continuing effect of GDEL4 (delivery beyond 41 weeks, RR 1.92 to 1.64, p .0022 to .021). WTGAIN1 (< 11 lb gain), by contrast, increased its effect on the infant (RR 2.49 to 2.93, p .0037 to .00088).

Among illnesses affecting gravidas, there was an impressive downward trend for DIS74 (syphilis) which had previously been shown to be a particularly strong adverse effect (RR = 41.49, p = .034); this was markedly reduced now and no longer statistically significant (RR = 8.70, p = .27). A similar trend, although not so clear-cut,

was found for DIS89 (pyelonephritis, RR 2.11 to 1.82, p .094 to .19). Enhanced effects were seen for DIS97 (other gynecologic disorders, RR 2.49 to 2.95, p .026 to .010), DIS107 (cholecystitis, RR 21.06 to 30.54, p .014 to .0052), and DIS140 (parasitic disease, RR 6.06 to 8.24, p .025 to .010).

The effects of the delivery variables were generally quite reduced relative to those encountered for the same factors when they had been studied by this analytical technique, but without taking any other variable into account (see Tables 24-7 and 24-11). The most impressive reductions were found for FORROT3 (very difficult forceps rotation), AUGMENT6 and AUGMENT9 (labor stimulation for amnionitis and placenta previa, respectively), all of which became statistically insignificant under this form of close scrutiny. The previously encountered strong impact for FORROT3 was no longer apparent (RR 5.41 to 1.28), although that for FORROT2 remained almost the same as it had been before (RR 9.36 to 8.27) and actually improved its degree of statistical significance (p .045 to .017). Both AUGMENT6 and AUGMENT9 were still associated with high relative risks, but were nevertheless obviously no longer significant (RR = 2.10, p = .54 for AUGMENT6; RR = 4.44, p = .31 for AUGMENT9).

Other delivery variables were less affected by the process, although a number crossed from levels of statistical significance to insignificance, including FORTRAC3 (very difficult forceps traction, RR 5.41 to 3.00), INDUCT6 (induction for amnionitis, RR 5.04 to 3.08), AUGMENT10 (enhancement for arrested labor, RR 1.91 to 0.93), CONTROL2 (uncontrolled delivery, RR 2.26 to 1.82), FUNDAL2 (moderate Kristeller pressure, RR 2.29 to 2.02), FUNDAL3 (strong pressure, RR 2.63 to 1.66), and PRES3 (occiput posterior, RR 1.97 to 1.79). Only BREECH3 (single footling) enhanced its effect, but it did not reach a statistically significant level (RR 5.73 to 6.86).

When the perinatal outcome data for offspring of multiparas were studied in the same way, the results of the logistic regression analysis for the full set of collective variables revealed only 23 of the original 57 factors to have retained their significant effects at the 5% probability level and only 28 at the 10% level (Table 25-5). The list of five labor progression variables was reduced to two, namely LAT3 and ACT3 (prolonged latent and active phase durations, respectively). DESC2 (protracted descent), which had previously proved to have a highly significant adverse effect (see Table 14-14), was no longer deleterious (RR 3.64 to 1.20, p 3.5×10^{-9} to .58). The effect of ARRS3 (arrest of descent) was similarly diminished (RR 2.88 to 1.63, p .0038 to .12).

Adjunctive drugs and anesthesias were almost totally without residual influence in this analysis, except for SPINAL (spinal anesthesia), which actually enhanced its previously detected marginally protective effect (see Table 18-15, RR 0.70 to 0.47, p .081 to .0069). Drugs that had shown strong effect earlier, such as OXYT1 (oxytocin for labor induction), OXYT3 (combined induction and augmentation), and GAS2 (continuous administration of inhalation anesthesia), were now shown to have negligible effect. Others retained some of their prior effects, but were not in the statistically significant range any longer, particularly AGT8 (streptomycin) and AGT27 (other antibiotics).

Many of the intrinsic variables were essentially unaffected by this close scrutiny (see Table 21-12). They included INST31 (enhanced protective effect, RR 0.35 to 0.20), INST71, MARIT5 (divorced), RACE3 (other than black or white), RHSENS (Rh disease, reduced effect but nonetheless still quite significant, RR 9.77 to 5.71), PIH1 (diastolic hypertension only), MALE (male infant), DIS37 (anemia responsive to iron therapy), and DIS80 (glomerulonephritis, markedly augmented effect, RR 28.54 to 40.48).

The effects of others were found to have been reduced to a statistically insignificant level, such as PARA2 (grand multipara), HGT2 (short stature), VAGBLD (early bleeding), VISIT4 (17-20 antepartum visits), DIS38 (sicklemia), and DIS49 (diabetes mellitus). The effect of DIS15 (active tuberculosis) was also reduced so that it was no longer statistically significant, but it retained a large magnitude of effect nonetheless (RR 16.60 to 9.78), as did DIS128 (hemorrhagic shock, RR 18.00 to 6.34) and DIS130 (supine hypotension, RR 6.44 to 4.91).

Contrary to the markedly reduced correlation of delivery factor effects with composite outcome (see above), the results for perinatal outcome showed that many delivery variables retained their deleterious effects. Whereas the magnitude of these effects may have been somewhat reduced in nearly every case (see Table 24-12), most of the delivery factors investigated by logistic regression analysis remained quite significantly related to adverse outcome.

In a few instances, the impact was actually augmented, namely for FORTRAC3 (very difficult forceps traction, RR 5.94 to 8.24, p .062 to .036), FORROT2 (difficult forceps rotation, RR 3.03 to 3.42, p .012 to .017), and CONTROL2 (uncontrolled delivery of head, RR 3.02 to 3.30, p .0045 to .0055). Those still significant even though associated with reduced relative risks were FORROT3 and FORROT4 (very difficult and failed forceps rotations, respectively), INDUCT4 (induction for diabetes), AUGMENT6 and AUGMENT10 (labor stimulation for amnionitis and arrested labor), BRDELIV3 (breech extraction), CSVAG (cesarean section after failed attempt to deliver vaginally), and SHOULD (shoulder dystocia). The high relative risks for each of these delivery variables, none of which was below 3.30, were worthy of emphasis.

Among those falling below acceptable significance levels were such previously relevant delivery factors as FORAPP1 (forceps application of average difficulty), INDUCT5 and INDUCT6 (induction for Rh disease and uterine infection), PRES3 (occiput posterior position), and ABRUPT (abruptio placentae). FORTRAC2 (difficult forceps traction), although still associated

Table 25-5
Logistic Regression Analysis of All Residual Variables in
Multiparas for Perinatal Outcome

Variable	Regression Coefficient	Standard Error	t-Statistic	Relative Risk	p-Value
LAT2	0.048	0.258	0.19	1.05	
LAT3	0.573	0.249	2.30	1.77	0.024
ACT3	0.874	0.448	1.95	2.40	0.052
DESC2	0.184	0.331	0.56	1.20	
ARRS3	0.490	0.311	1.58	1.63	
OXYT1	0.277	0.521	0.53	1.32	
OXYT2	-0.057	0.273	-0.21	0.94	
OXYT3	0.043	0.391	0.11	1.04	
SPINAL	-0.763	0.276	-2.76	0.47	0.0069
GAS2	0.266	0.221	1.21	1.30	
AGT8	1.435	1.002	1.43	4.20	
AGT23	-0.556	0.574	-0.97	0.57	
AGT27	2.796	1.727	1.62	16.38	
INST31	-1.609	0.654	-2.46	0.20	0.016
INST71	0.874	0.383	2.28	2.40	0.025
MARIT5	1.140	0.440	2.59	3.13	0.011
RACE3	0.818	0.266	3.08	2.27	0.0027
PARA2	0.273	0.229	1.19	1.31	
PPREM1	0.354	0.201	1.76	1.42	
HGT2	0.295	0.301	0.98	1.34	
RHSENS	1.742	0.662	2.63	5.71	0.0099
VAGBLD	0.588	0.311	1.89	1.80	
VISIT4	0.542	0.437	1.24	1.72	
PIH1	0.794	0.362	2.19	2.21	0.031
MALE	0.393	0.182	2.17	1.48	0.032
GRAV6	0.325	0.265	1.23	1.38	
DIS15	2.281	1.552	1.47	9.78	
DIS37	0.509	0.240	2.12	1.66	0.036
DIS38	0.968	0.598	1.62	2.63	
DIS49	1.221	0.665	1.84	3.39	
DIS80	3.701	0.859	4.31	40.48	3.8×10^{-5}
DIS126	0.345	0.229	1.50	1.41	
DIS128	1.847	1.124	1.64	6.34	
DIS130	1.592	0.953	1.67	4.91	
SDIS5	0.442	0.287	1.54	1.56	
FORTRAC2	0.981	1.009	0.97	2.67	
FORTRAC3	2.109	0.989	2.13	8.24	0.036
FORAPP1	-0.402	0.345	-1.16	0.67	
FORAPP3	1.567	1.069	1.47	4.79	
FORROT2	1.230	0.506	2.43	3.42	0.017
FORROT3	1.424	0.680	2.09	4.15	0.038
FORROT4	2.458	1.175	2.09	11.68	0.039
INDUCT4	2.067	0.873	2.37	7.90	0.020
INDUCT5	0.955	0.905	1.05	2.60	
INDUCT6	0.856	0.672	1.27	2.35	
AUGMENT6	3.915	0.899	4.35	50.15	3.3×10^{-5}
AUGMENT10	1.307	0.461	2.83	3.70	0.0056
BRDELIV3	2.117	0.700	3.02	8.31	0.0032
CONTROL2	1.195	0.421	2.84	3.30	0.0055
CSVAG	3.086	1.111	2.78	21.88	0.0065
PRES1	-5.343	7.086	-0.75	0.00	
PRES2	0.516	0.285	1.81	1.67	
PRES3	-0.999	0.627	-1.60	0.37	
PRES5-8	1.209	0.953	1.27	3.35	
PROLAP	0.776	0.559	1.39	2.17	
ABRUPT	0.750	0.515	1.45	2.12	
SHOULD	2.670	0.581	4.59	14.44	1.3×10^{-5}

with a high relative risk, was no longer statistically significant (RR 6.07 to 2.67, p .030 to .33). The same applied for FORAPP3 (very difficult forceps application, RR 8.53 to 4.79, p .0089 to .14) and PRES5-8 (breech presentation, RR 5.96 to 3.35, p .048 to .21).

Summary of Results for
Aggregated Variables

The foregoing logistic regression analyses have weighed the effects of all residual risk variables, considered together as an aggregated group but still stratified as to parity (nulliparas versus multiparas) and assessed according to two different indices of outcome (adverse perinatal versus composite results). The analyses were not precisely parallel because the lists of variables tested in each of the four logistic models were not exactly the same. This came about, as will be recalled, because the risk factors were essentially self-selected for each subset when they met three minimally necessary screening criteria. These criteria consisted of (1) the demonstration of significantly adverse or beneficial outcome by nonparametric bivariate Freeman-Tukey analysis, (2) nonredundant informational content as shown by cluster analysis, and

(3) further documentation of significant residual impact when tested by a logistic regression model consisting of all related factors from the specific labor, drug, intrinsic, or delivery variable group.

Among the many residual variables tested in each of the four parallel logistic regression analyses, a total of 86 were determined to be significant at the 10% probability level in at least one model and 75 at the 5% level (Table 25-6). These included 36 from the nulliparous-composite outcome group, 24 from the corresponding multiparous data, 27 from the nulliparous-perinatal outcome, and 22 from the remaining multiparous group. Since these add to 109, it must follow that many were shared between groups.

Only one variable was found to have significantly adverse relationships to outcome in all four analyses, namely MALE (male infant); the degree of statistical significance ranged from p = .032 in the multiparous-perinatal outcome group to p = 2.1 x 10^{-5} in the nulliparous-composite outcome series. The only factor showing significance in three logistic models was RACE3 (race other than black or white), but the results were inconsistent in that there were protective effects in both composite outcome analyses (p .00077 and .00013 for nulliparas

Table 25-6
Significant Residual Variables by Logistic Regression Analysis*

Variable		Composite Outcome		Perinatal Outcome	
		Nulliparas	Multiparas	Nulliparas	Multiparas
LAT3	Prolonged latent				1.77A
ACT2	Short active	1.29A		1.68A	
ACT3	Prolonged active			1.57	2.40
DESC3	Precipitate descent	0.71a			
OXYT2	Oxytocin augmentation			1.61A	
SPINAL	Spinal anesthesia				0.47b
GAS2	Continuous gas	1.39A		1.83A	
GAS3	Intermittent and continuous gas	1.61		2.05	
PUDEND	Pudendal block		1.26A		
PARAC	Paracervical block			2.04A	
IVD1	Intravenous anesthesia			3.39A	
AGT16	Vistaril	2.02A			
AGT24	Oxytocin	2.30A			
INST15	Institution 15		1.59A		
INST31	Institution 31				0.20a

358

Code	Description				
INST37	Institution 37	1.41A	1.33		
INST45	Institution 45			1.96A	
INST60	Institution 60	2.26F	1.76F		
INST71	Institution 71		2.29F		2.40A
MARIT5	Divorced				3.13A
RACE3	Other race	0.48d	0.57c		2.27C
AGE3	Age 25-29 yr.		0.81a		
PARA2	Grand multipara		1.42C		
POND2	Obese	1.46A			
WTGAIN1	Gain < 11 lb.			2.93D	
WTGAIN4	Gain 39 lb.+	1.38A			
WTGAIN5	Gain 48 lb.+	2.03C			
SES1	Index < 15		1.61B		
SES3	Index 25-34	1.28		1.81A	
SES4	Index 35-44		1.28A	2.45E	
SES8	Index 75-84	0.61a		1.99A	
SES9	Index 85+	0.27b			
BW2	2750-2999 g.	1.34A			
MALE	Male infant	1.55F	1.39E	2.00D	1.48A
SMOKE2	Duration 10+ yr.			2.39A	
SMOKE3	>1½ packs	2.65A			
VISIT1	< 7 visits		1.24A		
VISIT4	17-20 visits		1.79A		
RHSENS	Rh disease		3.02A		5.71B
LGA	Macrosomia			2.31A	
GDEL'4	>41 weeks		1.64A		
DIS37	Response to iron				1.66A
DIS48	Blood dyscrasia	16.62B			
DIS49	Diabetes mellitus		2.36B		
DIS63	Hyperthyroidism	4.32		21.05B	
DIS80	Glomerulonephritis		7.01B		40.48F
DIS87	GU tumor	52.44B			
DIS97	Other gyn disease			2.95B	
DIS100	Mental retardation	9.73F		13.10E	
DIS103	Neurological disease		2.08A		
DIS107	Cholecystitis			30.54B	
DIS111	Colitis, ileitis	11.17B	4.17		
DIS126	Late bleeding		1.34B		
DIS140	Parasitic infection			8.25B	
FORCEPS3	Class III forceps	8.65A			
FORAPP1	Application average	0.75a			
FORTRAC2	Traction difficult	2.16B			
FORTRAC3	Very difficult traction				8.24A
FORROT2	Rotation difficult			8.27A	3.42A
FORROT3	Very difficult rotation				4.15A
FORROT4	Failed rotation				11.68A
INDUCT3	Induction for PIH	2.15		3.30A	
INDUCT4	Induction for diabetes				7.90A
AUGMENT2	Stimulation for ROM		1.89B		
AUGMENT6	Amnionitis				50.15F
AUGMENT10	Arrested labor				3.70B
BREECH3	Single footling	4.99	3.98		
BRDELIV3	Extraction				8.31C
CONTROL2	Uncontrolled				3.30B
FUNDAL2	Moderate pressure	1.48A		2.02A	
FUNDAL3	Strong pressure	1.59B			
PROLAP	Prolapsed cord	2.71A			
SHOULD	Shoulder dystocia				14.44F
CSVAG	Failed delivery				21.88B
ROM11	Prolonged ROM	13.52	16.59		
PRES3	Occiput posterior			1.79A	
PRES5-8	Breech		32.71A		

* Relative risk shown. Probability code: A 0.05, B 0.01, C 0.005, D 0.001, E 0.0005, F 0.0001 or less; lower case protective, upper case adverse. Variables with no p-values at or below 0.05 have been suppressed; those with two or more below 0.10 are retained.

and multiparas, respectively) but adverse effects in the multiparous-perinatal data (p = .0027). These very significant but paradoxical results may be explained by a severely deleterious perinatal effect counterbalanced by a combination of the "cleansing effect" of a relatively high mortality rate—these individuals no longer being available for later assessment—followed by good late results.

In addition, 17 variables had significant effects in two of the analyses. In three of them (ACT3, GAS3, and ROM11), neither analysis yielded p values of .05 or less and in three others (SES3, DIS63, and INDUCT3), only one result was significant at the 5% level. This left ten in which both results were statistically significant and mutually supportive plus one in which they were both significant but inconsistent. This last variable was SES8 (socioeconomic index 75-84) with a protective effect in the nulliparous-composite data (p = .023) and an adverse effect in the nulliparous-

perinatal model (p = .046). Among the remaining 67 variables, 58 were significant at p = .05 or less; nine were protective (seven significantly so at $p < .05$) and 58 were adverse (51 with $p < .05$).

These 86 identified risk variables included four from the original master group of labor progression factors, 12 from the adjunctive drug and anesthesia group, 45 from among the intrinsic factors, and 25 from the delivery variable series. They constituted the residual list of variables to be studied further in regard to their impact on offspring from among the 129 left from all foregoing analyses of the subsets. At this point, relative ranking was in order for purposes of developing a score that would permit us to scale the variables so that they could be meaningfully compared. This was expected to provide a means for obtaining reliable measures of the relative risks of both the variables and various constellations of them.

CHAPTER 26

Ranking by Standardized Coefficient

Summary

In order to quantitate relative risk in a meaningful way, identified risk variables were examined by use of the standardized coefficient, a product of the logistic regression coefficient and the standard deviation of the variable mean. Aggregated variables were ranked according to the magnitude and sign of the standardized coefficient for both composite and perinatal adverse outcomes separately for nulliparas and multiparas. Comparison of ranking sequences showed good correspondence between groups. Parity subgroups were coalesced; all intrinsic variables were tabled for later study; a number of other variables were reintroduced to ensure against inappropriate deletion by prior confounding effects. The 112 remaining labor-delivery variables were subjected to logistic regression analysis; 11 were found significant for their effect on composite outcome and 26 for perinatal outcome. They were then ranked in order by standardized coefficient with good rank correlation.

Quantitation of the relative risk of any given variable was to be pursued next. Whereas rate ratios as estimators of relative risk had been obtained for all variables and their statistical significance ascertained, it was appreciated that the information thus derived was not truly comparable. Rate ratios based on different sample sizes, for example, may vary widely; those based on small numbers of cases are particularly unstable vis-à-vis their degree of reliability.

361

This makes comparisons suspect and the calculation of relative risk dubious. It was essential, therefore, to achieve comparability. To this end, we sought a method for scoring the impact of the variables on the basis of their position on a scale of effects ranging from very bad to very good. Assigning a uniform index of badness or goodness for this purpose, however, required transforming the risk indicator to a measurement that was homogeneously applicable and comparable among variables in terms of the importance of the contribution of each variable to the logistic probability (that is, risk).

The standardized coefficient is one such index. It is a signed (plus for adverse, minus for protective) but dimensionless quantity—that is, a pure number devoid of any unitage—obtained as a product of the multiplication of the logistic regression coefficient and the standard deviation of the variable itself. Thus, it provides a measure of the effect weighted according to both the frequency and distribution of the variable. We must stress that the standardized coefficient should not be misinterpreted as a true reflection or estimate of the relative risk of the variable. It merely serves for ranking to permit scoring the variables in an acceptable and logical manner.

Once the standardized coefficient has been obtained for each variable, all variables can be ranked in order from the largest positive value (most important adverse contributor to the logistic probability) to the largest negative value (most important beneficial contributor). Those falling midway can be said to have contributed least. The ranking order will allow a scale to be developed from the logistic function. In this way, a meaningful calculation of relative risk could be achieved for all items situated at any point along the scale.

Ranking Sequence for Collected Variables

Accordingly, the four groups of data, as formulated and assessed in chapter 25,

were re-examined. All variables were studied in each group, inclusive of those not previously determined to have statistically significant effects on outcome by logistic regression analysis (although they had been flagged earlier as potentially significant by bivariate analysis). This was done to give a more realistic overview of their relative standings on the full scale of effect without excluding those at the center of the spectrum where neither adverse nor beneficial impact is likely to be found. It was clear, of course, that many of those previously found to have little or no influence on the infant were truly neutral in regard to outcome—that is, their effect was not dissimilar from that expected for the population at large. Alternatively, some may actually have had some effect on outcome, but their effect was not capable of statistical substantiation because of the small numbers of cases exhibiting the variable.

Composite Outcome

Standardized coefficients were calculated for all 54 variables previously addressed in regard to composite outcome results in offspring of nulliparas (see Table 25-2). The variables were then ranked according to the magnitude and sign of their standardized coefficient (Table 26-1). The coefficients ranged from +0.220 to -0.396. They were concentrated between 0.114 and 0.040. This interval encompassed 38 or 70.4% of the variables under consideration, even though it occupied only 12.0% of the range of coefficients. Of the 16 variables falling outside this grouping, only four were located at the upper end of the scale, indicating a markedly skewed distribution. This was verified by the aforementioned concentration falling far from the center of the range (-0.088), by the observation that the mean (0.039 ± 0.105 SD) was distant from the modal (0.05) and median values (0.07), and by the large moment coefficients of skewness (-2.094) and kurtosis (8.199). It was clear that this distribution was not normal (gaussian); that it was probably bimodal did not become apparent until additional analyses were evolved (see below).

The three variables that fell above the eccentrically clustered group were MALE (male infant), INST60 (hospital 60), and DIS100 (mental retardation in the mother). Of these, DIS100 had the largest regression coefficient (2.275), an indication that its impact on outcome was likely to be strong.

MALE, by contrast, had a rather small regression coefficient (0.440), but the standard deviation was the largest encountered in the entire series (0.500). Given that the variable MALE could offer only two coding options (yes, no or 0,1) and that the offspring fell into each of them about equally often, it must follow that the stand-

Table 26-1
Rank Order of Aggregated Variables as Related to
Composite Outcome in Nulliparas

Rank Order	Variable Code	Regression Coefficient	Standard Deviation	Standardized Coefficient*
1	MALE	0.440	0.500	0.200
2	INST60	0.817	0.216	0.177
3	DIS100	2.275	0.059	0.133
4	GAS2	0.330	0.345	0.114
5	BW2	0.289	0.388	0.112
6	FUNDAL3	0.461	0.240	0.111
7	FORTRAC2	0.769	0.136	0.105
8	POND2	0.376	0.272	0.102
9	ACT2	0.257	0.391	0.100
10	FUNDAL2	0.392	0.239	0.094
11	SMOKE3	0.976	0.092	0.090
12	INST37	0.346	0.254	0.088
13	AGT16	0.701	0.124	0.087
14	STA1-2	0.306	0.278	0.085
15	PROLAP	0.996	0.085	0.085
16	WTGAIN4	0.320	0.264	0.085
17	SES3	0.249	0.330	0.082
18	DIS48	2.810	0.027	0.077
19	INST31	0.383	0.200	0.077
20	AGT24	0.832	0.092	0.076
21	GAS2	0.479	0.156	0.075
22	INDUCT6	1.044	0.070	0.073
23	DIS111	2.414	0.030	0.072
24	INDUCT3	0.765	0.090	0.069
25	DIS87	3.960	0.017	0.068
26	LGA	0.290	0.234	0.068
27	INST45	0.322	0.207	0.067
28	GRAV3	0.874	0.075	0.066
29	ACT13	0.554	0.115	0.064
30	FORCEPS3	2.157	0.024	0.053
31	BREECH3	1.607	0.032	0.052
32	INST71	0.234	0.221	0.052
33	DIS63	1.463	0.034	0.051
34	FORTRAC3	0.917	0.053	0.049
35	INDUCT1	0.381	0.125	0.048
36	AUGMENT6	1.373	0.035	0.047
37	ROM11	2.604	0.017	0.045
38	ACT3	0.118	0.378	0.045
39	FORROT2	0.238	0.176	0.042
40	FORROT1	0.129	0.319	0.041
41	AGT25	0.448	0.090	0.040
42	AGT2	0.084	0.229	0.019
43	WTGAIN2	0.709	0.170	0.012
44	SPINAL	0.022	0.491	0.011
45	DESC2	0.028	0.325	0.009

46	MARIT1	-0.091	0.452	-0.041
47	PWGT1	-0.650	0.155	-0.101
48	INST05	-0.241	0.436	-0.105
49	DESC3	-0.350	0.387	-0.135
50	FORAPP1	-0.286	0.494	-0.141
51	SES8	-0.495	0.287	-0.142
52	RACE3	-0.733	0.297	-0.217
53	MARIT5	-5.659	0.044	-0.249
54	SES9	-1.318	0.301	-0.396

* Standardized coefficient is obtained by multiplying the standard deviation of the variable by its logistic regression coefficient; this dimensionless quantity is especially useful for comparative ranking purposes.

ard deviation will be 0.500 in all instances.* The large standard deviation gives appropriate weight to the standardized coefficient of this variable (the product of the standard deviation and the regression coefficient) as a proper reflection of the population impact or relative importance of the variable in the study data. This is not meant to imply that the variable has no adverse effect on outcome for any given offspring; it is merely intended to caution against relying on its standing in the ranking sequence as necessarily reflecting its risk status to the individual rather than to the population as a whole.

At the protective end of the scale were seven variables that might be considered outliers on the distribution pattern because their standardized coefficients fell so far below the central tendency. They were, in order, SES9 (socioeconomic index 85+), MARIT5 (divorced), RACE3 (race other than black or white), SES8 (index 75-84), FORAPP1 (forceps application of average difficulty), DESC3 (precipitate descent), INST05 (hospital 05), and PWGT1 (prepregnancy weight 175 lb or more). Both FORAPP1 and INST05 had relatively small

regression coefficients (-0.286 and -0.241, respectively) counterbalanced by quite large standard deviations (0.494 and 0.436). The latter figures reflected the high relative frequencies of cases to which these variables applied. FORAPP1, for example, was coded in 13,596 NCPP records, representing 40.0% of the population or 92.2% of forceps applications (see Table 22-6); 24.6% of study gravidas delivered at INST05. Once again, any protective or beneficial effect these two variables might exert on outcome has to be weighed appropriately because the standardized coefficients have been influenced by the relatively large magnitude of these standard deviations.

The standardized coefficients were also calculated for the 55 variables previously studied in regard to the corresponding data for composite outcome in multiparas (see Table 25-3). They were ranked accordingly and found to be distributed over a much narrower range from +0.165 to -0.171 (Table 26-2). As with the nulliparous data, the distribution was not normal (gaussian), the mean (0.035 ± 0.079) falling somewhat below the modal (0.06) and median figures (0.06). The moment coefficients of skewness (-0.804) and kurtosis (2.776) were not so strongly indicative of an unusually skewed distribution as they had been earlier.

When the distribution of the standardized coefficients was plotted (Figure 26-1), however, it became very obvious that we were dealing here with a bimodal pattern. Two clearly distinctive groups of standardized coefficients surfaced, namely those in

*Standard deviation SD = $\{\Sigma d^2/n\}^{1/2}$ or SD = $\{n_1 \cdot n_0/n_0 + n_1\}^{1/2}$, where all values are either 0 or 1, n_0 is the total number of cases coded 0 and n_1 is the number coded 1. For the special case in which there are the same number of code 0 and code 1 cases, $n_0 = n_1$. The mean, m = $n_1/n_0 + n_1$, would then be 0.5 and each value must therefore deviate from the mean by 0.5. This yields d^2 = 0.25 for all cases. For any series of cases thus constituted, SD = $\{nd^2/n\}^{1/2} = \{d^2\}^{1/2}$ or SD = $\{0.25\}^{1/2}$ = 0.5. Alternatively, where $n_0 = n_1$ and n = $n_0 + n_1$, it must follow that $n_0 = n_1 = n/2$; thus, SD = $\{n/4/n\}^{1/2} = \{0.25\}^{1/2}$ = 0.5.

Table 26-2
Rank Order of Aggregated Variables as Related to
Composite Outcome in Multiparas

Rank Order	Variable Code	Regression Coefficient	Standard Deviation	Standardized Coefficient*
1	MALE	0.330	0.500	0.165
2	INST71	0.829	0.199	0.165
3	INST60	0.566	0.271	0.154
4	PARA2	0.352	0.359	0.126
5	PPREM1	0.268	0.402	0.108
6	DIS126	0.290	0.349	0.101
7	AUGMENT2	0.637	0.157	0.100
8	VISIT1	0.216	0.462	0.100
9	SES4	0.251	0.396	0.099
10	PUDEND	0.229	0.424	0.097
11	INST55	0.291	0.332	0.097
12	SES1	0.478	0.196	0.094
13	INST15	0.464	0.198	0.092
14	VISIT4	0.584	0.143	0.084
15	DEC2	0.267	0.301	0.080
16	DIS49	0.859	0.090	0.078
17	INST37	0.286	0.271	0.078
18	RHSENS	1.105	0.068	0.075
19	SES2	0.227	0.309	0.070
20	PIH1	0.378	0.184	0.069
21	HGT2	0.286	0.234	0.066
22	DESC2	0.227	0.291	0.066
23	PRES5-8	3.488	0.019	0.066
24	DIS100	1.048	0.062	0.065
25	DIS103	0.732	0.087	0.064
26	DIS80	1.947	0.033	0.063
27	SDIS5	0.242	0.245	0.059
28	DIS32	0.780	0.074	0.058
29	GRAV1	0.159	0.329	0.052
30	INDUCT6	0.678	0.076	0.051
31	DIS123	0.400	0.121	0.048
32	AGT27	2.488	0.019	0.047
33	DIS111	1.483	0.033	0.047
34	DIS128	1.510	0.031	0.046
35	PPMR1	1.220	0.038	0.046
36	BREECH3	1.381	0.033	0.045
37	ROM11	2.809	0.015	0.043
38	OXYT3	0.176	0.212	0.037
39	DIS75	2.283	0.015	0.035
40	OXYT1	0.219	0.125	0.027
41	FORTRAC3	0.047	0.455	0.021
42	SEC2	0.042	0.500	0.021
43	STATUS2	-0.210	0.255	-0.053
44	INST82	-0.200	0.280	-0.056
45	PABORT1	-0.177	0.426	-0.075
46	BW5	-0.215	0.382	-0.082
47	STA7	-0.272	0.305	-0.083
48	DIL3	-0.259	0.332	-0.086
49	SPINAL	-0.204	0.437	-0.089
50	AGT23	-0.509	0.185	-0.094
51	AGE3	-0.216	0.448	-0.097
52	AGT18	-1.158	0.085	-0.098
53	STA6	-0.559	0.188	-0.105
54	DIS21	-1.051	0.111	-0.117
55	RACE3	-0.564	0.304	-0.171

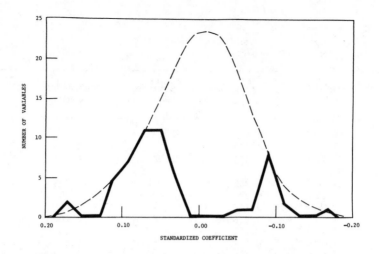

Figure 26-1. Distribution of standardized coefficients for variables based on standard deviation of the variable and the regression coefficent of the logistic regression analysis for the effects of the variable on composite outcome for offspring of multiparas. Bimodal distribution is clearly demonstrated. The broken line completes the normal distribution theoretically achievable by reinserting all deleted "neutral" variables. The horizontal scale is in increments of 0.02.

the positive range from 0.021 to 0.165 and the negative group between -0.053 and -0.171, with none between. That these two groups did not overlap at all was strong evidence of their origin from two distinct populations of variables. The neutral variables that should have been found between them (overlapping both of them to a degree) had been deleted by the foregoing preselection processes. Most of the 2441 variables originally considered for inclusion in this broad investigation had indeed been eliminated by virtue of their apparent lack of any demonstrable effect on outcome.

There were four variables with standardized coefficients outside the coalesced group of adverse variables, specifically MALE (male infant), INST71, INST60 (hospitals 71 and 60), and PARA2 (grand multiparity). The relatively small regression coefficients associated with MALE (0.330) and PARA2 (0.352) were magnified by their large standard deviations (0.500 and 0.359, respectively). At the opposite end of the spectrum, only one variable RACE3 (race

other than black or white), stood apart from the tightly clustered protective group. Its standardized coefficient resulted from a moderately sized regression coefficient coupled with a fairly large standard deviation.

Perinatal Outcome

A similar procedure was carried out for ranking variables according to their perinatal outcome effects. The standardized coefficients were calculated for the 53 variables previously identified as possibly significant for offspring of nulliparas (see Table 25-4). All of them were ranked in descending order according to sign and magnitude (Table 26-3). Coefficients ranged from +0.346 to -0.582, a much wider spectrum than any of the other analyses in this segment of the study. Analogous to the distribution of standardized coefficients for the nulliparous-composite outcome group, the pattern was markedly skewed to the high end of the scale as evidenced by the disparity between mean (0.074 ± 0.158), median

Table 26-3
Rank Order of Aggregated Variables as Related to
Perinatal Outcome in Nulliparas

Rank Order	Variable Code	Regression Coefficient	Standard Deviation	Standardized Coefficient*
1	MALE	0.693	0.500	0.346
2	SES4	0.895	0.355	0.318
3	WTGAIN1	1.075	0.219	0.235
4	GAS2	0.606	0.338	0.205
5	ACT2	0.517	0.394	0.203
6	GDEL4	0.497	0.406	0.202
7	SES8	0.690	0.292	0.201
8	LGA	0.838	0.232	0.195
9	OXYT2	0.476	0.407	0.194
10	SES3	0.592	0.326	0.193
11	ACT3	0.452	0.372	0.168
12	FUNDAL2	0.704	0.238	0.167
13	DIS97	1.082	0.153	0.166
14	PRES2	0.582	0.270	0.157
15	SMOKE2	0.871	0.178	0.155
16	PARAC	0.714	0.216	0.154
17	AGT1	0.407	0.366	0.149
18	INST45	0.673	0.208	0.140
19	DIS100	2.573	0.054	0.139
20	WTGAIN5	0.734	0.168	0.123
21	PRES3	0.438	0.280	0.122
22	DIS140	2.110	0.056	0.118
23	DIS107	3.419	0.034	0.116
24	WTGAIN4	0.431	0.265	0.114
25	IVD1	1.220	0.092	0.112
26	GAS3	0.719	0.155	0.111
27	DIS63	3.047	0.036	0.110
28	INDUCT3	1.193	0.090	0.108
29	POND2	0.390	0.265	0.103
30	RACE2	0.204	0.488	0.100
31	FORROT3	2.113	0.043	0.090
32	DIS86	0.598	0.148	0.088
33	CONTROL2	0.601	0.140	0.084
34	SEC3	0.353	0.224	0.079
35	INDUCT6	1.126	0.070	0.079
36	AGT22	1.825	0.043	0.078
37	FUNDAL3	0.508	0.119	0.061
38	BREECH3	1.926	0.029	0.055
39	FORTRAC3	1.099	0.050	0.055
40	DIS74	2.163	0.018	0.039
41	AUGMENT9	1.490	0.022	0.033
42	AUGMENT6	0.743	0.031	0.023
43	AUGMENT10	0.072	0.222	0.016
44	FORROT2	0.244	0.031	0.008
45	SEC2	-0.032	0.434	-0.014
46	DESC2	-0.225	0.314	-0.071
47	INST05	-0.256	0.440	-0.113
48	SPINAL	-0.276	0.490	-0.135
49	FORTRAC1	-0.290	0.484	-0.140
50	FORAPP1	-0.315	0.496	-0.156
51	SES9	-0.693	0.304	-0.211
52	DIS94	-5.821	0.066	-0.387
53	AGT26	-4.987	0.117	-0.582

(0.11), and modal values (0.11), and by the large moment coefficents of skewness (-1.916) and kurtosis (8.171).

The bimodality of distribution previously seen was also present here, although less clear-cut than before because there were so few protective factors under investigation. Nonetheless, standardized coefficients for all adverse factors except three were clustered between 0.008 and 0.205 (29 were between 0.055 and 0.168), while those relating to six of the nine protective factors fell between -0.071 and -0.211 (four were between -0.113 and -0.156). MALE (male infant), SES4 (socioeconomic index 35-44), and WTGAIN1 (weight gain 11 lb or less) were located in the tail of the distribution at the high end and AGT26 (magnesium sulfate), DIS94 (leiomyomata uteri), and SES9 (index 85+) were found in comparable positions at the low end.

Ranking the variables as related to perinatal outcome of the infants of multiparas followed the same paradigm. It addressed the 57 variables that had been studied as an aggregated group (see Table 25-5) to yield the ordered listing of variables shown in Table 26-4. The standardized coefficients ranged from +0.246 to -0.346 with the principal concentration around the value of 0.11, clustering mainly between 0.034 and 0.167. The mean (0.070 ± 0.117) differed from the modal and median values (0.09) about as expected for the degree of skewness which these distributions were heretofore shown to have. This was confirmed by the sizable moment coefficients of skewness (-2.381) and kurtosis (8.931) associated with these data. Since only six variables showed any degree of protective effect, the aforementioned bimodality of distribution could not be demonstrated well. Standardized coefficients for two factors fell into the high end tail, namely RACE3 (race other than black or white) and MALE (male infant); the three variables set apart at the low end were PRES1 (occiput anterior), INST31 (hospital 31), and SPINAL (spinal anesthesia).

Comparison of Ranking Sequences

The preceding material on rank order of all 137 potential risk variables for the four study groups (consisting of 54, 55, 53, and 57 factors, respectively) is compiled in Table 26-5. A total of 74 of the variables appeared only once. In general, those 63 variables tested in more than one analysis showed rather good consistency to agreement insofar as their relative position in the ranking order was concerned. There were five that were examined in all four studies:

SPINAL (spinal anesthesia)
MALE (male infant)
FORTRAC3 (very difficult forceps traction)
INDUCT6 (induction for infection)
DESC2 (protracted descent)

All but one showed very closely parallel ranks across the four analyses. The exception was DESC2, which was consistent except for the higher (more adverse) ranking associated with composite outcome in multiparas. Nine factors were ranked in three of the four study groups:

ACT3 (prolonged active phase)
GAS2 (continuous inhalation anesthesia)
INST71 (hospital 71)
RACE3 (race other than white or black)
DIS100 (maternal mental retardation)
FORAPP1 (forceps application of average difficulty)
FORROT2 (difficult forceps rotation)
AUGMENT6 (labor stimulation for infection)
BREECH3 (single footling breech)

Complete consistency was found in only two, namely BREECH3 and FORAPP1. Clear inconsistency occurred in only one, RACE3, which was far down the scale (protective) in both composite outcome subseries but at the extreme opposite end (adverse) in the multiparous-perinatal out-

Table 26-4
Rank Order of Aggregated Variables as Related to
Perinatal Outcome in Multiparas

Rank Order	Variable Code	Regression Coefficient	Standard Deviation	Standardized Coefficient
1	RACE3	0.818	0.301	0.246
2	MALE	0.393	0.500	0.196
3	LAT3	0.573	0.301	0.173
4	AUGMENT10	1.307	0.128	0.167
5	INST71	0.874	0.189	0.165
6	SHOULD	2.670	0.061	0.162
7	CONTROL2	1.195	0.134	0.160
8	DIS37	0.509	0.313	0.159
9	MARIT5	1.140	0.137	0.156
10	PIH1	0.794	0.182	0.145
11	PPREM1	0.354	0.402	0.142
12	FORROT2	1.230	0.109	0.134
13	VAGBLD	0.588	0.220	0.130
14	BRDELIV3	2.117	0.061	0.128
15	PRES2	0.516	0.247	0.127
16	DIS80	3.701	0.034	0.125
17	RHSENS	1.742	0.070	0.123
18	DIS126	0.344	0.350	0.121
19	AUGMENT6	3.915	0.030	0.112
20	ACT3	0.490	0.224	0.110
21	SDIS5	0.442	0.245	0.108
22	ARRS3	0.874	0.123	0.108
23	GRAV6	0.324	0.328	0.107
24	INDUCT5	2.067	0.052	0.107
25	DIS49	1.221	0.087	0.106
26	GAS2	0.266	0.380	0.101
27	PRES3	0.999	0.100	0.100
28	PARA2	0.273	0.358	0.098
29	ABRUPT	0.750	0.124	0.093
30	DIS38	0.968	0.095	0.092
31	DIS130	1.592	0.057	0.091
32	FORROT3	1.424	0.063	0.089
33	CSVAG	3.086	0.028	0.085
34	FORROT4	2.458	0.034	0.083
35	FORTRAC3	2.109	0.037	0.079
36	VISIT4	0.542	0.143	0.078
37	PROLAP	0.776	0.090	0.070
38	HGT2	0.295	0.232	0.068
39	INDUCT6	0.856	0.079	0.067
40	FORAPP3	1.567	0.041	0.064
41	AGT8	1.435	0.044	0.063
42	DIS15	2.281	0.025	0.058
43	INDUCT4	0.955	0.060	0.057
44	DIS128	1.847	0.030	0.055
45	AGT27	2.796	0.020	0.055
46	DESC2	0.184	0.285	0.053
47	FORTRAC2	0.981	0.048	0.047
48	PRES5-8	1.209	0.037	0.045
49	OXYT1	0.277	0.124	0.034
50	LAT2	0.048	0.364	0.017
51	OXYT3	0.043	0.214	0.009
52	OXYT2	-0.057	0.333	-0.019
53	AGT23	-0.556	0.187	-0.104
54	FORAPP1	-0.402	0.383	-0.154
55	SPINAL	-0.763	0.440	-0.336
56	INST31	-1.609	0.214	-0.344
57	PRES1	-5.343	0.065	-0.346

Table 26-5
Summary of Ranking Order for Aggregated Variables*

		Composite Outcome		Perinatal Outcome	
		Nulliparas	Multiparas	Nulliparas	Multiparas
LAT2	Short latent phase				50
LAT3	Prolonged latent phase				3
ACT2	Short active phase	9		5	
ACT3	Prolonged active phase	38		11	20
DEC2	Short deceleration phase		15		
SEC2	Short second stage		42	45	
SEC3	Prolonged second stage	17		34	
DESC2	Protracted descent	45	22	46	46
DESC3	Precipitate descent	49			
ARRS3	Arrest of descent				22
SPINAL	Spinal anesthesia	44	49	48	55
GAS2	Continuous gas	4		4	26
GAS3	Intermittent and continuous gas	21		26	
PARAC	Paracervical block			16	
PUDEND	Pudendal block		10		
IVD1	Intravenous anesthesia			25	
OXYT1	Oxytocin induction		40		49
OXYT2	Oxytocin augmentation			9	52
OXYT3	Induction and augmentation		38		51
AGT1	Demerol			17	
AGT2	Nisentil	42			
AGT8	Streptomycin				41
AGT13	Phenobarbital	29			
AGT16	Vistaril	13			
AGT18	Vesprin		52		
AGT22	Apresoline			36	
AGT23	Syntocinon		50		53
AGT24	Oxytocin	20			
AGT25	Sparteine sulfate	41			
AGT26	Morphine sulfate			53	
AGT27	Other antibiotics		32		45
INST05	Institution 05	48		47	
INST15	Institution 15		13		
INST31	Institution 31	19			56
INST37	Institution 37	12	17		
INST45	Institution 45	27		18	
INST55	Institution 55		11		
INST60	Institution 60	2	3		
INST71	Institution 71	32	2		5
INST82	Institution 82		44		
AGE3	Age 25-29 yr.		51		
MARIT1	Unmarried	47			
MARIT5	Divorced	53			9
STATUS2	Private patient		43		
RACE2	Black			30	
RACE3	Other race	52	55		1
GRAV3	Gravida 3	28			
GRAV6	Gravida 6+		29		23
PARA2	Grand multipara		4		28
SES1	Index < 15		12		
SES2	Index 15-24		19		
SES3	Index 25-34			10	
SES4	Index 35-44		9	2	
SES8	Index 75-84	51		7	
SES9	Index 85+	54		51	
VISIT1	< 7 visits		8		
VISIT4	17-20 visits		14		36

370

Code	Description				
BW2	2750–2999 g.	5			
BW5	3500–3749 g.		46		
LGA	Macrosomia	26		8	
MALE	Male infant	1	1	1	2
HGT2	Short stature		21		38
PWGT1	Weight 175+ lb.	47			
POND2	Obesity	8		29	
WTGAIN1	Gain < 11 lb.			3	
WTGAIN4	Gain 39 lb.+	16		24	
WTGAIN5	Gain 48 lb.+	43		20	
GDEL4	Delivery > 41 wk.			6	
VAGBLD	Early pregnancy bleeding				13
SMOKE2	Smoking > 10 yr.			15	
SMOKE3	Smoking > 30 per day	11			
PABORT1	Prior abortion		45		
PPREM1	Prior premature birth		5		11
PPMR1	Prior perinatal death		35		
RHSENS	Rh disease		18		17
PIH1	Diastolic hypertension		20		10
DIS15	Tuberculosis, active				42
DIS21	Tuberculosis, inactive		54		
DIS32	Low serum iron		28		
DIS37	Response to iron				8
DIS38	Sicklemia				30
DIS48	Blood dyscrasia	18			
DIS49	Diabetes mellitus		16		25
DIS63	Hyperthyroidism	33		27	
DIS74	TPI positive			40	
DIS75	Dark field positive		39		
DIS80	Glomerulonephritis		26		16
DIS86	Hematuria			32	
DIS87	GU tumor	25			
DIS94	Leiomyomata			52	
DIS97	Other gyn disorder			13	
DIS100	Mental retardation	3	24	19	
DIS103	Neurological disorder		25		
DIS107	Cholecystitis			23	
DIS111	Colitis, ileitis	23	33		
DIS123	Hydramnios		31		
DIS126	Late pregnancy bleeding		6		18
DIS128	Hemorrhagic shock		34		44
DIS130	Supine hypotension				31
DIS140	Parasitic disease			22	
SDIS5	Venereal diseases		27		21
FORCEPS3	Class III forceps	30			
FORTRAC1	Average forceps traction			49	
FORTRAC2	Difficult traction	9			47
FORTRAC3	Very difficult traction	34	41	39	35
FORAPP1	Average forceps application	50		50	54
FORAPP3	Very difficult application				40
FORROT1	Average forceps rotation	40			
FORROT2	Difficult rotation	39		44	12
FORROT3	Very difficult rotation			31	32
FORROT4	Failed rotation				34
CONTROL2	Uncontrolled delivery			33	7
INDUCT1	Elective induction	35			
INDUCT3	Induction for PIH	24		28	
INDUCT4	Induction for diabetes				43
INDUCT5	Induction for Rh				24
INDUCT6	Induction for infection	22	30	35	39
AUGMENT2	Stimulation for ROM		7		
AUGMENT6	Stimulation for infection	36		42	19
AUGMENT9	Stimulation for previa			41	
AUGMENT10	Stimulation for arrest			43	4
BREECH3	Single footling breech	31	36	38	
BRDELIV3	Breech extraction				14

Code	Description				
FUNDAL2	Moderate fundal pressure	10		12	
FUNDAL3	Strong fundal pressure	6		37	
PROLAP	Cord prolapse	15			37
ROM11	Prolonged membrane rupture	37	37		
SHOULD	Shoulder dystocia				6
ABRUPT	Abruptio placentae				29
CSVAG	Failed vaginal delivery				33
PRES1	Occiput anterior				57
PRES2	Occiput transverse			14	15
PRES3	Occiput posterior			21	27
PRES5-8	Breech presentation		23		48
DIL3	Cervix 3 cm.		48		
STA1-2	Station -1, -2	16			
STA6	Station +1		53		
STA7	Station +2 to +4		47		

* Numbers represent rank order standing of the variable according to the standardized coefficients for the parity-outcome group.

come group. Among the 49 variables assessed in two of the analyses, 29 were ranked quite consistently. Less uniformity was encountered among the remaining 20 variables, but only eight showed rankings that were paradoxically far apart:

OXYT2 (oxytocin augmentation of labor)
INST55 (hospital 55)
MARIT5 (divorced)
SES8 (socioeconomic index 75-84)
FORTRAC2 (difficult forceps traction)
CONTROL2 (uncontrolled delivery of fetal head)
AUGMENT10 (labor stimulation for arrested labor)
FUNDAL3 (strong fundal pressure)

Thus, ranking showed good to excellent correspondence in rank order for 53 variables or 84.1% of the 63 for which it was possible to determine consistency.

Focus on Labor-Delivery Variables

In order to proceed further, two additional modifications were felt needed. The first of these was a reduction in the complexity of subsequent analyses to be accomplished by diminishing the number of data subgroups. To this end, we first undertook to coalesce the index populations into a single large universe of gravidas by undoing the parity stratification. In order to ensure that parity effects, if any, would not be lost, parity was added to the list of possible independent risk variables to be tested. The case mix, previously composed of 6688 nulliparas and 8481 multiparas, now totalled 15,169 in all. The two outcomes were retained for measuring impact on offspring, namely adverse perinatal (death and severe neonatal depression) and composite (perinatal period to seven years) effects.

A second programmatic modification involved altering the relation between groups of variables. To this point, all risk variables were studied in regard to their possible effect on fetal and infant outcome. Despite the fact that the primary objective of this project was to determine the impact of labor and delivery factors on outcome, many prenatal and demographic variables have heretofore been included, with ample justification. However, as detailed in chapter 7, the intrinsic variables (plus others yet to be designated) can instead be considered potential predictors—that is, pre-existing (and potentially predisposing) conditions that might serve to forecast the appearance of those labor and delivery variables which place the offspring at risk in turn. Knowledge about such flagging predictors would help identify the gravida-at-risk.

As a first step, all 45 intrinsic variables were set aside. We also felt it appropriate at this juncture to reintroduce a number of labor and delivery variables that had been discarded earlier. Our intent here was to re-examine these factors one last time in order to provide another opportunity to demonstrate any adverse impact that might have remained undetected by virtue of dilutional or confounding effects. An additional rationalization was to insert some of the neutral factors back into the ranking scale so that the scoring system would be more representative of risks across the spectrum of risk. This could be expected to make calculation of relative risk more meaningful. The 70 variables introduced in this effort are listed in Table 26-6. They consisted principally of items of clinical interest. These were specifically chosen to reflect concerns among practitioners about deleterious effects. Such concerns are generally based on clinical impressions gained by experience. Some of them are widely held and most are incompletely or entirely unsubstantiated.

Logistic Regression Analysis

A logistic model was established for the entire collected series of 112 labor-delivery variables, excluding intrinsic factors but adding parity, as just described. It was applied once to assess the impact on composite outcome and again to measure perinatal outcome effects. As before, the logistic regression analysis was carried out to determine those variables within the model demonstrating significant levels of effect when the effects of all were being considered simultaneously. In all, for composite outcomes, there were 21 showing statistical significance at the 10% level and only 11 at 5% or less (Table 26-7). In ascending order, the latter included:

AUGMENT6 (stimulation of labor for infection)
FORTRAC3 (very difficult forceps traction)
FORTRAC4 (failed forceps traction)
SPINAL (spinal anesthesia, protective)
PROLAP (cord prolapse)

INDUCT3 (induction of labor for PIH)
FUNDAL3 (strong fundal pressure)
FORAPP2 (difficult forceps application)
DESC3 (precipitate descent, protective)
CONTROL3 (forceps control of delivery, protective)
PRES11 (brow presentation)

These findings were somewhat dissimilar from those previously encountered for the more generalized model (see Table 25-6). Seven of the variables had not been determined to be statistically significant in the earlier analyses, namely AUGMENT6, FORTRAC3, FORTRAC4, SPINAL, FORAPP2, CONTROL3, and PRES11, and many of those that had shown significance no longer did. The collapse of the parity stratification appeared to have caused little effect; the independent variable PARITY, introduced here to compensate and test for this effect, yielded almost no contribution to the logistic probability (regression coefficient -0.019, standard error 0.074, t = -0.251, RR = 0.98). Moreover, it will be apparent later (see below) that the standardized coefficient for this factor was essentially zero (-0.0093), indicating its near neutrality in regard to adverse or beneficial impact when all others were weighed concurrently.

The results of prior logistic regression analyses (see Tables 25-2 and 25-3) showed some interesting differences from these results. The very strong effects of a number of intrinsic variables were no longer present, of course, such as the adverse influences of INST60, INST71, MALE, and DIS100 or the protective forces of SES9 and RACE3. ACT2 (foreshortened active phase), previously significant in nulliparas but not in multiparas, failed to achieve statistical significance probably because the parity stratification had been undone. The same applied to DEC2 (short deceleration phase), significant in multiparas earlier, but no longer significant here. DESC3 (precipitate descent), by contrast, retained the statistically significant protective effect it had previously shown in nulliparas only,

Table 26-6
Test Variables for Exploratory Analysis of Labor-Delivery Factors*

Group Designation	Derived from Prior Analyses		Added for Reexamination	
Labor progression	LAT3	LAT2	DESC2	DESC2
	ACT2	DESC2	MAXS2	MAXS3
	ACT3	DEC3	ARRS3	
	DESC3	SEC2	ARRD3	
		SEC3		
Adjunctive drugs	SPINAL	GAS1	AGT18	
	PUDEND	OXYT1	AFT19	
	PARAC	OXYT3	AGT20	
	GAS2	AGT2	AGT23	
	GAS3	AGT6	AGT25	
	IVD1	AGT7	AGT26	
	OXYT2	AGT8	AGT27	
	AGT1			
	AGT13			
	AGT16			
	AGT22			
	AGT24			
Delivery variables	FORCEPS3	FORCEPS1	INDUCT1	BRDELIV1	PRES12
	FORTRAC2	FORCEPS2	INDUCT2	BRDELIV2	REACT1
	FORTRAC3	FORTRAC4	INDUCT5	BRFACH0	REACT2
	FORAPP1	FORAPP2	INDUCT6-9	BRFACH1	REACT3
	FORROT2	FORAPP3	AUGMENT1	BRFACH2	REACT4
	FORROT3	FORAPP4	AUGMENT3	BRFACH3	REACT5
	FORROT4	FORROT1	AUGMENT4	PRES1	ROM7
	CONTROL2	CONTROL1	AUGMENT5	PRES2	ROM8
	FUNDAL2	CONTROL3	AUGMENT11-18	PRES1-4	ROM9
	FUNDAL3	FUNDAL4	BREECH1	PRES9	ROM10
	PROLAP	ABRUPT	BREECH2	PRES10	
	CSVAG	PREVIA	BREECH4	PRES11	
	SHOULDER				
	INDUCT3				
	INDUCT4				
	AUGMENT2				
	AUGMENT6				
	AUGMENT10				
	BREECH3				
	BRDELIV3				
	PRES3				
	PRES5-8				
	ROM11				
	STA1-2				
	STA6				

* Excludes 45 intrinsic factors from the original 86 and adds PARITY as a variable plus 70 additional previously excluded variables for final reconsideration. This yields a total of 112 variables for further study.

Table 26-7
Logistic Regression Analysis of Collected Labor-Delivery Variables
for Composite Outcome*

Variable		Regression Coefficient	Standard Error	t-Statistic	Relative Risk	p-Value
DESC3	Precipitate descent	-0.156	0.074	-2.10	0.86	0.038
SPINAL	Spinal anesthesia	-0.279	0.094	-2.97	0.76	0.0037
AGT16	Vistaril	0.421	0.237	1.78	1.52	0.077
AGT23	Syntocinon	-0.346	0.200	-1.73	0.71	0.087
AGT24	Oxytocin	0.450	0.256	1.76	1.57	0.081
AGT27	Other antibiotics	1.587	0.898	1.77	4.89	0.080
FORTRAC2	Difficult forceps traction	0.511	0.295	1.73	1.67	0.087
FORTRAC3	Very difficult traction	1.159	0.350	3.31	3.19	0.0013
FORTRAC4	Failed traction	1.479	0.478	3.10	4.39	0.0025
FORAPP2	Difficult forceps application	0.263	0.118	2.23	1.27	0.028
FORAPP3	Very difficult application	0.337	0.206	1.64	1.40	0.10
CONTROL3	Forceps control	-0.670	0.341	-1.96	0.51	0.050
FUNDAL2	Moderate fundal pressure	0.239	0.126	1.89	1.27	0.060
FUNDAL3	Strong fundal pressure	0.272	0.120	2.27	1.31	0.025
PROLAP	Prolapsed cord	0.705	0.256	2.76	2.02	0.0069
CSVAG	Failed vaginal delivery	1.019	0.545	1.87	2.77	0.064
SHOULD	Shoulder dystocia	0.614	0.353	1.74	1.85	0.086
INDUCT3	Induction for PIH	0.809	0.343	2.36	2.25	0.020
AUGMENT6	Stimulation for amnionitis	2.458	0.581	4.23	11.68	5.2×10^{-5}
BRDELIV3	Breech extraction	1.678	0.941	1.78	5.36	0.077
PRES11	Brow presentation	1.189	0.607	1.96	3.29	0.050

* Variables with p-values less than 0.10 suppressed. Logistic model comprised 112 labor and delivery variables, excluding intrinsic factors and not stratified for parity; parity was added to the model as a test variable along with a number of other items previously deleted (see text). The test population included the offspring of a total of 15,169 gravidas.

375

although at a rate ratio closer to unity (from 0.71 to 0.86) and a weaker probability level (0.015 to 0.038). SPINAL, which had fallen short of significance in both prior logistic models (marginally in multiparas), was now significantly protective.

Similarly, FORTRAC3 (very difficult forceps traction) was now quite significant even though it had not been able to achieve a comparable level in the antecedent studies, perhaps because the numbers of cases were relatively small. The limitations of small relative frequencies (even within a large study series) undoubtedly also accounted for the impressively adverse effects now shown for FORTRAC4 (failed forceps traction), not previously uncovered (or examined for) in the parity subgroups. Furthermore, the fresh documentation of a significantly deleterious impact from FORAPP2 (difficult forceps application) had not been seen before. The effect of FUNDAL3 (strong fundal pressure), which was demonstrated earlier in nulliparas, was reconfirmed but at moderately reduced levels (RR 1.59 to 1.31, p 0.0089 to .025). The effects of INDUCT3 (induction for PIH) and AUGMENT6 (labor stimulation for infection) were magnified, the former previously showing significance in nulliparas only, the latter in neither parity group.

The results for the same procedure for a model containing all 112 labor-delivery factors as related to perinatal outcome demonstrated 26 variables with significant effects at p = .10 and 19 at p = .05 or less (Table 26-8). Those falling at or below the 5% probability level were (in order):

AUGMENT6 (labor stimulation for infection)
SHOULD (shoulder dystocia)
ABRUPT (abruptio placentae)
FORROT4 (failed forceps rotation)
SPINAL (spinal anesthesia, protective)
FORTRAC3 (very difficult forceps traction)
AGT27 (other antibiotics)
INDUCT6-9 (induction for other indications)

GAS2 (continuous inhalation anesthesia)
AGT1 (Demerol)
AGT22 (Apresoline)
FORTRAC2 (difficult forceps traction)
LAT3 (prolonged latent phase duration)
ACT2 (foreshortened active phase duration)
REACT3 (uterine hypertonus from oxytocin)
FUNDAL2 (moderate fundal pressure)
FUNDAL3 (strong fundal pressure)
FORROT2 (difficult forceps rotation)
CONTROL1 (manual control of head delivery, protective)

Comparison with those variables previously found significant in the model which included the intrinsic factors (see Table 25-6) showed four variables surfacing anew, namely ABRUPT, FORROT4, AGT27, and INDUCT6-9. PARITY was again found to have a negligible effect in the context of this analysis (regression coefficient -0.059, standard error 0.145, t = -0.404, RR = 0.94). As with the logistic model for composite outcome (see above), the standardized coefficient for this variable will prove to be small (see below), although not so vanishingly negligible as before, and somewhat protective (-0.029).

These findings differed somewhat from those obtained by the foregoing logistic regression analyses for perinatal outcome effects (see Tables 25-4 and 25-5). Good concurrence was encountered for ACT2 (foreshortened active phase) and FORROT2 (difficult forceps rotation), both of which had shown significant effects in both nulliparous and multiparous subseries; for GAS2 (continuous inhalation anesthesia) and FUNDAL2 (moderate fundal pressure), which had been significant among offspring of nulliparas; and for LAT3 (prolonged latent phase), SPINAL (spinal anesthesia), FORROT4 (failed forceps rotation), and SHOULD (shoulder dystocia), significant in multiparas before.

Discordant results were found for a number of variables that showed signifi-

Table 26-8
Logistic Regression Analysis of Aggregated Labor–Delivery Variables for Perinatal Outcome*

Variable		Regression Coefficient	Standard Error	t-Statistic	Relative Risk	p-Value
LAT3	Prolonged latent phase	0.447	0.199	2.25	1.56	0.027
ACT2	Short active phase	0.379	0.173	2.20	1.46	0.030
ACT3	Prolonged active phase	0.377	0.228	1.65	1.46	0.10
SPINAL	Spinal anesthesia	-0.625	0.182	-3.43	0.54	0.00088
PARAC	Paracervical block	0.499	0.263	1.89	1.65	0.062
GAS2	Continuous gas anesthesia	0.388	0.163	2.38	1.47	0.019
AGT1	Demerol	0.442	0.191	2.32	1.56	0.022
AGT22	Apresoline	2.315	0.998	2.32	10.13	0.022
AGT27	Other antibiotics	3.038	1.199	2.53	20.85	0.013
FORTRAC2	Difficult forceps traction	1.411	0.625	2.26	4.10	0.026
FORTRAC3	Very difficult traction	1.937	0.704	2.75	6.94	0.0071
FORROT2	Difficult forceps rotation	0.931	0.472	1.97	2.54	0.050
FORROT3	Very difficult rotation	2.012	1.186	1.70	7.48	0.091
FORROT4	Failed rotation	2.223	0.632	3.52	9.23	0.00065
CONTROL1	Manual control	-0.916	0.468	-1.96	0.40	0.050
CONTROL3	Forceps control	1.067	0.602	-1.77	0.34	0.079
FUNDAL2	Moderate fundal pressure	0.466	0.229	2.04	1.59	0.043
FUNDAL3	Strong fundal pressure	0.694	0.346	2.01	2.00	0.046
ABRUPT	Abruptio placentae	1.284	0.336	3.82	3.61	0.00023
CSVAG	Failed vaginal delivery	1.095	0.646	1.70	2.99	0.091
SHOULD	Shoulder dystocia	1.662	0.428	3.89	5.27	0.00018
INDUCT3	Induction for PIH	1.026	0.542	1.89	2.79	0.061
INDUCT6-9	Other indications	1.349	0.537	2.51	3.85	0.014
AUGMENT6	Stimulation for amnionitis	3.124	0.728	4.29	22.74	4.1×10^{-5}
PRES5-8	Breech presentation	1.402	0.837	1.67	4.06	0.098
REACT3	Uterine hypertonus	1.680	0.766	2.19	5.37	0.031

* Variables with p-values less than 0.10 suppressed among 112 factors tested in data from population of 13,933.

cant effects now in contradistinction to their earlier insignificant effects, including AGT1 (Demerol), AGT22 (Apresoline), AGT27 (other antibiotics), FORTRAC3 (very difficult forceps traction), FUNDAL3 (strong fundal pressure), AUGMENT6 (labor stimulation for infection), FORTRAC2 (difficult forceps traction), and ABRUPT (abruptio placentae). Several were found to have significant impact although they had not previously been tested, namely CONTROL1 (manual control of head delivery), INDUCT6-9 (induction for other indications), and REACT3 (uterine hypertonus).

Ranking Sequence for Labor-Delivery Variables

The entire sequence of 112 labor and delivery variables (excluding intrinsic factors) were subjected to further re-examination in order to provide appropriate information for ranking, as described above. The means and standard deviations of each variable were first obtained. The standardized coefficients were then derived by multiplying the regression coefficients which the logit model had yielded by the standard deviations. This permitted ranking in descending order by standardized coefficient from very adverse (largest positive coefficient) to very protective (largest negative coefficient) for both composite and perinatal outcome data.

The results for composite outcome are detailed in Table 26-9 for 100 items of relevance. Omitted from this list were a number of variables with results so unstable as to be uninterpretable; in general, most of them involved very rare events. Examining the spectrum of variables by deciles, a convenient but quite arbitrary division, we found all three of the adverse forceps traction variables (FORTRAC2, FORTRAC3, and FORTRAC4) in the top 10%, representing the highest-ranking deleterious factors. Moreover, they were associated with FORCEPS3 (class III midforceps delivery) and FUNDAL3 (strong fundal pressure) in regard to the ranking of

their effects. Both BRDELIV3 (breech extraction) and BREECH3 (single footling breech) appeared here as well. Interspersed among them were INDUCT3 (induction for pregnancy-induced hypertension), AUGMENT5 (labor stimulation for Rh isoimmunization), and AUGMENT6 (labor stimulation for infection).

The next decile, still quite high in the range of ranked effects, included one additional forceps operation variable, FORAPP3 (very difficult forceps application), plus FUNDAL3 (strong fundal pressure). The obstetrical crises of PROLAP (cord prolapse) and ABRUPT (abruptio placentae) occurred in this ranking location. AUGMENT4 (stimulation for diabetes) also ranked in this group as did AGT16 (Vistaril), AGT24 (oxytocin), and PUDEND (pudendal block anesthesia). The fetal malposition PRES2 (occiput transverse) and the labor disorder ACT3 (prolonged active phase) completed the subgroup.

In the third decile were found SHOULD (shoulder dystocia), PRES5-8 (breech presentation), PRES10 (face presentation), BRFACH2 (difficult forceps to the aftercoming head), along with SEC2 (foreshortened second stage) and ACT2 (short active phase). AGT13 (phenobarbital) ranked here with GAS2 (continuous inhalation anesthesia) and OXYT3 (oxytocin induction and stimulation of labor). AUGMENT2 (stimulation for ruptured membranes) was also present.

A number of drugs appeared in the fourth decile of ranked variables. This decile was noteworthy for the factors CSVAG (failed attempt at vaginal delivery), AUGMENT11-18 (stimulation for other indications), INDUCT6-9 (induction for other indications), LAT3 (prolonged latent phase), and REACT3 (uterine hypertonus from oxytocin). The fifth decile of variables included FORROT3 (very difficult forceps rotation), BREECH4 (double footling breech), and the abnormal labor patterns of DESC2 (protracted descent), MAXS3 (precipitate dilatation), and DEC3 (prolonged deceleration phase). Two variables dealing

Table 26-9
Ranking of Labor-Delivery Variables by Standardized Coefficient
for Composite Outcome

Rank Order	Variable		Regression Coefficient	Standard Deviation	Standardized Coefficient
1	FORTRAC2	Difficult forceps traction	0.381	0.494	0.1883
2	AUGMENT5	Stimulation for Rh disease	4.098	0.034	0.1411
3	BRDELIV3	Breech extraction	1.678	0.095	0.1245
4	FORTRAC4	Failed forceps traction	1.159	0.099	0.1143
5	FORTRAC3	Very difficult traction	0.511	0.195	0.0999
6	AUGMENT6	Stimulation for amnionitis	2.458	0.031	0.0773
7	FORCEPS2	Class III forceps	1.479	0.045	0.0678
8	FUNDAL3	Strong fundal pressure	0.272	0.245	0.0666
9	BREECH3	Single footling breech	0.691	0.095	0.0658
10	INDUCT3	Induction for PIH	0.809	0.081	0.0658
11	PROLAP	Cord prolapse	0.705	0.233	0.0627
12	FUNDAL2	Moderate fundal pressure	0.239	0.089	0.0557
13	AUGMENT4	Stimulation for diabetes	1.005	0.051	0.0515
14	FORAPP3	Very difficult forceps application	0.337	0.146	0.0493
15	AGT16	Hydroxyzine, Vistaril	0.421	0.115	0.0486
16	PRES2	Occiput transverse	0.173	0.258	0.0446
17	AGT24	Oxytocin	0.450	0.098	0.0443
18	ACT3	Prolonged active phase	0.144	0.308	0.0443
19	PUDEND	Pudendal block	0.106	0.402	0.0424
20	ABRUPT	Abruptio placentae	0.373	0.113	0.0422
21	SEC2	Shortened second stage	0.085	0.489	0.0415
22	SHOULD	Shoulder dystocia	0.614	0.067	0.0413
23	AGT13	Phenobarbital	0.433	0.094	0.0407
24	PRES5-8	Breech presentations	0.775	0.052	0.0402
25	PRES10	Face presentation	1.189	0.033	0.0398
26	GAS2	Continuous gas anesthesia	0.106	0.367	0.0390
27	ACT2	Shortened active phase	0.082	0.458	0.0378
28	AUGMENT2	Stimulation for ruptured membranes	0.204	0.177	0.0361
29	BRFACH2	Difficult aftercoming forceps	0.421	0.086	0.0360
30	OXYT2	Oxytocin induction and stimulation	0.173	0.203	0.0351
31	CSVAG	Failed vaginal delivery attempt	1.019	0.034	0.0351
32	AUGMENT11-18	Stimulation for other indications	0.315	0.101	0.0317
33	AGT27	Other antibiotics	1.587	0.020	0.0316
34	AGT25	Sparteine sulfate	0.326	0.092	0.0301
35	AGT22	Apresoline	0.800	0.037	0.0297
36	AGT8	Streptomycin	0.582	0.049	0.0287
37	LAT3	Prolonged latent phase	0.109	0.258	0.0282
38	REACT3	Uterine hypertonus	0.594	0.046	0.0273
39	INDUCT6-9	Induction for other indications	0.367	0.074	0.0270
40	AGT20	Atropine	0.207	0.126	0.0260
41	ROM11	Membranes ruptured >36 hr.	2.244	0.014	0.0258
42	FORROT3	Very difficult forceps rotation	0.555	0.046	0.0255
43	OXYT1	Oxytocin induction of labor	0.230	0.111	0.0255
44	AGT19	Scopolamine	0.090	0.265	0.0239
45	ROM10	Membranes ruptured 31-36 hr.	1.701	0.014	0.0239
46	PARAC	Paracervical block	0.127	0.189	0.0239
47	DESC2	Protracted descent	0.075	0.307	0.0230
48	MAXS3	Precipitate dilatation	0.058	0.377	0.0220
49	DEC3	Prolonged deceleration phase	0.065	0.329	0.0214
50	BREECH4	Double footling breech	0.620	0.335	0.0208
51	INDUCT1	Elective induction	0.144	0.141	0.0204
52	ARRS3	Arrest of descent	0.084	0.240	0.0203

53	FORCEPS2	Class II forceps	0.054	0.328	0.0176
54	FORAPP4	Failed forceps application	0.211	0.083	0.0174
55	FORROT2	Difficult forceps rotation	0.874	0.020	0.0174
56	REACT5	Tumultuous contractions	0.444	0.038	0.0169
57	LAT2	Shortened latent phase	0.042	0.384	0.0162
58	FORROT1	Forceps rotation of average difficulty	0.139	0.115	0.0161
59	FORAPP2	Difficult forceps application	0.304	0.051	0.0154
60	FUNDAL6	Failed fundal pressure	0.120	0.118	0.0142
61	GAS3	Intermittent and continuous gas anesthesia	0.053	0.184	0.0097
62	AGT6	Achromycin	0.149	0.060	0.0089
63	FORROT4	Failed forceps rotation	0.042	0.190	0.0078
64	DEC2	Shortened deceleration phase	0.025	0.303	0.0075
65	GAS1	Intermittent gas anesthesia	0.022	0.314	0.0070
66	AGT7	Penicillin	0.094	0.061	0.0057
67	BREECH2	Full or complete breech	0.119	0.037	0.0044
68	PRES3	Occiput posterior	0.015	0.278	0.0042
69	OXYT2	Oxytocin augmentation of labor	0.011	0.371	0.0041
70	PRES1-4	Vertex presentations	0.018	0.181	0.0032
71	FORCEPS1	Class I forceps	0.002	0.381	0.0009
72	AUGMENT10	Stimulation for arrested labor	0.001	0.180	0.0001
73	AGT18	Vesprin	-0.011	0.093	-0.0011
74	CONTROL2	Uncontrolled head delivery	-0.034	0.092	-0.0036
75	AGT1	Demerol	-0.013	0.355	-0.0044
76	IVD1	Intravenous anesthesia	-0.069	0.083	-0.0057
77	SEC3	Prolonged second stage	-0.040	0.192	-0.0077
78	REACT2	Sustained oxytocin contraction	-0.132	0.060	-0.0079
79	PARITY	Parity	-0.019	0.497	-0.0093
80	CONTROL1	Manual control of head	-0.104	0.109	-0.0113
81	ROM9	Membranes ruptured 25-30 hr.	-2.102	0.008	-0.0171
82	AUGMENT3	Stimulation for PIH	-0.202	0.086	-0.0173
83	INDUCT4	Induction for diabetes	-0.366	0.054	-0.0199
84	ARRD3	Arrest of dilatation	-0.081	0.347	-0.0282
85	MAXS2	Protracted dilatation	-0.081	0.371	-0.0299
86	REACT4	Abnormal fetal heart rate	-0.375	0.083	-0.3009
87	INDUCT2	Induction for ruptured membranes	-0.230	0.137	-0.0315
88	PRES1	Occiput anterior	-0.084	0.405	-0.0340
89	ROM7	Membranes ruptured 13-18 hr.	-3.018	0.014	-0.0424
90	ROM8	Membranes ruptured 19-24 hr.	-3.216	0.014	-0.0452
91	BREECH1	Frank breech	-0.887	0.060	-0.0528
92	AGT2	Nisentil	-0.301	0.202	-0.0608
93	PREVIA	Placenta previa	-1.316	0.047	-0.0622
94	AGT23	Syntocinon	-0.346	0.194	-0.0672
95	AUGMENT1	Elective stimulation of labor	-0.247	0.278	-0.0688
96	DESC3	Precipitate descent	-0.156	0.450	-0.0703
97	INDUCT5	Induction for Rh disease	-2.572	0.040	-0.1022
98	FORAPP1	Forceps application of average difficulty	-0.263	0.450	-0.1184
99	SPINAL	Spinal anesthesia	-0.279	0.491	-0.1370
100	CONTROL3	Forceps control of head	-0.372	0.498	-0.1852

with prolonged rupture of membranes were closely ranked here, namely ROM10 (31-36 hours) and ROM11 (more than 36 hours). PARAC (paracervical block) also ranked in this decile.

It should be noted that the concentration of adverse variables in the upper ranking order skewed the distribution so that the midpoint of the range did not represent neutrality of effect. As can be seen from Table 26-9, the point at which the standardized coefficients reached their nadir was at ranking order 72-73, where the coefficients converted from positive to negative. Thus, the fifth decile variables still possessed considerable adverse effect as did a number of the factors that ranked well below this group. The sixth decile of variables, for example, contained such items as FORCEPS2 (class II forceps), FORAPP4 (failed forceps application), FORROT1 (forceps rotation of average difficulty), and FORAPP2 (difficult forceps application), some or all of which may have exerted a deleterious impact on offspring. To this list might be added ARRS3 (arrest of descent) and LAT2 (shortened latent phase) as well as REACT5 (tumultuous contractions) and FUNDAL4 (failed fundal pressure).

At the protective end of the ranking range, the tenth decile included CONTROL3 (forceps control of head delivery), FORAPP1 (forceps application of average difficulty), SPINAL (spinal anesthesia), AUGMENT1 (elective stimulation of labor), AGT2 (Nisentil), and AGT23 (Syntocinon), all reflecting practices heretofore commonly undertaken for managing essentially normal labors in healthy gravidas. In contrast to the consistently adverse effects of other breech presentations and delivery methods, BREECH1 (frank breech presentation) ranked at this end of the scale. Similarly, PREVIA (placenta previa) appeared here, perhaps reflecting the good results from interventive surgical management policies for this disorder. Unexpected among this group were INDUCT5 (induction for Rh disease) and DESC3 (precipitate descent), contrasting with recognized

adverse effects of Rh isoimmunization and tumultuous labor (REACT5, see above).

The ninth decile signaled the protective effects of CONTROL1 (manual control of head delivery), INDUCT2 (induction for ruptured membranes), PRES1 (occiput anterior), and timely rupture of the membranes (ROM5, ROM6, and ROM8). Of interest, ARRD3 (arrest of descent) and MAXS2 (protracted dilatation), clinically associated with untoward results, appeared protective here; this suggested that any adverse effects from these factors may have been entirely accounted for or corrected by the delivery procedure or other practice used for therapy in these cases.

The ranking procedure was repeated for the entire series of labor-delivery variables as related to their perinatal outcome effects (Table 26-10). To a degree, the ranking order was comparable to that seen earlier for composite outcome (see above). Even though there were a number of inconsistencies in the positions of some variables, the ranking orders were very highly correlated. Applying Spearman's approach for assessing the correlation (agreement) of two rankings,* we found the correlation coefficient to be statistically quite significant ($r = .622$, $p < .001$) for the 100 factors ranked separately in Tables 26-9 and 26-10.

The three leading items in the rank listing for composite outcome data appeared among the first four in the perinatal outcome list, for example. Six of the variables in the top decile of the composite group were contained in the top decile of the perinatal group, namely FORTRAC2, AUGMENT5, BRDELIV3, FORTRAC4, FORTRAC3, and BREECH3. Among the first decile subset in the perinatal rank order, only AGT1 (Demerol) had not shown a strongly adverse rank in the com-

---

*Spearman's rank correlation is defined as:

$$r_s = 1 - \frac{6\Sigma d^2}{n(n^2-1)}$$

Spearman C: The proof and measurement of association between two things. *Am J Psychol* 1904; 15:72.

Table 26-10
Ranking of Labor-Delivery Variables by Standardized Coefficient
for Perinatal Outcome

Rank Order	Variable		Regression Coefficient	Standard Deviation	Standardized Coefficient
1	BRDELIV3	Breech extraction	6.709	0.072	0.4811
2	BREECH3	Single footling breech	5.050	0.090	0.4569
3	FORTRAC2	Difficult forceps traction	0.531	0.495	0.2629
4	AUGMENT5	Stimulation for Rh disease	6.717	0.033	0.2203
5	ACT2	Foreshortened active phase	0.379	0.460	0.1744
6	AGT1	Demerol	0.442	0.355	0.1568
7	FORTRAC3	Very difficult forceps traction	0.768	0.193	0.1483
8	ABRUPT	Abruptio placentae	1.284	0.111	0.1422
9	GAS2	Continuous gas anesthesia	0.388	0.363	0.1408
10	FORTRAC4	Failed forceps traction	1.411	0.096	0.1351
11	OXYT2	Oxytocin augmentation of labor	0.326	0.369	0.1204
12	LAT3	Prolonged latent phase	0.447	0.257	0.1149
13	FUNDAL3	Strong fundal pressure	0.466	0.245	0.1143
14	ACT3	Prolonged active phase	0.377	0.303	0.1142
15	SHOULD	Shoulder dystocia	1.662	0.065	0.1088
16	PRES2	Occiput transverse	0.402	0.257	0.1033
17	INDUCT6-9	Induction for other indications	1.349	0.075	0.1013
18	DEC3	Prolonged deceleration phase	0.298	0.326	0.0971
19	AUGMENT6	Stimulation for infection	3.124	0.031	0.0954
20	PARAC	Paracervical block	0.499	0.188	0.0936
21	FORCEPS2	Class II forceps	1.833	0.048	0.0878
22	INDUCT3	Induction for PIH	1.026	0.082	0.0844
23	FORROT3	Very difficult forceps rotation	2.223	0.038	0.0842
24	FORCEPS3	Class III forceps	1.937	0.043	0.0836
25	AGT22	Apresoline	2.315	0.036	0.0832
26	FUNDAL4	Failed fundal pressure	0.694	0.117	0.0811
27	REACT3	Uterine hypertonus	1.680	0.048	0.0804
28	GAS3	Intermittent and continuous gas anesthesia	0.403	0.185	0.0744
29	DESC2	Protracted descent	0.235	0.298	0.0701
30	ARRS3	Arrest of descent	0.294	0.237	0.0696
31	FORROT2	Difficult forceps rotation	0.931	0.071	0.0658
32	AUGMENT10	Stimulation for arrested labor	0.368	0.176	0.0649
33	PUDEND	Pudendal block	0.152	0.401	0.0611
34	INDUCT3	Induction for diabetes	1.125	0.052	0.0587
35	AGT27	Other antibiotics	3.038	0.019	0.0575
36	PROLAP	Cord prolapse	0.599	0.088	0.0525
37	LAT2	Foreshortened latent phase	0.129	0.384	0.0496
38	BRFACH2	Difficult aftercoming forceps	0.912	0.051	0.0463
39	PRES5-8	Breech presentation	1.402	0.032	0.0444
40	SEC3	Prolonged second stage	0.236	0.188	0.0443
41	OXYT1	Oxytocin induction	0.391	0.109	0.0428
42	AUGMENT11-18	Stimulation for other indications	0.423	0.100	0.0424
43	FORROT4	Failed forceps rotation	2.012	0.021	0.0417
44	AGT7	Penicillin	0.679	0.060	0.0410
45	AGT8	Streptomycin	0.868	0.047	0.0409
46	BREECH4	Double footling breech	0.454	0.089	0.0403
47	AGT20	Atropine	0.314	0.127	0.0398
48	CSVAG	Failed vaginal delivery attempt	1.095	0.034	0.0371

49	FORAPP3	Very difficult forceps application	0.227	0.145	0.0330
50	FORAPP4	Failed forceps application	0.371	0.080	0.0295
51	PRES3	Occiput posterior	0.095	0.275	0.0261
52	OXYT3	Oxytocin induction and augmentation	0.123	0.204	0.0251
53	FORROT1	Forceps rotation of average difficulty	0.158	0.153	0.0240
54	REACT5	Tumultuous contractions	0.582	0.037	0.0215
55	FUNDAL2	Moderate fundal pressure	0.078	0.233	0.0182
56	AGT16	Vistaril	0.144	0.117	0.0169
57	IVD1	Intravenous anesthesia	0.189	0.080	0.0151
58	AGT18	Vesprin	0.045	0.095	0.0042
59	FORAPP2	Difficult forceps application	0.009	0.383	0.0036
60	INDUCT2	Induction for ruptured membranes	0.010	0.138	0.0014
61	GAS1	Intermittent gas anesthesia	-0.005	0.316	-0.0017
62	AGT24	Oxytocin	-0.043	0.097	-0.0041
63	AGT25	Sparteine sulfate	-0.049	0.092	-0.0045
64	AUGMENT3	Stimulation for PIH	-0.168	0.086	-0.0146
65	FORCEPS1	Class I forceps	-0.269	0.057	-0.0153
66	PREVIA	Placenta previa	-0.342	0.046	-0.0159
67	AGT2	Nisentil	-0.080	0.206	-0.0164
68	AUGMENT1	Elective stimulation of labor	-0.062	0.282	-0.0176
69	SEC2	Foreshortened second stage	-0.045	0.488	-0.0220
70	DEC2	Foreshortened deceleration phase	-0.075	0.302	-0.0225
71	AUGMENT4	Stimulation for diabetes	-0.479	0.047	-0.0226
72	INDUCT1	Elective induction of labor	-0.166	0.141	-0.0234
73	ROM11	Membranes ruptured >36 hr.	-2.956	0.008	-0.0250
74	MAXS2	Protracted dilatation	-0.071	0.368	-0.0262
75	PRES1-4	Vertex presentation	-0.156	0.173	-0.0271
76	PARITY	Parity	-0.059	0.496	-0.0291
77	REACT4	Abnormal fetal heart rate	-0.394	0.081	-0.0321
78	AGT6	Achromycin	-0.735	0.060	-0.0440
79	MAXS3	Precipitate dilatation	-0.121	0.380	-0.0461
80	AGT13	Phenobarbital	-0.495	0.093	-0.0461
81	ARRD3	Arrest of dilatation	-0.150	0.344	-0.0517
82	DESC3	Precipitate descent	-0.120	0.453	-0.0543
83	ROM9	Membranes ruptured 25-30 hr.	-4.049	0.015	-0.0594
84	PRES10	Face presentation	-0.784	0.082	-0.0642
85	ROM10	Membranes ruptured 31-36 hr.	-4.400	0.015	-0.0646
86	REACT2	Sustained uterine contraction	-1.152	0.058	-0.0668
87	ROM7	Membranes ruptured 13-18 hr.	-5.862	0.012	-0.0702
88	AUGMENT2	Stimulation for ruptured membranes	-0.428	0.177	-0.0758
89	ROM8	Membranes ruptured 19-24 hr.	-5.213	0.015	-0.0765
90	AGT19	Scopolamine	-0.299	0.265	-0.0794
91	PRES1	Occiput anterior	-0.210	0.400	-0.0839
92	AGT23	Syntocinon	-0.479	0.195	-0.0936
93	CONTROL1	Manual control of head	-0.946	0.109	-0.1035
94	INDUCT5	Induction for Rh disease	-3.981	0.039	-0.1544
95	BREECH2	Full or complete breech	-5.249	0.035	-0.1832
96	FORAPP1	Forceps application of average difficulty	-0.577	0.454	-0.2620
97	BREECH1	Frank breech	-5.668	0.053	-0.2994
98	SPINAL	Spinal anesthesia	-0.625	0.492	-0.3076
99	CONTROL2	Uncontrolled delivery of head	-0.916	0.498	-0.4564
100	CONTROL3	Forceps control of head	-1.067	0.499	-0.5329

posite data; indeed, it had actually appeared somewhat protective earlier, albeit with a near zero standardized coefficient indicating neutrality of effect. The remaining three variables in the first decile of the perinatal list, ABRUPT, GAS2, and ACT2, had been found within the second or third deciles of the composite ranks. All but one of the factors listed in the first decile of the composite outcome ranking appeared in either the first or second decile of the perinatal list; the exception, FORCEPS3 (class III forceps), only ranked 24th in order.

Half the variables in the second perinatal decile had similarly been ranked earlier (first to third deciles). Discrepancies existed for the other half, but all fell on the positive side of the range of standardized coefficients. The most disparate was OXYT2 (oxytocin augmentation of labor), which had previously ranked 69th, but was now in 11th place. Greater inconsistencies occurred within the second decile of the composite list relative to their position here. This applied particularly to such factors as FORAPP3 (ranking 49th here), FUNDAL2 (55th), AGT16 (56th), and several which showed protective effects, such as AGT24 (62nd), and AUGMENT4 (71st). As has been apparent from several of the foregoing analyses, perinatal outcome results were not necessarily comparable to composite outcome results even though the latter measure of effect included the former. The observation confirmed the advantages of maintaining two separate sets of parallel analyses and continuing to utilize these two outcome indices to study risk effects.

CHAPTER 27

Scoring Risk

Summary

By summation of the regression coefficients of all labor-delivery risk factors operant in a given gravida, each case was scored quantitatively to yield an index of risk. The distribution of scores among the gravid population and the relationship of actual risk to magnitude of score were studied. Decile divisions were examined, but the summarization thus created was not found to fit the data in a sufficiently satisfactory manner. By permitting the outcome data to depict empirical cut points, we were able to establish a utilitarian model. It was shown to conform quite well to both perinatal and composite outcome data for the full array of labor, delivery, and drug risk variables. This provided the basis for assessing prelabor predictor variables for their impact on the risk-score effects which simultaneously accounted for the hazards of labor and delivery factors.

A scoring system was devised to help quantitate the risk inherent in a given set of labor-delivery factors acting concurrently in any individual gravida. Scores were assigned by summating the products of the regression coefficient (w_i) obtained from the logistic regression analysis for each operant risk variable and the variable measure itself (v_i):

$$\text{Score} = \sum_{i=1}^{n} w_i v_i$$

The score thus derived was dimensionless because the unit of measure for the regression coefficient was the inverse of that for the variable, making them mutually cancellable in the product. The risk variable measure for all labor, drug, and delivery variables was dichotomous, that is either 1 or 0; by contrast, many of the intrinsic variables (not considered for the purpose of the current exercise) were polytomous (capable of being multiply categorized).

A simple illustrative case may serve to elucidate the method. For a gravida presenting with a series of dichotomous risk factors (variable measure 1 if present, 0 if absent), the calculation of the score can proceed readily from the sequence of regression coefficients for composite outcome (see Table 26-9), as follows:

PRES1	Occiput anterior	-0.084
AGT1	Demerol	-0.013
LAT2	Short latent phase	0.042
FORCEPS1	Low forceps	0.002
CONTROL3	Forceps control of head	-0.372
PARAC	Paracervical block	0.127
	Risk score	-0.298

Even for more complicated cases, the calculation of risk score offers very little additional difficulty:

PRES2	Occiput transverse	0.173
AGT2	Nisentil	-0.301
AGT16	Vistaril	0.421
AGT24	Oxytocin	0.450
OXYT2	Labor augmentation	0.011
ACT3	Prolonged active phase	0.144
GAS2	Continuous gas anesthesia	0.106
FORCEPS2	Class II forceps	0.054
FORTRAC2	Difficult forceps traction	0.381
FORROT1	Forceps rotation, average	0.139
CONTROL3	Forceps control of head	-0.372
FUNDAL2	Moderate fundal pressure	0.239
	Risk score	+1.445

A further modification of the score, providing equivalent results, might take the form of the sum of the product of the standardized logistic regression coefficient (w_i^*) and the standardized variable measure (v_i^*):

$$\text{Score} = \sum_{i=1}^{n} w_i^* v_i^*$$

To this end, the distribution of the standardized variable v_i^* would have to be modified to a mean of zero and a standard deviation of one, where the mean and standard deviation of the original variable are v and s, respectively. Thus, for the individual variable, the transformation to the standardized variable would become:

$$v_i^* = \frac{v_i - \bar{v}}{\bar{s}}$$

All risk factors heretofore identified were standardized in this way for all 15,169 NCPP index cases. Summary scores were thereby derived for each gravida for both perinatal and composite outcomes. Scores for composite outcomes, for example, ranged overall from +1.65 to -6.38, mean -2.51 and standard deviation 0.464. Distribution was quite symmetrical around a modal value of -2.50 (which was also the median value). Less than 1% of the population studied had summary scores that actually fell into the positive range. The cumulative distribution curve is shown in Figure 27-1.

The range of scores was stratified into deciles for analytical purposes. Moreover, the extreme upper decile was further subdivided to focus on this end of the scale; three unequal groupings were formed, namely 91-95, 96-99, and the top 1 percentile (the 100th centile).

To make the decile limits more meaningful, the following landmark cut points are worth noting:

1st percentile score	-3.503
5th percentile score	-3.192
10th percentile score	-3.036
25th percentile score	-2.781
50th percentile score	-2.505

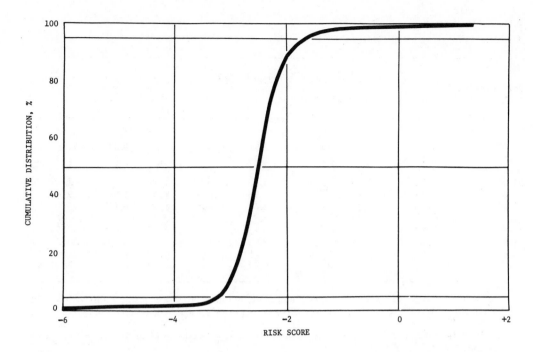

Figure **27-1.** Distribution of summary risk scores among 15,169 index cases, showing normal pattern with central tendency (mean) at -2.51. Overall, less than 1% had positive scores. Fifth percentile (-3.19), median (-2.50), and 95th percentile (-1.77) are indicated.

75th percentile score	-2.287
90th percentile score	-2.032
95th percentile score	-1.772
99th percentile score	-1.027

Distribution of Outcome Among Decile Risk-Score Strata*

The frequency of adverse outcomes was determined in each of the several scoring subsets thus formed. This was done to ascertain the utility of the score to predict an adverse outcome. Perinatal results (Table 27-1) were found, as expected, to be markedly skewed so that the best outcomes appeared in the low-score groups and the worst among those with high scores. Among the 323 identified bad perinatal out-

comes, 42.7% fell into the top decile (91-100 percentiles) and 35.2% in the top 5 percentile; this contrasted sharply with only 0.9% found in the bottom decile (0-10 percentiles). The distribution of these results by decile of risk score is depicted in Figure 27-2, which shows a stepped progression in concentration above the 70th percentile (6.5% to 10.9%, a 1.68 times enhancement) and a much greater one at the 90th percentile (13.9% to 42.7%, a 3.07-fold increment).

The frequencies of adverse perinatal results (death plus severe neonatal depression) within every scoring group were investigated (Table 27-1). Offspring of women whose scores fell into the lowest 10 percentiles did exceedingly well, only 0.22% having some demonstrable adverse perinatal effect. Between the 11th and the 70th percentiles, the rate was fairly consistent at a mean of 1.22% (the range for decile groups being 0.72% to 1.65%). The remaining three deciles (71-100 percentiles) averaged 5.23%, the decile group frequencies

---

*To distinguish these risk-score groups from those based on actual increments of risk ("incremental" groups), to be discussed later in this chapter, we have used the term "decile" here even though the uppermost decile group was further subdivided to yield 12 subsets of data.

Table 27-1
Perinatal Outcome by Risk Score

Percentile Score	Adverse Perinatal Results							
	Column%[a]	Row%[a]	RR[b]	t	p	RR$_1$[b]	t$_1$	P1
0-10	0.93	0.22	1.00	-	-	0.19	3.08	0.0034
11-20	4.95	1.15	5.23	2.98	0.0044	0.97	0.07	0.94
21-30	3.10	0.72	3.27	1.93	0.056	0.61	1.26	0.21
31-40	4.64	1.11	5.05	2.86	0.0062	0.94	0.17	0.35
41-50	5.26	1.18	5.36	3.08	0.0034	1.00	-	-
51-60	7.12	1.65	7.50	3.93	0.00026	1.40	1.06	0.29
61-70	6.50	1.51	6.86	3.69	0.00055	1.28	0.76	0.45
71-80	10.85	2.51	11.4	5.23	3.3×10^{-6}	2.13	2.62	0.010
81-90	13.93	3.21	14.6	6.13	1.4×10^{-7}	2.72	3.69	0.00055
91-95	7.43	3.48	15.8	4.60	2.9×10^{-5}	2.95	3.05	0.0037
96-99	21.05	12.21	55.5	8.61	$<1.0 \times 10^{-10}$	10.35	7.79	$<1.0 \times 10^{-10}$
>99	14.24	33.09	150.4	8.23	$<1.0 \times 10^{-10}$	28.04	7.98	$<1.0 \times 10^{-10}$

[a] Column % represents frequency of adverse outcomes for score group relative to total population outcome; row % refers to adverse outcome rates within the score groups.

[b] Rate ratio relative to referent rate of 0-10 percentile group (RR) or for 41-50 percentile group (RR$_1$).

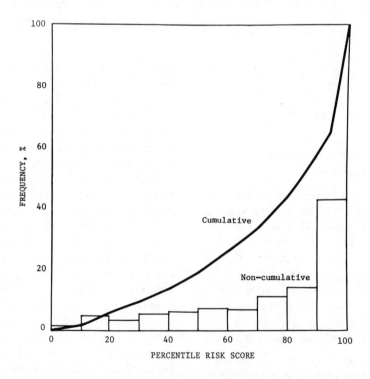

Figure **27-2.** Distribution of adverse perinatal cases across risk-score deciles. Concentration of bad outcomes is seen in the high score groups, especially above the 90th percentile.

increasing substantially in progressive fashion from 2.51% to 3.21% and 9.96%.

The greatest concentration of adverse perinatal effects was encountered in the uppermost 5 percentile of scores (12.21% incidence) and especially the top 1 percentile (33.09%). Relative to the 0-10 percentile referent rate (0.22%), all score groups (except 21-30 percentile) were statistically confirmed to have significantly increased rate ratios (p < .05), as shown in Table 27-1. When compared to a referent group more closely allied to both the mean rate and the median score group, such as that of the 41-50 percentile group (referent rate of adverse outcome 1.18%), the results for the 0-10 percentile group proved significantly protective, while those for all groups falling above the 70th percentile were significantly deleterious and increasingly so at higher score levels.

Composite outcome data (dealing with adverse results to offspring up to age seven years) among risk-score groups were also studied (Table 27-2). As with the perinatal outcome distribution, the 1239 adverse cases were largely concentrated at the upper end of the risk-score scale: 21.0% occurred in the top decile and 43.6% in the highest 30 percentiles. By contrast, only 4.3% fell into the lowest decile and 18.1% in

the lowest 30 percentiles. The pattern of case distribution paralleled that of the perinatal outcome data somewhat (see above). There was a moderate step-up at the tenth percentile (4.3% to 6.4%, a 1.49-fold increase), a larger one at the 60th percentile (8.9% to 11.9%, another 1.34-fold change or 2.77 times the lowest decile rate), and a most impressive one at the 90th percentile (11.9% to 21.0%, a 1.76-fold increment yielding a total of 4.88-fold increase over the range of score deciles).

Adverse Outcomes Within Decile Risk-Score Groups

Within-group frequencies of adverse composite outcome rose with advancing score. The best rates occurred at the low end of the scale (3.5% incidence in the 0-10 percentile score group). Although there was an almost uninterrupted trend for the rate to rise serially in subsequent groups, the frequency was more or less consistent at 5.2% to 7.3% through the 60th percentile (mean 6.6%). A substantive step-up to an average group rate of 9.4% followed for the next three deciles (range 8.8% to 9.7%) and another was seen in the top tenth percentile to 17.2%. Using the 0-10 percentile group rate as referent (3.5%), we determined that

Table 27-2
Composite Outcome by Risk Score*

Percentile Score	Adverse Composite Results								
	Column%	Row%	RR	t	p	RR_1	t_1	p_1
0-10	4.28	3.50	1.00	–	–	0.48	4.61	2.8×10^{-5}
11-20	6.38	5.22	1.49	2.32	0.024	0.72	2.33	0.022
21-30	7.43	6.15	1.76	3.40	0.0013	0.85	1.23	0.22
31-40	8.72	6.99	2.00	4.35	6.7×10^{-5}	0.96	0.30	0.77
41-50	8.88	7.27	2.08	4.61	2.8×10^{-5}	1.00	–	–
51-60	8.88	7.24	2.07	4.59	3.0×10^{-5}	1.00	0.03	0.98
61-70	11.86	9.70	2.77	6.93	7.1×10^{-9}	1.33	2.40	0.018
71-80	10.73	8.75	2.50	6.07	1.7×10^{-7}	1.20	1.50	0.14
81-90	11.86	9.69	2.77	6.92	8.9×10^{-9}	1.33	2.39	0.019
91-95	6.86	11.21	3.20	6.22	9.8×10^{-8}	1.54	2.97	0.0046
96-99	9.36	19.11	5.46	9.38	$<1.0 \times 10^{-10}$	2.63	6.85	1.2×10^{-8}
>99	4.76	39.07	11.16	8.90	$<1.0 \times 10^{-10}$	5.37	7.90	$<1.0 \times 10^{-10}$

*   See footnote, Table 27-1.

all other subset rates were statistically significant without exception (Table 27-2). When the rate in the median 41-50 percentile score group was used instead for the referent (7.3%), the 0-10 percentile and the 11-20 percentile group rates were found to be significantly protective, whereas those groups beyond the 90th percentile showed uniformly and strongly significant bad outcomes. In addition, statistical significance at p values of less than .02 were encountered for the 61-70 and 81-90 percentile groups, but inexplicably not for the intervening 71-80 percentile set.

Stratification of the uppermost decile as aforementioned (91-95, 96-99, and top 1 percentile) allowed us to appreciate the very impressive magnification of score effect on fetal-infant risk at these extreme levels (Tables 27-1 and 27-2, and Figure 27-3). Poor perinatal outcomes increased minimally from 3.1% in the 81-90 decile to 3.5% in the 91-95 percentile group, but jumped more than 3.5 times to 12.2% in the next subset (96-99 percentile) and a startling 9.5-

fold increase to 33.1% in the top 1 percentile. It was clear from these results that the risk scoring system thus devised might prove a powerful predictor of adverse outcome.

Infants whose mothers had scores from -1.027 (99th percentile) into the tail end of the positive range, for example, died perinatally or were severely depressed at birth in 33.1%, and 39.1% of the survivors had documentably bad outcomes. Although this small sample of NCPP index cases involved just 1% of the population (only 151 cases), they thus accounted for 14.2% of the adverse perinatal outcomes and 4.8% of the bad composite outcomes. Scores between -1.772 and -1.026 (96th to 99th percentiles) yielded 12.2% poor perinatal results and 19.1% composite. This 4% segment of the index population (607 cases) accounted for 21.2% and 9.4% of adverse perinatal and composite outcomes, respectively. Those 758 gravidas with scores between -2.032 and -1.771 (90th to 95th percentiles) delivered infants with 3.5% and 11.2% bad

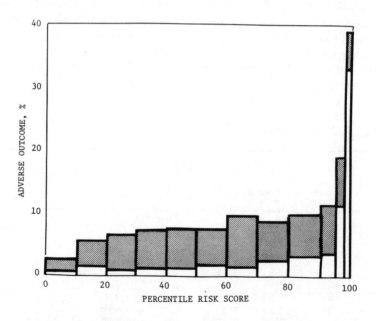

Figure 27-3. Incidence of adverse perinatal (white bars) and composite (white plus stippled bars) outcomes in successive risk score groups. The stepped increments at the 10th, 60th, 90th, 95th, and 99th percentiles confirm that the score is a utilitarian index for predicting bad fetal and infant results.

results (or 7.4% and 6.9% of all bad results). Altogether, scores above -2.031 (top decile) were associated with 10.0% adverse perinatal results and 17.2% bad composite results, accounting for 42.7% and 20.7% of the total of poor outcomes.

Goodness-of-Fit Between Logistic Model and Data

Before proceeding to assess whether any identifiable risk variable still possessed significantly unfavorable or beneficial impact not already accounted for by the risk score, we felt it important to ensure that the model fitted the data. The Freeman-Tukey deviates were determined for each subgroup based on the observed adverse outcome results and those expected according to the logistic model. Perinatal data were examined separately from composite data (Table 27-3) and the two sets of data were subjected to tests of goodness-of-fit. The analyses showed that the risk scoring system quite nicely satisfied the null hypothesis that the model fitted the data and was indeed able to predict the distribution of bad

outcomes. The chi-square values for goodness-of-fit clearly documented this fact in the overview for both sets of data. The p values obtained represented the conditional probability that the model was appropriate given the data at hand.

However, it should be noted that one composite decile group (61-70 percentile) and two perinatal groups (11-20 and 91-95 percentile) yielded Freeman-Tukey deviates suggesting a possible modelling irregularity. The observed outcome results were significantly different from those expected from the risk-score system. The most extreme example (the second decile for perinatal data) was significantly different from the expected rate at a 2% probability level. While this was somewhat unlikely to have been a chance occurrence, it was nonetheless considered a possibility because the lack of fit was not systematic in any regard. These subtle variations from a perfectly smooth fit may help explain some of the problems that were later disclosed (see below) when we pursued our detailed examination of each risk factor against outcome-specific referent data to ensure

Table 27-3
Assessment of Goodness-of-Fit for Decile Risk-Score-Group Model Fitting the Results[a]

Score Group, percentile	Perinatal Outcome				Composite Outcome			
	Observed	Expected	FTD	p^b	Observed	Expected	FTD	p^b
0-10	3	5.1	-0.894		53	57.4	-0.567	
11-20	16	8.9	2.083	0.020	79	75.0	0.480	
21-30	10	12.4	-0.620		92	86.7	0.584	
31-40	15	14.6	0.161		108	101.2	0.688	
41-50	17	18.4	-0.276		110	109.4	0.762	
51-60	23	21.1	0.447		110	118.8	-0.799	
61-70	21	25.3	-0.836		147	127.8	1.654	0.051
71-80	35	31.6	0.636		133	140.1	-0.589	
81-90	45	44.1	0.165		147	159.2	0.968	
91-95	24	35.1	-1.987	0.024	85	96.9	-1.214	
96-99	68	58.4	1.234		116	110.7	0.523	
Top 1	46	48.0	-0.259		59	56.0	0.427	

a   FTD, Freeman-Tukey deviates for 323 adverse perinatal outcomes and 1,239 bad composite outcomes among 15,169 index cases stratified by decile score group. Goodness of fit: for perinatal data, $\chi^2 = 14.09$, df = 10, p = 0.169; for composite outcome, $\chi^2 = 8.94$, df = 10, p = 0.537.

b   One-sided p-values.

that the risk-scoring system actually accounted for the cumulative risk in a meaningful and practical manner.

Residual Risk Effects in Decile Risk-Score Groups

To determine whether the effects of all identifiable risk factors had been suitably accounted for by the risk scores, we next examined each labor progression, drug, and delivery variable in detail. Parallel comparative groups were devised. One contained all cases exhibiting the variable under consideration and the other a designated referent population. In general, the referent chosen consisted of patients with a fetus in vertex presentation who were delivered by manual control of the fetal head (variable CONTROL1) and who did not exhibit the risk variable being studied. Both were stratified into the decile risk-score subgroups and the adverse outcome rates were determined for each cell of the matrix thus created. For every decile risk-score group, a cross-product (odds) ratio was calculated and the matching index and referent data were

compared statistically. In addition to the within-group examination, the entire set of comparative tables was investigated to derive an overview risk estimate that could be assessed in turn for statistical significance (by the Mantel-Haenszel chi-square test). In addition, the entire array was subjected to a test of homogeneity. Of importance here was the ability to derive the risk still inherent in the study variable after all risk factors had already ostensibly been taken into account by the risk-score. The confidence limits of risk were also made available by this approach.

Table 27-4 displays the matrix data for one such analysis involving a comparison of the composite effects of variable FORCEPS2 (class II midforceps) with those of the referent group (CONTROL1). It should here be recalled that the study subpopulation from which this material was derived had earlier been restricted to a more or less homogeneous selection of gravidas delivering infants free of serious anomalies and weighing between 2500 and 4000 g. The outcome results for each of the decile risk-score groups are shown together with

Table 27-4
Impact of a Risk Variable[a] on Adverse Composite Outcome Within Decile Risk Score Groups

Score Group, percentile	FORCEPS2			CONTROL1		OR[b]	p-Value
	No.	%	Expected	No.	%		
0-10	577	3.29	3.90	64	9.38	0.33	0.041
11-20	557	4.67	5.19	138	7.25	0.63	0.31
21-30	360	6.94	6.56	417	6.24	1.12	0.80
31-40	280	6.43	6.79	647	6.96	0.92	0.88
41-50	206	6.31	6.89	938	7.04	0.89	0.83
51-60	137	5.84	6.86	1133	6.97	0.83	0.75
61-70	103	4.85	9.71	1148	10.10	0.45	0.12
71-80	130	6.15	8.62	1022	8.90	0.67	0.37
81-90	124	13.71	9.84	849	9.31	1.55	0.17
91-95	100	14.00	12.40	303	11.88	1.21	0.70
96-99	82	24.39	20.61	175	18.86	1.39	0.39
Top 1	17	52.94	41.76	31	35.48	2.05	0.39
Overall	2673	6.81	7.01	6865	8.71	0.95	0.62

a   Risk variable FORCEPS2, Class II midforceps, compared to referent group consisting of cases with vertex presentation delivered under manual control, CONTROL1.

b   Cross-product (odds) ratio.

the cross-product (odds) ratio and the probability value of the difference having occurred by chance.

As expected, the frequencies of adverse outcomes increased markedly with increasing risk-score deciles. This applied to both the index series (FORCEPS2) and the referent. However, the serial rise was definitely greater in the former than in the latter as evidenced by the progressive augmentation of the odds ratio. A particularly abrupt increase was seen between the eighth (71-80 percentile) and the ninth (81-90 percentile) deciles where the odds ratio jumped from 0.67 to 1.55. Notwithstanding this apparent trend, the differences across decile risk-score groups were generally found to be insignificant. The single exception was the first decile (0-10 percentile) in which there was an appearance of a significantly protective effect. Overall, the analysis suggested good homogeneity with an odds ratio approaching and narrowly centered on unity (OR = 0.95). The summated combination of all two-by-two tables for the 12 risk-score subgroups (by Mantel-Haenszel chi-square statistics) yielded a large p value likewise indicating uniformity of the odds ratio over the range of the score (p = .62).

In order to probe further into the question of some undisclosed residual impact from the risk variable under study, we collapsed the risk-score groups by dichotomizing at the aforementioned point flagged by the trend in odds ratios, namely between the eighth and ninth score deciles. The resulting data on outcome for FORCEPS2

(Table 27-5) clearly documented the suggestion implied by those in the full data display by deciles (see Table 27-4). Among low-risk-score cases (0-80 percentile), we found a highly significant protective effect; by contrast, at the high-risk-score end of the scale (81-100 percentile), there was a counterbalancing deleterious effect which was of comparable magnitude and almost as statistically significant.

It was evident here that for this risk variable, the risk score model neither fit the data nor accounted completely for the full impact of the factor on the offspring. Although this deficiency applied to relatively few variables, it was nonetheless felt to be of sufficient importance to warrant revamping the way in which the scoring scale was divided (see below). Unless we could ensure that we had accounted for essentially all the effects of labor, drug, and delivery variables, we could not be confident that the final evaluations of the influence of intrinsic factors would be of value. It was only after this matter was corrected by means of incremental scoring (see below) that we were able to proceed.

Survey of Residual Risk Effects in Decile Strata

We have thus encountered one variable with substantive adverse effect incompletely accounted for by the risk-score model as constructed heretofore. We sought to determine if this was merely a chance event or reflected instead some per-

Table 27-5
Impact of a Risk Variable on Adverse Composite Outcome in
Low Versus High Risk Score Groups*

Score Group, percentile	FORCEPS2			CONTROL1		OR	p-Value
	No.	%	Expected	No.	%		
0-80	2350	5.19	6.92	5507	7.97	0.68	2.1×10^{-6}
81-100	323	18.58	13.03	1358	11.71	1.72	1.0×10^{-3}

* See footnote, Table 27-4 for risk factor and referent variable population. Decile score groups collapsed and dichotomized as shown to maximize effect.

vading weakness in the system itself. To this end, we subjected the entire spectrum of designated labor, drug, and delivery variables to the analytical paradigm just described.

The data for 55 selected delivery variables are shown in Table 27-6 for both perinatal and composite outcome results. Among those studied to disclose residual impact on adverse composite results, a number were found to have overall effects significantly greater than those already

Table 27-6
Risk-Enhancing Effects of Delivery Variables on
Decile Risk-Score-Stratified Outcome

Risk Variable		Perinatal Outcome		Composite Outcome	
		RR	95%CL	RR	95%CL
FORCEPS2	Class II midforceps	0.95	0.65-1.41	0.96[a]	0.78-1.17
FORCEPS3	Class III midforceps	0.96	0.64-1.42	0.95	0.76-1.19
FORTRAC2	Difficult forceps traction	0.97	0.72-1.30	0.96	0.82-1.11
FORTRAC3	Very difficult traction	1.30	0.78-2.16	1.03[a]	0.74-1.42
FORTRAC4	Failed forceps traction	2.01[a]	1.04-3.89	1.22	0.74-1.99
FORAPP2	Difficult forceps application	1.00	0.69-1.46	0.96	0.80-1.17
FORAPP3	Very difficult forceps application	1.46	0.84-2.54	1.13	0.79-1.62
FORAPP4	Failed forceps application	2.67	1.33-5.39[b]	1.46	0.79-2.69
FORROT2	Difficult forceps rotation	1.00	0.60-1.68	0.98	0.75-1.28
FORROT3	Very difficult forceps rotation	1.31	0.75-2.31	1.00	0.66-1.52
FORROT4	Failed forceps rotation	5.13	2.18-12.05[b]	1.78	0.82-3.90
CONTROL1	Manual control of head	1.02	0.79-1.31	1.01	0.89-1.16
CONTROL2	Uncontrolled head delivery	3.14	1.41-7.02[b]	1.33	0.83-2.14
CONTROL3	Forceps control of head	0.81	0.57-1.17	0.93	0.73-1.19
FUNDAL2	Moderate fundal pressure	1.25[a]	0.68-2.30	1.15[a]	0.85-1.56
FUNDAL3	Strong fundal pressure	1.31	0.77-2.23	1.27	0.96-1.68
PROLAP	Prolapsed cord	2.70	1.42-5.13[b]	1.66[a]	0.99-2.76
ABRUPT	Abruptio placentae	2.02	1.10-3.71[b]	1.26[a]	0.78-2.03
CSVAG	Cesarean after failed attempt	8.91	3.59-22.11[b]	3.38	1.45-7.90[b]
SHOULD	Shoulder dystocia	3.04	1.50-6.16[b]	1.75	0.93-3.30
PREVIA	Placenta previa	8.72	3.47-21.90[b]	3.63	1.28-10.28[b]
INDUCT1	Elective induction of labor	1.99	0.93-4.26	1.05	0.65-1.69
INDUCT2	Induction for ROM	1.89	0.87-4.10	1.10	0.71-1.72
INDUCT3	Induction for PIH	2.57	1.28-5.15[b]	1.44	0.83-2.50
INDUCT4	Induction for diabetes	6.37	2.70-15.03[b]	1.85	0.90-3.81
INDUCT5	Induction for Rh disease	8.70	3.39-22.35[b]	2.65	1.11-6.31[b]
INDUCT6-9	Induction for other indications	2.80	1.38-5.69[b]	1.50[a]	0.82-2.74
AUGMENT1	Elective stimulation of labor	1.08	0.67-1.72	0.89	0.66-1.21
AUGMENT2	Simulation for ROM	1.63	0.84-3.16	1.19	0.85-1.68
AUGMENT3	Stimulation for PIH	2.86	1.38-5.92[b]	1.35	0.76-2.39
AUGMENT4	Stimulation for diabetes	6.71	2.79-16.12[b]	1.95	0.97-3.91
AUGMENT5	Stimulation for Rh disease	9.47	3.66-24.52[b]	3.14	1.30-7.61[b]
AUGMENT6	Stimulation for amnionitis	13.21	5.12-34.04[b]	5.98	2.44-14.64[b]
AUGMENT10	Stimulation for arrested labor	1.60	0.97-2.65	1.05	0.75-1.48
AUGMENT11-18	Stimulation for other indications	2.16	1.13-4.11	1.32	0.80-2.19
BREECH2	Frank breech	2.08	1.05-4.13[b]	1.35	0.77-2.35
BREECH3	Complete breech	14.85	5.31-41.48[b]	3.14	1.32-7.46[b]
BREECH4	Single footling breech	5.91	2.54-13.75[b]	1.75	0.85-3.61
BREECH5	Double footling breech	2.62	1.29-5.35[b]	3.01	1.26-7.19[b]
BRFACH2	Difficult aftercoming forceps	3.19	1.48-6.90[b]	1.41	0.78-2.57
BRDELIV3	Assisted breech delivery	3.02	1.35-6.73[b]	1.41	0.80-2.47

BRDELIV4	Breech extraction	2.95	1.42-6.11[b]	1.41	0.79-2.50
PRES1	Occiput anterior	0.76	0.47-1.20	1.08	0.75-1.30
PRES2	Occiput transverse	1.05	0.71-1.58	1.00	0.78-1.27
PRES3	Occiput posterior	1.17	0.78-1.74	0.98	0.78-1.24
PRES5	Sacrum anterior	5.37	2.20-13.09[b]	1.97	0.90-4.31
PRES6	Sacrum transverse	7.34	2.95-18.27[b]	2.00	0.87-4.61
PRES7	Sacrum posterior	6.82	2.02-10.14[b]	3.76	1.37-10.33[b]
PRES1-4	Vertex presentation	0.14	0.06-0.35[b]	0.55	0.27-1.14
PRES11	Brow presentation	9.25	3.62-23.64[b]	3.12	1.30-7.46[b]
REACT1	No uterotonic response to oxytocin	3.20	1.46-7.03[b]	1.24	0.64-2.39
REACT2	Tetanic contraction from oxytocin	8.05	3.17-20.46[b]	2.05	0.93-4.49
REACT3	Uterine hypertonus from oxytocin	6.03	2.60-13.98[b]	2.62	1.14-6.05[b]
REACT4	FHR abnormality from oxytocin	3.15	1.51-6.57[b]	1.60	0.83-3.10
REACT5	Tumultuous labor from oxytocin	11.67	4.34-31.39[b]	2.81	1.19-6.65[b]

[a] Relative risk (RR) based on Mantel-Haenszel statistics combining all relevant 2 x 2 tables for risk score groups, and 95 percentile confidence limits (95%CL); those designated with asterisk show significantly enhanced relative risk at the high end of the risk-score scale.

[b] A range of 95 percentile confidence limits for risk that does not include 1.00 is by definition statistically significant at least at the 0.05 probability level.

taken into account by the model. There were 11 such variables in all, including CSVAG (cesarean section following failed attempt at vaginal delivery), PREVIA (placenta previa), INDUCT5 and AUGMENT5 (induction and augmentation of labor for Rh isoimmunization), AUGMENT6 (labor stimulation for amnionitis), BREECH3 (complete breech), BREECH5 (double footling breech), PRES5 and PRES7 (sacrum anterior and posterior), PRES11 (brow presentation), REACT3 and REACT5 (uterine hypertonus and tumultuous labor with oxytocin). Furthermore, six showed significantly enhanced risk at the upper end of the risk-score scale. In addition to FORCEPS2, described above, they included FORTRAC3 (very difficult forceps traction), FUNDAL2 (moderate fundal pressure), PROLAP (prolapsed cord), ABRUPT (abruptio placentae), and INDUCT6-9 (induction for all other indications). For perinatal effects, 33 of the 55 variables yielded significant results and two others significant high-end enhancement. All 11 of those that had shown significant effects in regard to composite outcome were also represented in this group showing perinatal effects.

Labor progression variables were examined in the same way by decile risk-score groupings (Table 27-7). In sharp contrast to the disparate findings seen with delivery variables, only one factor surfaced as potentially distinctive from the effects incorporated into the risk-score model, namely ACT3 (prolonged active phase). Although the analysis for this factor showed relatively good homogeneity overall, it did demonstrate significant augmentation of effect at the high end of the risk-score scale, analogous to that seen earlier for FORCEPS2. None of the 14 labor progression variables was found to have a significant combined effect (all decile-group effects considered concurrently).

Drug and anesthesia variables were also studied by this method (Table 27-8). Among the 26 analyzed factors, four showed residual effect on composite outcome and 13 on perinatal outcome. Since all four variables affecting composite results also appeared to influence perinatal outcome, the total number of risk factors identified was 13. The former were AGT7 (penicillin), AGT8 (streptomycin), AGT22 (Apresoline) and AGT27 (other antibiotics);

Table 27-7
Risk-Enhancing Effects of Labor Progression Variables on
Decile Risk-Score-Stratified Outcome

Risk Variable		Perinatal Outcome		Composite Outcome	
		RR	95%CL	RR	95%CL
LAT2	Foreshortened latent phase	1.00	0.70-1.44	1.04	0.87-1.25
LAT3	Prolonged latent phase	1.30	0.85-1.99	1.11	0.88-1.41
ACT2	Foreshortened active phase	1.00	0.71-1.41	0.99	0.84-1.17
ACT3	Prolonged active phase	1.01*	0.64-1.58	1.02	0.81-1.28
DEC2	Foreshortened deceleration phase	1.03	0.70-1.53	1.03	0.84-1.27
DEC3	Prolonged deceleration phase	0.99	0.68-1.45	1.02	0.83-1.24
SEC2	Foreshortened second stage	0.93	0.67-1.30	0.97	0.83-1.14
SEC3	Prolonged second stage	1.35	0.79-2.31	1.02	0.72-1.44
DESC2	Protracted descent	1.09	0.74-1.59	1.06	0.85-1.32
DESC3	Precipitate descent	0.92	0.65-1.29	0.92	0.77-1.10
MAXS2	Protracted dilatation	0.95	0.66-1.36	0.98	0.81-1.18
MAXS3	Precipitate dilatation	1.03	0.70-1.52	1.00	0.84-1.20
ARRS3	Arrest of descent	1.13	0.73-1.74	1.06	0.81-1.38
ARRD3	Arrest of dilatation	1.13	0.79-1.61	1.02	0.84-1.24

* Relative risk significantly enhanced in high-risk-score groups.

in addition to all of these, the latter included IVD1 (intravenous anesthesia), OXYT1 (oxytocin induction of labor), AGT6 (Achromycin), AGT13 (phenobarbital), AGT16 (hydroxyzine), AGT18 (triflupromazine), AGT24 (oxytocin), AGT25 (sparteine sulfate), and AGT26 (magnesium sulfate). Ten were noted to increase high-score risk significantly, eight for composite outcome and two for perinatal outcome. Because most duplicated those identified by overall testing, this added only three factors for consideration, namely PUDEND (pudendal block anesthesia), PARAC (paracervical block), and OXYT2 (augmentation of labor).

In all, 95 risk variables had thus been tested to ascertain whether their effects had been fully incorporated into the risk-score model. Of these, 46 proved to have significant residual effects (33 delivery and 13 drug variables, but no labor variables) and eight to have significant high-score effects (four delivery, one labor, and three drug variables). All overall composite effects were duplicated in the perinatal results, but not vice versa. It was clear from these analyses that the arbitrary decile cut points we had used for risk-score scalar di-

visions did not satisfy our basic needs. While gross overview tests of homogeneity may have indicated a good fit of the data to the model, this form of close scrutiny revealed unacceptable degrees of poor fit for our purposes.

Revising Risk-Score Strata to Reflect True Risk Impact

Means for correcting the misfit of model and data were sought by reassessing the way in which grouping stratifications had been done. Heretofore, we had merely divided the full risk-score scale into deciles and further subdivided the uppermost decile into three subsets. This had seemed logical at the time but, in retrospect, was found to be both arbitrary and inappropriate. It proved wrong because the adverse risks associated with the score were not a continuously increasing function of the magnitude of the score. Instead, there was a stepped relationship with greatly skewed concentrations at the high end of the score range.

By examining scores in increments of 0.2, we were able to show this important

Table 27-8
Risk-Enhancing Effects of Drug-Anesthesia Variables on
Decile Risk-Score-Stratified Outcome

Risk Variable		Perinatal Outcome		Composite Outcome	
		RR	95%CL	RR	95%CL
SPINAL	Spinal anesthesia	0.98	0.71-1.35	1.02	0.86-1.21
PUDEND	Pudendal block anesthesia	1.14[a]	0.81-1.61	1.09	0.92-1.29
PARAC	Paracervical block anesthesia	1.27	0.77-2.08	1.08[a]	0.78-1.50
GAS1	Intermittent inhalation anesthesia	1.05	0.70-1.58	1.03	0.84-1.25
GAS2	Continuous inhalation anesthesia	0.98	0.70-1.37	1.03	0.87-1.22
GAS3	Intermittent and continuous gas	1.40	0.85-2.33	1.07	0.78-1.46
IVD1	Intravenous anesthesia	2.76	1.43-5.35[b]	1.47	0.84-2.58
OXYT1	Oxytocin induction of labor	2.18	1.08-4.40[b]	1.18[a]	0.72-1.93
OXYT2	Oxytocin augmentation of labor	1.09[a]	0.77-1.55	0.98	0.81-1.19
OXYT3	Oxytocin induction and augmentation	1.21	0.71-2.08	0.99	0.72-1.35
AGT1	Demerol	1.01	0.71-1.44	0.97	0.80-1.16
AGT2	Nisentil	1.67	0.83-3.37	0.91	0.56-1.46
AGT6	Achromycin	7.46	2.93-18.95[b]	1.72[a]	0.82-3.60
AGT7	Penicillin	4.67	2.12-10.29[b]	2.02[a]	1.03-3.97[b]
AGT8	Streptomycin	6.39	2.77-14.74[b]	2.44[a]	1.17-5.09[b]
AGT13	Phenobarbital	3.02	1.34-6.83[b]	1.32[a]	0.77-2.26
AGT16	Hydroxyzine	2.36	1.10-5.09[b]	1.21[a]	0.76-1.93
AGT18	Triflupromazine	2.56	1.15-5.67[b]	1.27	0.66-2.43
AGT19	Scopolamine	1.04	0.62-1.74	0.94	0.74-1.21
AGT20	Atropine	1.86	0.99-3.48	1.16	0.76-1.79
AGT22	Apresoline	11.76	4.26-32.46[b]	2.91	1.21-6.99[b]
AGT23	Syntocinon	1.27	0.67-2.40	0.91	0.60-1.38
AGT24	Oxytocin	2.82	1.37-5.80[b]	1.31	0.80-2.14
AGT25	Sparteine	2.85	1.28-6.33[b]	1.44	0.84-2.46
AGT26	Magnesium sulfate	2.44	1.12-6.02[b]	1.23[a]	0.68-2.22
AGT27	Other antibiotics	19.54	6.60-57.80[b]	5.49	1.96-15.41[b]

a   Relative risk significantly enhanced in high-risk-score groups.

b   Statistically significant, $p < 0.05$.

feature quite clearly. For composite outcomes, for example, it was clear (Table 27-9) that there were no bad outcomes at all for cases with scores lower than -4.00 and very few up to -3.00; altogether, there were 3.77% such poor results in the 2310 offspring constituting this group. Among the 12,150 cases with scores between -2.99 and -1.80, somewhat less favorable outcomes were found, slowly increasing from 5.9% to 12.1% with an overall rate of 8.07%. Although still a relatively low rate, this reflected a 2.1-fold increase in impact over that seen associated with lower scores. A sharp increase was encountered at score -1.79, with 20.6% bad results. This seriously adverse level persisted to score -0.80, the inclusive group of 497 cases averaging 21.0% demonstrably poor composite outcomes; this was a further 2.6-fold increase over the prior score level and 5.6-fold over the lowermost level. From scores of -0.79 up through the positive tail of the distribution of the score range, results for the 41 infants were uniformly very bad at an average adverse rate of 48.8%. This reflected an additional 2.3-fold incremental impact over that of the prior score group and a grand total of 12.8-fold over the lowest score group.

Table 27-9
Distribution of Adverse Composite Outcome Across Risk-Score Scale*

Risk Score	Good Outcome No.	%	Bad Outcome No.	%	Risk of Bad Outcome	Cum%
-4.0 or less	30	0.22	0	0.00	0.000	0.20
-3.9 to -3.8	27	0.19	1	0.08	0.036	0.38
-3.7 to -3.6	71	0.51	3	0.24	0.041	0.87
-3.5 to -3.4	189	1.36	3	0.24	0.016	2.14
-3.3 to -3.2	565	4.06	25	2.02	0.042	6.03
-3.1 to -3.0	1341	9.63	55	4.44	0.039	15.23
-2.9 to -2.8	1725	12.38	109	8.80	0.059	27.32
-2.7 to -2.6	2485	17.84	190	15.33	0.071	44.95
-2.5 to -2.4	3408	24.47	303	24.46	0.082	69.42
-2.3 to -2.2	2141	15.37	219	17.68	0.093	84.98
-2.1 to -2.0	1002	7.19	104	8.39	0.094	92.27
-1.9 to -1.8	408	2.93	56	4.52	0.121	95.33
-1.7 to -1.6	208	1.49	54	4.36	0.206	97.05
-1.5 to -1.4	133	0.95	28	2.26	0.174	98.11
-1.3 to -1.2	71	0.51	18	1.45	0.202	98.70
-1.1 to -1.0	49	0.35	21	1.69	0.300	99.16
-0.9 to -0.8	36	0.26	11	0.89	0.234	99.47
-0.7 to -0.6	14	0.10	10	0.81	0.417	99.63
-0.5 to -0.4	14	0.10	10	0.81	0.417	99.79
-0.3 to -0.2	4	0.03	4	0.32	0.500	99.84
-0.1 to 0.0	3	0.02	4	0.32	0.571	99.89
+0.1 to +0.2	1	0.01	1	0.08	0.500	99.90
+0.3 to +0.4	3	0.02	1	0.08	0.250	99.93
+0.5 to +0.6	1	0.01	2	0.16	0.667	99.95
+0.7 to +0.8	1	0.01	1	0.08	0.500	99.96
+0.9 or more	0	0.00	6	0.48	1.000	100.00

*   Based on total series of 1,239 adverse outcomes among 15,169 index cases (8.17%).

These empirical incremental groupings, delineated according to actual risk for given risk scores, are summarized in Table 27-10. Without exception, the composite outcome result within each designated group is significantly different from that of all other groups, including adjacent groups (p < .001). The distribution of the scores by 0.2 increments and the composite outcome risks associated with each score are illustrated graphically in Figure 27-4. In addition, the envelopes of averaged risk for these five selected incremental risk-score groups is shown. This material provides documentation of the stepped increases in risk associated with increasing risk scores. Choice of cut points here was based strictly on the natural divisions of observed hazard rather than on arbitrary proportions of cases as in the foregoing decile divisions.

The same assessment was applied to the data for perinatal outcome as related to risk score. Table 27-11 displays the results by 0.2 increments of score, showing a stepped progression quite similar to that encountered for composite outcome. At or below a score of -5.50, all did well and there were few bad perinatal results up to score -4.70. This total subset of 3898 infants averaged only 0.62% adverse effects. From scores -4.69 to -2.90, the outcomes were somewhat worse in the range of 1.2% to 3.6%, with an overall group average of 1.92% for the 9122 cases included here. The rate represented a 3.1-fold increase in bad outcomes over that for offspring from the lowest score group. The stepped increase in adverse results at score -2.89 was impressive, persisting to score -1.90 at an average of 7.97% for the 665 cases. This represented

Table 27-10
Cut-Points for Composite Outcome Risk-Score Incremental Groups

Risk Score	Good Outcome		Bad Outcome		Risk of Bad Outcome	Population		
	No.	%	No.	%		No.	%	Cum%
-3.0 or less	2223	16.0	87	7.0	0.038	2310	15.2	15.2
-2.9 to -1.8	11169	80.2	981	79.2	0.081	12150	80.1	95.3
-1.7 to -0.8	497	3.6	132	10.7	0.210	629	4.2	99.5
-0.7 or more	41	0.3	39	3.2	0.488	80	0.5	100.0

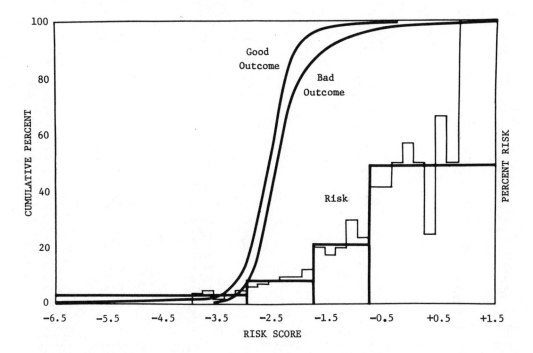

Figure 27-4. Cumulative distribution of risk scores for cases with adverse composite outcomes versus those with good results, showing that cases with bad outcomes generally had higher risk scores. The chance of a bad outcome for a given risk score is also illustrated in 0.2 score increments. The site at which stepped enhancements of risk appear serve to delineate cut points for designating principal risk-score groupings. The overall within-group risk is represented as well (heavy line).

a further increment of 4.2-fold over the next lower score group and 12.9-fold over the lowest score group. The next obvious step-up at scores of -1.89 through -0.70 yielded an overall rate of 22.0% for 200 cases, a 2.8-fold increase over the prior group and a remarkable 36.7-fold over the lowest score group. As expected, the highest scores of -0.69 or greater were associated with the worst perinatal results; these 48 cases had 56.3% bad results, 2.6 times higher than those with the next lower score and a startling 93.8 times that of the lowest score group.

The trends in these data are illustrated in Figure 27-5 as regards both the distribution of scores and the perinatal outcome vis-à-vis the risk score in 0.2 increments. The

Table 27-11
Distribution of Adverse Perinatal Outcome Across Risk-Score Scale*

Risk Score	Good Outcome		Bad Outcome		Risk of of Bad Outcome	Cum%
	No.	%	No.	%		
-5.5 or less	739	5.56	0	0.00	0.000	5.30
-5.4 to -5.3	673	5.07	4	1.24	0.006	10.16
-5.2 to -5.1	692	5.21	4	1.24	0.006	15.16
-5.0 to -4.9	713	5.37	12	3.72	0.017	20.36
-4.8 to -4.7	1057	7.96	4	1.24	0.004	27.98
-4.6 to -4.5	1441	10.85	17	5.26	0.012	38.44
-4.4 to -4.3	1660	12.49	20	6.19	0.012	50.50
-4.2 to -4.1	1585	11.93	26	8.05	0.016	62.06
-4.0 to -3.9	1345	10.12	24	7.43	0.018	71.89
-3.8 to -3.7	999	7.52	25	7.74	0.024	79.24
-3.6 to -3.5	766	5.77	29	8.98	0.036	84.94
-3.4 to -3.3	525	3.95	17	5.26	0.031	88.83
-3.2 to -3.1	356	2.68	10	3.10	0.027	91.46
-3.0 to -2.9	270	2.03	7	2.17	0.025	93.45
-2.8 to -2.7	217	1.63	10	3.10	0.044	95.08
-2.6 to -2.5	129	0.97	12	3.72	0.085	96.09
-2.4 to -2.3	117	0.88	15	4.64	0.114	97.04
-2.2 to -2.1	80	0.60	9	2.79	0.101	97.67
-2.0 to -1.9	69	0.52	7	2.17	0.092	98.22
-1.8 to -1.7	47	0.35	14	4.33	0.230	98.66
-1.6 to -1.5	29	0.22	8	2.48	0.216	98.92
-1.4 to -1.3	27	0.20	8	2.48	0.229	99.17
-1.2 to -1.1	26	0.20	1	0.31	0.037	99.37
-1.0 to -0.9	16	0.12	9	2.79	0.360	99.55
-0.8 to -0.7	11	0.08	4	1.24	0.267	99.66
-0.6 to -0.5	7	0.05	6	1.86	0.462	99.75
-0.4 to -0.3	4	0.03	4	1.24	0.500	99.81
-0.2 to -0.1	2	0.02	2	0.62	0.500	99.83
0.0 to +0.1	1	0.01	3	0.93	0.750	99.86
+0.2 to +0.3	2	0.02	4	1.24	0.667	99.91
+0.4 to +0.5	2	0.02	2	0.62	0.500	99.94
+0.6 to +0.7	0	0.00	1	0.31	1.000	99.94
+0.8 to +0.9	0	0.00	1	0.31	1.000	99.95
+1.0 to +1.1	2	0.02	2	0.62	0.500	99.98
+1.2 or more	1	0.01	2	0.62	0.667	100.00

* Based on a total of 323 adverse outcomes among 13,933 index cases (2.37%).

stepped progression in relative risk is shown together with the overall within-group risk for the five segments of risk score designated on the basis of empirically observed hazard. The summarized data for these five incremental score groups are tallied in Table 27-12. As with the composite outcome, the perinatal result for each of these groups is significantly different from that for all others, including adjacent sets (p < .001). Having now subdivided risk scores relating to composite outcome into four incremental groups and those for perinatal outcome into five groups according to dem-

onstrated risk, we were in a position to retest for residual risk effects of all labor, delivery, and drug variables to determine if the reconstructed model fit the data more precisely than before.

Survey of Residual Risk Effects in Incremental Strata

Using the same analytical paradigm devised for the decile groups, we examined two parallel populations for each risk variable, namely the one exhibiting the factor and another a selected referent subpopula-

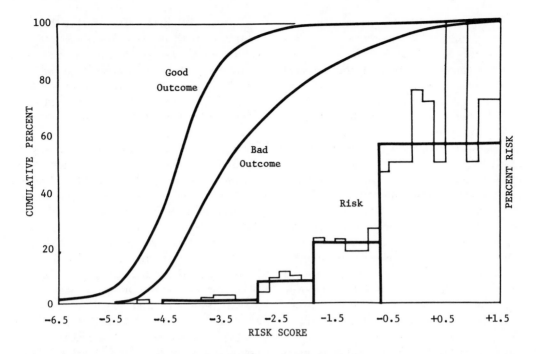

Figure **27-5.** Cumulative distribution of risk scores for adverse perinatal versus good outcome and incremental within-group risks of a bad perinatal result, analogous to Figure 27-4. The difference in distribution of scores here is much more impressive than for composite outcome. Similarly, the stepped sequence is more marked.

Table 27-12
Cut-Points for Perinatal Outcome Incremental Risk-Score Groups

Risk Score	Good Outcome		Bad Outcome		Risk of	Population		
	No.	%	No.	%	Bad Outcome	No.	%	Cum%
-4.7 or less	3874	28.46	24	7.43	0.006	3898	27.98	27.98
-4.6 to -2.9	8947	65.74	175	54.18	0.019	9122	65.47	93.45
-2.8 to -1.9	612	4.50	53	16.41	0.080	665	4.77	98.22
-1.8 to -0.7	156	1.15	44	13.62	0.220	200	1.44	99.66
-0.6 or more	21	0.15	27	8.36	0.563	48	0.34	100.00

tion. The latter, as aforementioned, was generally made up of cases in which delivery was by manual control of a fetus in vertex presentation (CONTROL1) and in which the variable being studied was absent. Both were stratified by the incremental risk-score subgroups and the results determined within each cell of the matrix thus formed for both composite and perinatal outcomes. Statistical comparisons were done across risk-score groups and the over-all collective residual risk was assessed for statistical significance. The entire array of data for each risk factor was also tested for homogeneity.

An example of the effect of one such variable, FORCEPS2 (class II midforceps), is shown for composite outcome in Table 27-13, formulated in exact parallel to the decile-group analysis of the same factor as displayed in Table 27-4. The cross-product (odds) ratio for each risk-score group is given together with the probability value representing the likelihood that the difference in rate of adverse outcomes (between the risk factor group and the referent group) was a chance event. We see the increase in bad outcomes in groups of cases with higher scores, as expected, both for index and control series. However, the increases are not exactly comparable, the FORCEPS2 cases showing a much greater enhancement than the CONTROL1 cases.

This nonparallel discrepancy is reflected in the increasing odds ratio. Nonetheless, only the difference in the lowest increment score group could be shown to be statistically significant and the overall analysis showed good homogeneity centering on a mean relative risk estimate of 0.87. There is the same high-end concentration of residual bad effect seen with the decile stratifications, suggesting that the model did not quite fit the data for this variable, even though the fit was somewhat better than it had been earlier. For low scores (-1.80 or less), the impact of FORCEPS2 was significantly less than that of CONTROL1 (5.93% versus 8.32%, OR = 0.69, p = .00011); for high scores (-1.79 or more), the reverse held true, but it did not prove significant (31.3% versus 22.4%, OR = 1.57, p = .11).

Further examination of the spectrum of risk variables for composite outcome results did show these findings to be exceptional in that very few others deviated so far from the reconstructed model. All delivery variables were studied in like manner

(Table 27-14). In sharp contrast to the prior findings with decile risk-score strata (see Table 27-6), the overall effects were almost uniformly centered on odds ratios of 1.00; the 95th percentile confidence limits fell on either side of unity in all cases and none showed statistically significant heterogeneity. Closer scrutiny across the risk-score subgroups showed that only 12 risk variables revealed any noteworthy fluctuations from the expected composite outcome results based on the risk-score model. Moreover, none of these 12 factors demonstrated a significant deviation in more than a single risk-score subgroup. Most showed protective effects confined principally to the low-end score group, including FORCEPS2 (as noted above), FORTRAC2 and FORTRAC3 (difficult and very difficult forceps traction), FORAPP2 (difficult forceps application), FORROT2 and FORROT3 (difficult and very difficult forceps rotation), AUGMENT1 (elective stimulation of labor, here in the midrange score group), AUGMENT10 (stimulation for arrested labor), and PRES1 (occiput anterior). Adverse effects were found in isolated instances, two in midrange score groups, specifically FUNDAL2 (moderate fundal pressure) and PRES3 (occiput posterior), and one at the low end (CONTROL1).

For labor progression risk variables (Table 27-15), there was very little information of relevance pertaining to deviations from the model for composite outcome. This confirmed goodness-of-fit both overall

Table 27-13
Impact of a Risk Variable* on Adverse Composite Outcome
Within Incremental Risk-Score Groupings

Score Range	FORCEPS2			CONTROL1		OR	p-Value
	No.	%	Expected	No.	%		
-3.0 or less	874	3.43	4.05	114	8.77	0.37	0.0065
-2.9 to -1.8	1706	7.21	8.08	6559	8.31	0.86	0.14
-1.7 to -0.8	85	27.06	22.00	174	19.54	1.53	0.17
-0.7 or more	8	75.00	57.50	18	50.00	3.00	0.23
Overall	2673	6.81	8.18	6865	8.71	0.87	0.19

* See footnote, Table 27-4.

402

Table 27-14
Incremental Risk-Score Groupings for Impact of Delivery Variables
on Composite Outcome*

Delivery Variable		Score Range				
		-6.4 to -3.0	-2.9 to -1.8	-1.7 to -0.8	-0.7 to +1.7	Overall
FORCEPS2	Class II midforceps	0.37b	0.86	1.53	3.00	0.87
FORCEPS3	Class III midforceps	0.56	0.89	1.06	1.02	0.88
FORTRAC2	Difficult forceps traction	0.39c	0.90	1.00	0.55	0.88
FORTRAC3	Very difficult traction	0.21a	0.92	1.64	1.82	0.98
FORTRAC4	Failed forceps traction	---	0.62	1.28	4.09	1.11
FORAPP2	Difficult forceps application	0.40b	0.89	1.17	0.82	0.86
FORAPP3	Very difficult application	3.60	1.34	0.66	2.46	1.20
FORAPP4	Failed forceps application	---	0.72	1.16	2.00	1.07
FORROT2	Difficult forceps rotation	0.42a	0.89	0.65	1.91	0.83
FORROT3	Very difficult rotation	1.45	0.61a	1.97	---	0.91
FORROT4	Failed forceps rotation	0.00	1.34	---	---	1.08
CONTROL1	Manual control of head	2.54C	1.06	0.85	1.22	1.07
CONTROL2	Uncontrolled head delivery	---	1.41	0.35	---	1.36
FUNDAL2	Moderate fundal pressure	0.31	1.10	3.24B	0.50	1.18
FUNDAL3	Strong fundal pressure	0.81	1.22	2.20	0.67	1.26
PROLAP	Prolapsed cord	---	1.19	1.67	0.39	1.31
ABRUPT	Abruptio placentae	0.59	1.04	1.14	1.82	1.06
CSVAG	Cesarean after vaginal delivery	---	---	0.85	0.91	1.30
SHOULD	Shoulder dystocia	---	1.21	1.00	---	1.21
PREVIA	Placenta previa	0.35	---	---	---	0.87
INDUCT1	Elective induction of labor	1.44	0.86	0.48	0.82	0.88
INDUCT2	Induction for ROM	0.41	1.03	1.04	1.80	0.95

INDUCT3	Induction for PIH	---	0.63	1.20	2.50	1.18
INDUCT4	Induction for diabetes	2.97	0.65	1.06	0.91	1.11
INDUCT5	Induction for Rh disease	---	---	1.07	0.89	1.06
INDUCT6-9	Induction for other indications	---	1.21	0.90	---	1.11
AUGMENT1	Elective stimulation of labor	0.62	0.85	0.23a	0.45	0.79
AUGMENT2	Stimulation for ROM	0.39	0.99	1.17	2.57	1.02
AUGMENT3	Stimulation for PIH	0.00	0.21	1.86	1.67	1.31
AUGMENT4	Stimulation for diabetes	---	---	1.24	1.82	1.29
AUGMENT5	Stimulation for Rh disease	---	---	1.07	0.89	1.30
AUGMENT6	Stimulation for amnionitis	---	---	---	2.06	2.66
AUGMENT10	Stimulation for arrested labor	0.29a	1.18	0.77	1.69	1.02
AUGMENT11-18	Stimulation for other indications	0.00	1.07	1.08	2.50	1.11
BREECH2	Frank breech	0.00	1.45	0.85	0.45	1.04
BREECH3	Complete breech	---	2.22	0.53	1.36	1.33
BREECH4	Single footling breech	0.00	0.79	1.88	0.46	1.09
BREECH5	Double footling breech	---	---	1.59	0.46	1.46
BRFACH2	Difficult aftercoming forceps	0.00	1.34	1.15	0.30	1.06
BRDELIV3	Assisted breech delivery	0.00	1.66	0.55	0.91	1.18
BRDELIV4	Breech extraction	---	0.77	1.36	0.61	1.06
PRES1	Occiput anterior	0.12d	1.02	0.77	0.21	0.91
PRES2	Occiput transverse	0.47	1.03	1.20	1.50	1.03
PRES3	Occiput posterior	0.77	0.86	1.90A	2.53	0.97
PRES5-8	Breech presentation	0.00	1.35	---	---	1.04
PRES1-4	Vertex presentation	1.00	2.09	0.80	1.00	0.84
PRES11	Brow presentation	1.00	1.83	0.27	1.00	0.54
REACT1	No uterotonic response to oxytocin	0.33	0.77	4.32	0.82	0.87
REACT2	Tetanic contraction from oxytocin	0.00	1.53	0.60	---	1.12
REACT3	Uterine hypertonus from oxytocin	---	1.86	0.61	0.81	1.43
REACT4	FHR abnormality from oxytocin	0.00	1.44	0.50	---	1.12
REACT5	Tumultuous labor from oxytocin	---	0.79	2.20	---	1.38

* Data shown are cross-product ratios which are estimates of relative risk. Probability code: $\underline{A}$ 0.05, $\underline{B}$ 0.01, $\underline{C}$ 0.005, $\underline{D}$ 0.001, $\underline{E}$ 0.0005, $\underline{F}$ 0.0001 or less; lower case protective. Omissions are instances where relative frequency was too small to compute statistics.

Table 27-15
Incremental Risk-Score Groupings for Impact of Labor Progression Variables
on Composite Outcome*

Delivery Variable		-6.4 to -3.0	-2.9 to -1.8	Score Range -1.7 to -0.8	-0.7 to +1.7	Overall
LAT2	Foreshortened latent phase	0.33b	1.08	1.26	0.87	1.05
LAT3	Prolonged latent phase	0.18	1.14	1.02	4.57	1.12
ACT2	Foreshortened active phase	0.46	1.09	1.01	0.56	1.05
ACT3	Prolonged active phase	0.30a	1.09	0.87	1.50	1.02
DEC2	Foreshortened deceleration phase	0.28a	1.21	0.98	0.64	1.13
DEC3	Prolonged deceleration phase	0.22d	1.07	0.73	1.16	0.98
SEC2	Foreshortened second stage	0.34b	1.07	1.20	0.36	1.03
SEC3	Prolonged second stage	0.30a	0.99	1.29	0.50	0.92
DESC2	Protracted descent	0.37	1.13	1.17	0.37	1.09
DESC3	Precipitate descent	0.50	0.84a	1.30	0.57	0.85
MAXS2	Protracted dilatation	0.28c	1.11	0.73	1.21	1.01
MAXS3	Precipitate dilatation	0.48	1.06	0.92	0.58	1.01
ARRS3	Arrest of descent	0.36	0.99	0.98	1.14	0.94
ARRD3	Arrest of dilatation	0.38a	1.02	0.97	0.96	0.97

* See Table 27-14 for probability code.

and within risk-score groupings. Nine of these variables showed protective effects, limited exclusively (with one exception) to the low-end risk-score segment: LAT2 (foreshortened latent phase), ACT3 (prolonged active phase), DEC2 and DEC3 (foreshortened and prolonged deceleration phases), SEC2 and SEC3 (foreshortened and prolonged second stage), DESC3 (precipitate descent, here in the moderately low score group), MAXS2 (protracted dilatation), and ARRD3 (arrest of dilatation). None showed any significantly adverse effects at all. Both LAT3 and ACT3 (prolonged latent and active phases) showed high-end enhancements, but neither of these proved statistically significant.

Data for composite outcome as related to drug and anesthesia variables conformed even more closely to the model (Table 27-16). Compared to decile-group data (see Table 27-8) in which a large number were found to deviate significantly from expected, there were no variables that fell far from a rate ratio of 1.00 and all showed good homogeneity. Significant low-end protective effects were found for three factors (GAS2 continuous inhalation anesthesia, OXYT2 oxytocin augmentation of labor, and AGT2 Nisentil) and adverse effects for only one (PUDEND, pudendal block anesthesia). Four others showed high-end enhancement (PARAC, paracervical block; OXYT2, oxytocin augmentation of labor; AGT13, phenobarbital; AGT16, hydroxyzine; and AGT24, oxytocin), but none could be shown to be statistically significant.

Perinatal outcome results were studied in the same way as well. Results for the full range of delivery variables proved remarkably consistent in regard to overall homogeneity and within-group fit (Table 27-17). Scattered odds ratios appeared either high or low, but none was found to be statistically significant except one, namely that for REACT3 (uterine hypertonus from oxytocin) and only for the moderately low risk-score group. Moreover, none of these findings duplicated those disclosed above

for the comparable analysis of composite outcome results (see Table 27-14). This suggested that these were merely chance occurrences. Paralleling the findings for composite outcome, however, were high-end enhancements encountered for FORTRAC4 and FORAPP4 (failed forceps traction and application), BREECH3 (complete breech), and PRES1 (occiput anterior), but all were determined to be insignificant when examined statistically. Two other risk variables, also not statistically significant, were found to have high-end enhancements, namely INDUCT5 and AUGMENT5 (induction and stimulation for Rh isoimmunization).

Similarly, perinatal outcome findings for the labor progression risk variables were determined to fit uniformly to the model (Table 27-18) without evidence of significant deviation from overall risk effects. The results across incremental score groupings were also rather good, except for four scattered significant within-group discrepancies. Three presented adverse effects, all within the moderately low risk-score level: these were LAT3 (prolonged latent phase), SEC3 (prolonged second stage), and MAXS2 (protracted dilatation). One other was protective at the moderately high level, namely ACT3 (prolonged active phase). The only risk variables that had also surfaced in the composite outcome analysis done earlier (see Table 27-15) were ACT3, SEC3, and MAXS2, but whereas the first of these showed a like effect (protective in both perinatal and composite data results), the other two showed opposite and contradictory effects. High-end enhancement was found for three factors, namely ACT2 (foreshortened active phase), ACT3 (prolonged active phase), and MAXS3 (precipitate dilatation), none of which was statistically significant. Only ACT3 paralleled the effect seen earlier with composite outcomes (likewise insignificant).

Perinatal outcomes for drugs and anesthesia were likewise analyzed using the newly developed model (Table 27-19). The results showed a very good fit of model to

Table 27-16
Incremental Risk-Score Groupings for Impact of Drug-Anesthesia Variables on Composite Outcome*

Delivery Variable		Score Range				
		-6.4 to -3.0	-2.9 to -1.8	-1.7 to -0.8	-0.7 to +1.7	Overall
SPINAL	Spinal anesthesia	0.60	0.86a	1.13	1.80	0.88
PUDEND	Pudendal block	0.18	1.20A	0.71	0.72	1.14
PARAC	Paracervical block	0.32	0.96	1.66	1.82	1.03
GAS1	Intermittent inhalation anesthesia	0.00	1.10	0.59	1.07	1.05
GAS2	Continuous inhalation anesthesia	0.00a	1.14	1.00	0.62	1.10
GAS3	Intermittent and continuous anesthesia	1.07	0.98	1.92	0.48	1.06
IVD1	Intravenous anesthesia	0.00	1.51	1.21	---	1.24
OXYT1	Oxytocin induction of labor	0.88	1.21	0.22	---	1.13
OXYT2	Oxytocin augmentation of labor	0.19f	0.99	1.01	1.75	0.93
OXYT3	Oxytocin induction and augmentation	1.41	0.93	0.87	0.89	0.95
AGT1	Demerol	0.65	0.95	1.25	0.55	0.95
AGT2	Nisentil	0.37a	0.98	1.13	---	0.76
AGT6	Achromycin	---	1.55	0.51	---	1.19
AGT7	Penicillin	---	1.31	1.80	---	1.33
AGT8	Streptomycin	---	1.66	1.43	---	1.45
AGT13	Phenobarbital	0.45	0.82	1.32	1.60	1.08
AGT16	Hydroxyzine	0.76	0.87	1.49	2.00	1.05
AGT18	Triflupromazine	0.44	0.51	2.06	---	0.87
AGT19	Scopolamine	0.00	1.02	0.78	---	0.93
AGT20	Atropine	0.00	1.16	0.99	0.90	1.10
AGT22	Apresoline	---	2.22	0.67	---	1.38
AGT23	Syntocinon	0.65	0.72	1.34	0.20	0.78
AGT24	Oxytocin	0.00	1.68	0.57	4.50	1.21
AGT25	Sparteine	---	1.44	0.74	0.36	1.22
AGT26	Magnesium sulfate	0.71	0.62	2.04	1.82	1.00
AGT27	Other antibiotics	---	---	0.00	1.00	1.89

* See Table 27-14 for probability code.

Table 27-17
Incremental Risk-Score Groupings for Impact of Delivery Variables
on Perinatal Outcome*

Delivery Variable		-4.7 or less	-4.6 to -2.9	Score Range -2.8 to -1.9	-1.8 to -0.7	-0.6 or more	Overall
FORCEPS2	Class II midforceps	1.06	0.82	1.36	0.69	0.00	0.96
FORCEPS2	Class III midforceps	2.47	1.16	0.88	0.47	0.20	1.01
FORTRAC2	Difficult forceps traction	1.37	1.04	1.04	0.76	0.30	1.02
FORTRAC3	Very difficult forceps traction	2.59	1.36	1.08	0.33	0.40	1.06
FORTRAC4	Failed forceps traction	0.00	0.00	1.31	0.63	2.40	0.88
FORAPP2	Difficult forceps application	1.33	0.96	1.05	0.63	0.33	0.95
FORAPP3	Very difficult forceps application	0.00	1.83	1.11	0.37	0.00	1.18
FORAPP4	Failed forceps application	0.00	0.00	2.16	0.24	2.25	0.90
FORROT2	Difficult forceps rotation	2.24	0.86	0.65	0.41	0.00	0.95
FORROT3	Very difficult forceps rotation	0.00	1.18	0.74	1.50	0.40	1.05
FORROT4	Failed forceps rotation	0.00	1.85	1.92	0.00	- - -	1.06
CONTROL1	Manual control of head	0.89	0.89	1.01	1.34	1.36	0.96
CONTROL2	Uncontrolled head delivery	0.00	1.02	0.00	- - -	- - -	0.88
FUNDAL2	Moderate fundal pressure	0.63	1.02	2.27	2.17	- - -	1.19
FUNDAL3	Strong fundal pressure	1.36	1.55	0.79	2.03	- - -	1.41
PROLAP	Prolapsed cord	0.00	2.19	1.99	1.04	0.20	1.12
ABRUPT	Abruptio placentae	0.00	1.56	0.97	0.92	0.80	1.08
CSVAG	Cesarean section after vaginal delivery attempt	- - -	- - -	0.00	1.42	0.60	0.88

Code	Description						
SHOULD	Shoulder dystocia	---	0.00	1.05	0.80	0.80	0.84
PREVIA	Placenta previa	0.00	3.38	0.00	0.00	---	0.93
INDUCT1	Elective induction of labor	0.00	1.69	0.00	---	---	1.03
INDUCT2	Induction for ROM	0.00	1.45	1.24	0.53	---	0.96
INDUCT3	Induction for PIH	0.00	1.16	1.28	0.73	0.75	0.93
INDUCT4	Induction for diabetes	0.00	4.51	0.00	1.20	---	0.91
INDUCT5	Induction for Rh disease	0.00	0.00	0.89	0.71	1.50	0.75
INDUCT6-9	Induction for other indications	0.00	0.00	0.74	1.20	---	0.97
AUGMENT1	Elective stimulation of labor	1.52	1.18	0.80	0.15	---	0.98
AUGMENT2	Stimulation for ROM	0.74	1.21	0.80	0.84	1.25	1.00
AUGMENT3	Stimulation for PIH	0.00	1.03	0.00	0.74	1.13	0.85
AUGMENT4	Stimulation for diabetes	0.00	0.00	0.00	1.50	---	0.75
AUGMENT5	Stimulation for Rh disease	---	0.00	0.00	0.71	1.50	0.76
AUGMENT6	Stimulation for amnionitis	---	---	---	1.41	1.33	1.38
AUGMENT10	Stimulation for arrested labor	2.49	1.55	1.13	1.10	0.22	1.20
AUGMENT11-18	Stimulation for other indications	0.00	0.73	0.77	1.55	1.00	0.98
BREECH2	Frank presentation	0.00	0.00	1.38	0.71	---	0.90
BREECH3	Complete breech	0.00	0.00	1.00	0.00	1.60	0.86
BREECH4	Single footling breech	0.00	4.13	0.00	1.13	0.30	0.83
BRFACH2	Difficult aftercoming forceps	0.00	1.49	1.05	0.57	0.60	0.81
BRDELIV3	Assisted breech delivery	0.00	0.99	1.15	0.00	1.44	1.03
BRDELIV4	Breech extraction	0.00	0.00	0.61	0.83	1.20	0.77
PRES1	Occiput anterior	0.00	0.75	1.13	1.51	4.00	0.95
PRES2	Occiput transverse	2.34	1.16	1.03	0.80	0.63	1.02
PRES3	Occiput posterior	2.23	1.30	1.19	0.58	1.00	1.18
PRES5-8	Breech presentation	0.00	1.99	0.00	---	---	0.93
PRES1-4	Vertex presentation	0.00	0.48	0.00	0.00	0.57	0.52
PRES11	Brow presentation	0.00	2.68	0.00	---	---	1.07
REACT1	No uterotonic response to oxytocin	0.00	2.57	0.00	0.00	0.00	1.08
REACT2	Tetanic contraction from oxytocin	0.00	5.42	0.00	0.00	---	1.07
REACT3	Uterine hypertonus from oxytocin	0.00	6.78A	0.94	0.58	0.60	1.04
REACT4	FHR abnormality from oxytocin	0.00	3.31	0.00	1.00	1.20	1.01
REACT5	Tumultuous labor from oxytocin	0.00	0.00	0.00	1.50	---	0.88

* See Table 27-14 for probability code.

Table 27-18
Incremental Risk-Score Groupings for Impact of Labor Progression Variables on Perinatal Outcome*

Delivery Variable	Score Range					Overall
	-4.7 or less	-4.6 to -2.9	-2.8 to -1.9	-1.8 to -0.7	-0.6 or more	
LAT	1.11	1.20	1.05	1.10	0.45	1.12
LAT3	2.43	1.74A	0.49	1.46	0.50	1.35
ACT2	1.93	1.04	1.60	0.76	2.50	1.11
ACT3	0.95	1.49	1.62	0.27a	5.20	1.28
DEC2	0.68	1.27	0.72	0.96	0.60	1.02
DEC3	0.00	1.46	0.74	0.56	1.00	1.10
SEC2	0.64	1.14	0.68	0.98	0.36	0.99
SEC3	0.00	2.04A	0.59	0.39	0.42	1.05
DESC2	1.52	1.55	0.69	0.94	0.20	1.12
DESC3	0.76	0.93	0.90	0.95	0.10	0.89
MAXS2	0.74	1.54A	0.60	0.61	1.39	1.16
MAXS3	1.40	0.89	0.52	2.02	1.75	0.98
ARRS3	3.74	0.84	1.42	0.81	0.43	1.03
ARRD3	1.57	1.34	1.01	0.56	0.31	1.11

Foreshortened latent phase
Prolonged latent phase
Foreshortened active phase
Prolonged active phase
Foreshortened deceleration phase
Prolonged deceleration phase
Foreshortened second stage
Prolonged second stage
Protracted descent
Precipitate descent
Protracted dilatation
Precipitate dilatation
Arrest of descent
Arrest of dilatation

* See Table 27-14 for probability code.

410

Table 27-19
Incremental Risk-Score Groupings for Impact of Drug–Anesthesia Variables on Perinatal Outcome*

Delivery Variable		Score Range					Overall
		-4.7 or less	-4.6 to -2.9	-2.8 to -1.9	-1.8 to -0.7	-0.6 or more	
SPINAL	Spinal anesthesia	2.42	1.06	0.86	0.65	2.40	1.03
PUDEND	Pudendal block	0.00	1.20	2.23	0.32a	1.80	1.15
PARAC	Paracervical block	0.00	1.54	0.74	0.98	0.50	1.13
GAS1	Intermittent inhalation anesthesia	1.15	0.91	1.11	0.56	0.50	0.87
GAS2	Continuous inhalation anesthesia	1.94	1.03	1.30	1.05	0.59	1.07
GAS3	Intermittent and continuous gas	0.00	1.24	0.71	1.91	0.75	1.13
IVD1	Intravenous anesthesia	0.00	4.01A	1.04	0.87	0.12	0.95
OXYT1	Oxytocin induction of labor	0.00	0.94	1.47	0.50	1.60	1.10
OXYT2	Oxytocin augmentation of labor	1.17	1.39	0.94	0.40	1.00	1.15
OXYT3	Oxytocin induction and augmentation	0.00	1.27	0.71	1.04	0.30	0.87
AGT1	Demerol	0.89	1.35	0.82	0.28a	1.00	1.04
AGT2	Nisentil	0.39	1.38	1.01	1.42	--	1.06
AGT6	Achromycin	0.00	2.98	0.00	0.00	--	0.91
AGT7	Penicillin	0.00	2.46	0.85	1.03	0.00	0.94
AGT8	Streptomycin	0.00	0.00	1.61	1.23	0.00	0.89
AGT13	Phenobarbital	0.00	0.00	2.51	0.00	0.00	0.88
AGT16	Hydroxyzine	2.94	0.46	2.46	0.00	0.00	1.20
AGT18	Triflupromazine	0.00	0.00	2.49	1.33	0.00	0.98
AGT19	Scopolamine	1.03	1.11	0.55	0.74	0.40	0.94
AGT20	Atropine	0.00	1.51	1.32	0.55	0.13	1.03
AGT22	Apresoline	0.00	0.00	1.89	0.00	1.75	0.96
AGT23	Syntocinon	1.11	0.77	0.84	0.63	2.00	0.85
AGT24	Oxytocin	0.00	2.97A	0.00	0.39	0.40	0.96
AGT25	Sparteine	0.00	0.60	3.06	0.00	1.60	1.09
AGT27	Other antibiotics	--	0.00	--	0.94	--	0.92

*   See Table 27-14 for probability code.

data. Whereas a total of 13 risk variables had previously surfaced as having residual effects unaccounted for by the scoring system (see Table 27-8), none did now. All risk variables showed smooth overall homogeneity and only four were noted to have isolated within-group discrepancies of significance. These latter outcome results were adverse at the moderately low score end in two (IVD1 intravenous anesthesia and AGT24 oxytocin) and protective at the moderately high end in the other two (PUDEND, pudendal block anesthesia; and AGT1, Demerol). Except for PUDEND, none of these had been seen earlier in the analysis of composite outcome data (see Table 27-16). Furthermore, the effect encountered here for PUDEND was opposite that found before both in effect (protective versus adverse) and in position on the risk-scoring scale (moderately high versus moderately low). High-end enhancement was seen in six: SPINAL (spinal anesthesia), PUDEND (pudendal block), OXYT1 (oxytocin induction), AGT22 (Apresoline), AGT23 (Syntocinon), and AGT25 (sparteine sulfate). Not only was none of these statistically significant, but none had shown a similar enhancing effect in the antecedent composite outcome analysis.

In summary, therefore, there was good consistency for both composite and perinatal outcome data for the entire range of labor, delivery, and drug variables with this reconstructed model. Of the 95 risk factors tested, outcome results for nearly all conformed closely to the expected frequencies of adverse results. None showed a significant residual overall effect. This was in contradistinction to the 46 that had deviated markedly from the expected results in the model using the decile stratification of risk-scores.

A number did show within-group disparate effects. They totalled 25 in the composite data analysis (12 delivery, nine labor, and four drug variables) and nine in the perinatal data analysis (one delivery, four labor, and four drug variables). They were nearly always of a protective nature (only ten were adverse in all) and primarily located in the lowest risk-score strata (only six appeared in high-end risk-score groups). Given the fact that there were 855 separate analyses done for within-group effects (95 risk variables tested in four composite risk-score subgroups totalling 380, and in five perinatal subgroups totalling 475), encountering 34 significant within-group discrepancies (for a total of 4.0% overall, 6.6% among composite analyses, and 1.9% among perinatal) would not be unexpected on the basis of chance alone.

There was essentially no consistency between composite and perinatal results in regard to the magnitude, direction, or location of the observed within-group effects nor among the specific risk variables affected. Since our principal interest was the adverse impact at the high end of the risk-score scale, we felt these deviations from the model would probably be of negligible importance. Where such deviations occurred, there was no pattern to indicate any undisclosed trend or serious distortion or deviation from the model.

Pervading consistency was found throughout in regard to the narrowly constricted overall risk of each of the risk variables subjected to such intense scrutiny. In addition, homogeneity both within and between groups was very good. We thus appeared to have satisfied the essential requirement of a risk scoring model that closely fit the data. This accomplished, we were ready to evaluate the effects of prelabor factors on outcome while all relevant intrapartum and delivery risk variables were being weighed simultaneously by the model.

CHAPTER **28**

Predictor Variables

Summary

A total of 369 factors were examined by application to both the decile risk score and the incremental strata models to determine their impact as predictor variables while the effects of all identified labor-delivery risk factors were being weighed simultaneously by means of the risk score. The variables studied in this way encompassed a range of demographic, historical, physical, socioeconomic, antepartum, and intercurrent health factors. Of these, 97 were found to exhibit significant effects on offspring. Inconsistencies of impact across the range of risk-score subgroups showed that the effects of 24 of these were not wholly reliable, leaving 73 as validated predictors of fetal-infant prognosis.

Analytical efforts to this point had been directed at providing a mechanism whereby all relevant labor-delivery risk factors could be identified and incorporated concurrently into a single quantitative formulation of risk. The mechanism took the form of a scoring system that defined the risk in a systematic and reproducible fashion. Without this basis, it would not have been feasible to proceed to assess the potential impact of prelabor factors that may themselves affect the outcome for offspring either directly or through the intermediary pathway by which they might influence the labor-delivery risk variables. The design concept underlying the resolution of this issue has been dealt with in some detail in chapter 7. Our aim here was to examine the indirect pathway, thereby identifying and quantitating the effect of the constellation of pre-existent risk factors from among the full panoply of variables available to study, taking each into account seriatim while simultaneously controlling for the influence of those affecting outcome during labor and delivery. In this way, we felt we could assess risk variables for their predictive effects insofar as they might serve to influence the development of the at-risk labor-delivery state.

We have already examined many of these intrinsic factors both in isolation and collectively in an integrated group (see chapters 19-21) as well as aggregatively in conjunction with all other labor-delivery risk factors (see chapter 25). However, we have not separated out their direct effects from their indirect interactional effects mediated by way of altered intrapartum management or complications. To illustrate, let us consider how a chronic illness such as maternal diabetes mellitus might impact on outcome. Its direct action is reflected in some of its adverse fetal effects in causing congenital anomalies, fetal keto-acidosis, hypoxemia, and hypoglycemia or hyperglycemia, as well as placental insufficiency and macrosomia or intrauterine growth retardation. Indirectly, it influences the development of hydramnios, cephalo-pelvic disproportion, and shoulder dystocia, and it may further serve to alter obstetric care so that uterotonic stimulation is used for induction and/or stimulation of labor, perhaps initiating premature labor and delivery, or invoking a midforceps operation or cesarean section. These latter yield secondary risk effects in turn because they carry their own inherent hazards to the fetus and infant. Unless we could distinguish and measure the latter indirect risks, we would not be able to determine the true magnitude of the former direct risks.

In the preceding chapter, we described a model risk-scoring system that was capable of weighing all identified relevant labor, delivery, and drug risk variables whenever they occurred alone or in combination with others in a given gravida. This made it possible to quantitate the risk to offspring. The objectivity it offered was felt to permit us to

proceed to investigate potential predictor variables in a meaningful way. How each such predictor variable might destabilize that system would help flag those with significant adverse (or beneficial) impact and provide the necessary information to measure its effect.

The analytical methods used here were the same as those for determining residual effects of labor and delivery risk variables on the risk scoring system, as detailed extensively in chapter 27. For each risk variable under consideration, two parallel populations were examined, one made up of cases with the factor in question and the other without the factor but limited to those delivering infants in vertex presentation by manual control. For multiply stratified variables, one subcategory was chosen as referent instead of choosing the absence of the study variable (INST05, for example, was selected as referent for the institutional variables because it represented the largest case load). Again, it is important to note that the index population being studied had been culled from the full NCPP database by limiting the investigation to cases in which there had been a child born who weighed between 2500 and 4000g and who had no identifiable congenital anomaly incompatible with survival or with normal growth and development. Comparable case groups for each predictor risk variable were stratified by the labor-delivery risk-score subsets previously established separately for composite and perinatal outcome results. The overall impact of the variable on the model was then evaluated. In addition, within-group assessments were made to determine the site or sites along the risk-score scale where the risk effect, if any, occurred.

The risk factors studied included all 271 of those intrinsic risk variables dealt with in foregoing analyses (see Tables 21-1 and 21-2) plus a number of others which had not previously been examined. These encompassed socioeconomic factors relating to per capita and family income, housing density, and the work history and work status of the gravida, her father, and the father of the baby. The gravida's place of birth, education, and religion were also reviewed. Gestational duration at the time she registered for antepartum care, her lowest hematocrit, and the outcome of her last prior pregnancy, among other obstetrical history and prenatal health factors, were investigated as well. In total, there were 369 predictor variables tested by this approach.

To reduce the complexity of this series of analyses, we arbitrarily subdivided the large number of factors being studied into six segments, specifically (1) demographic variables, (2) the physical characteristics of the gravida, (3) her obstetrical background, (4) the patient's socioeconomic milieu, (5) prenatal care variables, and (6) intercurrent, underlying, or pre-existing disease states identified in pregnancy. Each of these will be dealt with in turn, first as they may have affected the risk-scoring system designed to reflect decile risk-score groups and then as they affected the more satisfactory incremental risk-score group model.

Impact of Predictor Variables on Decile-Strata Model

Demographic Risk Variables

Decile risk-score divisions had been arbitrarily invoked as a means for grouping cases according to their location in the distribution of scores among the complete study series. Although it did not prove to be entirely satisfactory in regard to fitting the model to the data for labor-delivery risk variables, it did offer some useful insights. At the outset, therefore, we used this model to test the predictor risk variables for their effects. When the analytical paradigm was applied to the series of demographic variables (Table 28-1), a number yielded evidence of significant overall impact.

Institution. Among hospital units, for example, several were found to have had markedly unfavorable effects. All odds ratios fell on the high side of 1.00 relative to INST05, and seven were found to be statistically significant. Of these, one (INST10) showed only significantly adverse perinatal

outcome effects, two (INST37 and INST45) only composite outcome effects, and the remaining four both perinatal and composite effects (INST15, INST55, INST60, and INST71). Significant enhancement of the adverse risk effect at the high end of the risk-score scale was seen in many of these same variables, although not consistently, specifically five with perinatal data (excluding INST10 and INST71, but now including INST31 and INST37) and five with composite data (all those previously flagged, but not INST55). The probability levels for all the overall odds ratios were just marginal ($0.01 < p < 0.05$) for the perinatal outcomes, but considerably more significant for all the composite outcomes except one (INST55).

If these findings can be verified by the more reliable risk-score model in which incremental strata are utilized, the model will demonstrate that there were factors acting at these hospital units to influence fetal and infant outcome directly and by a mechanism distinct from that of the intrapartum and delivery risk variables already incorporated into the model. It is of confirming interest to note that all but INST10 had previously surfaced as potentially significant by logistic regression analysis of the entire spectrum of screened intrinsic variables considered collectively (see Table 21-13), and all but INST10 and INST55 were previously retained as significant contributors to adverse outcome by the comparable analysis of the full aggregation of labor, delivery, drug, and intrinsic factors (see Table 25-6).

Maternal Age. The effects of the mother's age (Table 28-1) appeared to alter the model somewhat when outcome results were compared with those of the median age subpopulation AGE2 (20-24 years). For perinatal outcomes, very young gravidas (AGE6 and AGE7, under 18 and 16 years) showed especially poor results even though all labor and delivery factors had been weighed by the scoring system simultaneously. Although there was some high-end enhancement of adverse effects for older

Table 28-1
Risk-Enhancing Effects of Predictor Factors on Decile Score Groups:
Demographic Variables

Risk Variable		Perinatal Outcome RR	95%CL	Composite Outcome RR	95%CL
INST10	Hospital 10	1.99	1.05-3.80A	1.17	0.81-1.70
INST15	Hospital 15	2.05*	1.08-3.92A	2.04*	1.47-2.85E
INST31	Hospital 31	1.21*	0.64-2.30	1.17	0.82-1.66
INST37	Hospital 37	1.56*	0.94-2.60	1.72*	1.32-2.26F
INST45	Hospital 45	1.60	0.93-2.76	1.60*	1.19-2.16C
INST50	Hospital 50	1.12	0.64-1.97	1.11	0.81-1.51
INST55	Hospital 55	2.02*	1.27-3.21A	1.24	0.96-1.60A
INST60	Hospital 60	1.73*	1.03-2.92A	2.63*	2.04-3.39F
INST66	Hospital 66	1.07	0.67-1.72	1.10	0.85-1.42
INST71	Hospital 71	2.21	1.22-4.00A	2.04*	1.50-2.76F
INST82	Hospital 82	1.30	0.75-2.26	1.24	0.93-1.63
AGE1	Maternal age under 20 yr.	1.19	0.88-1.62	1.23	1.06-1.43C
AGE3	Maternal age 25-29 yr.	1.04	0.73-1.48	0.91	0.76-1.09
AGE4	Maternal age 30-34 yr.	1.31*	0.86-1.99	1.23	1.00-1.52A
AGE5	Maternal age 35+ yr.	1.43*	0.91-2.24	1.00	0.77-1.31
AGE6	Maternal age under 18 yr.	1.41	0.98-2.04A	1.39	1.15-1.67D
AGE7	Maternal age under 16 yr.	2.17	1.30-3.61A	1.63	1.19-2.23A
STATUS1	Clinic service patient	0.61	0.35-1.06	1.22*	0.89-1.68A
MARIT1	Single status	1.36	1.02-1.83A	1.19*	1.02-1.39B
MARIT3	Common law	2.60	1.31-5.16A	1.13	0.70-1.82
MARIT4	Widowed	5.29	2.34-11.98A	1.71	0.85-3.41
MARIT5	Divorced	3.82*	1.96-7.45A	1.53	0.94-2.48
MARIT6	Separated	1.72*	1.05-2.83A	1.28*	1.00-1.63A
RACE2	Black	1.40*	1.08-1.81A	1.11*	0.98-1.26A
RACE3	Other race	5.32	2.27-12.46A	1.65	0.80-3.38
RELIG2	Catholic	1.10	0.86-1.41	0.83	0.73-0.94c
RELIG3	Jewish	1.02	0.53-1.95	0.52	0.35-0.78f
ORIGIN1	Place of birth: NY, NJ, PA	0.89	0.57-1.38	0.77	0.61-0.97b
ORIGIN2	MD to FL	1.06	0.71-1.58	1.15	0.94-1.41
ORIGIN3	KY, TN, AL, MS	0.83	0.48-1.43	0.93	0.72-1.20
ORIGIN4	AR, LA, OK, TX	1.66*	0.95-2.90	1.62*	1.24-2.12E
ORIGIN5	IL, IN, OH, MI, WI	1.29	0.57-2.92	0.89	0.54-1.45
ORIGIN6	MN, IA, MO, KA, NE, ND, SD	0.97	0.94-1.73	1.02	0.77-1.35
ORIGIN7	WY, ID, CO, MT, UT, NM, AZ, NV	3.43*	1.51-7.79A	1.21	0.66-2.21
ORIGIN8	WA, OR, CA	1.07	0.53-2.14	1.57	1.14-2.16B
ORIGIN10	Puerto Rico	1.47	0.89-2.42	0.68	0.50-0.91c
ORIGIN11	Other Atlantic islands	2.92	1.41-6.03A	1.26	0.75-2.10
ORIGIN12	Alaska and Canada	4.89	1.94-12.34A	1.93	0.94-3.94A
ORIGIN13	Central and South America			1.96	0.91-3.39
ORIGIN14	Pacific islands	8.69	3.27-23.07A	2.33	0.96-5.67
ORIGIN15	Europe	1.11	0.50-2.49	0.63	0.37-1.07b
ORIGIN16	Asia and Africa	3.16	1.33-7.51A	0.96	0.46-2.00

Risk-score-stratified relative risk (RR) data comparing outcomes for cases with intrinsic factor against those without it, using INST05 (hospital 05), AGE2 (20-24 yr.), STATUS2 (private patient), MARIT2 (married), RACE1 (white), RELIG1 (Protestant), and ORIGIN0 (New England) as referents, where applicable. Blanks indicate insufficient cases to provide meaningful analysis. Probability code: A 0.05, B 0.01, C 0.005, D 0.001, E 0.0005, F 0.0001 or less; lower case code designates protective effect.

* Relative risk significantly enhanced in high-risk-score groups.

parturients (AGE4 and AGE5, 30-34 and 35+ years), the overall odds ratios were not statistically significant.

For composite results, however, not only were the significantly adverse findings repeated in teenagers (AGE6 and AGE7), but they also appeared in those in categories AGE1 (under 20 years) and AGE4 (30-34 years). Only the protective effects of AGE3 (25-29 years) had been recognized by the earlier collective analyses of just the intrinsic factors (see Table 21-13) and of the entire aggregate of risk variables (see Table 25-6). These discrepant findings require resolution. For now, it is sufficient to note that the probability levels of the odds ratios pertaining to maternal age stratifications were marginal in all cases except those pertaining to composite outcomes for AGE1 and AGE6.

Hospital Status. Clinic status (STATUS1) was examined as a risk variable against the referent of STATUS2 (private care). Quite unexpectedly, the perinatal results suggested a protective effect, albeit not statistically significant. Contrariwise, there was a clear adverse effect in the composite outcome analysis, although only at a marginal level of significance and a relatively small magnitude of increase (OR = 1.22). In addition, there was further enhancement of adverse effect found to exist at the upper end of the risk-score scale for composite outcome data.

These findings had been supported earlier in the logistic regression analysis of all intrinsic variables studied collectively (see Table 21-13) by the observation that STATUS1 had no special adverse or beneficial effects when all other related intrinsic variables were considered simultaneously, but that STATUS2 was significantly protective in regard to composite outcome. When the full array of labor, delivery, drug, and intrinsic variables was considered simultaneously (see Table 25-6), however, neither of these variables was determined to have any significant residual effect on outcome. This remains to be retested by the more accurate incremental risk-score model.

Marital Status. The effects of the gravida's marital status on outcome were also studied in the same way (Table 28-1). Relative to the perinatal effects of MARIT2 (married), all other classifications showed significantly augmented risk without exception. Although none of these relationships was determined to be especially more significant than the others when tested statistically, the magnitude of effect for MARIT4 (widowed) and MARIT5 (divorced) was very large, indicating 5.3- and 3.8-fold enhanced effects, respectively. Moreover, both showed significant additional increments of effect at the high end of the risk-score range.

For composite outcome, only MARIT1 (single) and MARIT6 (separated) were determined to have effects that were significantly different from the referent within the risk-score model; high-end enhancement was seen for both of these as well. Although all the other related risk variables pertaining to marital status showed increases in adverse composite effect, they were not statistically significant.

In prior studies of intrinsic factors investigated collectively, in isolation or aggregatively with labor, delivery, and drug variables (see Tables 21-13 and 25-6), only MARIT5 had surfaced as having any significant residual effect when the effects of all others were weighed simultaneously. The overall influence of the absence of the baby's father (WORKF5) will later be seen as a highly significant adverse predictor for both adverse perinatal and bad composite outcomes (see Table 28-3), serving to confirm these findings.

Race. Maternal racial effects were similarly investigated by addressing the impact of race as a predictor variable while taking all labor and delivery factors into account by means of the risk-score model, as before (Table 28-1). In relation to the referent effects of RACE1 (white), other groups demonstrated significantly increased adverse perinatal outcome effects. RACE2 (black) showed high-end risk-score enhancement in addition. With regard to composite effects, however, only RACE1 yielded a significantly persistent long-term effect both overall and with high-risk-score augmentation.

These findings were consistent with those for the prior logistic regression analysis of the collective intrinsic factors (see Table 21-13) in which RACE2 was found to have significant adverse residual effects. However, RACE3 (other race) had previously been shown to have significantly protective effects. The latter relation for composite outcome was also confirmed by the earlier analysis involving the full aggregate of labor, delivery, drug, and intrinsic risk variables (see Table 25-6), although a contradictory adverse perinatal impact had been uncovered, limited to multiparas. The protective effect was not substantiated here. It will be re-examined later in regard to its effect on the incremental risk-score model.

Religion. Assessment of professed major religion as a risk variable had not been previously studied. It was not here refined as to denomination, practice, or orthodoxy. Analysis by the current paradigm showed no special perinatal effects distinct from those of the referent RELIG1 (Protestant), as shown in Table 28-1 by the overall odds ratios falling so close to 1.00. By contrast, composite outcome data revealed very significant protective effect for both RELIG2 (Roman Catholic) and RELIG3 (other, almost exclusively Jewish).

This finding cannot be readily explained except insofar as it may have reflected the socioeconomic make-up of many of the cases falling into the RELIG1 category. This latter group tended to include many in STATUS1 (clinic patient), for example, and perhaps reflected a concentration of other risk variables associated with poor nutrition and suboptimal obstetric care. At any rate, the observation clearly deserves to be studied in depth with the more reliable incremental risk-score model.

Birthplace. The geographic site of the gravida's birthplace was studied as a possible predictor variable. It, too, was a factor for which no prior examination had been done. ORIGIN0 (New England) was selected as referent because the plurality of cases represented led all others in the NCPP data base. National census tracts were subdivided into standard regional designations. When perinatal results were compared with those of the referent group adjusted by risk score (Table 28-1), most geographic subgroups showed essentially no residual impact. Among the contiguous United States regions, only ORIGIN7 (Western mountain corridor) showed a significant adverse effect with high-end enhancement. Offspring of those born in the South Central Gulf region (ORIGIN4) did not do well, but the increased odds ratio was not found to be statistically verifiable despite the significant enhancement of risk seen at the high end of the score range.

ORIGIN10 (Puerto Rico) yielded another insignificantly elevated effect, but those born on other Caribbean islands (ORIGIN11) had significantly adverse perinatal effects in excess of those encountered in the referent population. This was magnified still further among cases originating elsewhere, especially the Pacific Islands (ORIGIN14), Alaska and Canada (ORIGIN12), and Asia and Africa (ORIGIN16), in descending order of impact magnitude. European-born gravidas (ORIGIN15) showed contrastingly good results of the same order as the referent.

Composite outcome results did not confirm the adverse effect found in ORIGIN7 for the perinatal data. However, the ORIGIN4 effects were quite clearly verified and, moreover, this time they proved to be highly significant. ORIGIN8 (Northwest), not previously shown to have an adverse perinatal effect, was determined to have a decidedly deleterious one insofar as composite results were concerned.

There was a paradoxical and strongly protective effect in regard to composite outcome results for ORIGIN10 which contrasted sharply with the earlier suggestion of an adverse perinatal effect (statistically insignificant) from this risk variable. The bad perinatal impact of ORIGIN12 seen before was duplicated, although not to the same magnitude of effect, for the composite outcome data. However, neither ORIGIN14 nor ORIGIN16 showed the same effects here as had been encountered above for perinatal outcome. European birth (ORIGIN15) was decidedly protective in regard to composite outcome. Gravidas born in Latin America (ORIGIN13) appeared to subject their infants to excess composite outcome risk, but the increased odds ratio was not statistically significant and the numbers of cases were too small to permit a meaningful analysis of the perinatal effect of this demographic factor.

Past Obstetrical History

Gravidity. A number of different predictor factors relating to obstetrical history were investigated using the decile risk-score model. Gravidity, for example, was examined against a referent group chosen to represent the most numerous subpopulation, namely GRAV2 (gravida 2, one pregnancy completed prior to the present index pregnancy). Analogously, parity was studied by measuring effects against those of the referent PARA0 (nullipara prior to this pregnancy). As to perinatal outcome, no gravidity subset yielded any evidence of a significant impact not accounted for by the scoring system (Table 28-2). Only GRAV4 (gravida 4, including the current pregnancy) presented with an elevated odds ratio, but it was not statistically significant.

For composite outcome, only GRAV4 again surfaced as having a substantive risk-enhancing effect relative to that of the referent. Comparable results were not seen for GRAV5 and GRAV6, but those for PARA2 (grand multiparity, para 5+) were supportive in that both perinatal and composite effects were significantly enhanced over those of the referent. The odds ratio associated with excess of adverse perinatal results was especially impressive, indicating a three-fold augmentation of risk even when all labor and delivery factors were

already taken into account. This perinatal effect was mirrored, but to a lesser degree (although still statistically significant), in association with PARA1 (para 1-4); there was no comparable composite outcome effect for this variable, however.

Parity. As just noted, grand multiparity was shown to have a significant adverse impact on outcome when all other labor-delivery factors were simultaneously considered by means of the risk score. We had earlier maintained two parallel populations, one of nulliparas and the other of multiparas, in our exploratory analyses leading up to the full aggregative investigation of the entire array of variables under surveillance, as detailed in chapter 25. It was not until after we had developed the ranking of variables by standardized coefficients (chapter 26) that we felt we could safely abandon this stratification. In order to verify that our decision to coalesce the parity subgroups was correct, it was essential to assess whether parity per se retained any meaningful residual effects in regard to outcome for the fetus and infant.

When parity was subjected to the evaluative paradigm using the decile strata of risk scores (Table 28-3), it was determined that the overall odds ratios for both perinatal and composite outcomes fell almost precisely at 1.00 with narrow dispersion of the 95th percentile confidence limits on either side of unity. The absence of subtle hidden effects was further shown by the conformity of within-group odds ratios for each of the deciles of risk score, particularly insofar as the composite outcome data were concerned. Among perinatal data, there appeared to be some degree of protection at low-risk scores and adverse effect at high-risk score, but neither achieved statistical significance at the 5% probability level. Only the very topmost 1 percentile subgroup came even close (p = .062), but this did not significantly alter the overall lack of influence of parity as a predictor of risk.

Pregnancy Loss. Previous pregnancy wastage has been considered a factor for identifying gravidas who may place their

419

Table 28-2
Risk-Enhancing Effects of Predictor Factors on Decile Score Groups:
Physical Characteristics and Obstetric Background

Risk Variable		Perinatal Outcome		Composite Outcome	
		RR	95%CL	RR	95%CL
GRAV1	First pregnancy	1.00	0.60-1.38	1.02	0.62-1.36
GRAV3	Gravida 3	0.88	0.54-1.41	1.07	0.85-1.33
GRAV4	Gravida 4	1.39	0.87-2.21	1.36*	1.07-1.74B
GRAV5	Gravida 5	0.98	0.56-1.72	1.11	0.84-1.45
GRAV6	Gravida 6+	1.20	0.62-2.21	1.07	0.77-1.49
PARA1	Multipara, para 1-4	2.01	1.04-3.89A	1.35	0.92-1.99
PARA2	Grand multipara, para 5+	3.03	1.43-6.40A	1.42	1.12-1.80C
PABORT1	Prior abortion	1.12	0.79-1.59	0.95	0.79-1.13
PPREM1	Prior premature birth	1.54	1.07-2.21A	1.40*	1.17-1.69E
PSTILLB1	Prior stillbirth	1.48	0.88-2.40	1.17	0.89-1.53
PPMR1	Prior perinatal death	1.46	0.93-2.28A	1.30*	1.02-1.65A
PPMR2	Two prior deaths	3.61	1.60-8.16A	1.08	0.58-1.99
PPMR3	Three prior deaths	12.88	5.06-32.76A	3.21	1.30-7.93A
PRIOR0	No prior pregnancy	1.02	0.79-1.33	0.98	0.86-1.12
PRIOR1	Last outcome fetal death	1.49	1.00-2.23A	1.01	0.82-1.24
PRIOR2	Last died in first day	4.79	2.14-10.75A	1.46	0.71-3.01
PRIOR3	Last died in day 2-6	9.91	4.19-23.46A	2.04	0.95-4.34A
PRIOR4	Last died in day 7-27			3.47	1.35-8.93A
PRIOR5	Last died in month 2-12	6.48	2.71-15.52A	1.52	0.70-3.31
PRIOR6	Last died after first year			2.86	1.13-7.25A
HGT1	Maternal height > 68 in.	1.01	0.55-1.84	1.01	0.76-1.35
HGT2	Maternal height < 60 in.	1.94*	1.31-2.88B	1.25	0.99-1.58A
PWGT1	Prepregnancy weight < 175 lb.	1.43*	0.87-2.34	1.16*	0.88-1.53
PWGT2	Prepregnancy weight > 100 lb.	1.29*	0.79-2.13	1.27	0.99-1.62A
QI1	Ponderosity index lean	0.84	0.51-1.40	1.21	0.97-1.51A
QI2	Ponderosity index obese	1.12	0.81-1.54	1.13	0.97-1.33A
POND1	Ponderal index lean	1.20	0.64-2.22	1.31	0.97-1.78A
POND2	Ponderal index obese	1.31*	0.94-1.82A	1.24	1.05-1.46B
SMOKE2	Smoked > 10 yr.	1.26	0.88-1.78	0.95	0.78-1.15
SMOKE3	Smokes > 30 per day	2.71	1.29-5.68A	1.68	1.08-2.61A
SMOKE4	Smokes 10-30 per day	1.05	0.77-1.41	0.98	0.84-1.14
SMOKE5	Smokes > 10 per day	1.01	0.73-1.40	0.95	0.80-1.13
PELV2	Pelvis contracted	2.88	1.57-5.29A	1.41	0.90-2.22
PELV3	Pelvis borderline	1.68*	0.88-3.21	1.25	0.84-1.85

Referent variables: GRAV2 (gravida 2), PARA0 (nullipara), PABORT0, PREM0, PSTILLB0, PPMR0 (no prior fetal wastage or premature birth), PRIOR7 (last baby living and well), HGT3 (height 60-68 in.), PWGT3 (prepregnancy weight 100-175 lb.), QI3, POND3 (normal habitus), SMOKE0 (never smoked), and PELV1 (adequate pelvis). See Table 28-1 for probability code.

* Relative risk significantly enhanced in high-risk-score groups.

subsequent fetus at risk. It was, therefore, evaluated in two ways—first, by determining if there had ever been a prior fetal or infant loss and, second, by identifying the result for the last prior pregnancy. Those who had experienced one or more prior spontaneous abortions (PABORT1), for example, were compared with those who had not (PABORT0) using the decile risk-score model. Prior abortions failed to show

any residual adverse effect in terms of either perinatal or composite outcomes (Table 28-2).

In sharp contrast, having delivered a prior premature infant (PPREM1) carried significant excesses of perinatal and composite outcome risk compared to never having had a premature birth (PPREM0). These cases were found to have statistically very significant impact on both outcome

420

Table 28-3
Risk-Enhancing Effects of Parity on Decile Score Groups

Risk Score Percentile	Perinatal Outcome		Composite Outcome	
	OR	p-Value	OR	p-Value
0–10	0.67	0.74	1.13	0.67
11–20	0.49	0.21	0.97	0.89
21–30	0.48	0.28	1.14	0.52
31–40	1.09	0.87	1.14	0.53
41–50	0.71	0.49	0.87	0.48
51–60	0.72	0.44	0.73	0.13
61–70	0.99	0.98	1.04	0.82
71–80	0.74	0.38	1.16	0.44
81–90	0.87	0.64	0.90	0.56
91–95	0.68	0.35	0.82	0.40
96–99	1.86	0.18	1.21	0.36
Top 1	1.97	0.062	1.24	0.52
Overall	1.01	0.20	1.00	0.80
95% CL	0.80–1.29		0.88–1.14	

parameters and to carry additional high-end score enhancement as well. Some increase in perinatal risk accrued to those with prior stillbirths (PSTILLB1) as contrasted with their counterparts who had had none (PSTILLB0). However, this increase fell below the statistically significant level. The effect was even less apparent in regard to the composite outcome data for this factor.

Antecedent perinatal mortality (PPMR1) was clearly a significant predictor risk variable for both adverse perinatal and poor composite outcomes (Table 28-2). Two prior perinatal deaths (PPMR2) increased the deleterious effects on perinatal outcome more than 2.5 times over that for women who had not had this experience (PPMR0), to yield an impressive odds ratio of 3.61. The composite outcome effect, however, was inexplicably reduced to an insignificant level. Three prior deaths (PPMR3), although it affected only a small segment of the study population, was nonetheless found to have a 3.6-fold still more adverse impact on perinatal outcome than PPMR2 and 8.8 times more than PPMR1 with an odds ratio of 12.88 overall.

This was also mirrored in the composite outcome results with an equally significant odds ratio of 3.21, which was 2.5 times that

of PPMR1. Both PPREM1 and PPMR1 had been identified as adverse factors in the collective analysis of intrinsic factors alone (see Table 21-13), but not in the aggregative analysis of the labor, delivery, drug, and intrinsic variables (see Table 25-6). If these relationships are verified in the incremental risk-score model, there will be little remaining doubt that the factors pertaining to poor past obstetrical experience will be singularly important predictor variables for future untoward outcomes for fetus and infant.

Prior Pregnancy Outcome. Focusing on the outcomes of the last prior pregnancy, we compared the various subsets with a referent group (PRIOR7) in which the infants were known to have survived. Those with no prior pregnancy (PRIOR0) did just as well as the referent. However, those who had most recently had a stillbirth (PRIOR1) showed a significantly increased perinatal hazard, but without any apparent comparable demonstrated effect on composite outcome (Table 28-2). Gravidas whose last infant died during the immediate neonatal period, that is, during the first 24 hours (PRIOR2), showed a marked tendency toward perinatal death or severe neonatal depression as evidenced by the very large and statistically significant odds ratio of 4.79; just as with PRIOR1, however, this effect did not carry over into the composite outcome data.

Still more impressive were the findings for women who lost their newborn infants after the first day but during the first week of life (PRIOR3). Here, the adverse effects were significantly elevated for both perinatal and composite results; the odds ratio of 9.91 in the perinatal data was an especially remarkable observation. There were too few patients whose last infant had died after 1 week but within the first month after birth (PRIOR4) to permit a meaningful analysis of perinatal impact, but the results for composite outcome were nonetheless adequate to demonstrate a significantly deleterious effect of rather high magnitude (OR = 3.47).

Women whose prior infant had not lived beyond the first year (PRIOR5) had very poor results in the perinatal period of their current pregnancy, yielding a significant odds ratio of large magnitude (OR = 6.48). Although the composite outcomes for this group were worse than expected in the referent group (OR = 1.52), they could not be shown to be statistically significant. Late infant deaths beyond the first year (PRIOR6) also occurred too infrequently to provide enough data for the analysis to be done for subsequent perinatal death or neonatal depression, but there was a clearly significant adverse effect in the composite outcome data (OR = 2.86) for the next index pregnancy.

Physical Characteristics
Height. Maternal height was assessed as a risk predictor utilizing the decile risk-score model and the median height group HGT3 (60-68 in) as referent. Offspring of tall women in the HGT1 subset (>68 in) did just as well as those delivered of women in the referent series (Table 28-2), yielding odds ratios for both perinatal and composite outcomes almost precisely on the mark of unity (OR = 1.01). Contrastingly, short women in HGT2 (<60 in) showed significantly increased adverse effects for both

perinatal (OR = 1.94) and composite results (OR = 1.25). There was also some significant enhancement of effect at the high end of the risk-score range in the perinatal outcome data. HGT2 had similarly been determined to have significant adverse effects in the collective logistic regression analysis of intrinsic factors (see Table 21-13), but not in the more generalized aggregative analysis of all labor, delivery, drug, and intrinsic variables (see Table 25-6).

Weight. The risk predictor effects of prepregnancy weight were investigated in the same way, first without regard to its relation to body habitus or height. The median weight range of PWGT3 (100-175 lb) was selected as referent. When the decile risk-strata model was invoked, women in PWGT1 with large prepregnancy weight (>175 lb) increased their infant's perinatal and composite risks somewhat, but not significantly so in the overview. Nonetheless, there was some significant high-end enhancement of risk noted for both sets of outcome data.

Women in PWGT2, whose prepregnancy weight was low (<100 lb) similarly offered elevated adverse risk to their offspring. This achieved statistical significance for composite outcome results; although it was not significant insofar as perinatal data were concerned, the analysis revealed a significantly increased adverse effect focused at the upper end of the risk-score scale. No prepregnancy weight factor had previously been disclosed as a significant intrinsic risk factor in our foregoing logistic regression analyses of these factors either in isolation or together with all labor and delivery risk variables (see Tables 21-13 and 25-6).

Ponderal and Ponderosity Measures. Both ponderal and ponderosity (Quetelet's) indices were examined in an attempt to identify the impact of disordered height-weight relationships. These have been defined previously (see Table 21- 1). For purposes of this exercise, women with essentially normal body habitus were selected for the referent classes: POND3 (ponderal index between 13.734 and

11.891) and QI3 (Quetelet's index between 0.0260 and 0.0365). Offspring of those gravidas designated as lean by the ponderosity index (QI1) appeared to be somewhat protected against adverse perinatal outcome, but the low odds ratio was not found to be statistically significant (Table 28-2). Moreover, there was a small but significant increase in poor composite outcomes in this group. This latter effect was replicated in the composite data for lean women as defined by the ponderal index (POND1). For perinatal outcome, however, the slightly protective effects of QI1 were contradicted by a somewhat adverse effect here (also not significant).

Gravidas who began pregnancy in an obese state as measured by the ponderal index (POND2) subjected their infants to substantively excess risk in regard to both perinatal and composite outcome results. In addition to an overall increase in adverse perinatal impact well beyond that seen for the referent group when all labor and delivery risks were taken into account by the risk-score model (OR = 1.31), there was also significant high-end risk-score enhancement of effect seen.

POND2 had previously been recognized as a significant adverse risk factor in the collective logistic regression analysis of intrinsic factors (see Table 21-13), but its effect at that time appeared to be limited to composite outcomes only. The same applied for the parallel analysis of the full aggregate of labor, delivery, drug, and intrinsic variables (see Table 25-6). This suggested the possibility that the observation here for perinatal data may have been specious. It remained to be retested by the incremental risk-score model. As will be seen (see Table 28-7), it proved incorrect, demonstrating the importance of our having ensured proper goodness-of-fit for the scoring model to eliminate potentially erroneous conclusions about the impact of potential risk variables, wherever possible.

Tobacco Use. Smoking history and its effects were studied under this category of risk variables for want of a more appropriate one. As referent, we chose women who had never smoked (SMOKE0), applying the decile risk-score model paradigm, as detailed above. Duration of smoking appeared to be of far less importance to offspring than the intensity of the current smoking habit during pregnancy. Even long-term cigarette use exceeding ten years (SMOKE2) could not be shown to yield any excess of fetal/infant risk over that already dealt with by the risk score (Table 28-2).

By contrast, gravidas who smoked more than 30 cigarettes a day during pregnancy (SMOKE3) clearly placed their babies at substantially increased risk both perinatally (OR = 2.71) and later in terms of composite outcome results (OR = 1.68). Similar adverse findings were not encountered for lesser degrees of smoking habit during pregnancy. It is of interest to note that both SMOKE2 and SMOKE3 had been identified as relevant risk factors in the antecedent analysis involving just the collective intrinsic factors (see Table 21-13), but neither surfaced as such in the aggregative study of all the relevant variables under surveillance (see Table 25-6). Reexamination by the incremental risk-score model can be expected to resolve this apparent conflict in findings.

Pelvic Capacity. The adequacy of the maternal pelvis to accommodate to an average-sized fetus had been assessed clinically by careful digital examination in early pregnancy. All gravidas were classified according to their pelvic capacity. Those deemed to have a contracted pelvis (PELV2) were determined to have significantly worse perinatal results (Table 28-2) when studied against the risk-scoring paradigm (OR = 2.88). This adverse effect was not duplicated for composite outcome. Smaller degrees of effect were seen for cases with borderline pelvic contraction (PELV3), but the results were not statistically significant even though there was clear-cut enhancement of deleterious perinatal effects at the high end of the risk-score scale.

Socioeconomic Factors

The NCPP data resource was especially rich in information pertaining to socioeconomic factors. The socioeconomic index has been studied in the foregoing analyses. As will be recalled, it represented the combined mean of scores based on education and occupation of the head of gravida's household plus that for total annual family income (see chapter 5). As such, it was used as an overall rough guide reflecting the gravida's position on a scale ranging from indigency to affluence. We had available for more intensive evaluation a large number of additional diverse items relating in some detail to the gravida, the father of the baby, the gravida's family, and the offspring's siblings. Limitations of resources prevented our examining all of them, but several were studied in depth and yielded interesting data (Table 28-4).

Socioeconomic Index. The index itself was assessed first by comparing cases stratified by increments of ten index points against the median index group SES5 (socioeconomic index 45-54) within the framework of the decile risk-score model. In general, it was found that babies born to women with low indices fared particularly poorly while those with high indices showed decidedly protective effects (Table 28-4). This was especially evident in the composite outcome data analyses in which the trend from adverse (OR = 1.61) to beneficial (OR = 0.47) was smooth and unbroken in an almost perfect linear fashion.

The results in terms of deviation from the model, reflecting the impact of the risk variable, were statistically highly significant at both ends of the spectrum, most notably in SES1-SES3 (indices below 35) for adverse effects and in SES8-SES9 (indices of 75 or more) for protective effects. Less impressive and much more inconsistent findings were seen for perinatal data. There was some apparent adverse perinatal effect in all the low index groups, but they achieved statistical significance only in SES3 and SES4 (OR = 1.64 and 1.68). The protection associated with high indices encountered

with composite outcomes was not duplicated here.

Prior study of the socioeconomic index in conjunction with all other intrinsic variables (see Table 21-13) has shown similar adverse effects of low index, but produced paradoxical results for high index (somewhat adverse in SES8 and strongly protective in SES9). The more all-inclusive analysis involving labor-delivery variables plus intrinsic factors (see Table 25-6) confirmed both the adverse low index impact and the beneficial high index effect, although the symmetry was disturbed by one isolated discrepantly deleterious effect for perinatal outcome in SES8 limited to offspring of nulliparas.

Per Capita Income. To focus on the components of the socioeconomic index, per capita income of the gravida's immediate nuclear family unit was addressed next. The referent selected for comparative purposes in the decile risk strata model was the median group in INCOME3 ($1500-2249 per household member per year). The analytical results for perinatal outcome failed to show any significant deviations from the referent category (Table 28-4). While there was a suggestion of an adverse effect in the most indigent group, INCOME1 (less than $800) it was not statistically significant. The same level of effect (OR = 1.18) was shown to be significant for this risk variable in association with composite outcome.

A clear trend was found for the composite data in regard to increasing protection with increasing per capita income from the aforementioned significantly adverse effect of INCOME1 to the significantly beneficial effects in INCOME4 and INCOME5 ($2250 or more). However, the magnitude of the impact, both good and bad, was much smaller here than for the socioeconomic index variable cited earlier. Thus, per capita income was probably an important risk predictor, but it could only account for a modest proportion of the effect indicated by the SES variables.

Family Income. Probing further, we

Table 28-4
Risk-Enhancing Effects of Predictor Factors on Decile Score Groups:
Socioeconomic Factors

Risk Variable		Perinatal Outcome RR	95%CL	Composite Outcome RR	95%CL
SES1	Socioeconomic index < 15	1.47*	0.84-2.57	1.61*	1.22-2.12D
SES2	Socioeconomic index 15-24	1.27	0.77-2.09	1.31	1.04-1.64B
SES3	Socioeconomic index 25-34	1.64*	1.06-2.55B	1.29*	1.04-1.58B
SES4	Socioeconomic index 35-44	1.68	1.12-2.54B	1.18	0.96-1.44A
SES6	Socioeconomic index 55-64	1.09	0.66-1.79	0.86	0.67-1.09
SES7	Socioeconomic index 65-74	0.98	0.55-1.73	0.84	0.63-1.11
SES8	Socioeconomic index 75-84	1.15	0.61-2.14	0.60	0.43-0.85d
SES9	Socioeconomic index 85+	0.92	0.44-1.91	0.47	0.31-0.72f
INCOME1	Per capita income < $800/yr	1.19	0.81-1.74	1.18	0.97-1.43A
INCOME2	Per capita income $800-1499	0.97	0.64-1.46	0.92	0.75-1.13
INCOME4	Per capita income $2250-2999	1.06	0.64-1.77	0.79	0.60-1.03a
INCOME5	Per capita income $3000+	1.10	0.65-1.86	0.78	0.59-1.04a
FAMINC1	No family income	7.04	2.68-18.51A	2.39	1.15-4.99A
FAMINC2	Family income < $2000/yr	1.11	0.68-1.83	1.31	1.02-1.68B
FAMINC3	Family income $2000-3999	0.92	0.60-1.39	0.94	0.75-1.17
FAMINC4	Family income $4000-4999	0.82	0.51-1.30	0.80	0.62-1.02
FAMINC6	Family income $8000-9999	1.05	0.50-2.24	0.92	0.59-1.43
FAMINC7	Family income $10,000+	1.29	0.53-3.15	0.83	0.48-1.44a
HOUSE	Housing density 1.0+ person/room	0.98	0.74-1.29	1.15*	0.99-1.34B
EDUC0	No formal education	1.44	0.90-2.60	2.28	0.91-5.73A
EDUC1	Education < 7 yr.	1.31	0.88-1.97	1.46	1.19-1.80E
EDUC2	Education 8 yr.	1.46*	0.86-2.13	1.28	1.02-1.61A
EDUC3	Education 9-11 yr.	1.04	0.78-1.40	1.17	1.01-1.36A
EDUC5	Education 13-15 yr.	0.67	0.39-1.17b	0.64	0.47-0.87e
EDUC6	Education 16+ yr.	0.83	0.43-1.62a	0.39	0.24-0.63f
WORKG1	Gravida never worked	1.09	0.78-1.53	1.35	1.13-1.62E
WORKG2	Gravida white collar worker	0.61	0.42-0.89b	0.55	0.46-0.67f
WORKG3	Gravida blue collar worker	0.87	0.64-1.19	0.86	0.74-1.01
WORKF0	Father of baby never worked			2.65	1.11-6.32A
WORKF2	Father of baby in armed forces	2.60	1.19-5.68A	1.22	0.68-2.19
WORKF3	Father of baby student	1.31	0.70-2.45	0.73	0.47-1.13b
WORKF4	Father of baby unemployed	1.01	0.67-1.53	1.42	1.18-1.70E
WORKF5	Father of baby absent	1.69*	1.25-2.31D	1.51*	1.28-1.78F
WORKF6	Father of baby unknown	2.15	1.02-4.50A	1.68	1.07-2.65A
OCCUPF3	Father of baby blue collar worker	1.43*	1.02-1.98B	1.66*	1.40-1.97F

Referent variables: SES5 (socioeconomic index 45-54), INCOME3 ($1500-2249 per year per capita), FAMINC5 (family income $5000-7999), HOUSE0 (housing density < 1.0 person per room), EDUC4 (12 yr., high school graduate), WORKG0 (gravida not working now), WORKF (father of baby employed), OCCUPF2 (father of baby white collar worker).

* Relative risk significantly enhanced in high

examined gross family income using FAMINC5 ($5000-7999 per annum) as referent in the decile strata paradigm. Just as for the per capita income results, there was no objective evidence of an independent significant effect on perinatal outcome associated with this factor. For composite outcome, by contrast, the lowest family income groups, FAMINC1 (no income, OR = 2.39) and FAMINC2 (<$2000, OR = 1.31), were determined to have significantly adverse effects not accounted for by the risk-score model. At the high income end of the scale, FAMINC7 ($10,000+) was clearly protective and statistically significant insofar as composite outcome was concerned (OR = 0.83). Once again, however, the size of these effects was relatively small, indicating that they were merely contributory to a portion of the impact found earlier for the full socioeconomic index.

Housing Density. Housing density was another factor available for investigation. Although multiply stratified in the NCPP resource, most cases fell into either the referent HOUSE0 (less than 1.0 per dwelling room) or the adjacent HOUSE1 (1.0-3.0) with very few in more crowded circumstances. Accordingly, the analytical process was only capable of evaluating the effect of HOUSE1 against the referent within the decile strata system.

Perinatal outcomes were almost precisely the same in both categories (Table 28-4). Composite outcome results indicated a significantly adverse impact, however. Even though the magnitude of the effect was not large (OR = 1.15), it was determined to be quite significant when subjected to statistical testing. There was even a significant enhancement of effect in association with high labor-delivery risk scores. The small degree of adverse effect, although statistically significant, could only account for a minor proportion of the impact from low socioeconomic index found earlier (see above).

Education. Whereas the education of the head of the gravida's household had been weighed in the socioeconomic index, the gravida's own educational achievements were not. We examined this factor for its possible effect on the infant against the referent of EDUC4 (12 years' schooling completed, high school graduate). The study results almost precisely mirrored those of the socioeconomic index (Table 28-4), duplicating the effects previously encountered for both perinatal and composite outcomes insofar as direction and magnitude were concerned.

This was especially apparent for the composite data in which there was a clear inverse linear trend describing the fall in odds ratios with increasing educational exposure from 2.28 in EDUC0 (no formal education) at one extreme to 0.39 in EDUC6 (16+ years of education) at the other. Odds ratios for all groups on either side of the referent were determined to be statistically significant whether high and adverse with less education or low and protective with more education. These findings agree completely with those associated with the socioeconomic index series in which the odds ratios fell linearly from 1.61 to 0.47 and were equivalently significant in large measure above and below the median referent.

Analysis of perinatal data did not yield quite the same consistency of result, although there was a tendency for the effects to fall in parallel with those of the composite data—that is, adverse odds ratios with little education and beneficial ones with more education. The increased perinatal effect associated with minimal education here did not reach statistical significance, but the decrease with advanced education (EDUC5 and EDUC6) did. It will be recalled that the perinatal effects of the socioeconomic index variables were also far less clear-cut than the composite effects had been, perhaps reflecting the reduced statistical power of significance testing of smaller frequency series. In this regard, therefore, the EDUC variables seemed more valuable as a predictive factor.

Work History. The employment status of the gravida and of the father of the baby were detailed for purposes of identifying any adverse or beneficial effects associated with these factors. As referent for the gravida's occupational status, we chose WORKG0 to represent the most common situation in which the gravida was not currently working, although she had held a formal position in the past. When compared to the outcome results for this group (Table 28-4), those who had never worked had perinatal results about as expected (OR = 1.09) and distinctly worse composite outcome results (OR = 1.35). Gravidas continuing to work during pregnancy appeared to bestow some protective effects on their offspring. This applied regardless of the type of job, but the protection was statistically very significant for both perinatal (OR

= 0.61) and composite effects (OR = 0.55) among women employed as white collar workers.

The work history of the gravida's father failed to disclose information of interest, but data pertaining to the father of the baby did (Table 28-4). Against a referent group consisting of those currently employed in any capacity (WORKF1), if the baby's father had never worked (WORKF0), for example, the composite outcome was significantly adverse while taking all labor and delivery risk factors into account by the risk-score model (OR = 2.65). The small numbers of such cases precluded analysis for perinatal results. Where the father of the baby had previously worked but was unemployed (WORKF4) during the gravida's pregnancy, the results were also bad insofar as composite outcome was concerned; although the effect was not of the same magnitude (OR = 1.42), it proved considerably more significant by virtue of the fact that larger numbers of cases were involved. Perinatal outcome was unaffected, however.

A most impressive observation was the highly significant increased risk found when the father of the baby was absent (WORKF5) for both perinatal (OR = 1.69) and composite outcomes (OR = 1.51). The adverse effects were even greater, although of lesser statistical significance (because the group size was smaller), for cases in which the father of the baby was unknown (WORKF6). This again applied to both perinatal (OR = 2.15) and composite results (OR = 1.68). Absence of the baby's father may also have been reflected in the data for WORKF2 (father of baby in the armed forces), where significantly augmented poor perinatal outcome was encountered (OR = 2.60), an effect not repeated for composite outcome. Contrastingly, good composite outcome results were found for offspring of men who were designated students (WORKF3) during the course of the pregnancy (OR = 0.73). This perhaps reflected their available economic supports facilitating continuation of education concurrent with growing family responsibilities.

Among employed fathers, offspring of blue-collar workers (OCCUPF3) did not do well relative to the referent white-collar group (OCCUPF2). Quite significantly increased adverse perinatal (OR = 1.43) and composite effects (OR = 1.66) were seen accompanied by additional significant enhancement of these effects concentrated especially at the high end of the risk-score range. Although our analytical procedures did not stratify the preceding material on the father's work history by these occupational categories, it has to be recognized that the choice of referent we previously used (WORKF1, employed in any capacity) colored some of the other work group data favorably. If we had used the subcategory of white-collar worker instead, its more salutary effect on outcome would likely have raised the odds ratios of all those with adverse effects still further and may even have increased the effects of others to a significant probability level.

Antepartum Factors

Prenatal Care. An effort was made to determine the impact of prenatal care on outcome. To assess the time at which such care began, cases were stratified by gestational duration at registration into increments of four weeks. Those registering for prenatal care prior to the end of the first trimester (GREG1) were selected to serve as the referent group. Utilizing the decile risk-score model (Table 28-5), we were unable to uncover any adverse effects from late registration up to gestational age of 28 weeks (GREG2-GREG5). Those registering at the beginning of the third trimester (GREG6), however, did show adverse effects on their infants, especially evident in the significantly adverse composite results (OR = 1.28), notable for its high-end risk-score enhancement as well. Contradicting this finding were those results seen in cases registering still later in which no comparable adverse effects occurred. Dividing cases by trimester of registration and using first trimester registration as referent (TRIM-

427

EST1), we were able to confirm the significantly deleterious composite outcome influence of registration in the third trimester (TRIMEST3) and the lack of such an effect for midtrimester registration (TRIMEST2).

The number of antepartum office visits was expected to have a parabolic effect, that is, adverse at either extreme, reflecting minimal antepartum care at the low end and some intercurrent disorder necessitating many visits at the high end. With VISIT2 (seven to 14 visits, the median figure) as referent, the results were indeed as expected (Table 28-5). Cases with fewer than seven visits (VISIT1) showed significantly increased adverse composite outcomes (OR = 1.23). Those with 17 to 20 visits (VISIT4) had increased perinatal (OR = 1.65) and composite outcomes (OR = 1.42), but only the latter proved significant. Beyond 20 visits (VISIT5), the results were very impressively bad (perinatal OR = 7.16, composite OR = 2.91), but the analysis showed them to be just marginally significant because of the small numbers of cases affected.

It should be noted in passing that both VISIT1 and VISIT4 had been identified as risk variables when the intrinsic factors had been studied collectively (see Table 21-13) and in aggregate with all relevant labor and delivery variables (see Table 25-6). It was clear from the current analysis that they retained their impact as predictor variables while the risk-score model was operant. Whereas large numbers of antepartum visits were associated with bad infant results, it seemed likely that this factor served more as a marker of risk due to the condition that warranted the frequent return examinations rather than as a true peril in itself. Few visits might have functioned in the same way as an index of poor or absent obstetrical care.

Gestational Age at Delivery. The effect of premature delivery is incontestable. Our assessment, therefore, focused on the timing of delivery within a tightly constrained infant birthweight range. It will be recalled that this aspect of our research dealt with a population of gravidas who delivered babies weighing from 2500 to 4000 g only (and free of major anomalies). Gestational age based on menstrual dating was examined by the decile risk-score paradigm. Compared to those infants delivering at 38 to 41 weeks (GDEL0), who were selected as referent cases, nearly all delivering earlier or later were found to be at substantially increased excess risk as to both perinatal and composite results (Table 28-5). Increasingly poorer perinatal outcomes were seen the earlier the delivery occurred before 38 weeks. It rose to its highest level (OR = 3.59) in the group delivered under 34 weeks (GDEL1). This inverse progression of effect was not duplicated in the composite data, although the significantly adverse risk was present nonetheless.

Beyond term, both perinatal and composite outcomes worsened significantly, beginning at more than 41 weeks (GDEL4) with small but significant increments at each week beyond that to gestational ages of more than 43 weeks (GDEL6). The effects remained high beyond 44 weeks (GDEL7), but they lost their statistical significance in this subset. This appeared to come about for two reasons: First, the numbers of cases fell. Second, it was likely that there was some degree of dilution of the study material by cases in which pregnancy dating was erroneous by a factor of 1 month. Only GDEL4 had previously surfaced as a significantly adverse factor when studied among the intrinsic variables (see Table 21-13) and again when examined in concert with all other labor-delivery factors (see Table 25-6).

Birth Weight. Despite the narrow spectrum of infant weights in this series (2500-4000g), we examined birth weight effects against a median referent of 3250-3499g (BW4) in increments of 250g. There were no significant perinatal effects disclosed by the risk-score paradigm, although there was an apparent inverse trend toward increasingly adverse odds ratios with decreasing birth weights (Table 28-5).

Table 28-5
Risk-Enhancing Effects of Predictor Factors on Decile Score Groups:
Antepartum Factors

Risk Variable		Perinatal Outcome		Composite Outcome	
		RR	95%CL	RR	95%CL
GREG2	Registered at 12-15.9 wk.	0.73	0.44-1.20	0.90	0.70-1.16
GREG3	Registered at 16-19.9 wk.	1.05	0.67-1.66	1.04	0.81-1.34
GREG4	Registered at 20-23.9 wk.	1.08	0.69-1.70	1.06	0.83-1.36
GREG5	Registered at 24-27.9 wk.	1.09	0.68-1.74	1.13	0.88-1.45
GREG6	Registered at 28-31.9 wk.	1.24	0.76-2.02	1.28*	0.98-1.66A
GREG7	Registered at 32-35.9 wk.	0.82	0.46-1.48	1.14	0.86-1.51
GREG8	Registered at 36+ wk.	1.04	0.59-1.84	1.22	0.91-1.63
TRIMEST2	Registered in second trimester	1.22	0.90-1.66	1.17	0.99-1.38A
TRIMEST3	Registered in third trimester	1.15*	0.81-1.64	1.33*	1.11-1.59D
VISIT1	Prenatal visits < 7	1.07	0.81-1.42	1.23*	1.08-1.41C
VISIT3	Prenatal visits 15-16	1.12	0.69-1.84	1.05	0.80-1.39
VISIT4	Prenatal visits 17-20	1.65	0.94-2.88	1.42	0.99-2.04A
VISIT5	Prenatal visits 21+	7.16	3.01-17.05A	2.91	1.43-5.93A
GDEL1	Delivery at < 34 wk.	3.59*	2.03-6.34D	1.56*	1.09-2.21B
GDEL2	Delivery at < 36 wk.	3.02*	1.97-4.63F	1.63*	1.29-2.07F
GDEL3	Delivery at < 38 wk.	2.12*	1.52-2.96F	1.45*	1.23-1.73F
GDEL4	Delivery at > 41 wk.	1.63*	1.21-2.19D	1.13	0.96-1.32A
GDEL5	Delivery at > 42 wk.	1.63*	1.14-2.34B	1.22	1.01-1.49A
GDEL6	Delivery at > 43 wk.	1.76	1.13-2.74A	1.23	0.96-1.58A
GDEL7	Delivery at > 44 wk.	1.27	0.69-2.34	1.19	0.86-1.66
BW1	Birth weight 2500-2749 g.	1.49	0.95-2.34	1.25	0.99-1.59A
BW2	Birth weight 2750-2999 g.	1.29	0.87-1.89	1.28	1.06-1.55B
BW3	Birth weight 3000-3249 g.	1.12	0.78-1.61	1.20	1.01-1.44B
BW5	Birth weight 3500-3749 g.	0.94	0.62-1.43	0.92	0.75-1.13
BW6	Birth weight 3750-3999 g.	1.05	0.67-1.66	1.04	0.69-1.40
SGA	Small for gestational age	2.02	1.22-3.35A	1.23	0.91-1.65
LGA	Large for gestational age	1.25	0.83-1.87	1.15	0.92-1.42
MALE	Male infant	1.59	1.23-2.04F	1.39	1.23-1.59F
OBTYPE2	Resident in attendance	0.65	0.36-1.20	1.05	0.74-1.50
OBTYPE3	Intern in attendance	0.48	0.24-0.95a	1.27	0.89-1.81
OBTYPE4	Student in attendance	0.52	0.25-1.09	1.29	0.81-2.04
HCT1	Lowest hematocrit < 20%	19.50	7.46-50.43A	4.07	1.59-10.42A
HCT2	Lowest hematocrit 20-24.9	3.30	1.66-6.54A	1.37	0.83-2.27
HCT3	Lowest hematocrit 25-29.9	1.24	0.82-1.88	1.08	0.88-1.32
HCT4	Lowest hematocrit 30-34.9	1.05	0.79-1.41	1.01	0.87-1.16
RUP1	Amniotomy at delivery	0.86	0.57-1.30	0.99	0.82-1.19
RUP2	Amniotomy for induction	1.55	0.84-2.88	1.19*	0.76-1.86
RUP3	Amniotomy for augmentation	0.94	0.72-1.23	0.95	0.83-1.09
VAGBLD	First trimester bleeding	1.53*	1.03-2.28A	1.16*	0.90-1.50
RHSENS	Rh isoimmunization	9.56*	4.26-21.43A	2.78	1.35-5.73A
PIH1	Diastolic hypertension only	1.35*	0.65-2.77	1.46	0.93-2.28A
PIH2	Hypertension and proteinuria	1.32	0.53-3.33	1.42	0.77-2.59
PIH3	Proteinuria only	1.08	0.51-2.28	1.32*	0.82-2.10

Referent variables: GREG1 (registered for care prior to 12 weeks' gestational age), TRIMEST1 (registered in first trimester), VISIT2 (7-14 office visits), GDEL0 (delivery at 39-41 weeks), BW4 (3250-3499 g. birth weight), SGA0, LGA0 (neither small nor large for dates), FEMALE (female infant), OBTYPE1 (attending in attendance), HCT5 (lowest hematocrit 35.0+%), RUP0 (spontaneous rupture of membranes), VAGBLD0, RHSENS0, PIH0 (absence of condition).

* Relative risk significantly enhanced in high-risk-score groups.

Those in the lowest weight group (BW1, 2500-2749g) fared worst, but the result (OR = 1.49) was determined to fall just short of statistical significance at the 5% probability level.

For composite outcome data, all infant weight groups below the referent (BW1-BW3) yielded odds ratios which, although not of large magnitude (1.20-1.28), were found to be significantly in excess. Neither adverse nor beneficial effects were seen with the heavier infants. In the antecedent study of the collective array of intrinsic variables (see Table 21-13), BW2 had been shown to carry an adverse effect and BW5 an apparently beneficial one; neither retained these effects when examined in conjunction with the spectrum of labor and delivery variables (see Table 25-6).

We related birthweight to gestational age by identifying those cases falling above the 90th percentile (LGA, large for gestational age) or below the tenth percentile (SGA, small for gestational age) for the distribution of weights for a given gestational age (see Table 21-2). Both extremes were found to have adverse perinatal and composite effects (Table 28-5), but only the perinatal results were statistically significant in SGA.

The absence of greater impact from either factor was felt to be due at least in part to the narrowly constricted birth weight limits, excluding extremes of SGA and LGA infants from consideration. In addition, there were conflicting results in our prior studies of intrinsic factors taken collectively (see Table 21-13) and aggregatively with labor and delivery factors (see Table 25-6), in which only LGA was found to carry an adverse effect.

Fetal Sex. As demonstrated regularly before in these and other studies, boy babies did worse than girls. This was repeated here as regards both perinatal and composite outcome effects (Table 28-5). Relative to female offspring as the referent, male newborn infants fared consistently badly; although the increase in odds ratios was not large, the excess adverse effect was statistically very significant nonetheless. This pervasive effect had been shown strongly in the collective analysis of intrinsic factors (see Table 21-13) as well as in the aggregative study of all the relevant risk variables (see Table 25-6).

Obstetrical Attendant. The experience of the obstetrical attendant was also assessed. Designating the private attending obstetrician as referent (OBTYPE1), we were unable to show any adverse results by means of the decile risk-score system for any other attendant group (Table 28-5). Actually, most other groups showed some protective effects, reaching significant proportions among those cases cared for by interns (OBTYPE3), specifically for perinatal outcome. It was considered likely that this finding could be attributed to case selection biases given the probability that only (or principally) uncomplicated cases, and especially multiparas, would probably have been managed by this group of care givers in the participating NCPP hospital units. These factors had not previously surfaced as relevant risk indicators in our antecedent studies (see Tables 21-13 and 25-6).

Lowest Hematocrit. The maternal hematocrit is recognized to fall in pregnancy as blood volume increases and expanding red cell mass falls behind. Abnormally low hematocrit may serve as an index of iron and nutritional deficiency. Anemia will be examined later in more detail as an intercurrent medical condition (see Table 28-6, below). For now, we studied the simple variable of the lowest recorded hematocrit level in 5% increments against the referent of 35% or more (HCT5). When the decile risk-score paradigm was applied (Table 28-5), no effect was found in offspring of gravidas maintaining levels of at least 25% (HCT3 and HCT4). Significantly adverse perinatal effects were encountered below this level, odds ratios increasing from 2.10 in HCT2 (20%-24.9%) to 6.76 in HCT1 (under 20%). Composite outcome results were somewhat adverse as well, but not significantly so.

Rupture of Membranes. Membrane

status was reviewed here for want of a more appropriate site. Compared to cases in which the chorioamniotic membranes ruptured spontaneously (RUP0), only amniotomy for induction of labor (RUP2) was found to carry any adverse impact (Table 28-5), although it failed to reach statistically significant levels for either perinatal (OR = 1.55) or composite outcome (OR = 1.19), even though the latter was also associated with significant high-end risk-score enhancement of effect. Neither artificial rupture of the membranes for augmentation of labor (RUP3) nor that done at delivery (RUP1) was associated with any demonstrable increase in risk to the fetus or infant as evaluated by this approach.

Vaginal Bleeding. The full range of intercurrent illnesses will be dealt with below. Several conditions were looked at separately because they were peculiar to pregnancy. First trimester vaginal bleeding (VAGBLD) as recorded concurrently (or nearly so) on the NCPP data intake forms was examined, for example. This variable differed somewhat from DIS124 (see below) which consisted of a retrospective summary diagnosis recorded after delivery. Contrasted to infants born to women without this complaint (VAGBLD0), these cases showed significantly increased adverse perinatal effects (OR = 1.53) but no matching composite outcome residual (Table 28-5). This replicated what had been found in the collective analysis of intrinsic variables (see Table 21-13), but it was absent from the overall aggregative analysis (see Table 25-6).

Rh Sensitization. Rh isoimmunization (RHSENS), as expected, had also been previously determined to carry a serious risk. When this factor was studied using the decile risk-strata model, its seriously adverse effects were obvious (Table 28-5). It carried nearly ten times (OR = 9.56) excess of perinatal risk and almost three times (OR = 2.78) composite outcome risk of unsensitized cases, both statistically significant findings.

Pregnancy-Induced Hypertension. Pregnancy-induced hypertension was investigated in the same way using the criteria established in our foregoing investigatory project.* For these purposes all cases were classified according to the maximum recorded diastolic blood pressure and degree of proteinuria during the interval of pregnancy from 28 weeks to delivery: PIH1, only diastolic hypertension of 95 torr or more; PIH2, diastolic 85 torr or more and proteinuria 1+ or more; PIH3, only proteinuria 2+ or more. The referent consisted of cases with normal blood pressure levels (diastolic pressure no less than 65 torr) and no proteinuria.

When all labor and delivery risk factors were accounted for by the risk-score model, there were apparent increases in composite risk for all categories (Table 28-5), but these proved statistically significant only in PIH1 (OR = 1.46). Comparable risk also appeared for perinatal outcome in association with PIH1 and PIH2, but neither could be shown to be significant at the 5% probability level.

Intercurrent Disorders

The entire list of prescreened medical and surgical conditions to which pregnant women may fall heir were surveyed by the decile risk-strata model. For each of them, the absence of the specific disease or state was used as referent and the referent population was further reduced by including only cases in which manually controlled delivery of a fetus in vertex presentation had occurred. Once again, the parallel series of index and control gravidas were stratified by risk-score decile and the outcome results compared both within groups and overall.

The results (Table 28-6) demonstrated the significantly adverse effects of a number of these risk variables. Bad perina-

---

*Friedman EA, Neff RK: *Pregnancy Hypertension: A Systematic Evaluation of Clinical Diagnostic Criteria.* Littleton, Mass, PSG Publishing Co, 1977, p 172.

Table 28-6
Risk-Enhancing Effects of Predictor Factors on Decile Score Groups:
Intercurrent Disorders

Risk Variable		Perinatal Outcome		Composite Outcome	
		RR	95%CL	RR	95%CL
DIS1	Organic heart disease	2.66	1.36-5.22A	1.37	0.88-2.15
DIS7	Thrombophlebitis			1.99	0.83-4.79
DISi5	Active tuberculosis	23.23	8.38-64.37A	5.05	1.88-13.56A
DIS21	Inactive tuberculosis	2.22	0.97-5.11A	0.85	0.43-1.69
DIS22	Pneumonia	5.87	2.56-13.44A	1.35	0.61-2.99
DIS26	Bronchial asthma	2.03	0.98-4.20A	0.83	0.47-1.45
DIS31	Anemia	1.17	0.89-1.54	1.00	0.87-1.16
DIS32	Low serum iron	6.09	2.73-13.58A	2.59	1.36-4.97A
DIS37	Response to iron therapy	1.46	1.03-2.07A	1.13	0.94-1.36
DIS38	Sickle cell disease	3.99	1.99-8.33A	1.47	0.84-2.59
DIS48	Other blood disease			3.98	1.62-9.78B
DIS49	Diabetes mellitus	4.54	2.20-9.34A	2.29*	1.36-3.85B
DIS50	Hyperglycemia 200+ mg./dl.	6.77	3.05-15.04A	2.64*	1.41-4.96A
DIS51	Insulin therapy	6.85	3.13-15.00A	3.21*	1.78-5.77C
DIS54	Ketoacidosis			5.70*	2.02-16.04A
DIS57	Hypothyroidism	3.85	1.70-8.73A	1.50	0.73-3.05
DIS63	Hyperthyroidism	14.33	5.67-36.19A	3.27	1.36-7.88A
DIS74	Syphilis	24.31	8.63-68.50A	6.20	2.16-17.81A
DIS75	Chancre			8.95	3.01-26.64A
DIS76	Gonorrhea			2.27	1.12-4.62A
DIS80	Glomerulonephritis	21.93	8.65-55.59C	5.75	2.24-14.80B
DIS81	Urinary tract infection	1.15	0.83-1.59	1.04	0.88-1.22
DIS86	Hematuria	2.06	1.14-3.72A	1.26	0.85-1.86
DIS87	GU tumor			8.70	2.92-25.88A
DIS91	Incompetent cervix			3.86	1.50-9.89A
DIS94	Leiomyoma uteri	2.35	1.13-4.90A	1.42	0.79-2.55
DIS98	Convulsive disorder	5.29	2.29-12.25A	2.31	1.23-4.31A
DIS99	Convulsion in pregnancy	6.72	2.82-16.06B	2.96	1.52-5.79B
DIS100	Mental retardation	9.07	4.16-19.76B	6.93	3.76-12.77F
DIS103	Neurological disorder	4.66	2.18-9.97A	2.50	1.45-4.31C
DIS107	Cholecystitis	13.39	5.22-34.36A	2.91	1.18-7.17A
DIS111	Colitis, ileitis	16.50	6.38-42.65A	7.07	2.98-16.79D
DIS120	Hyperemesis gravidarum	1.55	0.72-3.34	1.07	0.64-1.80
DIS123	Hydramnios	2.69*	1.42-5.12A	1.83*	1.19-2.81A
DIS124	First trimester bleeding	1.47	0.91-1.96A	1.14	0.92-1.39
DIS125	Second trimester bleeding	1.13	0.70-1.85	1.08	0.85-1.39
DIS126	Third trimester bleeding	1.21	0.87-1.70	1.14	0.96-1.36
DIS128	Hemorrhagic shock	20.40	7.68-54.23B	3.98	1.59-10.00A
DIS130	Supine hypotension	7.44	3.34-16.57A	2.62	1.22-5.63A
DIS140	Parasitic disease	7.44	3.18-17.40A	1.65	0.75-3.65
SDIS5	Venereal diseases	1.79*	1.16-2.76A	1.42	1.11-1.80B

Referent variables consist of absence of disease variables under consideration.

* Relative risk significantly enhanced in high-risk-score groups.

tal and composite outcomes were found to be far in excess of those expected for many of these factors even though all labor and delivery risk had ostensibly been accounted for by the risk-score model. Most had previously been identified by the collective and aggregative analyses of intrinsic risk factors (see chapters 21 and 25). Only 13 of the disorders that had been flagged as significant by the study involving the intrinsic variables studied in isolation as a group (see Table 21-13) had also appeared in comparable roles when those same factors had been investigated in conjunction with the full array of labor, delivery, and drug variables (see Table 25-6). In the former analysis, eight additional disorders had been identified as possibly presenting significant hazard. We re-examined all 21 of these conditions plus a large number of others deemed potentially relevant to ensure against inadvertently overlooking some important and clinically meaningful relationships.

Among those intercurrent disorders previously shown to have significant adverse effects on offspring in the foregoing studies, all but one were verified to yield similar degrees of risk by means of the risk-score approach. That variable was DIS126 (third trimester bleeding); while the resulting odds ratios were somewhat increased with this variable, especially for perinatal outcome, they were no longer statistically significant when the impact of labor and delivery risk factors were being considered simultaneously by the risk score.

The magnitude of effect of some of the significant variables was rather impressive. Active tuberculosis (DIS15), for example, carried a remarkable 23-fold excess perinatal risk and a fivefold composite outcome hazard. Anemia as an otherwise unspecified diagnosis (DIS31) failed to survive this critical analysis as a risk factor (see HCT, above), but low serum iron (DIS32) did with a very high odds ratio of 6.09 for adverse perinatal effects, as did sickle cell disease (DIS38, perinatal outcome OR = 3.99).

Diabetes mellitus (DIS49) and its several markers of severity (DIS50, hyperglycemia; DIS51, insulin therapy; and DIS54, ketoacidosis; none of which had previously been flagged) showed similarly high levels of deleterious influence on the fetus and infant. Hyperthyroidism (DIS63), with odds ratios of 14.33 for perinatal and 3.27 for composite effects, was also especially noteworthy. Similarly, syphilis (DIS74), glomerulonephritis (DIS80), mental retardation (DIS100), cholecystitis (DIS107), colitis-ileitis (DIS111), and hemorrhagic shock (DIS128) were likewise found to yield uncommonly strong effects.

Probability values for most of these risk variables were found to be marginal at the 5% level, but the impact of a few factors was quite significant, such as that for DIS51 (diabetes requiring insulin), DIS80 (glomerulonephritis), DIS100 (mental retardation), DIS103 (neurologic disorder), and DIS111 (colitis-ileitis). Unless the more reliable incremental risk-score model (see below) was to reveal some unexpected flaw in our data, it is very likely that these intercurrent disease variables are indeed significantly deleterious to the infant. For the remaining variables, both the degree of effect and level of probability were such as to warrant closer scrutiny before accepting their risks as necessarily real.

Several of the tested factors yielded evidence of a significant excess of risk even though those effects had not been previously identified in antecedent analyses. Three have already been mentioned, namely DIS50, DIS51 and DIS54, as manifestations of severe diabetes. In addition, especially pertinent results were found for DIS22 (pneumonia), DIS57 (hypothyroidism), DIS75 (chancre), DIS91 (incompetent cervix), DIS98 (convulsive disorder), and DIS99 (seizure in pregnancy). A number of others showed lesser degrees of adverse effect, albeit nonetheless statistically significant, including DIS1 (cardiac disease), DIS21 (inactive tuberculosis), DIS26 (bronchial asthma), DIS76 (gonorrhea), DIS86 (hematuria), DIS94 (uterine fibroids), and DIS124 (first trimester bleeding, see VAGBLD, above).

Impact of Predictor Variables on Incremental-Strata Model

All the foregoing risk assessment of predictor variables utilized the risk-scoring model constructed on arbitrary decile stratifications of the distributions of scores among the study population. Some of the shortcomings of that approach were reviewed before (see chapter 27), particularly as regards the less-than-perfect fit of the model to the labor-delivery risk data. Thus, it was conceivable that a factor could be shown to have some residual effects not accounted for by the risk score when in fact those effects were due instead to one or more labor or delivery variables present in unexpected numbers in the subset under study as a consequence of maldistribution.

To ensure against that possibility, we had sought and found a model that would be more appropriate for our needs. It took the form of an incremental stratification of the risk-score range based on demonstrated serially stepped adverse effects. For perinatal outcome, four cut points were found which thereby yielded five incremental groups; for composite outcome, three cut points yielded four strata. Parallel subsets were selected for each predictor variable under consideration as previously described, the cases were stratified by the aforementioned risk-score strata, and the outcome results for each cell within the matrix thus created were compared statistically as before.

Demographic Risk Variables

The impact of the range of demographic variables was shown by invoking the incremental-strata model (Table 28-7). The results can be contrasted with those previously displayed for the decile risk-score model (see Table 28-1). What is immediately evident throughout is the absence of the significant high-end risk-score enhancement of effect so often found in the prior analyses. Because the model fit the data so much better, these high-end enhancements (undoubtedly often specious) no longer appeared. In addition, a number of variables, previously flagged as probably having significantly adverse effects, now showed up as being rather innocuous. Some occasionally even crossed over to the protective side. In the overview, nearly all the adverse odds ratios were of smaller magnitude (and therefore some proved less significant) and many of the protective ones became more protective (and correspondingly more significant).

Among collaborating institutions, for example, although the findings were generally about as they had been before, there were some important differences. The perinatal impact of INST10 and INST15 was considerably reduced and no longer statistically significant. Contrastingly, the composite outcome effect of INST31, not previously noted to be especially adverse, was now significantly so. Similarly, composite results for INST45 were worse both in magnitude of effect and degree of statistical significance. Effects of the other hospital units remained about the same as they had been earlier.

Maternal age effects were almost identical with those seen for the decile risk-score model, adverse influences concentrating particularly in the offspring of the youngest gravidas (AGE6 and AGE7). Clinic service status (STATUS1) still showed some increased composite outcome risk. In contrast, there were a number of changes found in regard to marital status. Whereas being single and never married (MARIT1) was just as adverse an effect as it had been before, MARIT3, MARIT4, and MARIT6 (common law, widowed, and separated) had all lost the deleterious perinatal impact disclosed earlier by the decile-strata analytical system.

Race was examined as a risk factor in the same way. RACE2 (black) was again confirmed to be associated with significantly adverse perinatal and composite outcomes (Table 28-7) at about the same magnitude and significance level as in the decile-strata system (see Table 28-1). The perinatal effect of RACE3 (other race), previously found to be significantly adverse, was no longer the case even though the odds ratio was still high (2.52 or less than half of what it had been earlier). RELIG2 (Roman Catholic) and RELIG3 (other religion, principally Jewish) still carried about the same strongly protective effects insofar as composite outcome was concerned.

The results for the mother's place of birth, however, were somewhat modified. ORIGIN2 (MD to FL), for example, which

Table 28-7
Risk-Enhancing Effects of Predictor Factors On Incremental Risk-Score Groups:
Demographic Variables*

Risk Variable		Perinatal Outcome		Composite Outcome	
		RR	95%CL	RR	95%CL
INST10	Hospital 10	1.72	0.90-3.29	1.03	0.72-1.48
INST15	Hospital 15	1.50	0.75-3.01	2.01F	1.44-2.76
INST31	Hospital 31	0.95	0.44-2.03	1.44A	1.04-1.99
INST37	Hospital 37	1.37	0.84-2.31	1.93F	1.49-2.50
INST45	Hospital 45	1.47	0.86-2.53	1.80F	1.36-2.39
INST50	Hospital 50	1.00	0.58-1.74	1.30	0.98-1.73
INST55	Hospital 55	1.75B	1.13-2.70	1.32A	1.03-1.69
INST60	Hospital 60	1.74B	1.05-2.89	2.79F	2.18-3.57
INST66	Hospital 66	1.12	0.71-1.78	1.23	0.96-1.57
INST71	Hospital 71	1.87A	1.04-3.37	2.17F	1.61-2.92
INST82	Hospital 82	1.13	0.65-1.96	1.32	1.00-1.73
AGE1	Maternal age under 20 yr.	1.25	0.93-1.69	1.23B	1.06-1.42
AGE3	Maternal age 25-29 yr.	1.02	0.72-1.45	0.92	0.77-1.10
AGE4	Maternal age 30-34 yr.	1.22	0.79-1.88	1.23A	1.00-1.52
AGE5	Maternal age 35+ yr.	1.33	0.84-2.11	1.03	0.79-1.34
AGE6	Maternal age under 18 yr.	1.44A	0.99-2.08	1.36C	1.12-1.63
AGE7	Maternal age under 16 yr.	1.97B	1.17-3.31	1.39A	1.03-1.89
STATUS1	Clinic service patient	1.01	0.46-1.43	1.43A	1.04-1.96
MARIT1	Single status	1.35A	1.00-1.81	1.19A	1.02-1.39
MARIT3	Common law	1.33	0.60-2.96	0.92	0.57-1.49
MARIT4	Widowed	2.37	0.75-7.42	1.48	0.71-3.06
MARIT5	Divorced	2.61B	1.22-5.59	1.44	0.88-2.36
MARIT6	Separated	1.41	0.84-2.39	1.28A	1.00-1.63
RACE2	Black	1.36B	1.05-1.76	1.14A	1.00-1.29
RACE3	Other race	2.52	0.74-8.59	0.87	0.38-2.01
RELIG2	Catholic	1.11	0.86-1.42	0.80d	0.71-0.92
RELIG3	Jewish	0.57	0.27-1.21	0.45f	0.30-0.67
ORIGIN1	Place of birth: NY, NJ, PA	0.90	0.58-1.42	0.82a	0.65-1.02
ORIGIN2	MD to FL	1.09	0.73-1.62	1.27B	1.04-1.54
ORIGIN3	KY, TN, AL, MS	0.74	0.43-1.30	0.96	0.75-1.23
ORIGIN4	AR, LA, OK, TX	1.44	0.80-2.57	1.70F	1.30-2.21
ORIGIN5	IL, IN, OH, MI, WI	0.69	0.26-1.83	0.87	0.53-1.41
ORIGIN6	MN, IA, MO, KA,NE, ND, SD	1.08	0.62-1.87	1.11	0.85-1.44
ORIGIN7	WY, ID, CO, MT, UT, NM, AZ, NV	1.98	0.69-5.69	0.98	0.52-1.86
ORIGIN8	WA, OR, CA	0.93	0.45-1.89	1.69D	1.24-2.30
ORIGIN10	Puerto Rico	1.41	0.86-2.31	0.67b	0.50-0.91
ORIGIN11	Other Atlantic islands	1.91	0.86-4.26	1.11	0.67-1.85
ORIGIN12	Alaska and Canada	1.92	0.50-7.38	1.43	0.59-3.49
ORIGIN13	Central and South America			1.56	0.80-3.04
ORIGIN14	Pacific Islands	2.84	0.75-10.76	1.03	0.32-3.35
ORIGIN15	Europe	0.70	0.27-1.86	0.58a	0.34-0.99
ORIGIN16	Asia and Africa	1.56	0.46-5.31	0.59	0.24-1.44

* See Table 28-1 footnote for referent variables and probability code.

had previously not shown any special impact, now showed significantly adverse composite outcomes. Contrariwise, a number of birthplace variables, significant before, were now devoid of any deleterious effects, including ORIGIN7 (WY to NV), ORIGIN11 (Caribbean islands), ORIGIN12 (Alaska and Canada), ORIGIN14 (Pacific islands), and ORIGIN16 (Asia and Africa). Some of these, such as ORIGIN11, ORIGIN12, and ORIGIN14, still displayed rather high odds ratios, especially for perinatal outcome, but they could not be shown to be statistically significant because of small relative frequencies. The rest remained at about the level they had been earlier with notably adverse composite outcome effects verified for ORIGIN4 (AR to TX) and ORIGIN8 (WA to CA) and protective composite effects for ORIGIN15 (Europe).

Past Obstetrical History

Risk factors pertaining to prior obstetrical experience were also studied by means of the incremental risk-score model and the results were generally confirmatory (Table 28-8) of those developed by the decile-strata model (see Table 28-2). The only exceptions were the aforementioned tendency for odds ratios to be somewhat less adverse on the high side of unity and more protective on the low side. Gravidity failed to show an alteration in risk effect. Only GRAV4 (Gravida 4) could be shown to have any sizable adverse impact. Statistical significance was limited to the excess effect on composite outcome only, even though the magnitude of risk was about the same for both perinatal and composite outcome results.

Grand multiparity (PARA2), which had previously been determined to expose the infant to significantly increased risk, was no longer found to have any residual signifi-

Table 28-8
Risk-Enhancing Effects of Predictor Factors on Incremental Risk-Score Groups:
Physical Characteristics and Obstetrical Background*

Risk Variable		Perinatal Outcome		Composite Outcome	
		RR	95%CL	RR	95%CL
GRAV1	First pregnancy	0.98	0.60-1.35	1.01	0.60-1.33
GRAV3	Gravida 3	0.86	0.54-1.37	1.06	0.85-1.32
GRAV4	Gravida 4	1.34	0.84-2.14	1.33A	1.05-1.69
GRAV5	Gravida 5	0.89	0.51-1.56	1.10	0.84-1.45
GRAV6	Gravida 6	0.91	0.44-1.86	1.06	0.77-1.47
PARA1	Multipara, Para 1-4	1.43	0.71-2.91	1.22	0.83-1.78
PARA2	Grand multipara, Para 5+	1.56	0.59-4.12	1.32	0.76-2.30
PABORT1	Prior abortion	1.03	0.73-1.44	0.93	0.78-1.11
PPREM1	Prior premature birth	1.55A	1.08-2.22	1.39E	1.16-1.67
PSTILLB1	Prior stillbirth	1.24	0.73-2.09	1.17	0.89-1.53
PPMR1	Prior perinatal death	1.27	0.80-2.00	1.28A	1.01-1.62
PPMR2	Two prior deaths	1.72	0.53-5.61	0.84	0.43-1.64
PPMR3	Three prior deaths	5.70A	1.49-21.89	2.01	0.57-7.03
PRIOR0	No prior pregnancy	1.07	0.82-1.39	0.95	0.83-1.08
PRIOR1	Last outcome fetal death	1.30	0.87-1.92	0.99	0.80-1.21
PRIOR2	Last died in first day	2.06	0.74-5.75	0.94	0.42-2.12
PRIOR3	Last died in day 2-6	3.71A	1.23-11.12	1.19	0.49-2.89
PRIOR4	Last died in day 7-27			1.53	0.34-6.81
PRIOR5	Last died in month 2-12	2.70	0.79-9.28	1.07	0.38-3.02
PRIOR6	Last died after first year			1.19	0.28-5.02
HGT1	Maternal height > 68 in.	0.76	0.39-1.45	0.97	0.73-1.30
HGT2	Maternal height < 60 in.	1.72A	1.16-2.55	1.23A	0.97-1.55
PWGT1	Prepregnancy weight > 175 lb.	1.25	0.74-2.10	1.07	0.81-1.40
PWGT2	Prepregnancy weight < 100 lb.	1.12	0.66-1.91	1.19	0.94-1.52
QI1	Ponderosity index lean	0.83	0.50-1.39	1.14	0.92-1.42
QI2	Ponderosity index obese	1.03	0.75-1.42	1.11	0.94-1.30
POND1	Ponderal index lean	1.00	0.51-1.96	1.22	0.91-1.65
POND2	Ponderal index obese	1.14	0.82-1.59	1.21A	1.02-1.43
SMOKE2	Smoked > 10 yr.	1.22	0.86-1.72	0.96	0.80-1.17
SMOKE3	Smokes > 30 per day	1.38	0.57-3.33	1.52A	0.98-2.34
SMOKE4	Smokes 10-30 per day	1.02	0.76-1.36	0.97	0.84-1.13
SMOKE5	Smokes < 10 per day	1.03	0.74-1.42	0.94	0.80-1.11
PELV2	Pelvis contracted	2.12A	1.08-4.16	1.36	0.87-2.13
PELV3	Pelvis borderline	1.11	0.49-2.51	1.18	0.80-1.76

* See footnotes in Table 28-2 for referent variables and Table 28-1 for probability code.

436

cant impact even though the odds ratios were still somewhat elevated. Similarly, PARA1 (para 1-4) could not be shown to retain the effect previously encountered in the composite outcome results examined by the decile risk-score model. The effect of parity itself as a risk variable was found to be uniformly distributed and not at all different from the referent for composite outcome (Table 28-9). As to perinatal data, however, there appeared to be some degree of protection (not statistically significant) at the low end of the risk-score-scale stratifications with a somewhat counterbalancing central and high-end adverse effect (highly significant). The overall impact of these diverse effects was negligible. The contradictory observations effectively cancelled each other out insofar as the goodness-of-fit analysis was concerned.

The adverse effects of a prior premature delivery (PPREM1) were reconfirmed here (Table 28-8) at almost precisely the magnitude of effect and degree of probability as had been seen before (see Table 28-2). Prior perinatal mortality, however, had less of an impact than it did earlier. Among cases with one previous loss (PPMR1), there was still some significantly deleterious composite outcome effect, but there was no longer any definable short-term perinatal effect. Those with two prior losses (PPMR2) did not show the significantly adverse perinatal effect that this factor had yielded in the preceding analysis. Offspring of gravidas

who had experienced three prior perinatal deaths were still at very increased perinatal risk (confirmed to be statistically significant). However, we could not verify the bad composite outcome effect seen before, even though the odds ratio remained high (but was no longer significant).

The outcome of the last prior pregnancy was considerably less of an adverse factor than it had been for the decile risk-score model. Only cases in which prior newborn infants had died within the first week but after the first day (PRIOR3) still revealed a significant excess of poor perinatal outcomes. Whereas all the other related prior outcome variables had shown similar bad effects for either perinatal or composite outcome—such as PRIOR1 (stillbirth), PRIOR2 (death in the first 24 hours), PRIOR4 (death in days 7-27), PRIOR5 (death in months 2-12), and PRIOR7 (death after the first year)—none of them repeated these effects here. Even PRIOR3 failed to yield outcome effects in the composite outcome data comparable to those which it was showing in the perinatal data (by the incremental model) or which it had previously shown (by the decile model). This clear revocation of the earlier findings suggested that the adverse effects associated with prior pregnancy wastage that we had disclosed before were probably more related to the influence of labor-delivery events and management than to the bad obstetric history per se.

Table 28-9
Risk-Enhancing Effects of Parity on Incremental Score Groups

Risk Score Level	Perinatal Outcome		Composite Outcome	
	OR	p–Value	OR	p–Value
Lowest	0.43	0.063	0.99	0.94
Low	0.76	0.072	1.03	0.71
Moderate	1.32	0.34		
High	3.34*	0.0007	1.21	0.34
Highest	1.51	0.49	1.11	0.81
Overall	0.98	0.90	1.04	0.54
95% CL	0.76-1.23		0.92-1.18	

* Statistically significant.

Physical Characteristics

The incremental risk-strata model quite competently supported our prior observations that short maternal stature (HGT2, under 60 in) was an adverse factor both as regards perinatal and composite outcome (Table 28-8). Children of tall mothers did about as expected, neither adverse nor beneficial effects having been found. The same lack of effect applied to the factor of prepregnancy weight. Both heavy (PWGT1) and light women (PWGT2) showed acceptably good outcome results. This negated the adverse composite outcome effect seen earlier for PWGT1 when it had been studied by the decile risk-score model (see Table 28-2). Relative parvitude (QI1 and POND1) or obesity (QI2 and POND2) was generally confirmatory in this regard; only POND2 (obese by ponderal index) showed any significant residual adverse effect, strictly limited to composite outcome and of marginal statistical significance.

Cigarette smoking had previously been shown to be bad for offspring only if continued during the current pregnancy at a moderately high intensity of habit (SMOKE3, more than 30 cigarettes per day). This relationship was duplicated here almost precisely for the composite outcome data (Table 28-8), but failed to reappear for perinatal data. No new information was forthcoming from the incremental strata model applied to the other variables relating to tobacco use.

Pelvic capacity as assessed by antepartum clinical pelvimetry was re-examined. The earlier observation that contracted pelvis (PELV2) was associated with significantly bad perinatal results was confirmed here (Table 28-8). The odds ratio for composite outcome results was found to be somewhat high, but it was not significant. Contrary to prior findings, moreover, borderline pelvis (PELV3) did not show any adverse effects even remotely suggesting it to be a clinically important risk factor.

Socioeconomic Factors

The socioeconomic index was subjected to analysis by the incremental risk-strata model for purposes of determining whether the findings from the decile model were correct. The study showed them to be almost entirely so (compare Tables 28-10 and 28-4). As before, there was a clear-cut unbroken inverse linear relationship between the socioeconomic index and the odds ratio for composite outcome. Although the within-group effect for SES4 (index 35-44) was no longer statistically significant, the adverse results at the low end of the index scale (SES1-SES3, indices below 35) and the good results at the high end (SES8-SES9, indices of 75+) were once again highly significant. Perinatal effects were about as they had been before with poor outcomes in all low socioeconomic groups with indices below 45, but the odds ratios achieved statistical significance only in SES3 and SES4 (indices 25-44). No comparable high index protection was encountered in regard to perinatal outcome.

Per capita income data fell almost precisely where they had fallen earlier. Low income (INCOME1, under $800 per person per year) was associated with significantly adverse composite outcome results, whereas high income (INCOME4 and INCOME5, $2250+ per person per annum) was clearly protective. There was only a suggestion (not statistically significant) of a bad perinatal effect from low per capita income, but no counterbalancing protective effect at the high end of the income range.

Gross family income, which had previously shown some strong low-end adverse impact (see Table 28-4), was now found to have similar low-end effects (Table 28-10), although they were less impressive in terms of magnitude and no longer statistically significant except in FAMINC2 (under $2000 per annum) for composite outcome. A new finding of considerable note was evidence of a clear-cut inverse linear trend signifying increasingly

Table 28-10
Risk-Enhancing Effects of Predictor Factors on Incremental Risk-Score Groups: Socioeconomic Factors*

Risk Variable		Perinatal Outcome RR	95%CL	Composite Outcome RR	95%CL
SES1	Socioeconomic index < 15	1.41	0.79–2.50	1.59D	1.21–2.08
SES2	Socioeconomic index 15–24	1.28	0.78–2.08	1.32B	1.05–1.66
SES3	Socioeconomic index 25–34	1.55A	1.00–2.41	1.29B	1.05–1.59
SES4	Socioeconomic index 35–44	1.68B	1.11–2.53	1.18	0.96–1.45
SES6	Socioeconomic index 55–64	1.00	0.61–1.64	0.85	0.67–1.08
SES7	Socioeconomic index 65–74	0.98	0.56–1.73	0.79	0.60–1.05
SES8	Socioeconomic index 75–84	1.07	0.58–1.97	0.58d	0.42–0.82
SES9	Socioeconomic index 85+	0.87	0.40–1.89	0.40f	0.27–0.61
INCOME1	Per capita income < $800/yr.	1.21	0.83–1.78	1.23A	1.02–1.48
INCOME2	Per capita income $800–1499	0.96	0.64–1.44	0.94	0.77–1.14
INCOME4	Per capita income $2250–2999	1.08	0.64–1.80	0.77a	0.59–1.01
INCOME5	Per capita income $3000+	1.17	0.68–2.00	0.78a	0.59–1.03
FAMINC1	No family income	2.65	0.72–9.74	1.93	0.87–4.29
FAMINC2	Family income < $2000/yr.	1.15	0.69–1.92	1.36B	1.07–1.74
FAMINC3	Family income $2000–3999/yr.	0.98	0.64–1.50	1.00	0.81–1.25
FAMINC4	Family income $4000–4999/yr.	0.86	0.53–1.38	0.85	0.67–1.08
FAMINC6	Family income $8000–9999/yr.	1.04	0.49–2.21	0.72a	0.47–1.10
FAMINC7	Family income $10,000+/yr.	0.76	0.28–2.09	0.61a	0.36–1.04
HOUSE1	Housing density 1.0+ person/room	0.95	0.72–1.26	1.19A	1.02–1.38
EDUC0	No formal education	1.32	0.82–1.98	0.90	0.21–3.89
EDUC1	Education 7 yr. or less	1.20	0.80–1.80	1.47E	1.20–1.81
EDUC2	Education 8 yr.	1.28	0.80–1.92	1.30A	1.03–1.63
EDUC3	Education 9–11 yr.	1.00	0.75–1.33	1.17A	1.01–1.36
EDUC5	Education 13–15 yr.	0.56a	0.31–1.01	0.60e	0.45–0.81
EDUC6	Education 16+ yr.	0.68	0.33–1.42	0.32f	0.19–0.53
WORKG1	Gravida never worked	1.15	0.82–1.62	1.41F	1.17–1.68
WORKG2	Gravida white collar worker	0.62b	0.42–0.89	0.55f	0.46–0.66
WORKG3	Gravida blue collar worker	0.86	0.63–1.17	0.89	0.76–1.04
WORKF0	Father of baby never worked			1.41	0.43–4.69
WORKF2	Father of baby in armed forces	1.13	0.41–3.14	0.99	0.54–1.81
WORKF3	Father of baby student	0.91	0.46–1.80	0.67b	0.43–1.03
WORKF4	Father of baby unemployed	0.90	0.59–1.37	1.40F	1.17–1.68
WORKF5	Father of baby absent	1.67E	1.22–2.28	1.54F	1.30–1.82
WORKF6	Father of baby unknown	1.27	0.53–3.06	1.40	0.89–2.21
OCCUPF3	Father of baby blue collar worker	1.36A	0.97–1.89	1.73F	1.45–2.05

* See footnotes in Table 28-4 for referent variables and Table 28-1 for probability code.

adverse effects with decreasing income. This was demonstrated by a high odds ratio of 1.93 in FAMINC1 (no income) at one extreme and a low odds ratio of 0.61 in FAMINC7 ($10,000+ per annum) at the other. Strongly significant high income protection against bad composite outcome was identified in FAMINC6 and FAMINC7 ($8000 or more).

A similar linear correlation was seen for perinatal effect, ranging from OR = 2.65 in FAMINC1 to OR = 0.76 in FAMINC7, the linearity being disturbed only in FAMINC6

(OR = 1.04). Notwithstanding this obvious relationship, neither extreme proved statistically significant for the perinatal outcome effects. While the gross family income variable had earlier appeared to contribute only in small measure to the effect mirrored in the socioeconomic index when examined by the decile-strata model, these new findings showed it to be an important component.

High housing density (HOUSE1) had been found to impact adversely on composite outcome in the decile risk-score analysis (see Table 28-4). When re-examined by the incremental-strata model, this effect was confirmed almost precisely (Table 28-10). Moreover, just as before, no perinatal effect could be shown. In regard to the gravida's education, a strong trend had previously been found for composite outcome results to be worse with less education and better with more (see Table 28-4). This was repeated here with especially intense protective effects seen at the high end as shown by significantly low odds ratios in EDUC5 and EDUC6 (more than high school education) and significantly high odds ratios in EDUC1-EDUC3 (below high school level). However, the finding of essentially no effect for EDUC0 (no formal education) was quite inconsistent with this trend. The less clear-cut, but nevertheless general tendency for perinatal results to parallel those of composite outcome, as seen in the decile-strata model, was reconfirmed here as well.

The impact of the gravida's work history was exactly as it had been before (compare Tables 28-10 and 28-4). Very highly significant adverse composite outcome effects accrued to offspring of women who had never worked (WORKG1). Equally strong protection existed among those delivered to women who functioned as white-collar workers (WORKG2). For perinatal data, only the protective effect associated with WORKG2 was determined to be significant, just as it had been before in the decile risk-score model.

As to the baby's father, there was still some adverse effect on composite outcome among children of men who had never been employed (WORKF0), but it was no longer statistically significant. The same applied to cases in which the identity of the baby's father was unknown (WORKF6) for both composite and perinatal outcome data. The deleterious composite outcome effect of a currently unemployed father (WORKF4) or an absent one (WORKF5) was verified at very strong levels of statistical significance. Furthermore, WORKF5 also had a very serious impact on perinatal results.

The adverse perinatal effect previously encountered in WORKF2 (father of baby in the armed forces) had vanished. The impressively beneficial effect of WORKF3 (student) on composite outcome was again present and had actually increased somewhat. Blue-collar employment (OCCUPF3) once more served as an indicator of excessively poor perinatal and composite outcome. The adverse effect previously seen in the decile-strata system for composite outcome with this variable was only slightly enhanced here, but at a very much lower probability level of it being merely a chance event.

Antepartum Factors

The effect of measurable prenatal care factors was reassessed using the incremental risk-score model in the same way it had been done for the decile-strata model (see Table 28-5). Results for cases registering late for antepartum care were found to be somewhat worse in regard to composite outcome. The adverse impact of GREG6 (registration at 28-31.9 weeks) was verified even more strongly than before. Moreover, now GREG5 (antepartum care beginning at 24-27.9 weeks) and GREG8 (at 36+ weeks) showed significantly deleterious effects not previously encountered. Just as before, however, no comparable perinatal effect could be demonstrated. By the trimester of pregnancy in which registration for antepartum care had occurred, the bad composite outcome effects of TRIMEST2 and TRIMEST3 (second and third trimester registration) were found to be greater both in magnitude (that is, to be associated with larger odds ratios) and in statistical significance.

As to the number of prenatal office visits, the parabolic relationship previously seen was confirmed (compare Tables 28-11 and 28-5). There was a very significantly adverse composite outcome effect found for VISIT1 (less than seven visits over the course of pregnancy). At the other end of the range of visit frequencies, the odds ratios for composite outcome were increased, as they had been with the decile

Table 28-11
Risk-Enhancing Effects of Predictor Factors on Incremental Risk-Score Groups:
Antepartum Factors*

Risk Variable		Perinatal Outcome		Composite Outcome	
		RR	95%CL	RR	95%CL
GREG2	Registered at 12-15.9 wk.	0.71	0.44-1.16	0.92	0.71-1.18
GREG3	Registered at 16-19.9 wk.	1.04	0.66-1.63	1.11	0.87-1.41
GREG4	Registered at 20-23.9 wk.	1.10	0.70-1.72	1.14	0.90-1.45
GREG5	Registered at 24-27.9 wk.	1.11	0.70-1.75	1.25A	0.98-1.60
GREG6	Registered at 28-31.9 wk.	1.14	0.70-1.85	1.39B	1.08-1.79
GREG7	Registered at 32-35.9 wk.	0.70	0.38-1.27	1.17	0.89-1.54
GREG8	Registered at 36+ wk.	0.92	0.52-1.62	1.30A	0.98-1.72
TRIMEST2	Registered in second trimester	1.22	0.90-1.66	1.22B	1.04-1.43
TRIMEST3	Registered in third trimester	1.08	0.76-1.54	1.38E	1.15-1.64
VISIT1	Prenatal visits < 7	1.00	0.75-1.31	1.25D	1.09-1.43
VISIT3	Prenatal visits 15-16	1.05	0.63-1.75	0.95	0.73-1.25
VISIT4	Prenatal visits 17-20	1.44	0.79-2.61	1.24	0.87-1.76
VISIT5	Prenatal visits 21+	2.22	0.64-7.68	2.03	0.91-4.57
GDEL1	Delivery at < 34 wk.	2.94E	1.62-5.33	1.49A	1.05-2.11
GDEL2	Delivery at < 36 wk.	2.75F	1.80-4.21	1.60F	1.26-2.02
GDEL3	Delivery at < 38 wk.	2.00F	1.44-2.78	1.45F	1.23-1.72
GDEL4	Delivery at > 41 wk.	1.60C	1.19-2.15	1.12	0.96-1.31
GDEL5	Delivery at > 42 wk.	1.67B	1.16-2.40	1.21A	1.00-1.48
GDEL6	Delivery at > 43 wk.	1.66A	1.06-2.61	1.20	0.93-1.54
GDEL7	Delivery at > 44 wk.	0.93	0.47-1.84	1.10	0.79-1.52
BW1	Birth weight 2500-2749 g.	1.48	0.94-2.32	1.22	0.97-1.54
BW2	Birth weight 2750-2999 g.	1.22	0.84-1.76	1.27A	1.06-1.54
BW3	Birth weight 3000-3249 g.	1.00	0.70-1.42	1.19A	1.00-1.42
BW5	Birth weight 3500-3749 g.	0.84	0.56-1.25	0.91	0.74-1.11
BW6	Birth weight 3750-3999 g.	0.96	0.61-1.52	1.01	0.80-1.28
SGA	Small for gestational age	1.94A	1.15-3.28	1.15	0.86-1.54
LGA	Large for gestational age	1.12	0.74-1.68	1.12	0.90-1.39
MALE	Male infant	1.64F	1.30-2.13	1.41F	1.25-1.59
OBTYPE2	Resident in attendance	0.82	0.44-1.53	1.20	0.84-1.71
OBTYPE3	Intern in attendance	0.65	0.33-1.25	1.43A	1.01-2.03
OBTYPE4	Student in attendance	0.55	0.25-1.19	1.30	0.83-2.03
HCT1	Lowest hematocrit < 20%	6.76A	1.79-25.52	2.05	0.60-7.02
HCT2	Lowest hematocrit 20-24.9%	2.10A	0.99-4.49	1.24	0.75-2.04
HCT3	Lowest hematocrit 25-29.9%	1.11	0.73-1.67	1.10	0.90-1.35
HCT4	Lowest hematocrit 30-34.9%	1.04	0.78-1.40	1.02	0.89-1.18
RUP1	Amniotomy at delivery	0.86	0.57-1.30	0.99	0.82-1.19
RUP2	Amniotomy for induction	1.09	0.52-2.27	1.02	0.65-1.59
RUP3	Amniotomy for augmentation	0.94	0.72-1.22	0.93	0.82-1.07
VAGBLD	First trimester bleeding	1.44A	0.95-2.16	1.13	0.88-1.46
RHSENS	Rh isoimmunization	3.65A	1.27-10.53	1.76	0.78-3.95
PIH1	Diastolic hypertension only	1.25	0.59-2.66	1.48A	0.96-2.29
PIH2	Hypertension and proteinuria	1.10	0.31-3.85	1.38	0.79-2.40
PIH3	Proteinuria only	1.06	0.48-2.33	1.27	0.81-1.99

* See footnotes in Table 28-5 for referent variables and Table 28-1 for probability code.

risk-score model, for VISIT4 and VISIT5 (17+ visits), but they could no longer be shown to be statistically significant. Perinatal effects were much weaker than they had been earlier. The very high odds ratio for excess adverse perinatal outcomes encountered previously for VISIT5 (21+ visits) was much reduced and, although still considerably increased, was not statistically significant any more.

The effects of gestational age at delivery were almost precisely what they had been before both as to magnitude of effect and probability level for perinatal and composite results over the entire range of GDEL variables (compare Tables 28-11 and 28-5). The only exceptions were the composite outcome effects of GDEL4 (delivery after 41 weeks) and GDEL6 (after 43 weeks) in which the odds ratios were no longer statistically significant even though still somewhat above unity. As before, the absence of any documentable adverse effects for GDEL7 (delivery beyond 44 weeks) was believed to be due to small numbers and inclusion of cases with erroneous pregnancy dating. Thus, despite the narrow birth weight constraints of this study population (2500-4000g), gestational age at delivery was clearly a decisive factor in regard to fetal and infant outcome.

Analogously, the birth weight effects were also duplicated almost exactly (Table 28-11). We found the same tendency for smaller infants to be associated with higher frequencies of adverse perinatal and composite outcomes as had been seen before (see Table 28-5). However, none of the odds ratios associated with perinatal data for the several birth weight variables proved statistically significant. For composite outcome results, only BW2 and BW3 (2750-3249g) were still shown to be significant, although only just below the 5% probability level. No high birth weight protection was verifiable. It must be reemphasized that these analytical results reflected the narrow range of birth weights included in this study, making interpretation difficult and extrapolation to a wider range of infant weights probably inappropriate.

Babies determined to be small for gestational age (SGA) on the basis of weight distributions specific for each week of gestation were again found to be at substantively increased perinatal risk (Table 28-11). This was just as it had been in the decile-strata model (see Table 28-5). The long-term composite effect of SGA was negligible in magnitude and not statistically significant. It must be kept in mind that the effects of all labor and delivery risk variables were being taken into account simultaneously by the mechanism of the risk-score paradigm and, perhaps much more important, the population under study did not include infants weighing less than 2500g for this aspect of the analysis. Macrosomic infants for gestational age (LGA), here excluding those over 4000g, failed to show any significantly excess perinatal or composite outcome hazard.

Fetal sex was reconfirmed as an important variable in regard to adverse outcome. Compared with female infants, boys showed increases in poor perinatal and composite results by the incremental-strata model (Table 28-11) of the same order of magnitude and significance as revealed earlier by the decile model (see Table 28-5). The impact of the variable MALE had been so consistently demonstrated that it could not be denied.

Evaluation of the obstetrical attendant as a risk factor proceeded as before. We had previously noted a significantly protective perinatal effect in association with OBTYPE3 (care rendered by intern) in the decile-strata model (see Table 28-5). Some degree of protection was still present here in the form of a low odds ratio, but it was no longer statistically significant. This suggested that our earlier contention that the effect was perhaps the effect of preferential case selection may have been correct. Countering this, however, was the new observation that the long-term composite outcome results were now significantly adverse. It is conceivable, of course, that this latter finding also reflected some inherent difference in population make-up for cases managed by OBTYPE3, probably heavily concentrated with indigent clinic service gravidas whose adverse long-term risks have already been demonstrated (see above).

Very low maternal hematocrit, especially HCT1 and HCT2 (under 25%), had previously been shown to be associated with markedly excessive perinatal peril (see Table 28-5), persisting in the composite outcome results for HCT1 (under 20%). The perinatal effect was replicated in the incremental risk-strata model analysis (Table 28-11), but the composite effects were not except for a suggestive increase in odds ratios which proved statistically insignificant. We have seen that the diagnosis of anemia alone (DIS31) did not carry a comparable risk, although specifically diagnosed forms of anemia did, such as DIS32 (low serum iron) and DIS38 (sickle cell anemia).

In this regard, it is clear that the subset of cases with a diagnosis of anemia, often made solely on the basis of hematocrit levels of 30% or less, was heavily weighted with gravidas in the subgroup HCT3 (lowest hematocrit 25% to 29.9%) whose offspring appeared to have done rather well as evidenced by our findings here. The adverse influence of anemia in pregnancy could not be shown to be present unless the hematocrit was less than 25% (HCT2), and it was most intense when in was under 20% (HCT1).

The status of the chorioamniotic membranes, particularly as regards when and why they were ruptured, could not be determined to have either good or bad effects on the fetus and infant by the prior analysis involving the decile risk-scale model (see Table 28-5), except perhaps for some insignificant adverse effect found in conjunction with RUP2 (amniotomy for labor induction). When repeated using the incremental-strata model, the analysis showed that even this effect vanished (Table 28-11). The results of this approach failed to show any residual impact of this set of variables at all, every odds ratio falling quite close to unity.

Vaginal bleeding in early pregnancy (VAGBLD) was once again determined to be followed by increased rates of adverse perinatal outcomes (Table 28-11). Although the odds ratio for the incremental model was somewhat smaller than it had been for the decile model (see Table 28-5), it retained its level of statistical significance below 5% probability of chance occurrence.

Rh isoimmunization (RHSENS) also duplicated the bad perinatal effect that had been encountered before. Although it was now at a much lower magnitude of impact (OR = 3.65) than in the decile model (OR = 9.56), the level of statistical significance remained the same. The composite outcome effect, however, was no longer statistically significant even though still increased well above unity.

Pregnancy-induced hypertension showed the very same range of effects seen before. Significant adverse effect was limited to PIH1 (elevated diastolic blood pressure of 95 torr or more) for composite outcome only. It was noted that statistically insignificant increases were also found for perinatal results in PIH1 and for composite data in both PIH2 (combined diastolic hypertension and proteinuria) and PIH3 (proteinuria only).

Intercurrent Disorders

When the decile risk-score model had been applied to an examination of the impact of intercurrent illnesses and conditions, a large number (35 in total) were demonstrated to have significantly adverse effects (see Table 28-6). In all but ten, the significance probability level was only between 1% and 5%. This meant that closer scrutiny with a more reliable model—specifically one in which the model fit the data better—might reveal that some of these variables were not truly meaningful as risk factors. For purposes of clarifying this issue, the incremental risk-score model was, therefore, invoked.

The results did indeed show that many of the intercurrent disease variables now failed to yield statistically significant effects

(Table 28-12). Among these were 17 that had previously been shown to have been associated with significantly increased fetal and infant risk. Whereas the odds ratios for 13 of them remained high, they could not be shown to be significant when tested statistically; they included DIS1 (cardiac disease), DIS22 (pneumonia), DIS37 (anemia responsive to iron), DIS38 (sickle cell disease), DIS48 (other blood diseases), DIS54 (ketoacidosis), DIS76 (gonorrhea), DIS86 (hematuria), DIS87 (genitourinary tumor), DIS91 (incompetent cervix), DIS94 (uterine fibroids), DIS123 (hydramnios), and DIS140 (parasitic disease). In the rest, the odds ratios fell to near 1.00, indicating that any prior effect had been completely negated by the model. This implied that the

Table 28-12
Risk-Enhancing Effects of Predictor Factors on Incremental Risk-Score Groups: Intercurrent Disorders*

Risk Variable		Perinatal Outcome		Composite Outcome	
		RR	95%CL	RR	95%CL
DIS1	Organic heart disease	1.70	0.82-3.52	1.30	0.83-2.03
DIS7	Thrombophlebitis			0.79	0.19-3.21
DIS15	Active tuberculosis	6.37A	1.47-27.68	2.18	0.50-9.41
DIS21	Inactive tuberculosis	0.89	0.24-3.33	0.55a	0.24-1.26
DIS22	Pneumonia	2.32	0.78-6.87	0.74	0.27-2.01
DIS26	Bronchial asthma	1.02	0.39-2.67	0.66	0.37-1.18
DIS31	Anemia	1.08	0.83-1.43	1.01	0.88-1.17
DIS32	Low serum iron	2.95A	1.11-7.84	2.12A	1.12-4.03
DIS37	Response to iron therapy	1.36	0.96-1.94	1.13	0.94-1.36
DIS38	Sickle cell disease	2.14	0.86-5.33	1.30	0.74-2.29
DIS48	Other blood disease			2.07	0.66-6.47
DIS49	Diabetes mellitus	2.21	0.97-5.03	1.83A	1.08-3.12
DIS50	Hyperglycemia 200+ mg./dl.	2.43	0.87-6.84	2.02A	1.01-4.04
DIS51	Insulin therapy	2.71A	1.09-6.72	2.75C	1.51-5.01
DIS54	Ketoacidosis			2.42	0.46-12.82
DIS57	Hypothyroidism	1.28	0.40-4.12	0.80	0.36-1.80
DIS63	Hyperthyroidism	4.46A	1.18-16.86	1.76	0.54-5.71
DIS74	Syphilis	6.92A	1.49-32.18	3.48	0.62-19.67
DIS75	Chancre			6.01A	1.03-35.06
DIS76	Gonorrhea			1.54	0.71-3.38
DIS80	Glomerulonephritis	9.32C	2.80-31.00	3.58A	1.09-11.72
DIS81	Urinary tract infection	1.04	0.76-1.43	1.01	0.86-1.19
DIS86	Hematuria	1.64	0.85-3.15	1.14	0.77-1.70
DIS87	GU tumor			5.13	0.95-27.60
DIS91	Incompetent cervix			1.70	0.39-7.43
DIS94	Leiomyoma uteri	1.36	0.52-3.58	1.09	0.58-2.07
DIS98	Convulsive disorder	1.58	0.48-5.23	1.95A	1.03-3.69
DIS99	Convulsion in pregnancy	2.53	0.66-9.67	2.57A	1.28-5.15
DIS100	Mental retardation	4.36A	1.70-11.18	6.86F	3.89-12.09
DIS103	Neurological disorder	2.81A	1.08-7.29	2.42C	1.41-4.17
DIS107	Cholecystitis	4.33A	1.17-16.05	1.68	0.44-6.37
DIS111	Colitis, ileitis	5.40A	1.38-21.14	5.66D	2.10-15.26
DIS120	Hyperemesis gravidarum	0.60	0.20-1.74	0.99	0.57-1.69
DIS123	Hydramnios	1.49	0.74-3.03	1.38	0.89-2.12
DIS124	First trimester bleeding	0.61b	0.39-0.98	0.87	0.71-1.07
DIS125	Second trimester bleeding	0.91	0.55-1.50	1.07	0.84-1.37
DIS126	Third trimester bleeding	1.09	0.78-1.53	1.13	0.95-1.35
DIS128	Hemorrhagic shock	6.56A	1.73-24.84	2.23	0.61-8.19
DIS130	Supine hypotension	3.26A	1.13-9.41	2.14	0.87-5.29
DIS140	Parasitic disease	2.21	0.70-7.03	0.92	0.31-2.69
SDIS5	Venereal diseases	1.47	0.94-2.28	1.42B	1.12-1.81

* See footnotes in Tables 28-6 for referent variables and Table 28-1 for probability code.

impact seen before for these variables had probably been related to some concurrent labor and delivery effect now corrected for by the risk-scoring system.

In two of these variables, not only had the antecedent adverse effect been erased, but an apparently protective one had unexpectedly replaced it. For DIS21 (inactive tuberculosis), for example, there was no longer any documentable adverse perinatal effect, but now there was a newly significant beneficial composite outcome effect (OR = 0.55) and a further suggestion of comparable protection (OR = 0.89) in regard to perinatal outcome (the latter not statistically significant). For DIS124 (first trimester bleeding), the earlier adverse perinatal effect was gone and a significantly protective one (OR = 0.61) was now present in its place, with a matching low but insignificant odds ratio (OR = 0.87) in the composite outcome data. These findings ran directly counter to those seen with the variable VAGBLD (see above) which showed persistently significant adverse perinatal effects. Since DIS124 was based on summary coding after delivery whereas VAGBLD was derived from interim prenatal history reports more concurrent with the event, the latter was more likely to be reliable. Given the questionable validity of DIS124, therefore, its discrepant results can probably be discounted in favor of those for VAGBLD (see Table 28-11).

Complete concurrence of analytical results, verifying both perinatal and composite outcome effects, was forthcoming for nine of these variables, namely DIS32 (low serum iron), DIS49 (diabetes mellitus), DIS50 (hyperglycemia over 200 mg/dL), DIS51 (insulin-requiring diabetes), DIS75 (chancre, but only composite outcome data were available for confirmation), DIS80 (glomerulonephritis), DIS100 (maternal mental retardation), DIS103 (neurologic disorder), and DIS111 (colitis-ileitis). Although the magnitude of the odds ratios fell somewhat in all but two of these (specifically, it did not decline in DIS100 and DIS103), they nonetheless remained signif-

icantly elevated and achieved about the same level of statistical probability as before.

Partial confirmation was obtained in nine others. In six of these, the perinatal effects were verified, but the composite outcome impact was not; these were DIS15 (active tuberculosis), DIS63 (hyperthyroidism), DIS74 (syphilis), DIS107 (cholecystitis), DIS128 (hemorrhagic shock), and DIS130 (supine hypotension). The reverse was the case (that is, only the composite outcome effect was verified) in the other three: DIS98 (convulsive disorder), DIS99 (seizure in pregnancy), and SDIS5 (venereal diseases). It should be stressed that in all nine, however, the odds ratios were still quite high even though they were not statistically significant.

For completeness and symmetry in reporting these data, we note that there were six disease variables, all of which had been considered potentially significant in prior exploratory studies but which had failed to be identified as such by the decile risk-score model, that were found to have no discernible impact on the fetus and infant by this incremental model. These were DIS7 (thrombophlebitis), DIS31 (anemia, see HCT above), DIS81 (urinary tract infection), DIS120 (hyperemesis gravidarum), and DIS125 and DIS126 (second and third trimester bleeding).

Within-Group Risk-Score Effects of Predictor Variables

All the foregoing material on the analytical results of the numerous applications of the risk-score paradigm had concentrated exclusively on the overall effects of the 369 predictor variables under surveillance without providing any of the details as to within-group risk effects—that is, as regards the impact of the factor being studied on the several delineated risk-score subsets of cases. The only exception was the variable of parity. The component effects of this variable, which had yielded no discernible overall effect, were displayed

(Tables 28-3 and 28-9) to show its very good homogeneity for composite outcome and interesting combination of counterbalancing high-end adverse and low-end protective perinatal effects. It was felt that similar data, if made available here, might help clarify some of the significant effects discussed above. For the 272 factors offering no objectively demonstrable overall adverse or beneficial impact, this exercise was deemed unnecessary because where statistically significant within-group effects were encountered among them, they tended to be isolated occurrences, probably specious in nature, arising as a chance event.

Parenthetically, it is necessary to point out that we should have expected 166 such chance developments by the incremental-strata model because we had accepted a probability level of 5% for statistical significance in a series of 3321 separate subgroup analyses involving 369 variables stratified into five perinatal and four composite risk-score strata. At the 1% probability level, only 33 chance associations would have appeared. By the decile-strata model, 443 chance associations could have been expected at the 5% level and 89 at 1% based on analyses of 12 risk-score subsets of perinatal and 12 of composite outcomes for the 369 variables, or 8856 separate examinations.

Detailed data for the 97 variables determined to deviate significantly from the refmined to deviate significantly from the referent in their overall fetal and infant effects (by Mantel-Haenszel chi-square testing) will, therefore, be dealt with here. Needless to say, many more of the within-group subset data were found to be significant. Most of the specious ones had been discounted by the summary testing for the significance of all subgroup data combined. Among the 97 predictor variables ultimately identified as significant by this means, chance association should have been uncovered in only 16 at the 5% level and three at 1% for 312 (78 x 4) composite outcome strata groups and 11 and two, respectively, for 225 (45 x 5) perinatal outcome groups. The actual numbers encountered were 96 and 53 for the composite data and 52 and 25 for the perinatal data.

Our purpose was to provide sufficient details of these variables to show whether the adverse or beneficial effects disclosed by the antecedent analyses were uniform across the risk-score scale (that is, independent of the labor and delivery risk effects) or were instead concentrated at the high (or low) end of the risk-score range (and were thus somehow differentially complementary or were modifiers of the labor-delivery risk). To this end, the odds ratios and associated probability levels, as determined for each of the incremental risk substrata, were assessed for all predictor factors found to have had significant residual overall impact on outcome. The data pertaining to 78 variables determined to have relevant effects on composite infant outcome results are shown in Table 28-13 and those for the 45 with documentable perinatal effects in Table 28-14. Since 26 of these variables appear in both tabulations, it follows that 52 predictor variables had a composite effect only and 19 a perinatal effect only. The 97 predictor variables constituted 26.3% of the total number surveyed.

Demographic Variables

In most cases, the within-group effects were more or less uniformly distributed over the risk-score spectrum, indicating that the influence of the predictor variables was pervasive and probably unrelated to the subsequent intrapartum or delivery complications, events, or interventions. This uniform consistency, for example, was seen for INST15 and INST60 in the composite outcome analyses and to a lesser degree for INST31 and INST71. General overall homogeneity with isolated discrepancies (always insignificant) was also found for some, such as INST37, INST45, and INST55. These observations pertaining to the institutions at which the infants were born were confirmed in the perinatal data. The impact of institutional factors could

Table 28-13
Details of Composite Impact of Significant Intrinsic Variables*

Risk Variable		Risk-Score Stratum			
		Lowest	Low	High	Highest
INST15	Hospital 15	2.03	1.93E	2.08	5.25A
INST31	Hospital 31	3.10	1.45A	1.02	1.75
INST37	Hospital 37	0.86	1.95F	1.89A	2.45
INST45	Hospital 45	1.63	1.83F	1.83	0.88
INST55	Hospital 55	1.41	1.33A	1.27	0.75
INST60	Hospital 60	3.36D	2.86F	1.76	5.25A
INST71	Hospital 71	1.02	2.21F	2.15	---
AGE1	Maternal age under 20 yr.	1.60A	1.29C	0.60A	1.02
AGE4	Maternal age 30-34 yr.	1.45	1.26A	0.87	2.27
AGE6	Maternal age under 18 yr.	1.79A	1.41D	0.71	0.78
AGE7	Maternal age under 16 yr.	1.50	1.49B	0.74	0.91
STATUS1	Clinic service patient	1.29	1.53A	1.31	1.03
MARIT1	Single status	1.19	1.19A	1.29	1.01
MARIT6	Separated	1.64	1.16	2.15A	5.17
RACE2	Black	1.55A	1.09	1.18	1.73
RELIG2	Catholic	0.89	0.80c	0.75	0.85
RELIG3	Jewish	0.59	0.47d	0.11c	0.23
ORIGIN1	Place of birth: NY, NJ, PA	1.05	0.80a	0.68	0.78
ORIGIN2	MD to FL	1.05	1.26A	1.54	1.04
ORIGIN4	AR, LA, OK, TX	3.64D	1.50C	1.94	3.33
ORIGIN8	WA, OR, CA	0.42	1.84E	1.15	0.83
ORIGIN10	Puerto Rico	1.01	0.63C	0.62	1.88
ORIGIN15	Europe	0.78	0.52A	0.71	---
GRAV4	Gravida 4	0.39	1.37B	1.71	0.60
PPREM1	Prior premature birth	0.68	1.34C	2.21C	2.35
PPMR1	Prior perinatal death	0.34	1.33A	1.14	1.06
HGT2	Maternal height < 60 in.	1.43	1.23	1.00	2.13
POND2	Ponderal index obese	1.45	1.15	1.37	2.71A
SMOKE3	Smokes > 30 per day	0.68	1.66A	1.16	---
SES1	Socioeconomic index < 15	2.73A	1.47B	2.40A	0.64
SES2	Socioeconomic index 15-24	1.84	1.21	2.47B	0.86
SES3	Socioeconomic index 25-34	1.09	1.31B	1.32	1.22
SES8	Socioeconomic index 75-84	0.78	0.50e	1.14	0.00
SES9	Socioeconomic index 85+	0.20c	0.44e	0.39	0.00
INCOME1	Per capita income < $800/yr.	1.04	1.35C	0.69	1.04
INCOME4	Per capita income $2250-2999	0.66	0.86	0.45A	1.25
FAMINC2	Family income < $2000/yr.	1.67	1.37A	1.25	0.96
FAMINC6	Family income $8000-9999 yr.	0.92	0.73	0.13A	0.86
FAMINC7	Family income $10,000+ yr.	0.69	0.58A	0.44	0.86
HOUSE1	Housing density 1.0+ person/room	1.37	1.18A	1.00	1.78
EDUC1	Education 7 yr. or less	2.43B	1.40C	1.38	2.85
EDUC2	Education 8 yr.	0.70	1.28A	1.62	3.67
EDUC3	Education 9-11 yr.	1.30	1.16A	1.26	1.00
EDUC5	Education 13-15 yr.	0.71	0.53e	1.11	0.00
EDUC6	Education 16+ yr.	0.48	0.27f	0.14a	1.22
WORKG1	Gravida never worked	1.75A	1.45E	0.97	1.50
WORKG2	Gravida white collar worker	0.32f	0.55f	0.72	2.86
WORKF3	Father of baby student	0.00b	0.74	0.00a	0.00
WORKF4	Father of baby unemployed	0.93	1.52F	0.83	0.66
WORKF5	Father of baby absent	2.28B	1.43F	1.97C	3.29A
OCCUPF3	Father of baby blue collar worker	1.64A	1.72F	1.72A	5.00A
GREG5	Registered at 24-27.9 wk.	0.82	1.34A	0.92	1.40
GREG6	Registered at 28-31.9 wk.	1.93	1.33A	1.14	4.90
GREG8	Registered at 36+ wk.	1.92	1.28	1.10	1.17
TRIMEST2	Registered in second trimester	0.83	1.31C	1.12	0.89
TRIMEST3	Registered in third trimester	1.49	1.41D	1.07	1.26

VISIT1	Prenatal visits < 7	1.93B	1.22C	1.05	1.49
GDEL1	Delivered at < 34 wk.	1.43	1.49A	1.75	---
GDEL2	Delivered at < 36 wk.	1.35	1.58E	2.08A	1.74
GDEL3	Delivered at < 38 wk.	1.43	1.43F	1.73A	1.16
GDEL5	Delivered at > 42 wk.	1.39	1.20	1.29	0.97
BW2	Birth weight 2850-2999 g.	1.76	1.23A	1.51	0.40
BW3	Birth weight 3000-3249 g.	0.99	1.24A	1.10	0.60
MALE	Male infant	1.48	1.38F	1.65B	1.56
OBTYPE3	Intern in attendance	1.62	1.47	1.02	0.50
PIH1	Diastolic hypertension only	2.07	1.31	2.64A	0.84
DIS21	Inactive tuberculosis	0.00	0.33a	1.90	---
DIS32	Low serum iron	0.00	2.24B	0.94	---
DIS49	Diabetes mellitus	2.86	1.94A	1.41	3.33
DIS50	Hyperglycemia 200+ mg./dl.	0.00	1.63	2.10	3.33
DIS51	Insulin therapy	0.00	4.37F	1.34	3.33
DIS75	Chancre	2.58	0.00	---	---
DIS80	Glomerulonephritis	8.61A	2.85	---	---
DIS98	Convulsive disorder	0.00	2.20B	0.75	---
DIS99	Convulsion in pregnancy	0.00	2.79C	0.00	---
DIS100	Mental retardation	8.61A	7.44F	0.00	2.14
DIS103	Neurological disorder	0.00	2.44D	3.83A	---
DIS111	Colitis, ileitis	0.00	6.35F	---	---
SDIS5	Venereal diseases	0.93	1.39B	2.34A	0.15a

* Expansion of odds ratio data from those variables found statistically significant in Tables 28-7 through 28-12 by 4 risk-score groupings for composite outcomes. Table consists of odds ratio estimates of relative risk. Omissions indicate cells with frequency of cases too small to compute odds ratio. See Table 28-1 for probability code.

thus be shown to be real—that is, they were not likely to be just chance occurrences.

Young maternal age, especially for teenagers, had been shown to have an unfavorable effect on offspring. Contrary to the homogeneous effect for the institutional variables, the stratified incremental risk-score data for AGE6 (maternal age under 18 years) and AGE7 (under 16 years) showed their effects to be concentrated at the low-risk end and middle of the risk-score range with some unexpected protective benefit at the high end for composite outcome results. Although not replicated precisely in the perinatal data, similar discrepancies were suggested by isolated findings of protective effects in the high (but not highest) risk-score subset.

These findings could be interpreted to signify a documentable adverse effect of AGE6 and AGE7 manifested most overtly among offspring of teenagers who did not subsequently develop labor and delivery problems. The effect was not seen in those who did have high-risk labor and delivery because the risk of the latter, which was being accounted for by the risk-score model, was not enhanced or compounded by the age effect. Alternatively (and clinically less likely to be correct), the age risk was somehow recognized and compensated for in the care rendered so as to improve outcome when high-risk labor and delivery problems arose.

Among the other demographic variables, STATUS1 (clinic service patient) showed relative homogeneity for composite outcome, approaching unity at the high end. MARIT1 (single status) did likewise, but was still more consistently adverse without exception for all perinatal subset data. MARIT5 (divorced) revealed pervasive effects except for some isolated insignificant low-end protection. MARIT6 (separated) was strongly and consistently deleterious in the composite outcome analyses.

RACE2 (black) was found to have a consistent effect across the entire range of the risk-score scale for both composite and perinatal outcomes. Unwavering protective effects were disclosed among the several risk-score subgroups for RELIG2 (Roman Catholic) and RELIG3 (other religion,

Table 28-14
Details of Perinatal Outcome Impact of Significant Predictor Variables*

Risk Variable		Risk-Score Stratum				
		Lowest	Low	Moderate	High	Highest
INST55	Hospital 55	2.51	1.53	3.32A	0.73	4.00
INST60	Hospital 60	4.38A	1.19	1.65	2.19	0.00
INST71	Hospital 71	1.18	1.66	2.48	2.50	---
AGE6	Maternal age under 18 yr.	1.58	1.50A	1.49	0.63	3.43
AGE7	Maternal age under 16 yr.	0.00	2.09A	2.54A	0.55	1.14
MARIT1	Single status	1.36	1.27	1.50	1.40	1.77
MARIT5	Divorced	0.00	2.27A	1.60	13.04C	---
RACE2	Black	2.65A	1.07	2.38B	1.21	2.32
PPREM1	Prior premature birth	1.74	1.23	2.17A	2.58A	1.39
PPMR3	Three prior deaths	0.00	0.00	10.64A	5.04	---
PRIOR3	Last died in day 2-6	0.00	3.72A	0.00	2.00	---
HGT2	Maternal height < 60 in.	0.00	2.11C	0.99	1.38	1.39
PELV2	Pelvis contracted	0.00	2.79B	0.63	0.00	1.73
SES3	Socioeconomic index 25-34	0.67	2.27C	0.75	1.20	1.13
SES4	Socioeconomic index 35-44	1.73	1.93B	1.33	1.71	0.94
EDUC5	Education 13-15 yr.	0.56	0.53a	0.28	1.33	0.00
WORKG2	Gravida white collar worker	0.46	0.54b	0.94	0.72	1.25
WORKF5	Father of baby absent	1.85	1.27	2.59C	1.96	7.44B
OCCUPF3	Father of baby blue collar worker	1.42	1.18	1.34	6.65C	1.77
GDEL1	Delivered in < 34 wk.	0.00	3.02D	2.90	8.29A	---
GDEL2	Delivered < 36 wk.	0.86	2.70F	4.36D	3.11	0.00
GDEL3	Delivered < 38 wk.	1.41	2.08E	1.96	2.66A	0.91
GDEL4	Delivered > 41 wk.	0.63	1.83D	1.88A	1.01	1.52
GDEL5	Delivered > 42 wk.	0.45	1.94C	2.07A	0.86	1.14
GDEL6	Delivered > 43 wk.	0.79	1.95B	2.13	1.28	0.23
SGA	Small for gestational age	5.66F	0.90	1.41	3.02A	0.00
MALE	Male infant	1.64	1.94F	1.36	1.37	0.68
HCT1	Lowest hematocrit < 20%	0.00	4.39A	19.11C	---	---
HCT2	Lowest hematocrit 20-24.9%	0.00	1.97	6.37C	0.65	0.00
VAGBLD	First trimester bleeding	0.99	1.52	1.31	1.29	2.16
RHSENS	Rh isoimmunization	0.00	2.14	3.90	5.63A	---
DIS15	Active tuberculosis	0.00	0.00	0.00	3.63A	---
DIS32	Low serum iron	0.00	3.30A	0.00	---	---
DIS51	Insulin therapy	0.00	4.91B	0.00	1.83	---
DIS63	Hyperthyroidism	0.00	3.42	---	---	1.81
DIS74	Syphilis	---	0.00	0.00	3.63A	---
DIS80	Glomerulonephritis	0.00	12.92F	---	---	---
DIS100	Mental retardation	0.00	4.44C	0.00	3.61	1.84
DIS103	Neurological disorder	0.00	2.50	0.00	7.43B	---
DIS107	Cholecystitis	28.03F	0.00	0.00	0.00	---
DIS111	Colitis, ileitis	0.00	4.67A	0.00	---	---
DIS124	First trimester bleeding	0.00	0.54a	0.96	0.60	0.53
DIS128	Hemorrhagic shock	0.00	0.00	0.00	7.38A	1.81
DIS130	Supine hypotension	0.00	3.97A	0.00	0.00	1.88

* Expansion of odds ratio data for statistically significant factors in Tables 28-7 through 28-12 by 5 risk-score groupings for perinatal outcome. See Table 28-1 for probability code.

449

mostly Jewish), clearly verifying their apparent benefit to fetus and infant.

The mother's place of birth was a uniformly adverse composite outcome variable only for ORIGIN4 (AR to TX) and to a lesser degree for ORIGIN2 (MD to FL). It was consistently protective only for ORIGIN15 (Europe). The presence of minor contradictory subset discrepancies did not appear to negate the significantly beneficial overall effect of ORIGIN1 (NY to PA). However, mounting divergence of within-group results at both ends of the risk-score range for ORIGIN8 (WA to CA) and ORIGIN10 (Puerto Rico) placed the findings for these variables (adverse for ORIGIN8 and beneficial for ORIGIN10) in serious doubt.

Past Obstetrical Background

The overall adverse effect that had surfaced earlier for GRAV4 (Gravida 4) in regard to composite outcome effects on infants could now be questioned on the basis of poor consistency of within-group results (Table 28-13). The significantly adverse effect in the low-risk subset was clearly counterbalanced by the apparent protection found at both extreme ends of the risk-score spectrum. It was worth noting that this variable was the only one in the entire group of factors relating to gravidity to show any effect and that its effect was neither consistent with nor mirrored any discernible trend with advancing gravidity. Given the heterogeneity of effect, it was very likely, therefore, that the findings for GRAV4 were specious.

PPREM1 (premature delivery in a prior pregnancy) showed strong and consistent within-group adverse effects over the entire range of risk score for perinatal outcome (Table 28-14) and only one isolated discrepant low-end subset protective effect for composite outcome data (Table 28-13). A somewhat less homogeneous pattern of composite outcome effects was seen with PPMR1 (one prior perinatal mortality), the subset effects ranging from moderately adverse (low risk score) to near unity (high end) to protective (in the lowest risk-score group).

Even greater heterogeneity existed in the perinatal data for PPMR3 (three prior perinatal deaths) with very adverse impact in moderate and high risk-score subgroups and no discernible adverse effect in those with low and lowest risk scores (Table 28-14). Despite these nonuniform effects, neither PPMR1 nor PPMR3 appeared to represent adverse predictor factors on the basis of these observations.

PRIOR3 (last prior infant a neonatal death in days 2-6) had been associated with significantly excess perinatal deaths overall in the index pregnancy. The effect was concentrated here in cases with low-risk scores and to a lesser extent high risk scores as well; lowest and moderate scores were paradoxically protective, although not significantly so. Nonetheless, this factor seemed to serve as a predictor variable of bad outcome.

Physical Characteristics

Short maternal stature HGT2 (under 60 in) was associated with an overall adverse composite and perinatal effect, although it did not show complete consistency among the several risk-score groups. For perinatal data (Table 28-14), the strongest adverse effect appeared in the low risk-score group and there were some additional insignificant increases in odds ratios for the high and highest subsets. The moderate-risk group showed neither good nor bad effect with an odds ratio of unity. Contrastingly, offspring of gravidas with lowest risk did uniformly well.

Composite outcome results for HGT2 (Table 28-13) were a good deal more supportive across the range of risk scores, although even here there was an odds ratio of 1.00 for the high-risk subset (but a substantially increased ratio for those with highest risk scores). Moreover, none of the subgroup results for composite outcome data proved statistically significant in their own right. Notwithstanding, the overview suggested that HGT2 was indeed probably an adverse risk factor.

POND2 (obese) showed entirely consistent adverse effects across the board for composite outcome subgroup results (Table 28-13). In addition, its presence as a predictor risk variable appeared to enhance the effect of labor and delivery risk considerably. This was seen by the increasing odds ratio with increasing risk score, especially notable in the highest risk-score group results.

This set of findings lent itself to interpretation as follows: POND2 placed the infant at increased hazard regardless of subsequent intrapartum risk. It further enhanced the peril of any labor and delivery risk that might subsequently arise. It was also conceivable, but could not be ascertained from these analyses, that POND2 might actually have increased the possibility that such labor and delivery risk problems would develop.

SMOKE3 (more than 30 cigarettes per day) showed adverse composite outcome effects in both midrange groups with low and high risk scores plus an isolated contradictory protective effect in the lowest risk group (Table 28-13). Unfortunately, because there were insufficient numbers of cases in the highest risk group to permit analysis, the issue could not be resolved satisfactorily. The conflicting results allowed us merely to conclude that there was probably an adverse effect from SMOKE3, but it needed confirmation.

Gravidas who were clinically deemed to have a contracted pelvis (PELV2) were found to show quite erratic perinatal subgroup data (Table 28-14). The very strong adverse odds ratio of the low risk-score group and less intense bad effect of the highest risk set was counterbalanced by somewhat apparently protective effects in all three of the other risk-score groups. This factor may, therefore, have a potentially deleterious impact on offspring in the overview.

Socioeconomic Factors

The socioeconomic index variables had previously been shown to be adverse at the low end of the index scale and protective at the high end, especially for composite outcome. Within-group results tended to be quite supportive of this trend. Complete concurrence across all subsets was found in the composite outcome data for SES3 and SES9 (Table 28-13) and nearly complete (as shown by a single, isolated, opposite but insignificant effect) for SES1, SES2, and SES8. In the perinatal data (Table 28-14), SES4 also showed almost perfect agreement. Only SES3 failed to meet the test of consistency. (Note that the formal statistical test had demonstrated satisfactory goodness-of-fit.) One subset showed a strong adverse effect, two were slightly deleterious, and two others rather beneficial. Even if we were to discount the validity of SES3, it would still leave the socioeconomic index variable as a very reliable predictor of risk.

The per capita income variables at either extreme of the income range had been shown to have significant effects on offspring inversely related to the amount earned. When examined by stratification of risk score, however, INCOME1 (less than $800 per person per annum) was shown to yield a significantly adverse effect only in one subset (low risk), essentially no effect in two others, and a protective effect in the fourth. INCOME4 ($2250-2999 per annum) was protective throughout except for a single discrepant finding in the highest risk-score group, whereas INCOME5 ($3000+) demonstrated perfect consistency in its strongly beneficial impact. The deleterious effect of low per capita income could not be upheld, but the protection afforded by high income was quite clearly demonstrated.

The family income variables FAMINC6 and FAMINC7 ($8000+ per year) showed the same very substantive confirmation of benefit to offspring with clear-cut evidence of homogeneity in all risk-score subsets without exception. Low family income, FAMINC2 (less than $2000 per year), was adverse in all risk-score groups except the highest in which the odds ratio approached unity. Thus, even though low per capita income had an inconsistent effect, low gross family income was obviously a deleterious risk factor. High housing density, HOUSE1 (1.0+ person per room), was also confirmed as an adverse variable, all but one risk subgroup showing bad results and the exception presenting with an odds ratio of 1.00.

The duration of maternal education had been shown to exhibit a marked inverse relationship to outcome. Within-group composite outcome data provided complete confirmation only for EDUC1 (less than seven years of education) with every subgroup showing clear adverse effects. Nearly complete verification was found for all the other EDUC variables. In none was there more than just a single risk-score subgroup with an odds ratio running counter to the general overall tenor of the effect exhibited by this variable. The within-group data, therefore, were very supportive throughout.

The effect of maternal work status was confirmed in regard to both composite and perinatal outcome results. WORKG1 (gravida never worked) had fairly consistent adverse effects among the several incremental risk-score groups (except for one odds ratio which fell close to unity) and WORKG2 (white collar worker) was almost uniformly protective (except in the highest risk group which was adverse for both perinatal and composite data).

There was perfect consistency across all risk strata for the variable WORKF3 (father of baby a student), strong protective composite outcome effects being found throughout WORKF5 (father of baby absent) was equally uniform in its strongly adverse composite and perinatal effects. This last variable also showed a trend toward increasing intensity in association with higher risk scores. OCCUPF3 (father of baby blue-collar worker) carried comparable uniformity of seriously adverse effects in all risk subgroups, again for both perinatal and composite results, and with an

apparent trend toward aggravation of effect with increasing risk score.

Antepartum Factors

Advanced gestational age at the time the gravida registered for antepartum care had been demonstrated to be significantly associated with adverse outcomes, especially at and beyond 24 weeks. The risk-score strata for GREG5 (registration at 24-27.9 weeks) for composite outcome were divided in their support of this observation, although there was an overall trend toward deleterious effect (Table 28-13). This relationship was further validated by the findings encountered for TRIMEST2 (registration in the second trimester).

Registration later in pregnancy, moreover, was also confirmatory as an adverse factor. Both GREG6 (28-31.9 weeks) and GREG8 (36+ weeks) showed uniformly increased odds ratios for all the risk-score subgroups. TRIMEST3 (registration in the third trimester) also yielded the same degree of homogeneity. Of interest in regard to the impact of these variables was the observation that the effect on the risk subgroups appeared to be independent of the risk score—that is, the hazard imposed on the fetus did not increase at higher scores.

This could be interpreted to mean that the peril of late registration was manifest through its direct effect (an unlikely conclusion) or through the intermedium of high-risk antepartum disorders (perhaps untreated or treated too late to avert fetal effects) rather than intrapartum problems. Except for GREG6, which did show a substantially increased odds ratio in the highest composite outcome risk-score subset (4.90), late registration did not appear to exaggerate the risk of labor-delivery factors as already accounted for by the risk-score model.

The contention that inadequate antepartum care carried serious risk was further supported by the finding of consistently bad results for cases with few prenatal visits, namely VISIT1 (fewer than seven visits).

Cases exhibiting this variable showed uniformly adverse outcomes without regard for risk-score category, again verifying the independence of this factor from labor-delivery risk.

Delivery before and after term had been associated with adverse outcomes when examined by the incremental risk-score model. Within-group results tended to be quite confirmatory for both composite and perinatal data analyses. Complete consistency across risk-score groups was found for all but one of the GDEL variables in regard to composite outcome (Table 28-13) and the exception, GDEL5 (delivery beyond 42 weeks), was almost entirely uniform with bad effects in three risk-score subgroups and an odds ratio near unity in the fourth.

For perinatal results (Table 28-14), only GDEL3 (delivery prior to 38 weeks) was homogeneously adverse. There was also close consistency in all subsets but one in association with GDEL1 (under 34 weeks) and GDEL4 (over 41 weeks). Despite their overall statistical homogeneity as attested to by analysis for goodness-of-fit, overtly discrepant results were found for GDEL2 (under 36 weeks), GDEL5 (beyond 42 weeks), and GDEL6 (beyond 43 weeks).

These last observations probed the pervasiveness of the adverse effects of postterm delivery. As previously discussed when we considered why GDEL7 (beyond 44 weeks) did not follow the same trend as other postdate pregnancies (see above), it was felt likely that these cases were "contaminated" with many in which dating of pregnancy duration was in error. Dilution of the at-risk postterm population by such gravidas, who were probably at term instead, weakened any real adverse impact and made it difficult to demonstrate such effect definitively.

Although this aspect of these investigations had been limited to a population of gravidas who delivered infants weighing 2500-4000g, the risk-score model had shown some significant adverse composite outcome effects for two birth weight groups. Review of the within-group results (Table 28-13) showed one of these, BW3 (3000-3249g), to have inconsistent odds ratios, two of the risk strata showing adverse effect, one no effect, and one protection. This heterogeneity suggested that the effect of the variable was not likely to be reliable. BW2 (2850-2999g) did show more uniformity, all but one of the risk-score subcategories presenting an adverse odds ratio; however, the ratio for the highest-risk group was quite protective. With this single exception, the birth weight effects on offspring were thus felt to be negligible, undoubtedly on the basis of the constraints imposed on case selection.

Male infants had regularly been shown to do worse than females. Display of the results for all the incremental risk-score subsets of the factor MALE verified this effect without exception in the composite outcome data (Table 28-13). The consistency in regard to magnitude of effect across the risk-score scale was also impressive. That the odds ratios fell narrowly between 1.38 and 1.65, with no indication of a trend related to increasing risk, implied that the effect of this factor was entirely independent of the labor-delivery risk inherent in the risk-scoring system. For perinatal outcome (Table 28-14), similar consistency was encountered except for the unexpected (insignificant and perhaps specious) protection found in the highest risk-score group.

Among the variables dealing with the obstetrical attendant providing care to the gravida, only OBTYPE3 (intern) had previously surfaced as likely to be significantly relevant insofar as adverse composite outcome was concerned. When examined for within-group effects (Table 28-13), it was clear that no risk-score subgroup yielded an odds ratio which proved significant in itself. Moreover, only two of the strata (both low risk) showed adverse effects; the third was neutral at unity and the last protective. The findings made it unlikely that this variable did indeed have any meaningful impact on offspring.

Very low maternal hematocrit in pregnancy had been demonstrated to give rise to unfavorable perinatal results. The within-group data for HCT1 (less than 20%), although not perfectly consistent, showed very strong confirmation in cases with low and moderate risk scores (Table 28-14); inadequate numbers prevented analysis of the higher score groups and those with lowest risk showed a protective effect. HCT2 (20%-24.9%) showed a similar trend, but with some degree of inconsistency. Again, there was clear adverse impact with low and moderate risk scores, but protection was found in all remaining categories of risk. These data suggested an adverse effect from low hematocrit manifested in inverse relation to the lowest level reached.

The adverse perinatal effects of both VAGBLD (early pregnancy bleeding) and RHSENS (Rh isoimmunization) were also confirmed by the nearly complete concurrence among the risk-score subgroups (Table 28-14). Uniformly increased odds ratios were encountered in all the subsets for VAGBLD except that for patients at lowest risk in whom the effect was neither good nor bad (OR = 0.99). For RHSENS, strongly unfavorable effects were seen rising progressively with increasing risk score. However, there were inadequate numbers in the highest risk-score group to permit meaningful analysis. Moreover, there was an unexpected protective effect in the group at lowest risk. PIH1 (diastolic hypertension), which had been associated with significantly increased overall untoward composite outcome effects, was confirmed to have such adverse impact across the range of risk scores (Table 28-13), except for the single spurious finding of protection (not statistically significant) at the highest risk levels.

Intercurrent Disorders

All 20 of the disease states verified as significant predictor variables by the incremental risk-score paradigm were examined for within-group concurrence, including seven with composite outcome effects only, seven with perinatal effects only, and six

with both. Eight showed clear-cut consistency across the range of risk-score groups in all or nearly all the subsets, namely DIS49 (diabetes mellitus), DIS50 (hyperglycemia), DIS51 (insulin therapy), DIS63 (hyperthyroidism), DIS80 (glomerulonephritis), DIS100 (mental retardation), DIS103 (neurologic disorder), and DIS124 (first trimester bleeding). The significantly protective effects of DIS124 contradicted those of VAGBLD, as previously noted; we have discussed a possible explanation for this discrepancy (see above).

In addition, there were 12 variables for which the within-group data did not uniformly support the antecedent effects derived for them from the overall assessment by the risk-score model. These factors included DIS15 (active tuberculosis), DIS21 (inactive tuberculosis), DIS32 (low serum iron, see HCT, above), DIS74 (syphilis), DIS75 (chancre), DIS98 (convulsive disorder), DIS99 (convulsion in pregnancy), DIS107 (cholecystitis), DIS111 (colitis-ileitis), DIS128 (hemorrhagic shock), DIS130 (supine hypotension), and SDIS5 (venereal diseases). Nonetheless, in all but one (DIS21), there were isolated risk-strata subgroup results which proved to be statistically significant.

DIS98 (convulsive disorder), for example, was found to be adverse for composite outcome in one subgroup and protective in two, but the deleterious effect was so strong (OR = 2.20, p = .0091) as to justify retaining it as probably significant. The same rationale applied to DIS99 (convulsion in pregnancy), where the single adverse risk-group impact was even more intense (OR = 2.79, p = .0042). It was appropriate for DIS111 (colitis-ileitis) as well, the very high odds ratio (6.35) was very strongly significant by statistical testing. For DIS107 (cholecystitis), both the magnitude and the significance of the odds ratio for perinatal outcome were impressive (OR = 28.03, p = 3.7×10^{-6}), even though the adverse impact could only be identified in a single risk-score group. These data suggested that the risk variables did indeed have some independent adverse impact on the fetus and infant.

CHAPTER 29

Gravida-at-
Risk

Summary

Attributable risk was quantitated in regard to perinatal and composite outcomes for all identified risk variables. Labor and delivery factors were considered separately from intrinsic factors, the former for their possible impact on obstetrical practices and the latter for their importance as predictor characteristics for identifying the gravida whose fetus is most likely to be at greatest risk of having a bad outcome. The constellation of attributes that describe the gravida-at-risk was detailed with specific reference to demographic features, past obstetrical history, physical factors, socioeconomic status, antepartum course, and intercurrent disorders.

Having evolved data to identify those labor-delivery factors that were significantly associated with adverse fetal and infant outcome and those prelabor conditions and characteristics that served to predict poor results, we were at last in a position to describe the gravida-at-risk. At the same time, it was felt necessary and feasible to quantitate the risk to offspring in more clinically meaningful terms than heretofore.

Attributable Risk

To this end, the attributable risk was determined for each of the relevant variables. The concept of attributable risk refers simplistically to that portion of the frequency of the bad outcome associated with a given factor which can be directly or indirectly attributed to the presence of that factor. In other words, attributable risk is the percentage of badness explained by exposure to a risk factor. This does not necessarily mean there is a direct or indirect causal connection, but there is nonetheless an implication of such. Actual proof of causation would demand a more formal demonstration of some direct mechanism of action. This often requires experimental work of a clinical or basic laboratory nature. Because we have taken the precaution to weigh confounding and interactional effects of so many factors simultaneously, however, there is a high degree of likelihood that many of the variables identified as having significant impact on offspring do indeed act by a direct pathway.

Attributable risk, objectively defined, is the difference between the risk found associated with a factor under study and the risk encountered in a referent population, the referent risk (rr). The referent population is chosen to reflect the index population except, of course, for the variable in question. Applicable referent groups have been created in the foregoing series of investigations for each of the variables and the incidence rates of bad outcomes were generated for both referent and index groups. The attributable risk (AR) can also be derived from the risk ratio (RR).

In this study, our prior analyses also permitted us to determine attributable risk data corrected for concurrent labor-delivery risk factors. Thus, we could substitute a more meaningful value for the crude attributable risk achievable by the more simplistic approach described above. This was made possible by the risk-scoring model derived earlier. The risk strata created by the model allowed us to give due weight to the impact of each risk factor according to coexisting constellations of risk factors. The weighted average of stratum-specific risk ratios, based on weighting by the number of unaffected index cases in each of the risk-score strata, yields the so-called *standardized morbidity ratio* (SMR). This is used in lieu of the overall risk ratio (for the data with all risk strata

collapsed into a single composite group) and it can be considered even better than the risk ratio obtained by means of the multivariate analytical approach (see Tables 26-7 and 26-8). Perhaps still better is the *standardized risk ratio* (SRR), another form of weighted average based on weighting by the number of unaffected referent cases in each risk stratum.

The attributable risk (AR), as stated, is the difference between the index risk (ir) for those cases exposed to a given risk variable and the referent risk (rr) for comparable unexposed cases, as shown by the equation

$$AR = ir - rr$$

The risk ratio (RR) describes the relationship between index and referent risks, as follows:

$$RR = \frac{ir}{rr}$$

Solving this last equation by substituting ir = AR + rr (from the prior equation) gives a derivation for attributable risk as related to the risk ratio and referent risk.

$$RR = \frac{rr + AR}{rr} = 1 + \frac{AR}{rr}$$

$$AR = (RR - 1)\, rr$$

While this approach may appear to be unnecessarily complex, it has a twofold rationale. First, it allows derivation of the attributable risk directly from the risk ratio resulting from the foregoing multivariate analyses. Second, it permits us to use the results of the risk-score model to derive a more reliable corrected attributable risk for each variable while simultaneously weighing the risks of all associated labor and delivery factors. Thus, replacing RR by the standardized morbidity ratio (SMR) or, even better, by the standardized rate ratio (SRR) provides an attributable risk corrected for all the risk factors which the risk-score model had taken into account.

An example will perhaps clarify the derivation. The composite outcome results for FUNDAL2 (moderate fundal pressure) and its referent group formed the following 2 x 2 table:

	Referent	Index
Normal	2487(a)	793(b)
Abnormal	201(c)	82(d)

The referent risk (rr) is estimated to be 7.48%, that is, $c/(a+c)$ or $201/(2487 + 201)$ = 0.0748. The index risk (ir) is 9.37% from $d/(b+d)$ or $82/(793 + 82)$ = 0.0937. The risk ratio (RR) is derived from

$$RR = \frac{ir}{rr} = \frac{0.0937}{0.0748} = 1.253$$

and the attributable risk (AR) from

$$AR = ir - rr = 0.0937 - 0.0748$$
$$= 0.0189 = 1.89\%$$

Alternatively, the AR could be estimated from the RR by

$$AR = (RR - 1)rr = 0.253 \times 0.0748 = 0.0189$$

We can also substitute the estimated RR derived from the earlier multivariate analysis (see Table 26-7) to give a partially weighted AR, as follows:

$$AR = (1.27 - 1)\, 0.0748 = 0.0202$$

Finally, we can invoke the risk-score model described and used so extensively in chapter 27 to ensure appropriate accountability for the concurrent risk of labor-delivery factors that are acting simultaneously. As will be recalled, the incremental risk-score system divided gravidas into five risk strata for perinatal outcome and four for composite outcome. The sample variable we are illustrating, FUNDAL2, thus breaks down into the following four 2 x 2 tables of adverse composite outcome:

Risk Stratum	Referent	Index	
Lowest	67(a)	44(b)	
	5	1	$RR_1 = 0.32$
Low	2360	707	
	185	61	$RR_2 = 1.09$
Moderate	58	38	
	8	7	$RR_3 = 2.55$
High	2	4	
	3	3	$RR_4 = 0.71$

These data provide the SMR as a mean of RRs for each risk-score weighted by the size of the unaffected index cell (b):

$$SMR = \frac{\Sigma\,(RR_i \times b_i)}{\Sigma\,b_i}$$

$$= \frac{(0.32 \times 44) + (1.09 \times 707) + (2.55 \times 38) + (0.71 \times 4)}{44 + 707 + 38 + 4}$$

$$= \frac{888}{793} = 1.12$$

From this, a weighted AR is obtained:

$$AR = (SMR - 1)rr = 0.86\%$$

Alternatively, SRR can be calculated in a similar fashion, weighting the RRs by unaffected referent cases (a):

$$SRR = \frac{\Sigma\,(RR_i \times a_i)}{\Sigma\,a_i}$$

$$= \frac{2743}{2487} = 1.10$$

$$AR = (SRR - 1)rr = 0.77\%$$

The confidence limits are based on the standard error of the AR. It is the square root of the variance, which is defined as the sum of the variances for the referent risk (RR) and index risk (ir). Each variance is derived from the weighted risk (R) level as a function of

$$Var = \frac{R\,(1-R)}{n}$$

The standard error (SE) for the foregoing data is 0.0102. The 95th percentile confidence limits are a multiple of 1.960 SE above and below the mean AR (0.0077 ± 0.0218) or -1.23% and 2.77%.

In effect, this can be interpreted to mean that the factor FUNDAL2 contributed 0.8%

additional hazard for the composite outcome to the 7.5% already present in comparable offspring at large in whom FUNDAL2 was not invoked (and in whom delivery was accomplished by CONTROL1, manual control of the head in vertex presention, a criterion used for selecting the referent series). If other labor-delivery risk factors had not been taken into consideration and confounding had not been controlled, the attributable risk calculation would have shown a 1.9% effect.

The attributable risk derived from the risk-score model data differed from that calculated for the overall data, signaling some degree of confounding and/or interactional effect from concurrent labor and delivery risk factors for this variable. Since the attributable risk for this variable was found to be different when corrected for other concurrent labor-delivery risk factors, it follows that the risk model recognized coexistent adverse effects and made appropriate corrections for them. These were perhaps the very conditions for which the Kristeller pressure was felt to be indicated and those additional interventive measures undertaken to help conclude an obstructed labor.

For variables that exhibited protective effects with risk ratios between zero and unity, the attributable risk will be negative. This comes about because the peril associated with the index group is less than that found in the referent. The attributable risk can then be interpreted as a measure of the ostensible benefit of the factor when exhibited in the population, the negative attributable risk being a quantitation of the proportion of the risk from which the offspring is protected. An example of this effect will be seen for both the composite and perinatal outcome results for SPINAL (spinal anesthesia). For composite outcome data, for example, the referent risk was 0.0860 and the risk ratio 0.75 to give an attributable risk of -0.0224. SPINAL, therefore, reduced the 8.60% inherent risk of a bad composite result by an uncorrected decrement of 2.24%. Correcting for coexistent labor-delivery risk constellations by

risk-score stratification yielded SMR = 0.82 and SRR = 0.89 for an adjusted attributable risk of -0.010 (95th percentile confidence limits -0.024 and 0.05). Thus, only 1.0% protective effect could be verified when other factors were accounted for simultaneously.

Survey of Attributable Risk Data

All variables previously identified as having significant impact on offspring were studied in this way. We were thereby able to quantitate the magnitude of the effect of each of them on the fetus and infant. To review briefly, the population being studied at this point was limited to those women delivering infants who weighed between 2500 and 4000 g and were free of anomalies incompatible with survival or normal growth and development. The outcome measures were adverse perinatal (death or severe depression) and composite results (abnormality by objective testing from the perinatal period through age seven years).

The factors studied for perinatal effect were those 26 labor-delivery variables found to have statistically verifiable effect, as listed in Table 26-8, when logistic regression modeling analytic methods had been applied to the 112 variables surviving analyses of the grand array of all significant variables studied in aggregate. In addition, quantitation of perinatal effect was done for 33 predictor variables left after careful assessment of residual impact and consistency by means of risk-score paradigms (see Tables 28-7 to 28-12). For composite outcome, there were 21 labor-delivery factors, shown in Table 26-7, and 64 predictor factors chosen from the same sources as those with perinatal effects.

Labor and Delivery Variables
Perinatal Outcome Data. Quantitation of attributable risk for the 26 relevant labor and delivery variables as regards their perinatal effects is shown in Table 29-1. Three labor progression risk variables have continued to show meaningful impact on

Table 29-1
Attributable Risk of Labor-Delivery Variables with Documented Impact
on Perinatal Outcome[a]

Variable		Attributable Risk, %			
		Crude	Multivariate	Weighted	95%CL
LAT3	Prolonged latent phase	2.03	1.06	1.04	-0.1 2.2
ACT2	Foreshortened active phase	0.94	0.86	0.80	-0.3 1.9
ACT3	Prolonged active phase	2.44	0.86	0.98	-0.3, 2.3
SPINAL	Spinal anesthesia	-0.59	-0.97	0.06	-0.6, 0.7
PARAC	Paracervical block	2.19	1.31	0.67	-0.9, 2.2
GAS2	Continuous inhalation anesthesia	2.25	0.98	0.24	-0.8, 1.3
AGT1	Demerol	0.91	1.11	0.32	-0.4, 1.0
AGT22	Apresoline	10.12	19.08	8.72	2.5 14.9
AGT27	Other antibiotics[b]	22.39	41.49	21.13	2.3, 39.9
FORTRAC2	Difficult forceps traction	6.12	6.54	4.05	1.3 6.8
FORTRAC3	Very difficult traction	10.68	12.53	5.32	2.0, 8.6
FORROT2	Difficult forceps rotation	3.21	3.25	3.01	1.1 4.9
FORROT3	Very difficult rotation	12.95	13.67	11.90	3.2 20.6
FORROT4	Failed forceps rotation	18.15	17.37	16.01	4.5, 27.5
CONTROL1	Manual control of head	-0.40	-1.50	0.03	-0.6, 0 7
CONTROL3	Forceps control	-0.75	-1.66	-0.30	-2.3, 1.7
FUNDAL2	Moderate fundal pressure	0.87	0.97	0.25	-0.9, 1.4
FUNDAL3	Strong fundal pressure	1.54	1.64	0.74	-0.4, 1.9
ABRUPT	Abruptio placentae	6.56	5.38	5.29	1.2, 9.4
CSVAG	Cesarean after failed vaginal attempt	11.88	4.20	3.40	2.0 4.8
SHOULD	Shoulder dystocia	13.00	8.80	6.61	1.0 12.2
INDUCT3	Induction for PIH	6.90	3.76	3.99	1.7, 6 3
INDUCT6-9	Induction for other indications[c]	7.45	5.90	4.64	1.2, 8.1
AUGMENT6	Stimulation for amnionitis	59.15	44.78	43.75	26.5, 61.0
PRES5-8	Breech presentation	6.19	4.35	4.73	1.8, 7.7
REACT3	Uterine hypertonus from oxytocin	11.91	9.09	7.80	1.0 14.6

a   See text for derivations: Attributable risk in multivariate column based on RR for data in
     Table 26-8 for 13,933 cases; weighted AR is obtained from SRR derived from risk-score model
     data.

b   Other than penicillin, streptomycin, achromycin, chloramphenicol or sulfa.

c   Other than elective, ROM, PIH, diabetes or Rh sensitization.

offspring through the long series of screening analyses to which we have subjected the spectrum of labor and delivery factors. They were LAT3 (prolonged latent phase), ACT2 (foreshortened active phase), and ACT3 (prolonged active phase). It should be recalled that ACT2 is essentially equivalent to MAXS3 (precipitate dilatation) and ACT3 to MAXS2 (protracted dilatation) in clinical terms. The referent risk for these variables was 1.86% to 1.89% as reflected in the adverse perinatal outcome data encountered in the referent groups, specifically those gravidas without the labor disorder who were delivered vaginally of a fetus in vertex presentation by manual control.

The crude relative risk for LAT3 was 2.08, yielding an attributable risk for this variable of 2.03%. Taking all concurrent labor and delivery risk variables into account by means of the risk-score paradigm described in chapter 27, we derived a weighted relative risk of 1.55. If this is applied to the calculation of the attributable risk, it produces a value for the weighted attributable risk of only 1.04%, nearly identical to the 1.06% derived from the multivariate analysis. This means that LAT3 contributed 2.03% to the adverse perinatal outcome results overall. Half of this effect, 0.99% or the difference between 2.03% and 1.04%, could be accounted for by other coexisting labor and delivery factors and the rest, 1.04%, could be attributed directly to the variable itself.

The same general association was seen for ACT3. Its large crude relative risk of 2.31 yielded an attributable risk of 2.44%, but the multivariate relative risk of 1.46 derived from the risk-score model reduced the attributable risk to 0.86%; this was reduced slightly to 0.80% by using the SRR instead. Thus, the total risk of 2.72% consisted of 1.92% for which other labor and delivery factors were accountable and only 0.80% attributable to ACT3 itself. The situation was somewhat different for ACT2 because the crude, multivariate and weighted relative risk values were all about the same (1.50, 1.46, and 1.43, respectively). Therefore, ACT2 was almost entirely responsible for all of the attributable risk of 0.94%; only 0.14% could be ascribed to other labor and delivery factors based on the corrected attributable risk of 0.80%.

Three anesthesia and three drug variables also survived the foregoing series of analyses, namely SPINAL (spinal anesthesia), PARAC (paracervical block anesthesia), GAS2 (continuous inhalation anesthesia), AGT1 (Demerol), AGT22 (Apresoline), and AGT27 (other antibiotics). The crude relative risk of 1.46 for AGT1 (and referent risk of 1.98%) produced an attributable risk of 0.91%. The relative risk derived from the multivariate analysis proved even larger at 1.56. It yielded an attributable risk of 1.11%. However, the weighted relative risk from the risk-score model (1.16) yielded the much smaller weighted attributable risk of only 0.32%. This implied that the series of index cases studied to ascertain the effect of AGT1 actually contained other adverse risk factors to enhance by confounding the impact of this agent by 0.59%. Taking all other labor and delivery factors into account simultaneously had thus disclosed an inappropriately magnified adverse effect from this risk variable.

The magnification was also present, but much less impressively, for AGT22 and AGT27. There was an already sizable attributable risk of 10.12% obtained from the crude relative risk of 5.84 for AGT22 (and referent risk of 2.09%). It was further increased by the multivariate relative risk of 10.13 to an impact of 19.08%, but it was reduced considerably by the weighted SRR of 5.17 to 8.72%. For AGT27, the attributable risk of 22.36% (from the crude relative risk of 11.70) was nearly doubled to 41.45% based on the multivariate relative risk of 20.85 and halved again to 21.13% by the SRR of 11.11.

The protective effect of SPINAL has been mentioned earlier (see above). The magnitude of its perinatal benefit was determined to be rather small on the basis of the crude relative risk of 0.72 which had resulted in an attributable risk of -0.59%. The much smaller relative risk of 0.54 derived from the multivariate analysis increased this protective fraction to -0.97%. The SRR of 1.03 from the risk-score model almost reduced the attributable risk to the vanishing point (0.06%), a phenomenon accomplished by the correction introduced by weighing the concurrent effects of labor-delivery factors.

The same general trend obtained for both PARAC and GAS2 because their adverse effects were reduced by taking the other labor-delivery factors into account. The crude attributable risk of 2.19% for PARAC, for example, fell to 1.31% when the derived multivariate relative risk value was used and to 0.67% by the SRR; the difference of 1.52% could thus be ascribed to factors other than PARAC. For GAS2, there was even a greater decline in attributable risk from 2.25% to 0.98% and 0.24%. Thus, nearly 90% of the original impact, 2.01%, was accounted for by other labor-delivery risk variables.

The remaining 17 factors were all delivery-related. Five dealt with forceps use, two of them for traction and three for rotation. FORTRAC2 (difficult forceps traction) had an uncorrected crude perinatal attributable risk of 6.12%. This represented the excess impact of this factor over the base or referent rate of 2.11% for a total of 8.23% associated adverse perinatal results. Substituting the multivariate relative risk of 4.10 in lieu of the crude relative risk of 3.90 increased the attributable risk to 6.54% for this risk variable, but the SRR of 2.92 reduced it to 4.05%.

At the next level of difficulty, FORTRAC3 (very difficult forceps traction), the attributable risk rose to 10.68% based on the crude relative risk of 6.06. This could be modified to 12.53% by the more reliable derived multivariate relative risk of 6.94, and markedly reduced to 5.32% by the SRR of 3.52. In both cases, it appeared there were other adverse factors present in the uncorrected data. When the confounding effects of these variables were controlled by the risk-score model, the relative risk decreased and the attributable risk was reduced in turn. Nonetheless, it was obvious that both the corrected and uncorrected data showed very serious effects from FORTRAC2 and even more so from FORTRAC3 insofar as perinatal outcome was concerned. This left little doubt at all as to their clinical relevance.

The three risk variables pertaining to forceps rotation showed a trend toward markedly increasing deleterious perinatal effects with increasing difficulty of rotation. Contrary to the data for forceps traction, however, there was little by way of adjustment of effect from substituting the multivariate or weighted relative risk for the crude relative risk. FORROT2 (difficult forceps rotation), for example, had a 3.21% attributable risk correctable only to 3.25% and 3.01%. The crude attributable risk increased fourfold to 12.96 for FORROT3 (very difficult rotation). This was upwardly modifiable to 13.67% by using the multivariate relative risk of 7.48 instead of the odds ratio of 7.14. The SRR of 6.64 reduced it somewhat to 11.90%.

The crude attributable risk increased

nearly half again for FORROT4 (failed forceps rotation) to reach 18.15% from the crude relative risk of 9.60. Even based on the lower multivariate relative risk of 9.23, the attributable risk was still impressively large at 17.37%. It fell slightly to 16.01% when the SRR of 8.59 was used instead. The failure of the risk-score model to influence the relative risk for these factors to any great degree suggested that no other coexistent labor-delivery factor was able to alter systematically their major impact on perinatal outcome; alternatively, no other factors coexisted in definable patterns in these data, a highly unlikely explanation given the nature of these variables and the conditions under which they are usually invoked.

Manual control of the delivery of a fetal head in vertex presentation (CONTROL1) was somewhat protective relative to spontaneous uncontrolled delivery, but the magnitude of benefit based on the raw odds ratio was small at an attributable risk of -0.40%. When corrected by the multivariate relative risk, its protective effect increased to -1.50%, but correction for concurrent labor and delivery factors by means of the SRR derived from the risk-score model reduced it to near zero (0.03%). Forceps control of delivery (CONTROL3) showed even greater protection with an attributable risk of -0.75% modified to -1.66% and -0.30% by the aforementioned corrections. Since the 95th percentile confidence limits for both CONTROL1 and CONTROL3 fell about equidistant on both sides of the AR scale (centering on zero), it may be concluded that the magnitude of their impact was probably negligible after all.

There was an apparent paradox of objective evidence of protection (slight at most, and clearly not adverse) from CONTROL3, on the one hand, and contrastingly serious harm from FORTRAC2-3 and FORROT2-4, on the other. This was clarified by recognizing that most forceps usage was limited to FORTRAC1 (traction of average difficulty) and FORROT0 (no rotation), neither of which had been found to be associated with bad results. Despite the poor out-comes seen with difficult forceps traction and rotation, their relatively small numbers precluded detection of any discernible over-all effect from forceps use in general.

Kristeller expression had been identified as having a significantly adverse perinatal impact in the foregoing studies. The magni-tude of this effect was determined to be 0.87% for FUNDAL2 (moderate pressure) and 1.54% for FUNDAL3 (strong pressure). Slight upward adjustments resulted from introduction of the derived multivariate rel-ative risk values to give attributable risks of 0.97% and 1.64%, respectively. The SRR from the risk-score model reduced these effects markedly to 0.25% and 0.74%. Thus, the risk-score model found some influence from other concurrent labor and delivery factors to account partially for the effects of fundal pressure.

Abruptio placentae (ABRUPT) is well recognized as a particularly serious late pregnancy and intrapartum obstetrical complication. This was clearly demon-strated by our sequence of analyses which showed a highly significant association with bad perinatal outcome. The attributable risk associated with the crude relative risk of 4.18 was 6.56%. With the multivariate relative risk, it was 5.38% and almost the same (5.29%) with the SRR. It was clear from these data that, even though ABRUPT carried a high risk for a poor perinatal result, 1.27% of the adverse impact was related to other labor and deliv-ery factors acting at the same time, perhaps including some undertaken specifically for managing the placental abruption.

Failed attempts to effect vaginal delivery leading to cesarean section (CSVAG) were likewise associated with increased frequen-cies of poor perinatal outcome. The attribu-table risk was determined to be 11.88% based on the crude relative risk of 6.64. However, this was correctable down to 4.20% when the smaller multivariate rela-tive risk of 2.99 was used, and further to 3.40% with the SRR derived from the risk-score model. The sizable 8.48% difference

in attributable risk was likely due to the fact that much of the effects of the prevailing adverse conditions and interventive mea-sures used during the unsuccessful attempts to accomplish vaginal delivery were accounted for by the factors included in the risk-score modeling and summariza-tion, among which were such seriously adverse factors as FORROT4 (failed for-ceps rotation, see above).

Shoulder dystocia (SHOULD) was still worse as a complicating delivery factor. Its crude attributable risk was 13.00%, correc-table to 8.80% and 6.61%. Again, the 6.39% decrease in attributable risk caused by sub-stituting the weighted SRR for the crude relative risk probably mirrored the kinds of labor and delivery disorders associated with (and perhaps predictive of) SHOULD. When their impact on offspring was taken into account by the risk-score system, the attributable risk fell to a level which was more likely to be a true reflection of the effect of this factor.

Induction of labor for pregnancy-induced hypertension (INDUCT3) had a crude attributable risk of 6.90% for perina-tal outcome. Although use of the multivar-iate relative risk and the SRR reduced this to 3.76% and 3.99%, respectively, thereby accounting for associated labor and delivery factors, even the modified attributable risk did not fully take into account the condition for which the induction was being done. In the preceding chapter, we addressed the rel-ative risk related to pregnancy-induced hypertension in its several clinically defined manifestations. Our examination there consisted of determining any residual effect after all labor and delivery effects had been accounted for by use of the risk-score model. Only PIH1 (diastolic hypertension) was shown to have a statistically significant residual adverse composite outcome effect. Both PIH1 and PIH2 (combination of ele-vated diastolic blood pressure and protein-uria) had increased perinatal risks, but neither proved statistically significant. We may now conjecture as to whether labor factors such as INDUCT3 and other measures invoked for managing preeclamptic patients might not have carried sufficient risk themselves so as to becloud the recognized bad effect of these disorders.

Labor inductions undertaken for a variety of conditions (INDUCT6-9) were also associated with significantly poor perinatal results. Specifically included here were inductions for amnionitis, pyelonephritis, abruptio placentae, and placenta previa, all conditions themselves associated with bad outcome. The uncorrected attributable risk for these cases was 7.45%, reduced to 5.90% and 4.64% by substituting the multivariate relative risk and the SRR. The reduction reflected the magnitude of the correction for associated labor and delivery factors. However, the residual attributable risk value may still have included some or all of the adverse influence of the underlying condition (except for abruptio placentae and placenta previa, both of which had been included in the risk-score assessment) rather than the induction per se. This is not meant to imply that the induction process was free of risk. Significant risk was clearly shown in earlier analyses in which all factors, including those for which the inductions were done, were examined simultaneously. It is just that we cannot be sure our quantitation of the attributable risk for these inductions accurately measured the magnitude of that risk.

Augmentation of labor by oxytocin for amnionitis (AUGMENT6) carried the highest measured attributable risk for perinatal bad outcome of all the risk variables investigated. As will be seen later, this substantive hazard persisted in the composite outcome results as well. The only other factors that even approached these levels were, in descending order, DIS100 (mental retardation), CSVAG (failed attempt at vaginal delivery), DIS111 (colitis-ileitis), AGT27 (other antibiotics), and FORTRAC4 (failed forceps traction). The attributable risk of AUGMENT6 was 59.15%, correctable for associated labor and delivery factors down to 44.78% by use of the derived relative risk and further to 43.75% by the SRR. The peril

from amnionitis itself could not be separated from the effect of the induction. It was clear, nevertheless, that the risk associated with this variable was devastating and possibly attributable in almost its entirety to the amnionitis. If induction for this condition enhanced the adverse effect of amnionitis, we were unable to demonstrate or to quantitate that enhancement here.

Delivery of a fetus in breech presentation (PRES5-8) was confirmed to be a serious hazard with a crude attributable risk of 6.19%. Substituting the multivariate relative risk and the SRR derived from the risk-score model decreased this somewhat to 4.35% and 4.73%. The difference of 1.46% represented the small degree of modification by coexisting labor-delivery factors in cases with PRES5-8. The magnitude of the risk associated with breech presentation was, therefore, documented to be sizable and apparently attributable directly to the risk factor itself.

The last of the risk factors assessed for attributable risk among the labor-delivery factors studied for perinatal effect was REACT3 (uterine hypertonus resulting from oxytocin stimulation). Analysis showed it to have an uncorrected attributable risk of 11.91%, reduced to 9.09% and 7.80% by the multivariate relative risk and the SRR. Just as for the other variables dealing with use of uterotonic agents (specifically INDUCT3, INDUCT6-9, and AUGMENT6), the downward correction of the attributable risk achieved by employing the multivariate and weighted relative risk—which weighed the effect of all other pertinent labor-delivery risk factors simultaneously—signified that we were undoubtedly seeing the impact here of other influences, most especially that of the condition for which oxytocin was given.

Composite Outcome Results. The attributable risk data for composite outcome were also studied among the 21 labor-delivery variables selected for this purpose because they had been found to retain strong relationships to adverse results even when examined in conjunction with all of the 112 risk factors in aggregate (see Table 26-7). The results are shown in Table 29-2. Only one labor-delivery progression variable, DESC3 (precipitate descent), is represented along with one anesthesia factor, SPINAL (spinal anesthesia), and four drug factors, namely AGT16 (Vistaril), AGT23 (Syntocinon), AGT24 (Pitocin), and AGT27 (other antibiotics). Of these, only SPINAL and AGT27 had surfaced among those with equivalent perinatal effects (see above).

Five were related to forceps use: FORTRAC2-4 (difficult, very difficult, and failed forceps traction) and FORAPP2-3 (difficult and very difficult forceps application). Although FORTRAC2 and FORTRAC3 had earlier shown adverse perinatal effects, the others had not. Moreover, the serious effects of FORROT2-4 did not persist in the composite outcome results, perhaps

because they were subsumed by those of difficult forceps traction and/or application.

CONTROL3 (forceps control in vertex delivery) reappeared as a protective factor, but CONTROL1 (manual control) did not. ABRUPT (abruptio placentae) was not represented, but CSVAG (cesarean section after failed attempt to deliver vaginally) and SHOULD (shoulder dystocia) were. As before, INDUCT3 (labor induction for pregnancy-induced hypertension) and AUGMENT6 (stimulation of labor for amnionitis) were strongly adverse factors. However, INDUCT6-9 (induction for other indications) was no longer a contender.

In place of PRES5-8 (breech presentation), BRDELIV (delivery by breech extraction) stood to reflect the most relevant of the breech-related risk factors insofar as poor composite outcome was concerned. It was joined by PRES11 (brow presentation), not previously identified

Table 29-2
Attributable Risk of Labor-Delivery Variables with Documented Impact on Composite Outcome*

Variable		Attributable Risk, %			
		Crude	Multivariate	Weighted	95%CL
DESC3	Precipitate descent	-2.10	-1.27	-1.09	-2.5 0.3
SPINAL	Spinal anesthesia	-2.25	-2.06	-0.95	-2.4, 0.5
AGT16	Vistaril	3.49	4.48	3.45	0.5, 6.4
AGT23	Syntocinon	-2.13	-2.52	-2.18	-4.4, 0.5
AGT24	Oxytocin	7.32	4.92	4.40	-0.4, 9.2
AGT27	Other antibiotics	37.01	33.69	34.64	5.4, 63.9
FORTRAC2	Difficult forceps traction	3.26	5.81	2.86	0.8, 4.9
FORTRAC3	Very difficult traction	10.30	19.03	9.39	3.6, 15.2
FORTRAC4	Failed forceps traction	28.68	29.43	24.15	7.0 41.3
FORAPP2	Difficult forceps application	2.17	2.35	2.02	0.2, 3.8
FORAPP3	Very difficult application	4.53	3.48	3.52	2.0 5.0
CONTROL3	Forceps control of delivery	-1.11	-3.76	-1.46	-3.5 0.6
FUNDAL2	Moderate fundal pressure	1.89	2.02	0.77	-1.2, 2.8
FUNDAL3	Strong fundal pressure	2.66	2.32	1.94	0.5 3.4
PROLAP	Prolapsed cord	12.86	8.76	7.30	-1.1, 15.7
CSVAG	Cesarean after failed vaginal attempt	49.43	15.36	9.75	-2.6, 22.1
SHOULD	Shoulder dystocia	6.83	7.35	6.14	0.6, 11.7
INDUCT3	Induction for PIH	12.55	10.78	9.57	2.7, 16.4
AUGMENT6	Stimulation for amnionitis	52.28	46.08	44.14	25.1, 63.2
BRDELIV3	Breech extraction	23.72	18.92	16.84	7.6, 26.1
PRES11	Brow presentation	11.86	9.94	9.16	2.0, 16.3

* Derivations same as for Table 29-1: Multivariate AR based on RR for data in Table 26-7 for 15,169 cases; weighted AR from SRR from risk-score model data.

464

among adverse perinatal factors, REACT3 (uterine hypertonus from oxytocin), shown above to have a major adverse perinatal effect, was not equally adverse in its composite outcome effect, possibly because any effect it might have had was already incorporated into that of AGT24.

DESC3 (precipitate descent) appeared to be a protective factor with an attributable risk of -2.10%, correctable to -1.27% and -1.09% by use of the multivariate relative risk and the SRR derived from the risk-score model which took all concurrent labor-delivery risk variables into account. There were clinical reasons to doubt that DESC3 could actually be beneficial to the fetus because rapid descent through the birth canal can sometimes be quite traumatic and, especially if associated with tumultuous uterine contractions, may even cause hypoxic damage. The high referent risk frequency of 9.10% poor composite results suggested a problem in proper selection of the referent group against which to compare the index subset. All other referent risks ranged between 7.48% and 8.70%, but the weighted attributable risk obtained using even the lowest of these would still be -0.90%.

Logical explanations could include the following: (1) The clinical impression was wrong (rather unlikely given the documentation in isolated cases); (2) there were strongly protective associated labor-delivery factors not recognized by these studies (also unlikely given the care and detail of foregoing analyses) or there were prelabor factors that were not accounted for here (plausible); and (3) all or most of the adverse effects felt to be associated with this factor were attributable to other co-existing variables (also possible, especially for predictive factors). In all probability, a combination of the last two of these mechanisms was acting here to obfuscate the adverse effect of this factor. Furthermore, its deleterious impact was probably manifested in a relatively small proportion of cases and thus was readily counterbalanced by the much more favorable situation of the very commonly seen rapidly progressive second stage labor in otherwise healthy, uncomplicated multiparas. The 95th percentile confidence limits overlap somewhat into the positive range of the attributable risk scale, lending support to this contention.

SPINAL was associated with an attributable risk of -2.25%, negligibly corrected to -2.06% and -0.95%. Although this composite outcome benefit was considerably larger than it had been for perinatal outcome, it was about the same or smaller in relative terms when viewed from the vantage point of the referent risk which was more than four times larger here (8.60% versus 2.11%). Nevertheless, in absolute terms, there was a protective component to this variable that could not be readily explained away on the basis of concurrent labor and delivery factors, especially since such factors were being weighed in the balance by the risk-scoring system we used. It should be noted, of course, that the protective effect might conceivably have been related to the coexistence of favorable predictor factors. Against this argument were the prior findings of significant residual benefit even when such prelabor variables were considered simultaneously by logistic modeling techniques (see chapter 25).

Vistaril (AGT16), which had not been shown earlier to have a documentable effect on perinatal results, was found to be associated with a large crude attributable risk of 3.49% in regard to composite outcome. This increased to 4.48% when the multivariate relative risk was substituted and returned to 3.45% by the SRR. In light of the common clinical practice of administering both AGT16 and AGT1 (Demerol) together for their synergistic analgesic-ataractic action, it was perhaps worth reflecting on the complementary nature of their effects. In the parallel analysis of the perinatal data, AGT1 had a crude attributable risk of 0.91%, corrected to 0.32% and AGT16 did not surface as relevant at all. In the composite outcome data, AGT16 had about the same level of relative risk but much higher attributable risk values due to the larger referent risk rate, and AGT1 failed to appear.

These observations suggested that one may represent the obverse of the other, both acting in concert to affect the infant adversely. If this deleterious impact is real (and it did seem to be for AGT16 at least), it was apparently not additive—that is, there was no evidence that the effect of one increased the effect of both acting together. We would have expected both to surface at the same time if there were such independent cumulative effects from them. Alternatively, their failure to appear simultaneously may have been due to inadequate numbers of instances in which one was administered without the other.

Both AGT23 (Syntocinon) and AGT24 (Pitocin) appeared here and paradoxical actions were observed for them. AGT23, for example, showed a protective attributable risk of moderate magnitude (-2.13%, corrected to -2.52% and -2.18%), whereas AGT24 demonstrated a rather sizable adverse attributable risk (7.32%, corrected to 4.92% and 4.40%). The large downward correction seen for AGT24 with the multivariate relative risk and the SRR clearly reflected the effects of labor-delivery risk variables concurrent with (and perhaps motivating factors for) use of oxytocin. The absence of any such correction for AGT23, by contrast, would support a contention that this agent was probably used preferentially in patients who did not have such adverse risk factors present—that is, they were likely to have been given the agent electively for induction or stimulation of labor.

Thus, the proprietary uterotonic preparation chosen probably served as a marker of concurrent risk: low risk cases for AGT23 and high risk for AGT24. In regard to the hazard measured for AGT24, some portion of it was clearly attributable to the aforementioned labor-delivery factors and perhaps some additional component to the prelabor conditions for which it may have been used. Whether some residual attributable risk could be ascribed to the agent itself is unlikely (although tempting to consider) in face of the apparent protective effect (or at least absence of harm) from use of AGT23.

The strongly adverse impact of AGT27 (other antibiotics) replicated that seen for the perinatal outcome data, but at a much larger magnitude of attributable risk (37.01%, corrected to 33.69% and 34.64%). Thus, more than 40% of infants whose mothers had an infection of such serious nature as to warrant receiving one of these agents suffered death, depression, or damage (comprising 33%-37% attributable to this factor plus nearly 9% background rate). There were obvious major effects associated with the risk variable, but we could not quantitatively distinguish those of the condition from those of the agent.

The very bad perinatal impact of difficult forceps traction was found for composite outcome at a somewhat lower degree of effect. FORTRAC2 (difficult forceps traction) was previously associated with a crude attributable risk of 6.12% (corrected to 6.54% and 4.05%) and it now had one of 3.26% (corrected to 5.81% and 2.86%); for FORTRAC3 (very difficult traction), it went from 10.68% (12.53% and 5.32% adjusted) to 10.33% (19.03% and 9.39% adjusted). To these was added the factor of FORTRAC4 (failed forceps traction) which had an attributable risk of 28.68% (modifiable to 29.43% and 24.15%). Its havoc was reminiscent of that seen with CSVAG, a risk factor which encompassed nearly all cases of failed forceps but was not mutually congruent with failed forceps. The magnification of effect with increasing difficulty of traction supported the view that this risk variable constituted a real peril to offspring.

Difficult and very difficult forceps applications also had measurable attributable risks: 2.17% for FORAPP2 (corrected to 2.35% and 2.02%) and 4.53% for FORAPP3 (corrected downward to 3.48% and 3.52%). Just as difficult forceps rotation appeared to have discriminatingly inherent adverse effects separate from those of difficult forceps traction in the perinatal data (see above), difficult forceps application also seemed to have a separate effect from difficult traction. The increase in attributable risk for FORTRAC2-4 seen when the multivariate relative risk was applied suggested that there had been a concurrent protective effect, but this was countered by the SRR-derived attributable risk data. The resulting decrease reflected correction for adverse factors, perhaps those relating to difficult forceps traction, with which difficult application was so often associated, or to difficult application in cases with difficult traction.

CONTROL3 (forceps control in vertex delivery) was again significantly protective relative to spontaneous uncontrolled delivery. The magnitude of the protection afforded, as reflected in the attributable risk of -1.11% (correctable up to -3.76% and -1.46%), was larger than it had been for the perinatal results (-0.75%, -1.66% and -0.30%). We have already addressed (see above) the apparent contradiction of these beneficial findings and the adverse effects of the more difficult and less frequently invoked forceps operations involving traction and rotation (to which application can now be added as well).

The composite outcome effects of FUNDAL2-3 (moderate and strong Kristeller expression) were greater than the perinatal effects had been. The attributable risks for FUNDAL2 increased from 0.87% (0.97% and 0.25% corrected) to 1.89% (2.02% and 0.77%); for FUNDAL3, 1.54% (1.64% and 0.74%) to 2.66% (2.32% and 1.94%). The large diminishing effect from the corrections for labor and delivery factors in the perinatal analysis was duplicated here for both FUNDAL2 and FUNDAL3. In both, there appeared to have been some degree of adverse impact attributable to risk variables other than fundal pressure. Despite this, however, there was still a residual adverse effect that could not be ignored and that appeared to be attributable directly to this factor, especially for strong fundal pressure.

Prolapse of the umbilical cord (PROLAP) had not previously appeared among conditions contributing significantly to perinatal problems, perhaps because its well-recognized harmful impact was incorporated into other variables such as those pertaining to the procedures done for intervention. Moreover, since fetuses dying before labor had been excluded from consideration in these analyses for the obvious reason that no labor or delivery factor could logically be deemed to have affected them on a retrograde basis, perinatal mortality from prelabor cord prolapse had been eliminated. Nevertheless, PROLAP was found to be a strongly adverse factor for composite outcome results. The crude attributable risk associated with it was 12.86%, reduced to 8.76% through the use of the relative risk derived from the multivariate analysis and 7.30% by the SRR from the risk-score model. The sharp reduction in attributable risk by about one third confirmed that, in addition to the powerful impact of this risk variable, other labor-delivery factors were indeed acting simultaneously to augment its adverse effect considerably.

The major perinatal effects of CSVAG (cesarean section after failure to accomplish vaginal delivery) had been well documented and were repeated for composite outcome to an even greater degree. The attributable perinatal risk, which had been 11.88% (corrected down to 4.20% and 3.40%), was now 49.43% (corrected to 15.36% and 9.75%). The marked reduction in the attributable risk when all concurrent labor and delivery risk factors were weighed by risk scores was noteworthy. It accounted for more than 80% of the adverse effect (the difference of 29.68% constituted 80.3% of the overall impact of this variable on composite outcome). Thus, much of the influence of CSVAG could be attributable to identifiable labor-delivery variables. There was, in addition, an impressively sizable residual effect associated with

CSVAG, warranting our recognizing it as among the most serious of the risk variables we have been able to identify.

Shoulder dystocia (SHOULD), which had been determined to be an even greater offender than CSVAG in regard to its perinatal impact (attributable risk 13.00%, corrected to 8.80% and 6.61%), was found to have a somewhat lower, but still substantive, attributable risk for bad composite outcome (6.83%, increased by the multivariate relative risk to 7.35% and reduced again to 6.14% by the SRR). Because substitution of the standardized relative risk derived from the risk-score model did not reduce the attributable risk in the major way it had for the perinatal data, the analysis served as a convincing demonstration of the strong effect of SHOULD as an adverse risk variable acting almost independently of other factors insofar as its influence on composite outcome was concerned.

Induction of labor for pregnancy-induced hypertension (INDUCT3) enhanced the large effects encountered before with perinatal results and reconfirmed them in the composite outcome series. The attributable risk rose sharply from 6.90% (corrected to 3.76% and 3.99%) to 12.55% (10.78% and 9.57%). This was a clear confirmation of the significantly adverse effect of this risk variable.

AUGMENT6 (labor stimulation for amnionitis) was just about as devastating here as it had been for perinatal effects according to the uncorrected attributable risk (59.15% before, 52.25% now). Correcting for concurrently acting labor and delivery factors by use of the multivariate relative risk and the SRR obtained from the risk-score system reduced the attributable risk for adverse composite outcome to 46.08% and 44.14%, again about the same as for perinatal data. AUGMENT6 had already been identified earlier as the most seriously deleterious risk variable in terms of the magnitude of its influence on perinatal results. It is patently obvious that its greatly damaging effects

persisted in large measure among surviving infants, nearly half showing some objective evidence of permanent residual effect.

Breech extraction (BRDELIV3) was found to carry a major uncorrected attributable risk of 23.72%. Correcting for concurrent labor-delivery factors, we obtained attributable risks of 18.92% and 16.84%. Although the composite outcome risk associated with BRDELIV3 could not be compared directly with the perinatal hazard of PRES5-8 (breech presentation), these findings do suggest a possible relationship. It could be interpreted to signify that a major fraction of the adverse risk encountered during the perinatal period for babies presenting by the breech continues in later life, especially among those delivered by breech extraction. Conversely, the deleterious perinatal impact of breech presentation may not persist except in those cases sustaining the greatest damage, specifically among those subjected to breech extraction. Our analytical approach could not distinguish between these two contentions.

Brow presentation (PRES11) was the last of the risk factors with significant composite outcome effects among the labor and delivery variables for which the attributable risk was quantitated. It measured 11.86%, adjusted downward to 9.94% and 9.16% by the multivariate relative risk and the SRR, respectively. It was not immediately clear why this variable, which was so transparently a harmful one with regard to its late effects, should not have been able to exhibit a similar impact perinatally. Closer examination actually did show a highly adverse perinatal effect, but we were reminded of the relatively few fetuses with brow presentation who had actually experienced labor and were delivered vaginally. Because the expected rate of death and severe damage was also low, both numerator (cases with adverse effect) and denominator (subpopulation under study) were too small to raise the level of perinatal impact to that of acceptable statistical significance. This was an instance in which being unable to prove an adverse effect significant did not mean the effect was not real, but simply that it could not be statistically verified.

Predictor Variables

Perinatal Outcome Data. Among the 33 predictor risk factors studied for perinatal impact were eight pertaining to demographic characteristics, one to prior obstetric experience, one physical attribute, six socioeconomic status, ten antepartum conditions, and seven intercurrent diseases. The effects of all but nine of these surfaced again in the composite outcome analyses (see below). Attributable risk was calculated as before for each of these variables to quantitate its measurable perinatal effect on offspring (Table 29-3). These data were further correctable for the influence of concurrent labor and delivery factors by use of the relative risk derived from the risk-score model.

Three institutions had been determined to have residual impact on the fetus or infant when all other relevant predictor and labor-delivery variables were being simultaneously considered, namely INST55, INST60, and INST71. Their uncorrected perinatal attributable risks ranged from 1.55% to 1.98%. All were downwardly modified by substituting the multivariate and the standardized relative risk (SRR) statistics. Although these latter attributable risk values were somewhat smaller, they nonetheless indicated that some other factor or factors, as yet not fully accounted for by the analytical investigations completed thus far, were still acting at these hospital obstetrical units to alter outcome adversely.

It was not at all clear what these factors might be in view of the apparent wide differences among the population (and perhaps the clinical practices) at these institutions. Patients at INST71, for example, were mostly black and those at INST60 primarily white, whereas those at INST50 were drawn from a population admixture consisting principally of black and Puerto Rican women. Just these racial differences alone would suggest that there was probably no easily recognized commonality in background to explain the persistent residual attributable risk at these units.

Pregnancy during the teenage years was clearly an important risk factor for fetus and infant. AGE7 (under 16 years) and, to a lesser degree, AGE6 (under 18 years) had been determined to be significantly adverse variables. The crude attributable risk associated with AGE6 was found to be 0.93%, essentially unaffected by concurrent labor and delivery risk factors, only being reduced to 0.77% by use of the SRR. Much more impressive was the crude attributable risk of 2.44% for AGE7. It still remained high at 1.92% and 1.45% when corrected, indicating the strong impact of this factor, effectively doubling the underlying risk of an adverse perinatal result.

Marital status had also showed its effects when studied in depth. In particular, MARIT1 (single, never married) and MARIT5 (divorced) were identified as bad. Quantitatively, MARIT1 had an attributable risk of 0.90% (correctable down to 0.72% and 0.62%) and MARIT5 3.78% (3.32% and 2.39%). Even though MARIT5 was not encountered often as a risk variable in this study (160 cases in all), its perinatal effects were nevertheless so strong that they retained their statistical significance throughout. Moreover, although the factor failed to remain statistically significant in regard to composite outcome (it was the only demographic factor to behave in this way), its impact continued to be felt at equivalently high levels.

RACE2 (black) had an uncorrected attributable risk of 1.06%, downwardly correctable to 0.62% and 0.86%. Thus, while still a significant factor insofar as the perinatal outcome data were concerned (because the size of the black population was so large), RACE2 had only a small vestige of adverse impact left after all other identifiable associated labor and delivery risk vari-ables were taken into account.

A past history of a premature delivery (PPREM1) was the only factor among the variables relating to obstetrical experience

Table 29-3
Attributable Risk of Predictor Variables with Documented Impact
on Perinatal Outcome*

Variable		Attributable Risk, %			
		Crude	Multivariate	Weighted	95%CL
Demographic Factors					
INST55	Hospital 55	1.55	1.15	1.12	0.0, 2.2
INST60	Hospital 60	1.98	1.13	1.38	-0.1, 2.9
INST71	Hospital 71	1.62	1.33	1.10	-0.1, 2.3
AGE6	Maternal age < 18 yr.	0.93	0.87	0.77	0.1, 1.4
AGE7	Maternal age < 16 yr.	2.44	1.92	1.45	0.4, 2.5
MARIT1	Single status	0.90	0.72	0.62	0.0, 1.2
MARIT5	Divorced	3.78	3.32	2.39	0.5, 4.3
RACE2	Black	1.06	0.62	0.86	0.0, 1.7
Past Obstetrical Background					
PPREM1	Prior premature birth	1.08	1.16	0.92	-0.1, 1.9
Physical Characteristics					
HGT2	Maternal height < 60 in.	2.04	1.64	1.23	0.3, 2.2
Socioeconomic Factors					
SES3	Socioeconomic index 25-34	1.11	1.08	0.91	0.0, 1.8
SES4	Socioeconomic index 35-44	1.15	1.34	1.16	0.2, 2.1
EDUC5	Education 13-15 yr.	-1.11	-0.99	-1.06	-2.0, -0.1
WORKG2	Gravida white collar worker	-1.38	-1.10	-0.77	-1.3, -0.2
WORKF5	Father of baby absent	1.84	1.43	1.24	0.0, 2.5
OCCUPF3	Father of baby blue collar worker	0.91	0.53	0.31	-0.1, 0.7
Antepartum Factors					
GDEL1	Delivery at < 34 wk.	2.43	3.34	2.75	0.4, 5.1
GDEL2	Delivery at < 36 wk.	2.41	3.01	2.64	0.9, 4.4
GDEL3	Delivery at < 38 wk.	1.69	1.72	1.93	0.2, 3.7
GDEL4	Delivery at > 41 wk.	1.36	1.03	0.86	-0.2, 1.9
GDEL5	Delivery at > 42 wk.	1.56	1.15	1.02	0.1, 1.9
SGA	Small for gestational age	1.17	2.13	1.61	0.5, 2.7
MALE	Male infant	1.26	1.08	0.91	0.3, 1.5
HCT1	Lowest hematocrit > 20%	10.22	11.69	12.01	1.7, 22.3
VAGBLD	Early pregnancy bleeding	2.31	0.97	0.79	-0.2, 1.8
RHSENS	Rh isoimmunization	10.24	6.07	4.69	0.4, 9.0
Intercurrent Disorders					
DIS51	Insulin-dependent diabetes	9.07	3.92	4.44	0.5, 8.4
DIS63	Hyperthyroidism	5.83	7.99	8.04	0.9, 15.2
DIS80	Glomerulonephritis	13.98	19.22	18.89	5.2, 32.6
DIS100	Maternal mental retardation	11.04	7.76	7.88	2.3, 13.5
DIS103	Neurological disorder	3.59	4.16	3.56	1.2, 5.9
DIS107	Cholecystitis	2.57	7.69	4.03	0.9, 7.2
DIS111	Colitis-ileitis	5.20	10.16	9.63	0.2, 19.1

* Based on data from Tables 28-7 to 28-12, deleting those with inconsistent or unstable
within-group risk-score results, as shown in Table 28-13.

that retained its adverse impact when weighed in conjunction with other predictor variables. This was found to apply quite consistently to both perinatal and composite outcome results. For the perinatal data, its raw attributable risk was ascertained to be 1.08%, increasing slightly to 1.16% by substitution of the multivariate relative risk and down again to 0.92% by the SRR derived from the risk-score model which took labor-delivery variables into account. As will be seen later, the magnitude of the attributable risk for composite outcome effect of PPREM1 was found to be still greater, confirming its seriously adverse short- and long-term impact.

The only maternal characteristic with an objectively definable deleterious effect on offspring was short stature in the form of the variable HGT2 (less than 60 in). The crude attributable risk found associated with it was 2.04%. It fell to 1.64% and 1.23% when corrected as described earlier. This was not an inconsequential degree of bad perinatal effect, especially when viewed in light of the fact that much of the adversity resulting from any associated labor disorder or difficult delivery procedure had already been accounted for by the risk-scoring system.

Just as poverty and indigency were deleterious to the fetus and infant, so the indices of prosperity were beneficial. Low socioeconomic index variables, SES3 and SES4 (indices 25-34 and 35-44), had crude attributable risks of 1.10% (correctable to 1.08% and 0.91%) and 1.15% (1.34% and 1.16%), respectively. SES4 did not reappear on the list of significant composite outcome variables (see below), but it was replaced by a number of other similar variables with equivalent or even greater effect. By contrast, EDUC5 (13-15 years of education) and WORKG2 (gravida worked as a white-collar employee), as markers of affluence, were clearly protective at attributable risks of -1.11% (adjustable to -0.99% and -1.06%) and -1.38% (-1.10% and -0.77%). It deserves to be emphasized that these last two items were the only protective factors to appear on this list of significant predictor variables for perinatal outcome.

Cases in which the father of the baby was absent (WORKF5) constituted another serious risk group. The attributable risk found for them was 1.84%, diminished somewhat to 1.43% and 1.24% when the effect of concurrent labor and delivery factors were discounted. For offspring of gravidas whose father was a blue-collar worker (OCCUPF3), the crude attributable risk was 0.91%. This was reduced to 0.53% by use of the multivariate relative risk and still further to 0.31% by the SRR, signifying that the effect of this factor was probably rather small in the overview, even though imposing some small degree of perinatal risk.

Both preterm and postterm delivery are well accepted in clinical practice as adverse factors. The magnitude of their effects was assessed. The results obtained, however, must be interpreted only with the full understanding of the birth weight limits (between 2500 and 4000 g) imposed by constraints of case selection in these studies. These limits notwithstanding, offspring delivered prior to 38 weeks (GDEL3) had an uncorrected attributable risk of 1.69%, essentially unaffected (except for some enhancement) by correction for coexistent labor and delivery risk factors (to 1.72% and 1.93%). With diminishing gestational age at delivery, attributable risk increased even though birthweight remained essentially fixed. This was reflected in attributable risks of 2.41% and 2.43% for GDEL2 (less than 36 weeks) and GDEL1 (less than 34 weeks). Both were enhanced by correction for labor and delivery risk factors acting simultaneously. These last large upward corrections implied the presence of modifying labor and delivery variables acting concurrently in the relevant subsets.

For advanced gestational age, both GDEL4 (delivery beyond 41 weeks) and GDEL5 (beyond 42 weeks) showed significant attributable risks of 1.36% (corrected downward to 1.03% and 0.86%) and 1.56% (1.15% and 1.02%). In regard to overt birth weight and gestational age discordance, SGA (small for gestational age) was found to be statistically significant despite the limited range of infant weights included for investigation. It was associated with an attributable risk of 1.17%, increasing to 2.13% and 1.61% when corrected for the concurrent labor-delivery protective effects by use of the multivariate relative risk and the SRR derived from the risk-score model. In passing, it should be noted that neither GDEL4 nor SGA reappeared in the parallel analyses for composite outcome results (see below).

The consistently encountered adversity related to male infants (MALE) was examined to measure the effect of this risk variable. Despite its great statistical significance, the crude attributable risk was only 1.26%. It could be further reduced to 1.08% and 0.91% by appropriate corrections. Thus, although MALE clearly had a deleterious effect on the infant, the magnitude of that impact was not particularly great in either relative or absolute terms.

Severe anemia as manifested in very low hematocrit, specifically below 20% (HCT1), was determined to be a very strong risk factor. The uncorrected attributable risk for bad perinatal outcome was determined to be a very impressive 10.22%. Further augmentation to 11.69% and 12.01%, achieved by substituting the multivariate relative risk and the SRR, attested to the serious nature of this condition which could thus be shown to impact unfavorably on about every eighth affected pregnancy (1:8.3). Of almost the same degree of effect was Rh isoimmunization (RHSENS) with a crude attributable risk of 10.24%, although it was diminished considerably by the correction factors to 6.07% and 4.69%. A much smaller influence was demonstrable from first trimester bleeding (VAGBLD) at an attributable risk of 2.31%, modified greatly down to 0.97% and 0.79%. None of these risk variables reappeared among the significant composite outcome factors (see below).

Of the remaining seven intercurrent disorders flagged as important in regard to their adverse perinatal effects, DIS80 (glomerulonephritis), DIS100 (mental retardation), and DIS51 (diabetes mellitus) carried the greatest apparent degrees of risk. For DIS80, the attributable risk was 13.98%, adjusted upward to a startling weighted attributable risk frequency of 19.22% and 18.89% (every fifth fetus or infant harmed); for DIS100, 11.04% corrected down to 7.76% and 7.88%; for DIS51, 9.07% to 3.92% and 4.44%. Two others carried similar high levels of risk, namely DIS63 (hyperthyroidism) with an uncorrected attributable risk of 5.83% (increased to 7.99% and 8.04% by adjustment) and DIS111 (colitis-ileitis) with an attributable risk of 5.20% (increased to

10.16% and 9.63%). In addition, DIS107 (cholecystitis) and DIS103 (neurologic disorder) showed major effects. DIS107 had an attributable risk of 2.57% (corrected to 7.69% and 4.03%) and DIS103, 3.59% (4.16% and 3.56%). Of these, only the effects of DIS63 and DIS107 failed to persist into the composite outcome series.

Composite Outcome Results. The 64 predictor factors for which significant composite outcome effects had been documented were divisible as follows: 19 demographic, one obstetrical background, three physical trait, 21 socioeconomic, 11 antepartum, and nine intercurrent illness variables. In all, 24 had just been encountered among the 33 factors examined in the foregoing perinatal outcome analyses and the remaining 40 were new. The magnitude of the attributable risk was calculated for each of them (Table 29-4).

Institutional deviations were encountered for seven units with crude attributable risks ranging from 2.01% to 11.38%. Correcting these for the effects brought to bear by concomitant labor and delivery variables, we narrowed the range somewhat to 1.70% to 9.50% for multivariate relative risk and 1.29% to 8.18% for SRR. The weighted effects of all but one were at moderate levels below 5%. The greatest impact was found for INST60 (crude attributable risk 11.38%, corrected to 9.50% and 8.18%) and, to a lesser extent, INST71 (7.25% to 6.21% and 4.51%), both reflecting similar adverse perinatal results earlier (see above). INST55, which had also yielded significantly bad perinatal results before, was now actually near the bottom of the list of obstetrical units represented here.

Teenage pregnancy was again identified as a risk factor. Attributable risk frequencies of moderate proportion were found, increasing from 1.75% (unchanged by the multivariate relative risk or SRR) for AGE1 (under 20 years) to 2.74% (also not correctable by the adjustment procedures) for AGE6 (under 18 years) and 3.54% (adjustable to 2.95% and 2.65%) for AGE7 (under 16 years). Except for the AGE1 effect, this set of results mirrors the impact determined above for such cases in regard to perinatal outcome. At the other extreme, offspring of older gravidas were also at risk. For AGE4 (30-34 years), for example, the attributable risk was 2.10%, modified downward by the multivariate relative risk to 1.74% and by the SRR to 1.59%.

The hospital status had not previously surfaced as a significant risk variable in the prior perinatal data analysis. For composite outcome, however, STATUS1 (clinic ser-

vice) was clearly deleterious with a 4.17% crude attributable risk. Although reduced to 1.97% by substitution of the multivariate relative risk and to 1.78% by the SRR, the magnitude of the attributable risk was still large enough to make this an important demographic variable with an effect on the infant worthy of note. Single marital status (MARIT1) was again relevant as a minor risk factor with an attributable risk of 1.78% (correctable to 1.47% and 1.31%). Although MARIT5 (divorced) did not reap-

Table 29-4
Attributable risk of Predictor Variables with Documented Impact on Composite Outcome*

Variable		Attributable Risk, %			
		Crude	Multivariate	Weighted	95%CL
Demographic Factors					
INST15	Hospital 15	7.74	5.36	4.51	0.2, 8.8
INST31	Hospital 31	3.58	2.34	1.29	-1.1, 3.7
INST37	Hospital 37	6.98	4.94	3.45	-0.5, 7.4
INST45	Hospital 45	5.84	4.25	3.16	-0.4, 6.7
INST55	Hospital 55	2.01	1.70	1.59	0.2, 3.0
INST60	Hospital 60	11.38	9.50	8.18	4.2, 12.2
INST71	Hospital 71	7.25	6.21	4.51	1.7, 7.3
AGE1	Maternal age < 20 yr.	1.75	1.74	1.71	0.9, 2.5
AGE4	Maternal age 30-34 yr.	2.10	1.74	1.59	0.4, 2.8
AGE6	Maternal age < 18 yr.	2.74	2.73	2.35	1.0, 3.7
AGE7	Maternal age < 16 yr.	3.54	2.95	2.65	0.1, 5.2
STATUS1	Clinic service patient	4.17	1.97	1.78	0.3, 3.3
MARIT1	Single status	1.78	1.47	1.31	0.4, 2.2
MARIT6	Separated	2.58	2.16	2.01	0.0, 4.0
RACE2	Black	1.79	1.08	1.08	0.1, 2.1
RELIG2	Roman Catholic	-2.12	-1.82	-1.64	-2.8, -0.5
RELIG3	Jewish	-5.39	-5.02	-4.92	-7.1, -2.7
ORIGIN1	Place of birth NY to PA	-1.32	-1.33	-1.26	-2.2, -0.3
ORIGIN15	Place of birth Europe	-3.38	-3.11	-3.04	-4.7, -1.4
Past Obstetrical Background					
PPREM1	Prior premature birth	3.28	3.08	2.45	0.3, 4.6
Physical Characteristics					
HCT2	Maternal height < 60 in.	2.39	1.88	1.88	1.0, 2.8
POND2	Ponderal index obese	2.41	1.67	1.43	0.0, 2.9
SMOKE3	Smokes > 30 per day	3.92	4.27	3.78	1.8, 5.8
Socioeconomic Factors					
SES1	Socioeconomic index < 15	5.17	4.76	4.19	1.3, 7.1
SES2	Socioeconomic index 15-24	2.63	2.58	2.34	0.2, 4.5
SES3	Socioeconomic index 25-34	2.57	2.34	2.10	0.3, 3.9
SES8	Socioeconomic index 75-84	-3.67	-3.39	-3.47	-5.5, -1.4
SES9	Socioeconomic index 85+	-5.45	-4.84	-4.11	-5.7, -2.5
INCOME4	Per capita income $2250-2999	-2.33	-1.79	-1.48	-2.8, -0.2
INCOME5	Per capita income $3000+	-2.22	-1.71	-1.66	-4.4, 1.1
FAMINC2	Family income < $2000/yr.	3.66	2.86	2.54	0.6, 4.4
FAMINC6	Family income $8000-9999/yr.	-3.16	-2.22	-2.06	-3.3, -0.8
FAMINC7	Family income $10,000+/yr.	-4.02	-3.10	-2.62	-3.7, -1.5
HOUSE1	Housing density 1.0+ person per room	1.90	1.31	1.17	0.3, 2.0

EDUC1	Education 7 yr. or less	4.32	3.56	3.33	1.3, 5.4
EDUC2	Education 8 yr.	2.92	2.27	2.25	0.7, 3.8
EDUC3	Education 9-11 yr.	1.80	1.29	1.21	0.1, 2.3
EDUC5	Education 13-15 yr.	-3.26	-3.03	-3.03	-3.9, -2.2
EDUC6	Education 16+ yr.	-5.45	-5.15	-5.00	-6.9, -3.1
WORKG1	Gravida never worked	2.89	2.46	2.22	0.1, 4.3
WORKG2	Gravida white collar worker	-5.01	-4.59	-4.08	-5.6, -2.6
WORKF3	Father of baby a student	-3.74	-2.47	-3.06	-5.9, -0.2
WORKF5	Father of baby absent	4.62	4.03	3.66	1.8, 5.5
OCCUPF3	Father of baby blue collar worker	4.21	3.59	3.20	2.0, 4.4

Antepartum Factors

GREG6	Registered at 28-31.9 wk.	3.40	2.62	2.56	0.4, 4.7
GREG8	Registered at 36+ wk.	3.26	2.02	2.09	-0.1, 4.3
TRIMEST3	Registered in third trimester	3.09	2.49	2.23	1.1, 3.4
VISIT1	Prenatal visits < 7	2.27	1.90	1.75	0.7, 2.8
GDEL1	Delivery at < 34 wk.	3.29	3.56	3.19	0.1, 6.3
GDEL2	Delivery at < 36 wk.	4.65	4.36	3.70	1.3, 6.1
GDEL3	Delivery at < 38 wk.	3.84	3.27	2.83	1.0, 4.7
GDEL5	Delivery at > 42 wk.	2.06	1.52	0.73	-0.6, 2.1
BW2	Birthweight 2750-2999 g.	1.95	2.03	1.80	0.5, 3.1
MALE	Male infant	2.92	2.78	2.51	1.2, 3.8
PIH1	Diastolic hypertension	3.14	3.94	3.12	0.6, 5.6

Intercurrent Disorders

DIS49	Diabetes mellitus	14.33	6.71	6.80	2.5, 11.1
DIS50	Hyperglycemia 200+ mg./dl.	16.89	8.32	7.37	4.2, 10.5
DIS51	Insulin therapy	19.67	14.19	13.65	6.3, 21.0
DIS80	Glomerulonephritis	16.89	21.05	14.68	5.5, 23.9
DIS98	Convulsive disorder	7.65	7.73	7.01	2.9, 11.1
DIS99	Convulsion in pregnancy	11.55	12.78	10.10	3.0, 17.2
DIS100	Maternal mental retardation	51.44	47.17	45.54	26.8, 64.3
DIS103	Neurological disorder	10.49	11.52	10.13	2.6, 17.7
DIS111	Colitis-ileitis	37.79	37.93	30.38	4.0, 56.8

* See footnote, Table 29-3.

pear here, MARIT6 (separated) showed up in its place; its attributable risk was 2.58%, adjusted to 2.16% and 2.01%.

RACE2 (black) carried a crude attributable risk of 1.79% (modified down to 1.08% for both correction manipulations), comparable to that observed earlier for the perinatal data. Unexplained protective effects, not previously seen, were encountered for the factors of RELIG2 (Roman Catholic) and RELIG3 (other, primarily Jewish) which were associated with uncorrected attributable risks of -2.12% (reduced to -1.82% and -1.64%) and -5.39% (decreased to -5.01% and -4.92%), respectively. Two other unexpectedly beneficial variables were ORIGIN1 (gravida born in NY, NJ or PA) and ORIGIN15 (born in Europe); they had attributable risks of -1.32% (or -1.33% and -1.26%) and -3.38% (-3.11% and -3.04%).

A past obstetrical history of premature delivery (PPREM1) carried a risk for poor composite outcome comparable to that seen earlier for perinatal results. The attributable risk was 3.28%, decreasing slightly to 3.08% and 2.45% when corrected for concurrent labor and delivery factors. As before, this was the only risk factor determined to be consistently and significantly adverse in regard to its effect on the current fetus and infant among those variables concerned with prior obstetrical experience.

Short maternal stature (HGT2, height under 60 in) was again associated with an excess of bad results, totalling 2.39% (1.88% corrected) in attributable risk for composite outcome. Obesity, as reflected in the ponderal index (POND2), had not previously been shown to have an unfavorable effect on perinatal results. In regard to composite data, however, it proved a significant

474

adverse risk variable with an attributable risk of 2.41% (1.67% and 1.43% adjusted). An even greater impact was found for a moderate smoking habit in pregnancy, namely more than 30 cigarettes per day (SMOKE3). It yielded an attributable risk of 3.92%, increasing to 4.27% when the multivariate relative risk was substituted and to 3.78% when the SRR derived from the labor-delivery risk-score model was introduced.

The socioeconomic index was even more closely correlated with composite outcome than it had been with perinatal outcome. Cases with low indices did very badly. The lower the score, the worse the attributable risk. For SES1 (index under 15), the attributable risk was 5.17% (4.76% by the multivariate relative risk and 4.19% by SRR); for SES2 (index 15-24), it had already decreased to 2.63% (2.57% and 2.34%) and for SES3, it fell further to 2.57% (2.34% and 2.10%). On the high index side, the trend continued with protective attributable risks of -3.67% (-3.39% and -3.47%) and -5.45% (-4.84% and -4.11%) for SES8 (index 75-84) and SES9 (index 85+), respectively.

Income data confirmed these trends. The per capita income variables of INCOME4 ($2250-2999) and INCOME5 ($3000+) showed comparable protection with attributable risks of -2.33% (-1.79% and -1.48%) and -2.22% (-1.78% and -1.66%). Extremes of family income were equally contrasting, low figures being associated with adverse effect and high figures with benefit. FAMINC2 (under $2000 per year) had an adverse attributable risk of 3.66% (2.86% and 2.54%), whereas FAMINC6 ($8000-9999 per year) and FAMINC7 ($10,000+ per year) had protective values of -3.16% (-2.22% and -2.06%) and -4.02% (-3.10% and -2.62%). Similarly, high housing density (HOUSE1, 1.0+ person per room), while not quite so strong a factor, nonetheless yielded an attributable risk of 1.90% (1.31% and 1.17%).

The duration of the gravida's education also correlated inversely and linearly with the effect on the fetus and infant. The shor-

ter the education, the greater the risk, ranging from EDUC1 (seven years or less) with 4.32% (3.56% and 3.33%) attributable risk, at one extreme, to EDUC6 (16+ years) with -5.45% (-5.15% and -5.00%) attributable risk, at the other. There was good agreement between the perinatal effect seen for the variable WORKG2 (gravida a white-collar worker) and composite outcome results; both showed a beneficial influence, now much stronger with an attributable risk of -5.01% (-4.59% and -4.08%). The referent group selected for this analysis was fortuitously made up of cases with unusually bad overall risk, the resulting referent risk (10.20%) being the largest encountered in this segment of the program. As a consequence, the magnitude of the protection attributable to this factor was probably unduly large. Nevertheless, if the referent risk had fallen more in line with others, which clustered between 6.55% and 8.22%, the crude attributable risk of WORKG2 would have been -0.77% to -2.44%—that is, still protective, but to a lesser degree.

The employment status of the father of the baby was also consistent in its composite outcome effects with those exhibited earlier for perinatal outcome. If he was a blue-collar worker (OCCUPF3), the attributable risk was 4.21% (3.59% and 3.20% corrected). Again, one should note here the outlying referent risk at the low end of the range (4.92%); if this had fallen closer to the median, the crude attributable risk would necessarily have been much smaller (2.60% to 0.93%), albeit remaining significantly adverse. Comparably bad results were found when the baby's father was absent (WORKF5), as documented by the attributable risk of 4.62% (4.03% and 3.66%). This contrasted with the protective attributable risk of WORKF3 (student) at -3.74% (-2.47% and -3.06%).

Registration for antepartum care late in pregnancy at or after 28 weeks was deleterious to offspring in terms of their composite outcome. This relationship had not been encountered previously for perinatal results. The attributable risk for GREG6 (registration in the seventh month of pregnancy) was 3.40% (2.62% and 2.56%) and for GREG8 (registration in the last month), it was 3.26% (2.02% and 2.09%). Collectively, those who registered in the third trimester (TRIMEST3) had an attributable risk of 3.09% (2.49% and 2.23%). Along similar lines, gravidas who had fewer than seven visits before delivery (VISIT1) showed their adverse effects in the attributable risk of 2.27% (1.90% and 1.75%).

While the VISIT1 risk variable may have reflected inadequate prenatal care, it may also have been an index of preterm delivery. Despite the birth weight constraints imposed here (2500-4000 g), premature delivery did occur in these cases and was clearly recognizable as a deleterious influence on outcome. Paralleling the findings for the perinatal effects of early delivery, those for composite outcome were uniformly bad. The most intense effect was seen for GDEL2 (delivery prior to 36 weeks), where an attributable risk of 4.65% (4.36% and 3.70%) was found. Postterm delivery after 42 weeks (GDEL5) was also significantly adverse with an attributable risk of 2.06% (1.52% and 0.73%), although not to so great a level as preterm delivery had been.

Male infants (MALE) continued to show their disadvantage. Just as for the perinatal data, the attributable composite outcome risk for MALE was substantive at 2.92% (2.78% and 2.51%). Inexplicably, one birth weight subset showed untoward effects, namely BW2 (2750-2999 g) which had an attributable risk of 1.95% (2.03% and 1.80%). This may well have been a chance occurrence given the large number of analyses done here, but it was included for completeness.

Whereas severe anemia (HCT1), early pregnancy bleeding (VAGBLD), and Rh isoimmunization (RHSENS) had all shown significantly bad impact in the perinatal parameters, they were no longer related to an adverse composite outcome. In their place, diastolic hypertension (PIH1) appeared with an uncorrected attributable

risk of 3.14%, increased to 3.94% by inserting the multivariate relative risk and back to 3.12% by the SRR derived from the labor-delivery risk-score model.

Very high levels of adverse effect were also verified for the collective variable of diabetes mellitus (DIS49), which had an attributable risk of 14.33% (6.71% and 6.80% corrected). Focusing on those diabetics in poor control with documented hyperglycemia above 200 mg/dL (DIS50), we found the attributable risk rose to a formidable 16.89%, but returned by correction to 8.32% and 7.37%. The attributable risk for insulin-dependent diabetics (DIS51), as distinct from those with just abnormal glucose tolerance tests, was still greater at 19.67% (remaining high at 14.19% and 13.65% when corrected). Thus, one in four or five children was affected directly by this disorder when it was present. Adding the referent risk frequency (that is, the underlying background rate of 8.1%) meant that more than one in five offspring delivered of these gravidas was harmed overall.

Glomerulonephritis (DIS80), the most seriously adverse perinatal risk variable in regard to the magnitude of its attributable risk, persisted as one of the strong offenders here. Although not the worst, its crude attributable risk for composite outcome was nonetheless quite high at 16.89%, adjustable to 21.05% and 14.68% when concurrent labor and delivery factors were accounted for in the multivariate relative risk and the SRR derived from the risk-score model. Thus, more than one quarter of such infants were adversely affected (after adding the 8.2% referent rate).

Two new intercurrent disorders, not found among those with significant perinatal effects, showed a major impact on composite outcome, namely DIS98 (convulsive disorder) and DIS99 (seizure in pregnancy) with attributable risks of 7.65% (7.73% and 7.01%) and 11.55% (12.78% and 10.10%). The remaining conditions had all surfaced as adverse in regard to the perinatal outcome, but their influence on composite results was greatly magnified. DIS100 (mental retardation), for example, had had an already impressive perinatal attributable risk of 11.04% (corrected to 7.76% and 7.88%); now it was a startling 51.44% (47.17% and 45.54% corrected), well above any risk level attained in these studies. It reflected the fact that half or more of the offspring of mentally retarded mothers did poorly. Those with DIS111 (colitis-ileitis) did only slightly better, their attributable risk reaching 37.79% (37.93% and 30.38%). DIS103 (neurologic disorder) trailed at an attributable risk of 10.49% (11.52% and 10.13%), which was still quite high. In view of the much lower (but not inconsequential) attributable risks encountered for these variables in the perinatal outcome data, it was clear that their late effects on the surviving infant were substantial.

Identifying the Gravida-at-Risk

As a result of the foregoing series of analyses, we were able to identify a number of prelabor, intrapartum, and delivery variables which individually and collectively had significant influence on fetal and infant outcome. Moreover, we quantitated the magnitude of the effect of these variables. In a very practical sense, this constellation of factors should be able to help identify those pregnant women who place their offspring at special hazard. The information on intrinsic and antepartum risk factors ought to prove useful to the practicing obstetrical attendant for distinguishing pregnancies at serious potential risk.

Once these cases are identified, close surveillance and specialized attention may serve to avert some or all the peril to which the babies are exposed. The value of corrective antepartum intervention was not specifically addressed in these studies, however, so we are unable to elucidate the degree of benefit such measures might contribute. Nonetheless, it is an acceptable medical premise—derived on both an intuitive basis and as a consequence of clinical experience—that some good, perhaps considerable at times, can be expected to result.

Suffice it to say at this point, objective measurement of these benefits had not yet been done in the same depth as reported here.

While the labor and delivery perils are central to the objectives of this investigation, it is the spectrum of adverse demographic, historical, physical, socioeconomic, antepartum, and intercurrent disease characteristics that may be most helpful for anticipating and avoiding problems which in turn will harm the fetus and infant. If properly alerted to the prevailing risk in a given patient, the physician can take appropriate measures for assiduous observation, aggressive study, learned consultation, and ameliorative treatment as needed. Subsequently in labor, knowledge about the risks associated with labor progression disorders, drugs, anesthesias, delivery practices, and complications will aid in modifying management to optimize outcome results. Needless to say, this goal is applicable to all cases, but it is perhaps most especially to be sought after in gravidas whose fetuses are at significantly increased risk. The additive hazards associated with certain labor and delivery conditions and procedures can be expected to create a particularly devastating peril for them.

Demographically, the gravida at greatest risk for an adverse perinatal outcome is the single black teenager (see Table 29-3). Although we are constrained from adding attributable risks because there may be interrelated effects, when all three of these risk factors occur in the same patient, the risk of a bad perinatal outcome undoubtedly increases considerably. Those under 16 years of age are uniquely vulnerable, the total perinatal risk for them increasing even more. If an untoward institutional effect also pertains, as it did at three of the collaborating study hospitals, the risk for the offspring of these young women could be still higher, all without any consideration being given to coexisting risk variables representing illnesses or conditions that might add even more risk.

The same demographic characteristics also affect late outcome results adversely (see Table 29-4). Single black teenagers expose their infants to a large excess risk of bad composite outcomes. For those under 16 years of age, the overall risk rises further. If the gravida is also a clinic patient, more composite outcome hazard is added as well and, if relevant, still more depending on the prevailing institutional risk.

Other demographic factors of importance for identifying the gravida-at-risk include marital separation or divorce. Separation increases the late composite risk by 2.0% (corrected data), while divorce augments perinatal risk by 2.4% (relative to a stable marriage), both substantially worse than being single (1.8% enhanced composite risk as an isolated risk factor). Just as early youth constitutes a hazard, advanced age does as well. Women undertaking pregnancy at age 30 or more increase composite outcome risk by 1.6%. The perinatal impact of advanced age (not described in the foregoing analyses) is 0.8% for age 30-34 years and 1.6% for 35+ years, but neither can be shown to be statistically significant.

The only information pertaining to obstetrical experience in prior pregnancy that shows a consistently bad effect on the current pregnancy is a premature birth in the past. This increases perinatal risk by 0.9% and composite outcome risk by 2.5%. Even in the absence of other coexistent adverse factors, therefore, one can expect exposure risks of 3.0% and 9.4%, respectively, when the background risk is added. If superimposed on one or more of the aforementioned demographic risk variables, the cumulative hazard becomes still greater. This is an important observation because premature birth occurs so often in association with some of them. An unmarried black gravida who has had a prior premature delivery, therefore, may add as much as 2.4% excess risk to the perinatal outcome (total 4.5%) and 4.8% to the composite outcome (total 12.7%); if still a teenager, her risks may tally to 3.2% and 7.2% (totalling 5.3% and 15.1%); and if also a clinic patient, the composite outcome could increase further to 9.0% (total 16.9%). One must be

cautioned again, however, that in reality these effects are not necessarily additive.

Short stature is a significant adverse physical characteristic which should alert the care provider to the increased risks that are likely to occur. Women who are less than 60 inches tall add 1.2% perinatal risk and 1.9% composite outcome risk to that which already exists, bringing the total for cases with this factor alone to 3.4% and 10.1%. Obesity, based on ponderal index, augments late composite hazard significantly by an additional 1.4%, but it does not appear to affect perinatal outcome. The 0.8% perinatal attributable risk associated with this factor was not found to be statistically significant. Those gravidas who smoke more than 30 cigarettes per day subject their infants to a burden of 3.8% bad composite outcomes. Any other concurrent risk factor may add to these, of course.

Socioeconomic factors are also helpful for recognizing the gravida-at-risk, especially in regard to those variables reflecting indigency. Gravidas with a low socioeconomic index, below 35 for example, enhance perinatal risk by 0.9% and composite outcome risk by 2.3%, for overall totals of 2.9% and 10.3% inclusive of background risk. Still lower indices raise the composite hazard, but not the perinatal, to 4.2% for those with an index of less than 15 (for a total composite outcome risk of 12.2%). As before, this adverse factor seldom occurs in isolation. Therefore, the perils attributable to accompanying risk factors may be cumulative. Thus, a 15-year-old single, black, clinic patient who has a socioeconomic index of 30 exposes her fetus to sizable hazards of bad perinatal and composite outcome.

Other poverty-related socioeconomic features that help identify the at-risk patient all impact principally on the composite outcome and, by implication, the developing infant. This does not mean they have no perinatal effect, but rather only that such effect as they have is not strong enough to be statistically significant. Low family income, for example, adds 2.5% to adverse composite outcome, high housing density 1.2%, and less than a grade school education 3.3%. Moreover, if the gravida had never been gainfully employed, another 2.3% risk is disclosed. If the baby's father is absent (deserted as distinct from formally separated, see above), the risk rises 3.7%. This is only slightly greater than if he is present but works in a blue-collar trade (3.2%). Both these last descriptors of the baby's father also have a demonstrably bad perinatal effect, although of a much smaller magnitude: 1.2% for absence and 0.3% for blue-collar employment.

Among antepartum factors, the patient who begins her prenatal care late identifies herself as being at risk. Those who appear for care at or beyond 28 weeks are particularly so, increasing the frequency of bad composite outcomes by 2.6%. Including background risk, the total hazard would be 9.3% for gravidas with this factor alone, but women who register late are often those with other risk factors prevailing, especially of a socioeconomic nature. The deleterious effect of late registration is not reflected in the perinatal results.

Analogously, gravidas who have not had at least seven antepartum visits for obstetrical care before delivery also increase the composite outcome risk to their infant. As discussed earlier, this often relates to late registration and/or early delivery; it may also come about because the patient fails to keep her appointments, being neglectful of her health over the course of pregnancy. While we have not separated out the differential impact of these several possibilities, it is clear that few antepartum visits alone increase composite outcome hazard by 1.8% (9.4% total), an effect independent of and perhaps additive to the risk attributable to late registration or premature delivery.

Delivery before term is a well recognized infant risk factor, of course. Its deleterious effect is generally ascribed to the small size and immature functional development of the infant. However, our data show that even infants who are ostensibly term-sized do not do well if delivered prematurely. As

will be recalled, we limited our final study population to those producing infants weighing between 2500 and 4000 g. Despite these tight birth weight constraints, delivery prior to 38 weeks increased perinatal risk by 1.9% (3.6% total) and composite outcome risk by 2.8% (10.1% total); prior to 36 weeks, by 2.6% and 3.7% (4.3% and 10.9% total). That delivery at still earlier gestational age, prior to 34 weeks, did not further increase the peril suggests dilution of the data by cases with erroneous dating.

A similar paradoxical effect had been seen earlier for postterm deliveries, those occurring beyond 44 weeks essentially losing the adverse influence clearly documented for women who deliver after 41 or 42 weeks, probably on the same basis (that is, misdating). Nonetheless, both perinatal and composite outcome risks are significantly increased by 1.0% (2.7% total) and 0.7% (7.9% total) for offspring of gravidas delivered beyond 42 weeks. After 41 weeks, only perinatal results confirm this adverse effect (0.9%, total 2.6%). Thus, both preterm and postterm labors serve as signals of high risk.

While low birth weight is an obvious risk factor for bad outcome, its specific impact was not assessed in this study by virtue of the aforementioned limits imposed for case selection. Within those limits, only one birth weight group showed some adverse composite effect (see above); as noted, it may merely have been a specious finding. Evidence of intrauterine growth retardation constitutes an overt risk factor for poor perinatal result (1.6%, total 3.8%). Given the current ultrasonographic capability to diagnose small-for-gestational-age infants before delivery, finding it serves as a useful index for identifying the gravida-at-risk. Similarly, recognizing that the fetus is male serves the same function for both perinatal (0.9%, total 2.6%) and composite outcome risk (2.5%, total 9.3%).

The medical problems to which pregnant women fall heir are legion. We have tried to learn which of them are most influential insofar as their effects on offspring are concerned. In the course of these studies, relatively few retain significant effects when all other concurrently acting risk variables are weighed in the balance. They fall into ten groups which, in descending order by magnitude of effect (based on weighted attributable risk data), are:

Central nervous system disorders
Colitis-ileitis
Glomerulonephritis
Diabetes mellitus
Severe anemia
Hyperthyroidism
Rh isoimmunization
Cholecystitis
Diastolic hypertension
Vaginal bleeding in early pregnancy

Among conditions affecting the maternal central nervous system, the worst infant impact is encountered consistently with mental retardation. One can expect 7.8% perinatal effect (10.1% in all after the base risk is added) and an astonishing 45.5% composite outcome effect (53.5% total) from this single factor alone. Convulsive disorders, including seizures in pregnancy, and other neurologic disorders primarily affect composite outcome (from 10.1% for pregnancy convulsions to 7.0% for epilepsy and other convulsive disorders). Inflammatory bowel disease is also a strong indicator of both perinatal (9.6%, total 12.1%) and composite outcome risk (30.4% total 38.5%). Glomerulonephritis follows with a remarkable 18.9% adverse perinatal effect (21.2% total) and a comparably large bad composite outcome risk (14.7%, total 22.9%).

Untoward fetal and infant effects of maternal diabetes have been well documented in the past, although the magnitude of the effects and how they are specifically altered by different clinical features may not have been so clear. Our findings may help in this regard. As expected, the presence of overt diabetes (other than gestational or chemical diabetes) carries a rather high risk, amounting to 4.9% for perinatal (a large figure, but

not statistically significant) and 6.8% for composite outcomes (total 7.2% and 14.9%). Those requiring insulin for metabolic control have 4.4% perinatal and 13.7% composite outcome effects; if out of control, as evidenced by substantive hyperglycemia, the superimposed risk is 6.8% and 7.4%, respectively (plus added base risk).

Severe maternal anemia with hematocrit levels below 20% yields a 12.0% perinatal effect, although it does not appear to have a comparable composite effect of either great magnitude or statistical significance (3.2%). Hyperthyroidism is also principally associated with bad perinatal results (8.0%) without a similar significant effect on composite outcome (3.0%). The effect of Rh isoimmunization varies, of course, according to its severity and the time in pregnancy when it arises. Overall, it causes 4.7% perinatal and 10.0% composite effects (the latter not statistically significant), obviously a major impact. Diastolic hypertension in late pregnancy appears to exert its action almost exclusively on composite outcome (3.1%), whereas the effects of cholecystitis and vaginal bleeding are seen primarily in the perinatal results (4.0% and 0.8%, respectively).

These then are the risk factors to which one should be alerted for purposes of identifying the gravida who places her fetus and infant in peril in advance of labor. The attributable risk data can be of additional value for determining the magnitude of the danger in terms of the chances of a bad outcome for both perinatal (death and severe depression) and composite measures (adverse result from the perinatal period to age 7 years). The relevant frequencies (weighted for concurrent labor-delivery risk factors) are shown in Table 29-5. For assessing a given patient, one could merely summate the risks pertaining to each risk variable she presents with and then add the base rate for the population at large. This latter is the referent risk which remains unaccounted for by the risk factors being weighed and to which all patients are, therefore, exposed. To the result of this calculation can also be added the intrapar-

Table 29-5
Identification of Gravida-at-Risk by Adverse Effects of Predictor Variables*

Risk Variable		Perinatal Risk %	Composite Risk %
AGE1	Maternal age < 20 yr.	(0.6)	1.7
AGE4	Maternal age 30-34 yr.	(0.7)	1.6
AGE6	Maternal age < 18 yr.	0.7	2.4
AGE7	Maternal age < 16 yr.	1.5	2.7
STATUS1	Clinic service patient	(1.0)	1.8
MARIT1	Single status	0.6	1.3
MARIT5	Divorced	2.4	(4.3)
MARIT6	Separated	(0.9)	2.0
RACE2	Black	0.9	1.1
RELIG2	Roman Catholic	(0.0)	-1.6
RELIG3	Jewish	(-1.0)	-4.9
ORIGIN1	Place of birth NY to PA	(0.0)	-1.3
ORIGIN15	Place of birth Europe	(-0.9)	-3.0
PPREM1	Prior premature birth	0.9	2.5
HGT2	Maternal height < 60 in.	1.2	1.9
POND2	Ponderal index obese	(0.8)	1.4
SMOKE3	Smokes > 30 per day	(0.3)	3.8
SES1	Socioeconomic index < 15	(1.1)	4.2
SES2	Socioeconomic index 15-24	(0.5)	2.3
SES3	Socioeconomic index 25-34	0.9	2.1
SES4	Socioeconomic index 35-44	1.2	(1.4)
SES8	Socioeconomic index 75-84	(-0.3)	-3.5
SES9	Socioeconomic index 85+	(-1.2)	-4.1
INCOME4	Per capita income $2250-2999	(-0.2)	-1.5
INCOME5	Per capita income $3000+	(0.0)	-1.7
FAMINC2	Family income < $2000/yr.	(0.4)	2.5
FAMINC6	Family income $8000-9999/yr.	(-0.7)	-2.1
FAMINC7	Family income $10,000+/yr.	(-1.3)	-2.6
HOUSE1	Housing density > 1.0 person per room	(0.1)	1.2
EDUC1	Education 7 yr. or less	(0.9)	3.3
EDUC2	Education 8 yr.	(0.7)	2.3
EDUC3	Education 9-11 yr.	(0.2)	1.2
EDUC5	Education 13-15 yr.	-1.1	-3.0
EDUC6	Education 16+ yr.	(-1.2)	-5.0
WORKG1	Gravida never worked	(0.4)	2.2
WORKG2	Gravida white collar worker	-0.8	-4.1
WORKF3	Father of baby a student	1.2	-3.1
WORKF5	Father of baby absent	(1.8)	3.7
OCCUPF3	Father of baby blue collar worker	0.3	3.2
GREG6	Registered at 28-31.9 wk.	(0.7)	2.6
GREG8	Registered at 36+ wk.	(0.2)	2.1
TRIMEST3	Registered in third trimester	(0.3)	2.2
VISIT1	Prenatal visits < 7	(0.1)	1.8
GDEL1	Delivery at < 34 wk.	2.8	3.2
GDEL2	Delivery at < 36 wk.	2.6	3.7
GDEL3	Delivery at < 38 wk.	1.9	2.8

GDEL4	Delivery at > 41 wk.	0.9	(1.1)
GDEL5	Delivery at > 42 wk.	1.0	0.7
BW2	Birth weight 2750-2999 g.	(0.4)	1.8
SGA	Small for gestational age	1.6	(0.9)
MALE	Male infant	0.9	2.5
HCT1	Lowest hematocrit < 20%	12.0	(3.2)
VAGBLD	Early pregnancy bleeding	0.8	(1.8)
RHSENS	Rh isoimmunization	4.7	(10.0)
PIH1	Diastolic hypertension	(0.7)	3.1
DIS49	Diabetes mellitus	(4.9)	6.8
DIS50	Hyperglycemia 200+ mg./dl.	(6.8)	7.4
DIS51	Insulin therapy	4.4	13.7
DIS63	Hyperthyroidism	8.0	(3.0)
DIS80	Glomerulonephritis	18.9	14.7
DIS98	Convulsive disorder	(0.6)	7.0
DIS99	Convulsion in pregnancy	(0.1)	10.1
DIS100	Maternal mental retardation	7.9	45.5
DIS103	Neurological disorder	3.6	10.1
DIS107	Cholecystitis	4.0	0.9)
DIS111	Colitis-ileitis	9.6	30.4

* The data are the weighted attributable risks for each variable. Figures in parentheses represent risk levels for factors not found to be statistically significant. Positive values are adverse; negative are protective.

tum and delivery risk, as defined by the attributable risk information shown earlier in this chapter, according to the types of problems that develop or the intervention one anticipates undertaking.

The result of this process cannot be considered to represent the actual risk to which the fetus is exposed, of course, but rather an estimate of the impact if there were no confounding or interactional effects between variables. In order to obtain a more correct quantitative summation of attributable risk for a series of risk variables, it would be necessary to return to the logistic regression coefficient for each variable, such as those listed in Tables 26-7 and 26-8 for labor-delivery factors. These can be added together, as needed. The natural antilog gives the relative risk which can then be substituted in the formula for attributable risk

$$AR = (RR - 1)rr$$

where RR is the newly derived relative risk and rr is the base rate or referent risk. Empirical comparative testing of this calculation against the more simplistic summation of the weighted attributable risks shows the former to be somewhat larger in all cases. This means that merely adding the attributable risk values together in a given case gives a conservative estimate of the true risk to the fetus, again assuming no confounding among variables.

CHAPTER 30

Impact on Clinical Practice

Summary

The attributable risk data on labor-delivery risk variables, as derived in the preceding chapter, were reviewed in detail. These dealt with definable labor course pattern abnormalities, pharmacologic agents and anesthesias, specific delivery interventions, such as forceps operations, delivery control, Kristeller pressure, and labor induction and augmentation, as well as malpresentation and complications. Knowledge about the magnitude of the risks of each of these variables in regard to outcome was shown to be useful for purposes of modifying obstetrical practices to ensure appropriate risk-benefit balance in favor of the fetus and infant, whenever possible.

In the course of these complex analyses, it was essential to avoid losing sight of the original objectives of the investigational program. Our intent was to determine which labor and delivery factors were associated with significant impact on the offspring when the effects of all others were being considered simultaneously. We pursued this aim assiduously and have been able to show that the goal was not completely elusive, no matter how difficult to reach. Along the way, we delved into issues pertaining to the effects on outcome of labor progression disorders, drugs and anesthesias, and the broad array of delivery events and interventions. In addition, we examined a spectrum of intrinsic characteristics and prelabor conditions for purposes of providing information for recognizing the gravida who is likely to place her fetus and infant at risk independent of subsequent labor and delivery hazards.

Having now identified those risk factors and measured the magnitude of their adverse impact, we could take the opportunity to suggest how obstetrical practice might be altered so as to improve outcome. In its least adorned form, such advice might consist merely of an admonition to avoid all those risk variables documented to expose the fetus to peril. The list includes the range of items shown in Table 30-1. Also displayed is the degree of excess risk that can be expected from each factor acting alone—that is, the percentage increase in adverse perinatal and composite outcome above the background or underlying base risk for the population of gravidas at large.

In the real world of clinical practice, however, things are seldom so simple. Some

Table 30-1
Summary of Adverse Effects of Labor-Delivery Risk Variables*

Risk Variable		Perinatal Risk %	Composite Risk %
LAT3	Prolonged latent phase	1.0	(1.3)
ACT2	Foreshortened active phase	0.8	(0.7)
ACT3	Prolonged active phase	1.0	(1.1)
DESC3	Precipitate descent	(-0.6)	-1.1
SPINAL	Spinal anesthesia	0.1	-1.0
PARAC	Paracervical block	0.7	(1.0)
GAS2	Continuous inhalation anesthesia	0.3	(1.7)
AGT1	Demerol	0.3	(0.3)
AGT16	Vistaril	(1.0)	3.5
AGT22	Apresoline	8.7	10.4`
AGT23	Syntocinon	(0.1)	-2.2
AGT24	Oxytocin	(2.5)	4.4
AGT27	Other antibiotics	21.1	34.6
FORTRAC2	Difficult forceps traction	4.1	2.9
FORTRAC3	Very difficult forceps traction	5.3	9.4
FORTRAC4	Failed forceps traction	(21.0)	24.2
FORAPP2	Difficult forceps application	(2.6)	2.0
FORAPP3	Very difficult forceps application	(6.9)	3.5
FORROT2	Difficult forceps rotation	3.0	(2.1)
FORROT3	Very difficult forceps rotation	11.9	(4.0)
FORROT4	Failed forceps rotation	16.0	(8.0)
CONTROL1	Manual control of head	0.0	(1.0)
CONTROL3	Forceps control of head	-0.3	-1.5
FUNDAL2	Moderate fundal pressure	0.3	0.8
FUNDAL3	Strong fundal pressure	0.7	1.9
ABRUPT	Abruptio placentae	5.3	(2.6)
PROLAP	Prolapsed cord	(7.2)	7.3
CSVAG	Cesarean after failed vaginal attempt	3.4	9.8
SHOULD	Shoulder dystocia	6.6	6.1
INDUCT3	Induction for PIH	4.0	9.6
INDUCT6-9	Induction for other indications	4.6	(4.6)
AUGMENT6	Stimulation for amnionitis	43.8	44.1
PRES5-8	Breech presentation	4.7	(5.1)
BRDELIV3	Breech extraction	(9.7)	16.8
PRES11	Brow presentation	(4.9)	9.2
REACT3	Uterine hypertonus from oxytocin	7.8	(7.0)

* These data are weighted attributable risks for each variable. Figures in parentheses represent risk levels for factors not found to be statistically significant. Positive values are adverse; negative are protective.

risks are clearly unavoidable insofar as they consist of complications that are not under the control of attendant personnel, such as dysfunctional labor, cord prolapse, abruptio placentae, and fetal malpresentation. There are times when circumstances require intervention even though the treatment itself carries risk. Essentially every medical management decision must, therefore, balance the risk of the therapeutic measures invoked for a given condition against the risk of not administering it or against the risk of alternative means. Too often, when called upon to make such critical decisions, physicians do not have all the necessary information they need, especially as regards accurate quantitation of the risk of the procedure or of the drug under consideration. The data presented here should go far toward correcting that deficiency.

Labor Progression Risk Factors

When labor progression variables were examined as a group in isolation from other labor, drug, anesthesia, delivery, and intrinsic influences (chapter 14), eight were found to have substantive adverse effects on offspring and one appeared protective. These nine retained residual impact even after intensive analysis by a series of studies involving bivariate screening, cluster analysis, and several forms of logistic regression analysis, all done to ensure against confounding or interactional effects. Bad perinatal outcome (death or severe depression) was determined in this way to be significantly associated with LAT2 (foreshortened latent phase), LAT3 (prolonged latent phase), ACT2 (foreshortened active phase), ACT3 (prolonged active phase), SEC3 (prolonged second stage), DESC2 (protracted descent), and ARRS3 (arrest of descent) and adverse composite outcome (perinatal to 7 years) with ACT2, ACT3, and DEC3 (prolonged deceleration phase). Only DESC3 (precipitate descent) showed significantly good results, limited to composite outcome. After the more all-encompassing analyses of the full aggregate of all relevant risk factors were undertaken to deal with the issue of interaction (chapter 25), only four labor progression variables were left with persistent effect, three adverse (LAT3, ACT2, and ACT3) and one still protective (DESC3).

It should be re-emphasized at this point that others may also have some effect on fetal well-being, but those effects could not be substantiated statistically in the body of data at hand. This failure to be verified could have come about because the effects were not strongly manifested (either there was actually a small magnitude effect or perhaps a large one associated with an extremely rare event) or were subsumed by the effects of coexisting factors, including those of the measures undertaken to treat them.

For example, the adverse perinatal effect of DESC2 had been quite sizable in its earliest occurrence in this study. This was especially the case in multiparas among whom it had a risk ratio of 2.55 (see Table 14-11), rising to a highly significant 3.64 in the step-up logistic regression model (see Table 14-14). Nonetheless, when all other factors were taken into account simultaneously (see Table 25-5), its risk ratio fell to an insignificant 1.20. (Note that it retained some degree of risk, 20% in excess of that expected, but that risk was no longer statistically verifiable.)

One explanation for this deflation is that a component of the factor's adverse effect was being incorporated into the risk of associated conditions and interventive measures, such as uterotonic stimulation, forceps rotation and delivery, Kristeller pressure, or cesarean section after failed attempt to effect vaginal delivery, all seriously adverse factors in their own right. Thus, while the factors we have identified as significantly affecting outcome are clearly those with the strongest and most consistent influences, others should not necessarily be assumed to be risk-free.

Prolonged Latent Phase. The labor disorder of prolonged latent phase (LAT3) carries an excess adverse perinatal impact of

1.0% (2.0% if concurrent labor and delivery risk factors are not considered simultaneously) and bad long-term outcome of 1.3% (the latter not statistically significant). While it is an unavoidable complication of labor insofar as we know at this juncture, clinicians should be aware of its associated hazard and conduct themselves accordingly. Management principles have been expounded in the past for purposes of minimizing both maternal and fetal complications.* Emphasis was placed on timely recognition of the problem and its relatively benign nature if handled appropriately, namely by prescribing a program of therapeutic rest in the form of morphine sulfate. Alternatively, if any delay in effecting delivery is unacceptable—an unusual situation—and conditions are propitious (that is, the cervix is favorable, the vertex is presenting and well engaged, and there is no disproportion), oxytocin stimulation could be invoked instead.

To proceed with aggressive intervention in the face of unfavorable conditions tends to be inappropriate in most cases whether by uterotonic stimulation or amniotomy. These measures may unnecessarily expose the mother and the fetus to the perils of a long, difficult labor perhaps sometimes complicated by such serious conditions as amnionitis, arrested labor, cord prolapse, abruptio placentae, uterine rupture, and others.

It seems likely that the associated complications or interventions account for some or all the hazard of this labor aberration because past data have not shown a comparably bad effect from it when managed conservatively. When one realizes that a substantial proportion of cases with prolonged latent phase are actually in false labor, one can begin to appreciate how illogical it is to consider undertaking aggressive and potentially hazardous intervention in a condition of this nature, unless clearly indi-

cated. There can be little justification in terms of counterbalancing benefit otherwise.

Precipitate Labor. Earlier, we recognized that ACT2 (foreshortened active phase) and MAXS3 (precipitate dilatation) were interchangeable variables, describing essentially the same phenomenon of abnormally rapid progression of the cervical dilatation pattern in the active phase of first stage labor. Their effect on the fetus and infant is small in absolute terms at 0.8% perinatal and 0.7% composite risk (only the former being statistically significant), but it cannot be ignored. The fetal hazard of precipitate labor is generally agreed to be associated with hypoxia caused by excessively frequent and forceful uterine contractions and/or the trauma resulting from unduly rapid descent through the birth canal (so-called compression-decompression or "blast" effect). This condition may result from use of uterotonic agents, especially if associated with excessive uterine contractility or tumultuous labor.

Our inability to demonstrate a parallel adverse effect from precipitate descent (DESC3) or foreshortened second stage (SEC2) goes counter to this concept. Indeed, rapid descent was shown to be somewhat protective in regard to composite outcome, but negligibly so in its perinatal effect. Furthermore, if we return to the raw data for outcome by slope of descent, uncorrected for confounding by concurrent labor disorders (see Table 11-13), we find a rather clear association between rapid descent and bad outcomes. While confounding is a possible explanation for this discrepancy, it may also be that precipitate descent patterns do occur spontaneously, often in otherwise normal multiparas. In such cases, any adverse effect might be counterbalanced (if not overcompensated for) by the good results ordinarily expected in uncomplicated cases. Moreover, the deleterious impact of concurrent oxytocin and uterine hypercontractility is accounted for separately in these analyses (see below). Similarly, the adverse effect of precipitate

*Friedman EA: Labor: Clinical Evaluation and Management, ed 2. New York, Appleton-Century-Crofts, 1977, p 369.

dilatation, clearly demonstrated, may itself be a confounding factor insofar as the effect of precipitate descent is concerned because the two patterns are so often concurrent in the same labor.

These conjectural considerations probably do not explain the paradoxical observations in a completely satisfactory manner. This holds especially since the protective composite effects shown for precipitate descent were noted exclusively in nulliparas rather than multiparas (see Tables 14-15 and 25-6). In the overview then, precipitate dilatation is probably deleterious as demonstrated. Precipitate descent, however, may not be unless it is associated with or caused by factors which carry adverse effects themselves.

In practical terms, a diagnosis of precipitate dilatation occurring spontaneously without uterotonic stimulation may or may not give the clinician sufficient time and opportunity to intervene with regional conduction block anesthesia (peridural) or less preferably with heavy sedation or β-adrenergic agents to diminish the contractility and thereby inhibit the rapid progress, averting potential damage in consequence. If stimulation by oxytocin infusion is the cause, the drug must be stopped at once. Given the short half-life of circulating oxytocin (three minutes), its effect can be expected to subside in short order provided it was being administered as a dilute solution by the IV route. Because administration by other routes (intramuscular, buccal, and intranasal) are not amenable to this kind of rapid reversal, they cannot be condoned.

Moreover, even oxytocin by intravenous infusion has to be given in a most carefully controlled manner to avoid overstimulation which can lead in turn to precipitate labor. This entails constant monitoring of uterine response and fetal well-being by trained personnel backed by physicians who are immediately available in the event of complications and who are knowledgeable about how to diagnosis, evaluate, and manage such complications expeditously. Use of

a pump mechanism is far superior to a drip for accuracy and control.

In addition, it is essential that patients be evaluated before they are given oxytocin to determine if they may be prone to develop precipitate labor. Gravidas who have a prior history of precipitate labor or rapid uncontrolled delivery, for example, are not appropriate candidates. If oxytocin must be used under such circumstances, one might consider giving a peridural anesthesia first, thereby ensuring some degree of inhibition in advance of the oxytocin.

Protraction Disorder. Just as a short active phase stands as the alter ego for precipitate dilatation, so prolonged active phase (ACT3) substitutes for protracted active-phase dilatation (MAXS2). Abnormally slow active phase progress yields a 1.0% excess adverse perinatal effect (2.4% uncorrected) and a 1.1% composite effect (the latter statistically insignificant). This impact applies regardless of the presence or absence of other coexistent risk factors, implying an adverse influence from the labor pattern itself.

The pathogenetic mechanism of the hazard may be related to unrecognized associated hypoxia or perhaps to the trauma of accompanying interventive measures. Since the effects of the latter measures are not entirely accounted for in these abnormal labors by our analytical approach, it must follow that the labor predisposes to bad outcomes above and beyond that which can be expected under less stressful circumstances. In other words, the risk factors act in a complementary or synergistic fashion. Because the adverse effects of the more difficult procedures are dealt with and flagged here, it is also likely that some of the residual effects seen with protraction disorders are related to the unmeasured impact of less difficult operations, which are probably innocuous except in conjunction with these labor disorders and perhaps with other adverse influences as well.

The same probably applies to protracted descent (DESC2) as well. This disorder had been shown objectively to be bad in regard to its effect on offspring in the raw data dealing with the relation between outcome and low slopes of the descent process (see Table 11-13). These data were obtained without consideration for the concurrent effects of other labor disorders. When such effects were considered, protracted descent continued to show highly significant adverse effects (see Table 14-15). Although the effect was still present to some extent in the full aggregative analysis that had taken into account coexistent labor and prelabor factors (see Tables 25-3 and 25-5), the effect of the factor of protracted descent was no longer statistically significant. This meant that whatever effect this factor had had was related to or subsumed or counterbalanced by concurrent variables, including those pertaining to interventions undertaken to treat the condition (oxytocin, for example) or to accomplish the delivery (such as forceps rotation and traction).

There is little one can do to improve progress in labor when the disorder of protracted dilatation or protracted descent exists. Stimulation has not been shown to be effective and may only complicate the situation by adding the risks of the oxytocin. Nonetheless, it is obviously important for the obstetrical attendant to recognize when the labor aberration develops so that all necessary evaluation can be undertaken and management can be modified accordingly. The association between protraction disorders and cephalopelvic disproportion makes it mandatory to rule out bony dystocia first. If disproportion can be documented, it gives one adequate justification to proceed with cesarean section. If not, the patient must be followed carefully in labor with close surveillance by electronic fetal heart rate monitoring for evidence of fetal distress.

Moreover, it is important to avoid giving medication or anesthesia that is likely to inhibit the already dilatory progress of labor. These patients are especially sensitive to the delaying effects of both narcotic analgesics and peridural anesthesia. Of even greater concern, one must guard against invoking interventions which are potentially harmful to the fetus as a consequence of trauma, most notably operative instrumentation with forceps to effect vaginal delivery. The seriously adverse effects of difficult forceps procedures (see below) are undoubtedly magnified in a patient who has had a protraction disorder. Similar enhancement of adverse effect may convert a forceps operation that cannot otherwise be shown to be harmful under ordinary clinical circumstances into a potentially hazardous one if done in the presence of protracted dilatation or protracted descent.

Arrest Disorder. None of the arrest disorders was significantly associated with adverse residual effect when all other factors were weighed simultaneously. Once again, this does not mean that these conditions are free of risk. It will be recalled that both prolonged deceleration phase (DEC3) and arrest of descent (ARRS3) were found to be significantly harmful factors when examined alone or in conjunction with other labor progression variables (see Tables 13-22 and 14-15). Their significance faded, however, in the aggregative analysis, indicating that almost all their impact could be accounted for or attributable to other concurrent variables in large measure, although some statistically insignificant residual effects could still be detected (see Table 25-5).

The implication of these findings is that it is not necessarily the arrest that causes the damage, but rather some factor associated with arrested labor, most probably related to management. Uterotonic stimulation and instrumental manipulation for achieving (or attempting to achieve) vaginal delivery are likely candidates for this role. Not only do some evoke clearly demonstrated inherent deleterious effects, but it is probable that similar effects arise from more benign manipulation done concurrently with (that is, as treatment for) an arrest disorder. If such risk factors are not imposed, however, an arrest disorder does not appear to carry very much demonstrably bad impact on its own.

From the clinical point of view, arrest disorders should conjure an image of cephalopelvic disproportion. Since about half the cases are associated with disproportion, the clinician has a positive obligation to evaluate the cephalopelvic relationship before proceeding. If disproportion is present, cesarean section is clearly warranted; if not, uterotonic stimulation will often prove successful in causing additional progress in dilatation and/or descent so that atraumatic vaginal delivery can eventuate. Careful fetal monitoring is critical during such augmentation of labor to detect any evidence of hypoxia and thereby to ensure against fetal compromise.

Moreover, one must maintain close vigil on maternal status in order to recognize when the oxytocin is not accomplishing any further progress or the progression in dilatation or descent is so slow as to suggest that there may be an insurmountable obstruction which had not been correctly diagnosed earlier. Of special concern because of its serious associated risk is the error of interpreting the advancement of fetal station due to molding as if it were true descent. Proper diagnosis requires verification that the caudally advancing forward leading edge of the fetal head, as observed by serial vaginal examinations, is true descent. This can be done by noting comparable advancement of the base of the fetal skull by periodic suprapubic palpation. Failure to recognize that the fetal head is fixed in the pelvis and that descent is not occurring despite uterotonic stimulation exposes the fetus to great danger from the trauma to its intracranial contents from excessive molding. If a difficult forceps procedure is superimposed in addition, this risk is considerably aggravated. This enhanced risk applies whether the attempted delivery procedure is successful or not, as our data clearly demonstrate (see below).

Adjunctive Drug and Anesthesia Risk Factors

Isolated examination of the wide array of drugs and anesthesias which are administered to parturients in labor had shown a limited number, 45 in all, to be associated with fetal and infant effects. When all were considered collectively by cluster and logistic regression analyses, 17 emerged as retaining a strongly, statistically verifiable relationship to outcome (chapter 18). Five dealt with oxytocin use (induction, augmentation, and both induction and augmentation, plus Syntocinon and Pitocin), six with anesthesia (spinal, pudendal, and paracervical block, continuous inhalation anesthesia, combined intermittent and continuous gas, and intravenous anesthesia) and six with various drugs used in labor. All but three showed adverse effects. The three protective variables were spinal, Nisentil, and Syntocinon. When reexamined in conjunction with the full assembly of other labor, delivery, and intrinsic factors (chapter 25) to account for confounding and interactional effects, only nine were left. They included all six anesthesias, two oxytocin variables (OXYT2, augmentation and AGT24, Pitocin), and one drug (AGT16, Vistaril). The same caveats expressed earlier for labor progression variables also apply here. Other adjunctive drugs and anesthesias may also carry risk, but the method of analysis identified and measured the effects of only those with the most pervasive influence.

Anesthesia. Administration of spinal anesthesia (SPINAL, rarely more than saddle block effect) was largely protective, reducing attributable composite risk by 1.0% (2.3% uncorrected) and enhancing perinatal risk negligibly (0.1%). Uncorrected perinatal data showed a protective effect of 0.6%. The apparent benefits of this form of anesthesia are probably related to patient selection. The anesthesia was (and in some places, continues to be) used by the saddle block technique and was very commonly invoked to provide pain relief in the last few moments of a normally progressive labor in an otherwise healthy woman without serious delivery complications. The outcome in such cases should, therefore, have been expected to be quite good. Thus, the ostensible protection associated with spinal anesthesia can probably be discounted as specious. Moreover, even if the anesthesia did have any potentially bad fetal or infant effect (for example, from the hypotension and diminished uterine blood flow that may occur), its duration of action prior to birth was probably too short in most cases for the effect to have any real or lasting impact.

Paracervical block (PARAC), by contrast, had a 0.7% deleterious perinatal effect (2.7% uncorrected) despite the common practice of administering it to a similar population of otherwise uncomplicated cases usually in the last minutes of labor. Although the patient selection bias should have yielded a protective effect, the result was adverse. This contradictory finding suggests the probability that PARAC is actually worse in regard to its perinatal effect than it was determined to be by these analyses. The seriously adverse influence of this form of anesthesia on the fetus has been shown by a number of prior published studies.* Intense bradycardia may result. Although it is usually transient in nature, the infant may be born in an asphyxic condition and succumb. Some have demonstrated that the effect may reflect the type of anesthetic agent used,† rather than the technique. Nevertheless, the perinatal risk to the fetus shown here is entirely supportive of the earlier clinical studies which demonstrated overriding risk. Unless newer data can show PARAC to be devoid of hazard, that risk appears to outweigh the benefits of this anesthetic method over alternative local or regional block anesthesias.

---

*Freeman RK: Fetal cardiac response to paracervical block anesthesia. *Am J Obstet Gynecol* 1977; 113:583; Ralston DH, Shnider SM: The fetal and neonatal effects of regional anesthesia in obstetrics. *Anesthesiology* 1978; 48:34; Morishima HO, Covino BG: Bradycardia following paracervical block in the fetal baboon. *Anesthesiology* 1980; 53:S318.
†Weiss RR, Halevy S, Almonte RO, et al: Comparison of lidocaine and 2-chloroprocaine in paracervical blocks: Clinical effects and drug concentrations in mother and child. *Anesth Analg* 1983; 62:168.

General inhalation anesthesia administered on a continuous basis (GAS2) had been distinguished from those given intermittently (GAS1) either by an anesthetist or self-administered by the patient. Although the latter could not be shown to carry any special hazard by our foregoing investigations, GAS2 did. It enhanced perinatal risk significantly by 0.3% (2.3% uncorrected). Trends in obstetrical anesthesia have diminished use of this mode over the years, perhaps with good reason. Women increasingly desire to be awake so as to experience the birthing process and to participate actively in infant bonding. To this end, many go through labor with little or no analgesia and accomplish delivery only with some local or regional block or even with no anesthesia. This gratifying development has certainly yielded fewer depressed babies at birth and may have contributed other advantages insofar as parenting is concerned. At minimum, the degree of risk exposure occurring as a consequence of GAS2 is thereby averted.

Analgesia for Labor. Meperidine (AGT1, Demerol) and hydroxyzine (AGT16, Vistaril, Atarax) were rather commonly given in combination for pain relief in labor. Both were shown to carry fetal and infant risk: AGT1 0.3% perinatal and AGT16 3.5% composite. We have already alluded to the declining use of analgesic and ataractic agents over the years for relieving the pain of labor. Any associated fetal and infant risk can be expected to fall in parallel.

The paradox of adverse effects from AGT1 and lack of adverse (and better than average) effects from AGT2 can only be explained in two ways. First, the effects may be real and these two closely related agents might actually have opposite actions on the fetus, a most unlikely postulate. Second, the patient populations to whom the drugs were given may have differed in some major ways. The latter is a much more plausible hypothesis. It assumes the differences in population make-up were not completely accounted for by the logistic regression models we employed. AGT2 was introduced and administered preferentially to healthy private patients, for example. Contrariwise, AGT1 was widely used among clinic patients. Given the strong impact of socioeconomic status, income, and education, the outcome results should, therefore, have been somewhat better for those receiving AGT2 than for the general unmedicated population and considerably better than for those getting AGT1. The relatively small and equivalently counterbalancing attributable risks for two agents with such similar pharmacologic effects suggest their fetal and infant effects are on average negligible, but there may be some nontrivial risk in high-risk labors (see Table 27-19), nonetheless.

Uterotonic Agents. The same or similar logic probably applies to the conflictual findings in regard to the composite outcome effects of AGT23 (Syntocinon) and AGT24 (Pitocin). The former was protective with an attributable risk of -2.2%, the latter adverse at 4.4% (7.3% uncorrected). There is even greater similarity between these two products than between Nisentil and Demerol. Their structure and function are identical; only the methods of manufacture differ. Thus, it is just not reasonable to ascribe the difference in effect to differential drug actions (although it is remotely possible, of course, perhaps as a consequence of the action of preservatives or contaminants). A difference in the characteristics of the patients and the patterns of drug use in clinical practice is more likely to account for some of the difference instead, as implied for analgesic effects.

However, contrary to the small and roughly equivalent risk and benefit attributable to AGT1 and AGT2, those associated with AGT23 and AGT24 were very dissimilar. This could be interpreted to mean that population make-up differences were not evenly balanced. Alternatively and more likely, there was indeed an adverse drug effect associated with both drug variables, but it was heavily overclouded by the protective factors prevalent in the population subgroup of patients to

whom AGT23 was given and perhaps made worse by the associated deleterious characteristics of women given AGT24.

Furthermore, we have already seen that many, if not all, of the bad outcome results found with oxytocin use were related to the indication for which it was invoked. The powerful residual effects of INDUCT3 (induction of labor for pregnancy-induced hypertension) and AUGMENT6 (stimulation for amnionitis) confirm this observation (see below). Whether other uses of oxytocin also carry substantive risk, particularly the more common elective use for induction (no longer condoned) or augmentation, cannot be stated with confidence, but neither can they be said to be entirely risk-free in view of the impressive outcome data for AGT24. It must follow, therefore, that oxytocin use should be limited to those situations in which its benefits will clearly counterbalance any hazard inherent in the drug or its use.

Other Drugs. The hypotensive agent, hydralazine (AGT22, Apresoline), has a seriously deleterious perinatal effect on offspring, enhancing bad outcomes by 8.7% (10.2% uncorrected). Needless to say, the drug is not invoked in labor except to treat very severe hypertension. Our analyses did not permit us to separate out the effect of the drug, if any, from the effect of the condition for which it was used. However, a prior comparable study* had demonstrated that cases in which antihypertensive drugs employed for treating specific types of pregnancy hypertension had between two and four times the fetal mortality of those who were untreated. Although cases were similar in regard to the presence or absence of diastolic hypertension and/or proteinuria, it was still possible that the drug served as a marker for the most severely affected cases.

In a similar vein, AGT27 (other antibiotics) could also have merely represented a variable for designating the most serious

---

*Friedman EA, Neff RK: *Pregnancy Hypertension: A Systematic Evaluation of Clinical Diagnostic Criteria.* Littleton, Mass, PSG Publishing Co, 1977, p 201.

infections—that is, those which did not respond readily to the more commonly used antibiotics. Its attributable perinatal and composite risks were extreme at 21.1% and 34.6%, respectively. Whether the more powerful antibiotics carry any serious risk above and beyond that of the infection for which they have to be given cannot be answered from these data. Given the life-threatening nature of resistant or fulminating infections, the issue is not too relevant. When one weighs the risk-benefit relationship under such circumstances, there is usually little argument that the peril of the condition to mother and fetus generally far outweighs the risk of the agent, unless there is a safer alternative option.

Delivery Factors

Of the original 1980 delivery variables we investigated collectively (chapter 24), 47 still showed significant effects on fetus and infant after they had been screened and studied by our series of probing analyses. When further examined in aggregate with all other labor, drug, and intrinsic variables (chapter 25), 25 continued to show evidence of significant impact on the fetus and surviving infant. Except for two variables that showed protective effects (CONTROL1 and CONTROL3, manual and forceps control of the fetal head at delivery, as contrasted with spontaneous, uncontrolled delivery), all were significantly deleterious in regard to their association with outcome to offspring.

The largest affinity subgroup of variables consisted of 15 related to actual delivery intervention procedures, namely nine dealing with forceps use, two with fundal pressure, three with control of the fetal head at vaginal vertex delivery, and one with cesarean section after failed attempt to achieve vaginal delivery. Four addressed induction or stimulation of labor and the patient's reaction to uterotonic stimulation. Three represented fetal malpresentation (two for breech and one for brow). The last three risk factors dealt with the major delivery complications of abruptio placentae, cord prolapse, and shoulder dystocia.

Forceps Operation. All nine of the forceps-use risk factors related to procedures that were considered difficult, very difficult, or failed forceps operations. To put this information in perspective, it will be recalled that this study used disinterested (not uninterested), trained observers to record their observations in as objective a manner as feasible while the procedure was being performed. Assessment of the degree of difficulty in application, traction, or rotation of forceps, therefore, should neither have been influenced by the outcome in hindsight nor have reflected the subjective impression of the obstetrical attendant. Absent actual physiologic measurements of the forces exerted, this approach was felt to be as reliable as could be attained.

Midforceps (FORCEPS3, applied at station 0 to +2) had been found to be a very strong determinant of bad outcome. This was especially apparent in regard to composite results in nulliparas who showed a remarkable relative risk of 8.7 (see Table 25-6). When parity subgroups were collapsed and the impact of this variable was examined in concert with other labor and delivery variables, most notably those dealing with difficulty assessments, its adverse effect was no longer verifiable as statistically significant. It is rather likely that its effect was subsumed by the factors which describe the difficulty associated with the different components of forceps operations, namely application, traction and rotation. The latter in turn not only applied to midforceps procedures, but appeared to be equally relevant to forceps employed at lower pelvic stations as well.

Our data show a bad impact from forceps placed at high station related principally, but not exclusively, to difficult or failed procedures. Similarly, difficult or failed forceps operations carry serious risk. Perinatal hazard, for example, is increased 4.1% by difficult forceps traction (FORTRAC2) and 5.3% by very difficult traction (FORTRAC3); the attributable risk is 6.1% and

10.7% if coexistent labor-delivery risk factors are not considered. Moreover, these operations add 2.9% and 9.4% (3.3% and 10.3% uncorrected) to the composite risk, respectively, whereas failed forceps traction (FORTRAC4) is associated with a startling 21.0% and 24.2% attributable risk for adverse perinatal and composite outcome (the perinatal risk is not statistically significant).

Difficult forceps application was shown to affect perinatal outcome, but not significantly so (2.6% difficult, 6.9% very difficult); nonetheless, it did add significantly to poor composite outcomes: 2.0% if difficult and 3.5% if very difficult (2.2% and 4.5% uncorrected). Forceps rotation, which had been shown to have a deleterious overall effect regardless of difficulty, was shown to have a very unfavorable perinatal impact with a 3.0% attributable risk if difficult, 11.9% if very difficult, and 16.0% if failed (3.2%, 13.0%, and 18.2% uncorrected). The composite outcome risks were also high, but did not reach levels necessary for statistical verification.

Whether the effects of high station and of difficulty are additive or synergistic could not be determined, but it is clear that those risks pertaining to the several component actions are. Each has been shown to retain statistically significant adverse effects even when those of the others are taken into account simultaneously. One of the more impressive findings of these analyses is that for cases in which cesarean section had to be undertaken after all attempts to achieve vaginal delivery had failed (CSVAG), including—but not limited to—failed forceps operations. The 3.4% perinatal and 9.8% composite risks (11.9% and 49.4% crude) associated with this factor stand as testimony to its very serious nature.

These observations need not be interpreted as condemnation of all forceps use. We have seen an apparently protective effect from forceps control of the delivery of the fetal head (CONTROL3, see below). While the seemingly paradoxical benefit can be readily explained on the basis of patient selection, it does at least suggest that most forceps procedures are not harmful. The protection appears to apply only in regard to preventing the damage from uncontrolled delivery; the same benefit accrues to controlled manual delivery. Those forceps procedures deemed to have been difficult or to have failed can be shown to impose a substantive risk on the fetus and infant. They must, therefore, be avoided.

If one can anticipate that such difficulty will be encountered, one should reconsider the wisdom of undertaking the forceps procedure. Under these circumstances, one has to weigh the risk of any prevailing fetal condition against benefits and risks of expectant delay (that is, allowing the labor to continue under appropriate surveillance), or of labor stimulation, or of an alternative delivery method (for example, cesarean section). Unless there is some strong, documentable argument favoring forceps intervention over a less hazardous option, proceeding to use forceps when it is likely to be difficult (and therefore perilous) is unacceptable.

The range of conditions under which difficulty of application, traction, or rotation is likely to be encountered includes those associated with or indicative of the presence of cephalopelvic disproportion. Numbered among them are the major aberrations of labor, particularly the patterns of protraction and arrest of dilatation or descent, and other indices of obstructed labor, such as persistent malposition or maladaptation of the fetal head to the maternal pelvis, especially if occurring in a woman with a large infant and/or a small pelvis. The obstetrical team has to be alert to such manifestations signaling a possible impediment to an atraumatic vaginal delivery. One must recognize and carefully consider the risks to which the fetus is exposed if a forceps procedure were to be undertaken.

Delivery Control. In cases with vertex presentation, uncontrolled precipitate delivery of the fetal head (CONTROL2, to be contrasted with precipitate dilatation or precipitate descent with which it is often, but not invariably, related) constitutes an adverse risk factor. In contradistinction, both manual and forceps control (CONTROL1 and CONTROL3) are protective, although only to a rather small extent (the largest effect being -1.5% composite outcome risk for CONTROL3). For clarity, it should be noted that manual control referred here almost exclusively to the modified Ritgen maneuver and forceps control most often to so-called prophylactic low or "outlet" forceps procedures (see above).

These markedly polarized observations (of bad results with CONTROL2 and good outcomes with CONTROL1 and CONTROL3) make it important, therefore, to ensure good control of the delivery of the fetal head over the perineum. The risk of trauma from the rapid sequence of compression-decompression associated with uncontrolled precipitate delivery can thus be avoided. Frequent, close nursing observations of the labor process can help in this regard by anticipating when a gravida is approaching readiness for delivery. Being alert to patterns of precipitate cervical dilatation and especially precipitate descent is very important in this regard.

Kristeller expression of even moderate degree (FUNDAL2) is associated with some adverse results. It enhances poor perinatal outcome by 0.3% and composite by 0.8% (0.9% and 2.1% uncorrected). Strong fundal pressure to aid delivery (FUNDAL3) makes matters worse with 0.7% perinatal and 1.9% composite outcome risk (1.5% and 2.7% uncorrected). While these data are not exceptionally bad, they do show that moderate or strong fundal pressure is not so innocuous as it is considered by some. Restrictions on its use are, therefore, probably warranted.

Indeed, fundal pressure is likely to carry the greatest hazard when it is most needed (although not necessarily most appropriately indicated), namely in cases in which the progress of second stage labor has stopped, perhaps as a consequence of bony or positional dystocia. If the Kristeller pressure is then used to overcome the obstruc-

tion, traumatic damage could be expected to result. Just as for the more serious risk variables of difficult and failed forceps use (see above), one must weigh the hazard to be expected from fundal pressure against its possible benefit, if any. Without the counterbalancing advantage of such definable benefit, it is best to refrain.

Labor Enhancement. Induction of labor for pregnancy-induced hypertension (INDUCT3) results in increased perinatal risk of 4.0% and composite outcome risk of 9.6% (6.9% and 12.6% uncorrected). Similarly, inductions for special indications (INDUCT6-9, including uterine infection, pyelonephritis, abruptio placentae, and placenta previa) yield 4.6% (7.5% uncorrected) for both perinatal and composite outcomes (the latter not statistically significant). Extremely bad results also occur after uterotonic augmentation of labor for amnionitis (AUGMENT6), about half the fetuses and infants showing evidence of damage. This is reflected in the startling 43.8% perinatal and 44.1% composite risk levels associated with this variable (59.2% and 52.3% if other labor-delivery factors are not also considered).

As stated earlier in regard to the risk of oxytocin use (AGT23 and AGT24, see above), it is difficult to separate the effect of the drug from that of the indication for its use. The magnitude of the impact seen here, however, is so much larger than that for oxytocin itself, even though all were weighed concurrently, that it is clear that these variables must be designated as critically important. Nonetheless, it is not possible to declare whether their adverse action is due to the condition, the drug, or a combination of both related to some special adversity associated with use of uterotonic stimulation in these cases.

The occurrence of uterine hypertonus in response to oxytocin administration (REACT3) results in seriously increased risk to the fetus and infant. It is associated with 7.8% perinatal (11.9% uncorrected) and 7.0% composite effects (the latter not statistically significant). This impact was determined to exist independently of (and concurrently with) that of oxytocin use in general and the aforementioned especially adverse indications in particular. It is logical to assume, therefore, that the adverse effects of AGT24 are either unrelated or only tangentially related to this complication of its use. Similarly, the hazards associated with the several induction-augmentation risk variables are distinct from and perhaps complementary to this one. That there may be an additive effect cannot be determined, although it seems likely.

In passing, it should be noted that uterine hypertonus from uterotonic stimulation may characteristically develop in the presence of cephalopelvic disproportion. The uterus under these circumstances appears to be particularly sensitive to even small doses of oxytocin. The hypertonic reaction, therefore, may serve as another index of obstructed labor. We were unable to differentiate such cases from those in which the hypertonus resulted from inadvertent overstimulation by oxytocin. Furthermore, the duration of hypertonus, an obviously important aspect insofar as fetal hypoxia from reduced uterine blood flow is concerned, could not be examined separately. Notwithstanding these deficiencies, it is clear that uterine hypertonus carries a major risk. It warrants a recommendation favoring electronic fetal heart rate monitoring as well as concomitant objective surveillance of uterine contractility whenever oxytocin is used.

Fetal Malpresentation. Breech presentation was associated with poor outcome. The 4.7% perinatal risk (6.2% uncorrected) for infants delivered as a breech (PRES5-8) was matched by the 5.1% (statistically insignificant) composite outcome risk. Most were delivered vaginally by assisted breech maneuvers (partial extraction), a procedure which did not have any detectable additional adverse effect. However, some were subjected to total breech extraction (BRDELIV3) and the results for them were especially bad at 9.7% attributable risk perinatally (not significant) and a very note-

worthy 16.8% (23.7% uncorrected) adverse composite outcome. The current trend away from vaginal delivery of fetuses in breech presentation, with special aversion against difficult breech deliveries, is strongly supported by these data.

The results for brow presentation deliveries (PRES11) are also bad with 4.9% perinatal (insignificant) and 9.2% composite risk (11.9% uncorrected). Brow presentation is recognized to be commonly associated with two problems, both important as deleterious factors in their own right, namely fetal prematurity and cephalopelvic disproportion. Since consideration of premature delivery of a small infant was precluded in this study by birth weight limitations imposed on case selection, bony dystocia was undoubtedly a frequently related factor in these cases.

The malpresentation then may have served as still another flag indicating the presence of an obstructed labor and its associated fetal and infant hazard. The obstetrical attendant should, therefore, be on guard to recognize the situation. If recognized, one can avoid invoking the aforementioned risk and compounding it by ill-advised attempts to effect vaginal delivery when it may not be feasible to do so without substantially enhanced peril.

Delivery Complications. Three major delivery complications were identified as contributing adversely to fetal and infant outcome. Abruptio placentae yielded 5.3% (6.6% uncorrected) perinatal risk and an insignificant 2.6% composite outcome risk. Prolapse of the umbilical cord was associated with 7.2% perinatal hazard (not statistically significant) plus 7.3% (12.9% uncorrected) composite risk. Equally bad were the large 6.6% perinatal risk and the 6.1% rate of bad composite outcomes resulting from shoulder dystocia (13.0% and 6.8% crude).

While abruptio placentae and cord prolapse are not ordinarily avoidable complications, it should be obvious that some of the fetal hazard associated with them can be minimized by expeditious diagnosis and intervention. Current management principles accept an attempt to augment labor and effect vaginal delivery in cases with abruptio placentae, provided maternal status and fetal condition permit and neither mother nor baby is likely to be jeopardized as a consequence.

Careful and astute fetal surveillance is essential, of course, so that operative intervention by cesarean section can be undertaken rapidly, if needed. Any delay in effecting operative delivery after the fetus begins to show manifestations of hypoxia cannot be condoned. Moreover, use of potentially traumatic forceps procedures for vaginal delivery under these circumstances is inappropriate.

Cord prolapse generally requires a much more aggressive approach. Given the documented perils of difficult forceps operations for vaginal delivery (see above), cesarean section is preferable in these cases if the fetus is alive and viable (that is, sufficiently mature in development to survive) at the time the diagnosis is made. Heroic efforts to deliver vaginally by forceps when conditions are suboptimal can be expected to add the effects of trauma to those of hypoxia from the cord complication.

The risk of shoulder dystocia, by contrast, might be avoidable if it were possible to predict when it is likely to occur. Unfortunately, there is as yet no reliable objective means available to help assess the fetal bisacromial diameter or the plasticity of the shoulder girdle to accommodate to the maternal pelvis. Nonetheless, there are some signals that warrant attention because they may help predict that shoulder dystocia will occur.

Shoulder dystocia occurs principally at the delivery of a large infant. Although ultrasonographic techniques are still somewhat limited in regard to assessment of large fetuses, fetal weight can be more accurately determined today by this means than heretofore. Cesarean section may indeed be indicated in order to prevent shoulder dystocia in a patient with a very large fetus, say one with an anticipated birth weight over 4500 g. This is particularly relevant if the gravida is diabetic (and therefore at special risk for fetal macrosomia), has small pelvic dimensions or distorted pelvic architecture, or exhibits labor manifestations indicating the likelihood of cephalopelvic disproportion, as detailed earlier in regard to forceps use (see above).

These cases aside, the complication of shoulder dystocia can still occur without forewarning. In view of its associated substantive risk, it is imperative for clinicians to become thoroughly knowledgeable about the technical skills needed for dealing with it and to develop competency in carrying out the appropriate maneuvers expeditiously and atraumatically. Furthermore, since shoulder dystocia may occur unexpectedly in the course of an uncontrolled precipitate delivery when a physician may not be present or readily available, other obstetrical personnel should also be familiarized with emergency measures.

CHAPTER **31**

Summary and Conclusions

A comprehensive investigation was undertaken to identify the fetal and infant risk factors of labor and delivery and to quantitate the degree of risk associated with each of them. In pursuit of these objectives, special attention was paid to confounding and interactional effects between variables. The data base used for this purpose was derived from a population of 58,806 gravidas and their offspring studied prospectively in great detail to yield information pertaining to a wide range of pregnancy-related factors as well as long-term follow-up of the child's growth and development.

The variables we examined encompassed 2441 factors in four discrete categories, namely (1) labor progression, (2) adjunctive pharmacologic agents, (3) intrinsic maternal, fetal, and pelvic factors, and (4) delivery procedures, conditions, and complications. Outcome measures used to test the risk of these variables ranged from perinatal death and neonatal depression through eight-month mental and motor scores, one-year neurologic examinations, and three-year speech, language, and hearing evaluations to four- and seven-year intelligence assessments.

The base population was reduced to 45,142 index cases by limiting analysis to those with complete records and adequate follow-up. Among them, there were 17,935 with detailed labor data for purposes of reconstructing an adequate dilatation pattern and 14,357 with sufficient information for a comparable descent curve. The data files constructed from these cases were surveyed in depth for reliability by cross-validation with the original patient records. They proved quite acceptable as reflected in a very low rate of error (1.1%). After those

497

of no clinical significance were discounted, the error rate was determined to be 0.05%.

The sequence of analyses involved three separate steps for each group of variables. Factors were first explored in isolation to learn their frequency and distribution and then to determine their possible association with bad outcomes. Bivariate testing was done to ascertain whether there were statistically significant associations with adverse results. Next, all significant factors in each group were subjected to hierarchical cluster analysis to find any bearing the same informational content as others, thereby to detect redundancy and reduce the number of variables for further consideration. Finally, all remaining factors were subjected to a probing series of logistic regression analyses. This last step was necessary to control for confounding and interactional effects. Those 129 variables retaining statistical significance after this series of analyses were thus shown to have effects on the fetus and infant while the effects of all others in the goups were being accounted for simultaneously.

The four groups of residual variables were then again subjected to cluster and logistic regression analyses, but this time all 129 were studied collectively and concurrently as a single group. This operational sequence reduced the total to 86 significant factors. Of those remaining, four pertained to the labor course, 12 to drugs and anesthesias, 45 to intrinsic characteristics and conditions, and 25 to the delivery process.

Parity subgroups were coalesced and case material was constricted to include only those producing infants weighing 2500-4000 g and free of congenital anomalies incompatible with survival or normal growth and development. This left a homogeneous study population of 15,169 gravidas and offspring. In addition, intrinsic factors were set aside in order to quantitate the risk associated with the labor-delivery factors. A number of other variables, previously not found to be statistically significant, were reintroduced for study to avoid the possibility that they had been deleted

inappropriately on the basis of confounding effects. Reassessment of 112 labor-delivery variables by logistic regression analysis revealed 16 to have significant perinatal impact and 11 a comparable composite effect (composite referring to any documentably adverse effect from the perinatal period to age 7 years).

All relevant labor-delivery variables were ranked according to the magnitude and sign of the standardized coefficient, a product of the logistic regression coefficient and the standard deviation of the variable. Summating the logistic regression coefficients for all labor and delivery risk factors in a given case allowed us to score each gravida by her index of risk. The distribution of scores and the relationship of the scores to outcome results were studied in order to develop a model that could be used to categorize patients by the labor-delivery risk. Decile divisions did not prove satisfactory, but an incremental system did. This involved allowing the outcome data to define empirical cut points.

This accomplished, we were able to use the risk-score model to assess prelabor variables as predictors of bad outcome while weighing the labor and delivery hazards simultaneously. A total of 369 factors were thus studied to ascertain their predictor effects. Among them, 97 retained significant effects on outcome. Discounting some with unstable relationships left 73 as verifiable prognostic variables in regard to fetal and infant outcome.

For each variable thus identified as carrying significant hazard, the attributable risk was calculated. This provided a quantitation of the degree of risk that could be directly or indirectly attributed to that factor regardless of the presence of other risk variables. The attributable risk data for intrinsic prelabor factors formed the basis for objectively detailing the constellation of descriptive factors for purposes of identifying the gravida-at-risk whose fetus and infant is likely to be in jeopardy.

Special emphasis was placed on recognizing patients with certain demographic characteristics as needing intensive assessment and management. Single black teenagers stood apart as being particularly vulnerable. A prior premature birth also served as a flag to forewarn of future problems. Similarly, women of short stature were found to be at risk. Strongly adverse effects were documented for patients with a low socioeconomic index, low family income, high housing density, and limited education. If the father of the baby was absent, the results tended to be worse.

Patients who began prenatal care late placed their fetus at serious risk as well. Moreover, those who were neglectful of such care did, too, particularly women who only had a small number of antepartum visits for obstetrical observation and management. Premature and postdate delivery adversely affected outcome, as did intrauterine growth retardation. Male fetuses were consistently in greater peril than females.

A variety of medical problems were confirmed to be hazardous. These included diabetes mellitus, pregnancy-induced hypertension, and Rh isoimmunization. Perhaps less well recognized hitherto was the demonstrably deleterious impact of inflammatory bowel disease, maternal mental retardation and other neurologic disease, glomerulonephritis, severe anemia, hyperthyroidism, and cholecystitis. Vaginal bleeding in early pregnancy was also associated with significantly bad results.

A number of labor factors were shown to have adverse effects on the fetus and infant. Most notably among labor aberrations were prolonged latent phase and protraction disorders. Arrest disorders of labor were also deleterious, but their effects could be accounted for largely by concurrent factors, perhaps most importantly related to interventive measures invoked to attempt to effect vaginal delivery.

Among adjunctive agents used in labor, paracervical block and general inhalation anesthesia carried potentially serious risk. Narcotic analgesics had contradictory results suggesting a negligible effect on offspring at most. Uterotonic agents also showed inconsistent effects, but they nevertheless did seem to have some untoward action overall. This applied more particularly to inductions of labor for pregnancy-induced hypertension and a variety of other indications and stimulation of labor for amnionitis. When uterine hypertonus occurred, the results with uterotonic stimulation were much worse.

Hydralazine was associated with serious risk but its effect, if any, could not be distinguished from that of the hypertensive condition for which it was used. The same applied in regard to the severe risks occurring with use of some antibiotics, the effects of which might instead have reflected those of the serious infection for which they were given.

Delivery factors were of importance with regard to outcome. The hazard of midforceps was ascribable to several component features of operative vaginal delivery procedures. Particular note was taken of the peril related to difficult or failed forceps application, traction, and rotation. The more difficult the operation, the greater the risk. Cases in which cesarean section had to be done because all attempts to achieve vaginal delivery had failed did very badly indeed.

Despite the poor results associated with the more difficult forceps manipulations, the overall results with forceps control of the delivery of the fetal head in vertex presentation (consisting mostly of uncomplicated low forceps procedures in otherwise healthy patients) were quite good relative to uncontrolled delivery. Thus, not all forceps use was necessarily bad. Moreover, precipitate delivery without good control constituted a risk factor. In addition, invoking Kristeller pressure of moderate or strong intensity was also associated with a high incidence of untoward effects.

Not unexpectedly, breech births proved hazardous and the risk was markedly enhanced by the more difficult form of breech delivery, namely breech extraction. Brow presentation was likewise shown to have a deleterious effect on the fetus, perhaps because of its association with prematurity and, more importantly, with cephalopelvic disproportion. The complications of abruptio placentae and cord prolapse were demonstrated to be associated with poor outcomes, also as expected. Similarly, shoulder dystocia carried a high risk.

The results of these studies should help obstetrical attendants identify those gravidas at greatest risk. Once flagged, such women deserve special attention and care directed toward preventing the anticipated adverse result. This may be accomplished by optimizing maternal and fetal status and perhaps by providing special expertise, as needed, in the form of knowledgeable personnel who can offer skilled attention in well-equipped facilities where intensive surveillance is readily available and expeditious interventive management can be accomplished without delay if it should become necessary. Such cases also deserve the advantages that can be offered by institutions capable of intensive neonatal resuscitation and support.

In addition, the data show the need to modify some obstetrical practices, particularly insofar as delivery procedures are concerned. The information pertaining to quantification of specific attributable risk permits one to weigh the hazards of a given interventive measure against its ostensible benefit. The latter is usually a reflection of the risk of the condition for which the procedure is being undertaken. Thus, the magnitude of the benefit is the degree of risk that can be avoided by intervention. This applies in those situations in which the risk of the condition is felt to indicate the procedure. Without a clearly documentable counterbalancing justification in the form of a risk-benefit assessment that favors the fetus, any procedure that exposes the fetus or infant to substantive risk (in excess of benefit) cannot be considered acceptable.

INDEX

logistic regression 140-144, 350, 353, 354, 358, 360, 373, 376, 377
magnesium sulfate 178-180
mental score 72, 80
motor score 72, 80
neonatal death 66, 68, 72, 80
neonatal depression 66-67, 68-69, 72, 80-81
neurological abnormality 72, 80-81
nonparametric analysis 80-81
normal limits 86-87
outcome effect 80-81, 97-104, 131-145, 485-489
oxytocin 153, 181-183
parity 58-61
perinatal death 66, 80-81
protraction 487-488
race 56
reconstruction 20, 52
risk rank 368, 370, 382, 384
risk score 395, 396, 405, 406, 410
standardized coefficient 363, 367, 369, 378-380
stillbirth 66, 80
summary data 55
tranquilizer 172-176
uterotonic agents 181-183
variable 23
Actuarial variable *See* Intrinsic factor
Adjunctive agent *See* Drug
Age, gestational *See* Gestational duration
Age, maternal 19, 39, 499
attributable risk 469, 470, 472-473, 477-478, 481
characteristics 57-58, 203-204
cluster analysis 249-250
code 241
definition 22
distribution 17, 17, 204
labor 57-58
logistic regression 251, 253, 256, 263, 352, 359
outcome effect 216-217, 229, 243, 244, 251, 253, 256, 263
parity 57-58
predictor variable 415, 416, 434, 435, 447-449
risk rank 370
standardized coefficient 365
stratification 55
Aggregative hierarchical cluster *See* Cluster analysis
Aims, research 5-8, 10, 35
Alcoholism 210, 230, 232
Alphaprodine 150, 152
cluster analysis 193, 194, 195, 346, 347
code 187
logistic regression 195-201, 349, 350, 354
outcome effect 157-159, 160, 192, 489, 490-491, 499
risk rank 370, 383
risk score 397, 406, 407, 411

standardized coefficient 363, 380, 381
temporal effect 171-172, 183
Amnionitis 310, 311, 324, 335, 346, 347, 354-357, 359, 368, 371, 373, 375-379, 382, 394, 395, 404, 459, 463, 464, 468, 484, 486, 491, 494, 499
Amniotomy 2, 6, 39
See also Membranes, chorioamniotic
frequency 271
latent phase 486
outcome effect 313, 314, 320, 322, 323, 327, 328
predictor variable 429, 430-431, 441, 443
variable 266, 267, 318
Analgesic agent 6, 24, 59, 146, 148-153
See also Alphaprodine; Meperidine; Morphine
code 187
latent phase 486
outcome effect 157-159, 192-201, 499
protraction disorder 488
temporal effect 166-172, 183
Analysis
adjunctive agents 38, 185-201
delivery factors 39-40, 277-315
design overview 36-37
drug data 185-201
intrinsic factors 39, 213-239, 240-264
labor data 37-38, 127-145
methodology 40-47
projects 6, 35-36
sequence 36, 128
Anemia 204, 209, 499
attributable risk 470, 472, 476, 480, 482
frequency 207, 208
logistic regression 252, 253, 257, 261, 263, 352, 356, 357, 359
outcome effect 230, 231, 233, 234, 247, 248, 252, 253, 257, 261, 263
predictor variable 429, 430, 432, 433, 441, 443-445, 448, 449, 454
risk rank 371
standardized coefficient 365, 369
Anencephaly 129, 212
Anesthesia
accident 211, 232, 235
agents 13, 24, 146-149, 154
attributable risk 459, 460, 484
cluster analysis 193, 194, 195, 346, 347
code 187
delivery 275
level 13
logistic regression 195-201, 349, 350, 352-358
outcome effect 189-193, 232, 247, 489-492, 499
response 13
risk rank 370, 382-384
risk score 396, 397, 406, 407, 411, 412
risk variables 36, 186
route 13, 150, 153-155

shock 211, 232, 235, 236, 247
standardized coefficient 363, 365, 367, 368, 378-380
survey 153-155
time 13
type 13, 150, 153-155
Anomaly, fetal *See* Malformations, congenital
Antepartum visit *See* Prenatal care
Antibiotic 146, 148-153, 499
attributable risk 459, 460, 464, 466, 484
code 187
cluster analysis 193, 194, 195
logistic regression 195-201, 352, 353, 356, 357, 375-378
outcome effect 162, 192, 491-492, 499
risk rank 370, 382
risk score 395, 397, 407, 411
standardized coefficient 365, 369, 379
temporal effect 178, 179, 183
Anticonvulsant agent 149, 248
Antidepressant 149
Antihistamine 149, 151
Antihypertensive agent 149, 162-163, 178-180, 187, 491, 499
See also Hydralazine; Reserpine
logistic regression 195-201
Antipyretic agent 148-153
Antitussive 149
Apgar score 14, 20, 21, 23
See also Neonatal depression
Appendicitis 208, 210, 230, 235, 236
Apresoline *See* Hydralazine
Architecture, pelvic *See* Pelvic variable
Arrest of descent
augmentation 274, 275, 320, 322, 324, 333, 354-357, 359, 371, 372, 380, 402, 404
cesarean 275, 276
cluster analysis 136-139, 346-348
code 128
computer diagnosis 51, 105
cut points 128
definition 52, 115-116
distribution 106, 109
duration 107, 108-112
forceps 274-276, 293-294
frequency 106, 116, 117
intelligence quotient 113-116
level of station 108, 110, 111
limit 128
logistic analysis 140-144, 356, 357
neonatal death 113-116
neonatal depression 112-116
neurological abnormality 113-116
outcome effect 112-114, 122, 125-126, 131-145, 293, 294, 485, 488-489, 499
risk rank 370, 371, 372, 382
risk score 396, 404, 405, 410
standardized coefficient 369, 379, 381
study population 106, 116-117, 120

transverse 293, 294
Arrest of dilatation
algorithm 51
augmentation 274-276, 402, 404
Bayley score 121-126
code 128
communication disorder 121-126
computer diagnosis 51, 105
cut points 128
definition 51, 115-116
degree of dilatation 107, 110, 111, 117-120, 120-121
distribution 106-108, 117, 118
duration 107-110, 118-124
frequency 106, 116, 117
intelligence quotient 121-126
limits 128
neonatal death 121
neonatal depression 112-116, 121-126
neurological abnormality 121-126
outcome effect 112-114, 120-121, 123-124, 131-145, 499
risk rank 383
risk score 396, 404-406, 410
standardized coefficient 380, 381
stillbirth 121
study population 106, 116-117, 120
Arrested labor *See* Arrest of descent; Arrest of dilatation
Asthma, bronchial 208, 209, 211
outcome effect 231, 232, 234, 246-248
predictor variable 432, 433, 444
Asynclitism 6, 23, 39
Ataractic agent *See* Tranquilizer
Atropine 150, 152
cluster analysis 193, 194
code 187
logistic regression 196-201
outcome effect 163, 192-193
risk rank 383
risk score 397, 407, 411
standardized coefficient 379
temporal effect 180-181, 183
Attendant, obstetrical
cluster analysis 346-348
definition 24, 318
frequency 270-271
outcome effect 294-296, 317, 320, 322, 327, 332, 337, 342
predictor variable 429, 430, 441-443, 448, 453
type 270-271
variable 266, 318
Attitude, fetal *See* Breech presentation
Attributable risk
confidence limits 457
defined 455-458
formula 456, 457, 482
impact on practice 483-496
labor-delivery variables 458-469

logistic regression 254, 258-260, 264, 354, 355, 359
outcome effect 232, 235, 254, 259
predictor variable 432-445, 449, 454
risk rank 371
standardized coefficient 367
Gantrisin 150, 187, 192-193
Gastrointestinal disease 208, 210
logistic regression 253
outcome effect 230-232, 235, 236, 238, 253
Gender, fetal *See* Sex, fetal
General anesthesia 154, 187
attributable risk 459, 460, 484
cluster analysis 194, 195, 346, 347
logistic regression 195-201, 349, 350, 354-358, 360, 376, 377
outcome effect 189-193, 489, 490, 499
risk rank 368, 370, 382, 384
risk score 397, 406, 407, 411
standardized coefficient 363, 367, 369, 378-380
Genetic data 11
Genitourinary disorder 210, 232, 235, 247
See also Glomerulonephritis; Urinary tract infection
logistic regression 252, 253, 255, 264, 350, 354, 355, 359
outcome effect 253, 255, 264
predictor variable 432, 433, 444
risk rank 371
standardized coefficient 363, 367
Gestational duration 6, 39, 499
attributable risk 470, 471, 474, 476, 479, 481-482
cluster analysis 249-251
code 242
definition 23
distribution 17, 18, 203, 204, 205
logistic regression 251, 254, 258, 259, 263
outcome effect 223-224, 228, 229, 245, 246, 251, 254, 259, 263
postterm pregnancy 224
predictor variable 428, 429, 441, 442, 448, 449, 453
Gestational variable 39
Global score 23
See also Bayley developmental scale
Glomerulonephritis 208, 210, 499
attributable risk 470, 472, 474, 476, 480, 482
logistic regression 252-254, 257, 261-262, 263, 352, 353, 356, 357, 359
outcome effect 230, 232, 235, 247, 248, 252-254, 257, 261, 263
predictor variable 432, 433, 444, 445, 448, 449, 454
risk rank 371
standardized coefficient 365, 369
Glucose tolerance test 13, 209, 232, 233, 237
Gompertz function 40, 64, 75

Gonorrhea *See* Sexually transmitted disease
Goodenough test 15
Graham-Ernhart block sort 14
Gravida-at-risk 6, 35, 372
attributable risk 455-458
identification 477-482
labor-delivery variables 458-469
predictor variables 469-477, 498
Gravidity 6, 39, 204
code 241
logistic regression 252, 255, 257, 350, 352, 357
outcome effect 243, 245, 252, 255, 257
predictor variable 419, 420, 436, 447, 449, 450
risk rank 370
standardized coefficient 363, 365, 369
Growth measurement 14
Gynecologic disorder 12, 208, 210, 231, 232, 235, 237, 238, 254, 259, 264
See also Incompetent cervix; Leiomyomata uteri; Vaginitis
logistic regression 354, 355, 359
risk rank 371
standardized coefficient 367

Halothane 154
Head, fetal *See also* Forceps; Midforceps; Vacuum extractor
attributable risk 464, 467, 484
control 273, 280, 318, 346-348, 354-357, 359, 367, 369, 371-373, 375, 376, 378, 381, 383, 394, 403, 408, 459, 461, 492, 493- 494, 499
delivery 13, 266, 273, 499
extended 306
risk referent 392, 401
Hearing *See* Communication disorder
Heart disease *See* Cardiac disease
Height, maternal 39, 204, 251
attributable risk 470-471, 473, 474, 478, 481
code 242
definition 24
logistic regression 252-254, 256, 262, 263, 352, 356, 357
outcome effect 219-220, 243, 245, 252-254, 256, 261, 263
predictor variable 420, 422, 436, 438, 447, 449, 450
risk rank 371
standardized coefficient 365, 369
Hematocrit 13, 24, 429, 430, 441, 443, 470, 472, 476, 480, 482
See also Anemia
Hemoglobin 13, 14, 24
Hemorrhage 211, 232, 235, 236, 247, 253, 254, 257, 258, 261-262, 264, 352, 356, 369, 371, 432-445, 449, 454
See also Shock
Hepatitis 208, 210
outcome effect 230, 232, 235, 236
Hiatus hernia 210, 232

Hierarchical clustering *See* Cluster analysis
Hierarchical lexicon patterns 96-97
High-risk criteria 6, 35
Historical variable 39
Hormone 149
Hospital *See* Institution
Housing 15, 499
  attributable risk 473, 475, 479, 481
  definition 24
  density 24, 425, 426, 439-440, 447, 452
  variable 39
Hydatidiform mole 17, 18
Hydralazine 151, 180
  attributable risk 459, 460, 484
  code 187
  logistic regression 195-201, 354, 355, 376-378
  outcome effect 162-163, 491, 499
  risk rank 370, 382
  risk score 395, 397, 407, 411, 412
  standardized coefficient 379
Hydramnios 39, 204, 208, 210, 211
  code 243
  logistic regression 257, 258, 352
  outcome effect 226, 228-231, 235, 236, 245, 246, 257
  predictor variable 432, 444
  risk rank 371
  standardized coefficient 365, 378, 379
Hydrocephalus 129, 212
Hydrochlorothiazide 151
Hydroxyzine pamoate 150, 151
  attributable risk 464-466, 484
  cluster analysis 193, 194, 364, 367
  code 187
  logistic regression 195-201, 349, 350, 358, 375
  outcome effect 160-161, 192-193, 489, 490
  risk rank 370, 383
  risk score 397, 406, 407, 411
  standardized coefficient 363, 367
  temporal effect 172-174, 183
Hyoscine *See* Scopolamine
Hyperemesis gravidarum 208, 210, 211
  outcome effect 232, 235, 236, 248
  predictor variable 432, 444, 445
Hypotensive agent 149
  code 187
  logistic regression 195-201
  outcome effect 162-163
  temporal effect 178-180, 183
Hypoxia, fetal 487, 489, 490, 496

Ideal labor 59
Ileitis, regional *See* Inflammatory bowel disease
Income 15, 218, 499
  attributable risk 475, 478-479, 481
  per capita 424, 425, 438, 439, 447, 451-452, 473
  score 24-25
  variable 39

Incompetent cervix 204, 208, 210
  outcome effect 230, 231, 233, 235
  predictor variable 432, 433, 444
Incrementation process 62, 64
Index population 17-18, 21, 49, 186, 497
Indication
  amniotomy 266
  augmentation of labor 266, 274, 275
  breech delivery 267
  cesarean section 267, 275, 276, 319
  forceps 267, 274-276, 318
  frequency 274-276
  induction of labor 266, 274, 275, 308-311
  vacuum extractor 267
Induction of labor *See also* Amniotomy; Oxytocin; Sparteine
  agent 153, 167
  amniotomy 313, 314, 429-431
  attempts 308, 309
  attributable risk 459, 462-464, 468, 484
  cluster analysis 193-195, 344
  complication 271
  defined 23
  frequency 271
  indication 308, 310, 311
  logistic regression 195-201, 350, 352-357, 359, 360, 373, 375-378
  method 271
  outcome effect 189-193, 306-312, 317, 320, 322, 324, 327-329, 331, 333-342, 489, 491, 494, 499
  reaction 311-312, 319, 321, 323, 327, 344, 380, 383, 409, 494
  risk rank 368, 370, 371, 382, 383
  risk score 394-397, 403-404, 406, 407, 409, 411, 412
  standardized coefficient 363, 365, 367, 369, 378-380, 381
  variable 266-267, 318
Infant death *See* Neonatal death; Perinatal mortality; Stillbirth
Infection 211, 233, 235, 236, 492, 499
  See also specific infection
Infertility history 12, 24, 204, 206
  code 242
  outcome effect 225, 226, 232, 233, 235, 246
Inflammatory bowel disease 208, 210, 232, 247, 499
  attributable risk 463, 470, 472, 474, 477, 480, 482
  cluster analysis 249-250
  logistic regression 252, 253, 255, 257, 258, 264, 350, 352, 359
  outcome effect 247, 248, 252, 253, 255, 257
  predictor variable 432, 433, 444, 445, 448, 449, 454
  risk rank 371
  standardized coefficient 363, 365
Information processing 12

Nisentil *See* Alphaprodine
Nitrous oxide 154
Noncore patients 17, 18
Nonparametric analysis 40-41, 44, 46, 55, 64, 498
  aggregated risk factors 343-344
  arrest disorder 112-114
  definition 40-41
  delivery factors 277-315, 317-329
  distribution 40
  drug data 156-165, 166-184, 186-193
  interpretation 40-41
  intrinsic factors 213-239, 240-249
  labor data 75-87, 91-104, 112-114, 127-145
  lexical analysis 91-104
  risk score 391-392
Nonregressive entry 19, 20
Novocaine 154
Nuchal arm 273, 306
Nuchal cord 24, 319
Nullipara *See* Parity
Nupercaine 154

Obesity *See* Ponderal index
Obstetrical trend 4, 59
Obstetrical experience 7, 24, 39, 204, 206, 251
  See also Abortion; Neonatal death; Premature
    delivery; Stillbirth
  code 241
  labor 59, 61
  outcome effect 221-223, 228, 229, 243, 245
  predictor variable 419-422, 436-437
Obstetrician 24, 266, 270-271, 294-296, 317, 318, 320, 322, 327, 332, 337, 430, 441, 442, 445, 453, 500
Occupation 24, 218, 425, 427, 439, 440, 447, 449, 452
  See also Work
  attributable risk 470, 471, 474, 475, 479, 481
Odds ratio 392-393
Onset of labor *See also* Augmentation of labor; Induction of labor
  code 187
  frequency 271
  outcome effect 189-193, 306, 307, 317, 320, 322, 324, 327-331, 333-338, 340, 342
  variable 266, 318
Origin *See* Birthplace
Outcome variable 20, 21
  See also specific outcomes
  composite 130, 186, 190, 241, 344
  perinatal 130, 186, 241, 344
Overview 7, 8, 36-37
Oxygen 14
Oxytocin 3, 6, 23, 24, 59, 146, 148, 150-153, 186
  See also Augmentation of labor; Induction of
    labor
  arrest disorder 488-489
  attributable risk 464-466, 484
  cluster analysis 193-195, 344, 346-348

  code 187
  latent phase 486
  logistic regression 195-201, 349-352, 354-358, 375
  outcome effect 163-165, 188-193, 306-312, 489, 491, 494-495, 499
  precipitate labor 486-487
  protraction disorder 488
  reaction 311-312, 319, 326, 329
  risk rank 370, 372, 382-384, 406, 407, 411, 412
  risk score 396, 397
  standardized coefficient 363, 365, 367, 369, 378-381
  temporal effects 166, 181-182, 183
  variable 266, 267

Pallor 14
Papanicolaou smear 13
Paracervical block 154
  attributable risk 459, 460, 484
  cluster analysis 194, 346, 348
  code 187
  logistic regression 195-201, 354, 355, 358, 377
  outcome effect 186, 188, 189-193, 489-490, 499
  risk rank 370, 382
  risk score 396, 397, 406, 407, 411
  standardized coefficient 367, 379, 381
Parasitic disease 13, 211, 233, 254, 259, 264, 354, 355, 359, 367, 371, 432, 444
Parity 6, 19, 39, 373, 498
  age 57-58
  code 241
  definition 22
  distribution 17, 18, 203, 205
  grand multipara 57
  labor 58-60
  lexical analysis 95
  logistic regession 253, 254, 256, 261, 263, 352, 353, 356, 357, 359, 373, 376
  outcome effect 218-219, 228, 229, 243, 245, 253, 254, 256, 261, 263
  predictor variable 419, 420, 421, 436-437
  risk rank 370, 383
  standardized coefficient 365, 366, 369, 380
  stratification 55
Pathology 11, 14
Patient characteristics 16-17
Patient status 39, 204
  attributable risk 473, 478
    weighted 481
  cluster analysis 249-251, 344, 346, 347
  code 241
  definition 24
  logistic regression 251, 257, 258, 263, 352, 353
  outcome effect 217, 218, 229-230, 243, 244, 251, 257, 263
  predictor variable 416, 417, 434, 435, 447, 448
  risk rank 370
  standardized coefficient 365

demographic factors 415-419, 434-436, 446-450

impact on risk score 415-445

intercurrent disorder 431-433, 443-445, 454

obstetrical history 419-422, 436-437, 450

physical characteristics 422-423, 438, 450-451

prenatal factors 427-431, 440-443, 452-454, 498

socioeconomic factors 424-427, 438-440, 451-452

Preeclampsia *See* Pregnancy-induced hypertension

Pregnancy-induced hypertension 204, 211, 248, 499

attributable risk 459, 462-463, 464, 468, 474, 476, 480, 482, 484

augmentation 274, 275, 320, 329, 383, 394, 404

cesarean section 275, 276

cluster analysis 249, 346, 347

code 242

forceps 275, 276, 293, 294

induction 274, 275, 310, 311, 320, 324, 329, 333, 359, 360, 371, 375-378, 394, 404, 484, 491, 494, 499

logistic regression 252-254, 256, 261-263, 352, 356, 357, 359, 360, 375-377

outcome effect 245, 246, 252-254, 256, 261, 263, 310, 311, 328

predictor variable 429, 431, 441, 443, 448, 454

risk rank 371, 382, 383

standardized coefficient 363, 365, 369, 378-380

Premature delivery 129, 219, 225, 499

attributable risk 469-470, 473, 474, 478, 479, 481

brow presentation 495, 500

forceps 275

frequency 203, 204, 207

infertility 233

leiomyomata uteri 236

logistic regression 253, 254, 256, 261, 263, 352, 353, 357

outcome effect 223-224, 243, 245, 253, 256, 261, 263

predictor variable 420-421, 436, 437, 447, 449, 450

prior 39, 204, 207, 218, 229, 241, 253, 254, 256, 261, 263, 352, 353, 357, 365, 371, 420

risk rank 371

standardized coefficient 365, 369

Prenatal care 11, 13, 204, 499

attributable risk 474, 476, 479, 481

cluster analysis 251

code 242

logistic regression 253, 254, 256-258, 261-263, 352, 353, 356 357, 359

outcome effect 224-225, 228, 229, 243, 245, 253, 254, 256, 257, 261, 263

predictor variable 428, 429, 440-443, 448, 452-453

risk rank 370

standardized coefficient 365, 369

Prentice model 41

Presentation, fetal 13, 211, 219, 485

See also Breech presentation; Brow presentation; Face presentation

frequency 271-273

outcome effect 6, 320, 322, 327, 493

variable 23, 39, 266-267, 318

Prinadol *See* Phenazocine

Prior pregnancies 24

Private care *See* Patient status

Probit scale 62, 63

Prochlorperazine 150, 160

Progestational agent 149

Prolapsed cord 24, 39, 204, 211, 227-230, 267, 319, 485, 486

attributable risk 464, 467, 484

logistic regression 350, 357, 359, 373, 375

management 496

outcome effect 321, 323, 326, 327, 329, 331, 334, 336, 340, 342, 495-496

risk rank 372, 382

risk score 394, 395, 403, 408

standardized coefficient 363, 369, 378, 379

Prolonged deceleration phase *See* Deceleration phase

Prolonged latent phase *See* Latent phase

Promazine 150, 152

code 187

outcome effect 159-161

temporal effect 172-173, 183

Promethazine 150, 152

code 187

outcome effect 160-161, 192-193

temporal effect 172-174, 183

Propiomazine 150, 152

code 187

outcome effect 160-161, 192-193

temporal effect 173, 175, 183

Protocols 10

Protracted descent *See* Maximum slope of descent

Protracted dilatation *See* Maximum slope of dilatation

Psychiatric history 24, 204, 208, 210, 211, 232, 248

Psychological examination 11, 14, 20

Pudendal block 154

cluster analysis 193, 194, 195

code 187

logistic regression 195-201, 352, 353, 358

outcome effect 189, 489

risk rank 370, 382

risk score 396, 397, 406, 407, 411, 412

standardized coefficient 365, 378, 379

Puerperal events 11, 13

Pulmonary disease 39, 204, 208, 209

logistic regression 254

outcome effect 231, 232, 238, 247, 248, 254
standardized coefficient 369
Pyelonephritis 247, 248, 254, 259, 275, 494
induction 310, 311, 324
logistic regression 354, 355

Quetelet's index *See* Ponderal index

Race 6, 16, 19, 39, 499
attributable risk 469, 470, 473, 474, 477-478, 481
characteristics 56-57, 203, 205
cluster analysis 249-250, 344, 346-348
code 241
definition 22
distribution 17, 18, 203, 205
labor 56-57
logistic regression 251-256, 258-261, 263, 350, 352-359, 373
outcome effect 217-218, 228, 229, 243, 245, 251-256, 259, 261, 263
predictor variable 416-418, 434, 435, 447-449
risk rank 368, 370
standardized coefficient 364-370
stratification 55
Radiation exposure 12, 13, 204
code 242
frequency 207
outcome effect 225, 226, 228, 229, 246
Rank correlation 381
Ranked variable *See* Standardized coefficient
Rectification process 19-20, 48
Registration 11, 12, 17
See also Walk-in patient
attributable risk 474, 475-476, 479, 481
code 242
distribution 203, 204, 205
late 225
logistic regression 258
outcome effect 215, 229, 245, 246
predictor 427-428, 429, 440, 441, 447, 452
Reliability of data 19, 34, 497
Religion 15, 24, 416, 418, 434, 435, 447-450, 473, 474, 481
Repeat pregnancy 18
Reproductive history 12
Research design *See* Experimental design
Reserpine 151, 162-163, 180, 187, 197
Resident *See* Attendant
Resuscitation 14, 500
Rheumatic fever 208, 211, 232, 234
Rh sensitization 13, 14, 24, 204, 499
attributable risk 470, 472, 476, 480, 482
augmentation 274, 275, 379, 394, 395, 404, 406, 409
cesarean section 267, 275
code 242
induction 274, 275, 310, 311, 371, 380, 383, 394, 404, 406, 409
logistic regression 252-254, 256, 258, 261,

263, 352, 353, 356, 357, 359
outcome effect 245, 246, 252-254, 256, 261, 263, 310, 311, 324, 327
predictor variable 429, 431, 441, 443, 449, 454
risk rank 371, 383, 406, 409
standardized coefficient 365, 369, 378-381
Risk factor *See also* Attributable risk; Predictor variable
adverse 484
assessment 41-46
diagnostic 36
drug 185-201
identification 5
interrelation 5
intrinsic factor 240-264
labor course 127-145
objective 5
outcome effect 36
predictor variable 36
synergism 5
Risk score
cut point 398, 399, 401
decile strata 387-396, 498
defined 385-386
distribution 386-387, 398-401, 498
formula 385, 386
goodness-of-fit 391, 392
incremental strata 396-412, 498
outcome effect 387-391, 397-400, 498
range 386
residual effects 392-396
Rotation, forceps *See* Forceps rotation
Rotation, manual 39, 266, 270, 282, 299, 318
outcome effect 319, 320, 322
Ruptured membranes *See* Membranes, chorio-amniotic
Ruptured uterus *See* Uterine rupture

Sampling 16
Scopolamine 150, 152
code 187
outcome effect 163, 192-193
risk rank 383
risk score 397, 411
standardized coefficient 379
temporal effect 180-181, 183
Secobarbital 150, 152
code 187
outcome effect 161-162, 192-193
temporal effect 176, 177, 183
Second stage
age, maternal 57
analgesia 167-172
antibiotics 178, 179
barbiturates 176-178
Bayley score 85
belladonna alkaloids 180-181
calculation 50-51, 55
cluster analysis 136-139, 346-348
code 128